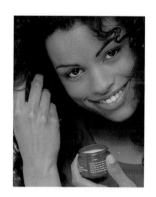

# natural
# health &
# beauty

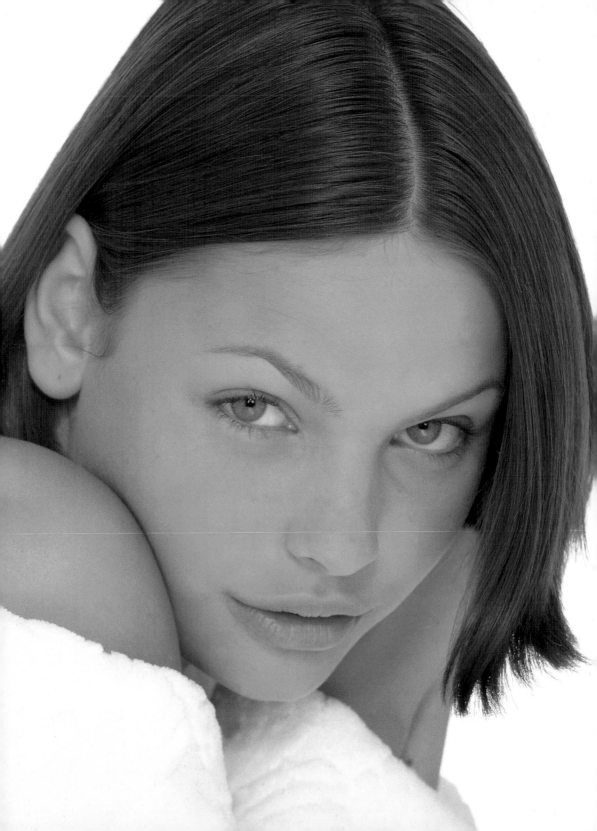

# natural
# health &
# beauty

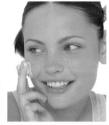
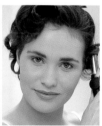
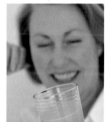

All-natural treatments, therapies and makeovers for a sensational complexion, vibrant hair and complete body cleansing

CONSULTANT EDITOR:
## Helena Sunnydale

H·H
HERMES
HOUSE

This edition is published by Hermes House

Hermes House is an imprint of Anness Publishing Ltd
Hermes House, 88-89 Blackfriars Road, London SE1 8HA
tel. 020 7401 2077; fax 020 7633 9499
www.lorenzbooks.com; info@anness.com

A CIP catalogue record for this book is available from the British Library.

Publisher: Joanna Lorenz
Editorial Director: Helen Sudell
*Skincare and Make-up* written by: Sally Norton and Kate Shapland
*Haircare and Styling* written by Jacki Wadeson
*Introducing Pilates* written by: Emily Kelly
*Healing Aromatherapy* written by: Shirley Price
*Ayurvedic Beauty* written by: Janet Wright
*Aging Naturally* written by: Jennifer Amerena
Photography: Simon Bottomley, Nick Cole, Michelle Garrett, Christine
Hanscomb, Alistair Hughes and Liz McAulay
Designer: Design Principals
Make-up: Debbi Finlow, Vanessa Haines, Liz Kitchiner and Paul Miller
Additional Make-up: Bettina Graham
Hair: Debbi Finlow and Kathleen Bray, assisted by Wendy M B Cook
Exercise advisor: Dean Hodgkin
Exercise and Diet Consultant: Dr Naomi Lewis
Illustrators: Cherril Parris (hair), David Cook (pilates)
Models: Amanda, Christiana, Carley, Laura, Emily, Frieda, Hannah, Juliet, Sarah,
Zonna, Cheryl, Jane, Joanna and Stacey

Previously published in 5 separate volumes: *The Ultimate Beauty Book*,
*Aromatherapy for Women*, *Ayurvedic Beauty*, *Commonsense Pilates* and
*Aging Naturally*

10 9 8 7 6 5 4 3 2 1

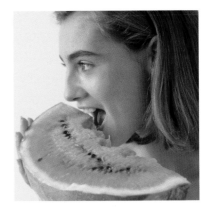

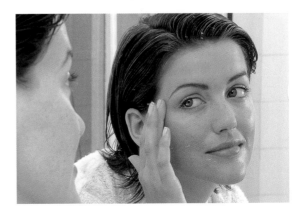

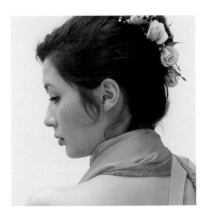

# Contents

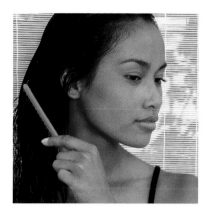

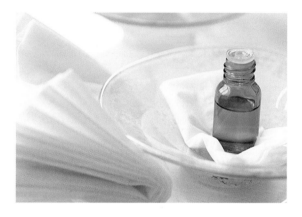

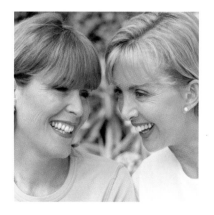

# Introduction

Since time began human beings have sought to improve their health and well-being through ingenious use of the materials around them. Natural medicines were probably the first discoveries in this field, but it wasn't long before people looked for ways of doing more than just survive. They used the natural healing properties of herbs and flowers as preventative treatments too.

Our ancestors were using herbal powders and creams thousands of years ago — we know because they were buried with these valuable items beside them for use in the afterlife. They may have started out using an oil to help an injury heal, then discovered that it left their skin feeling more supple or protected it from the weather. If the sheen highlighted their cheekbones, all the better. Health, beauty and well-being were beginning to be developed hand in hand.

Over the centuries we've discovered ever more sophisticated ways of improving our health, enhancing our looks and staying youthful. The range of products now at our disposal would bewilder even our grandmothers. We can conquer infections or delay the menopause with drugs they had never

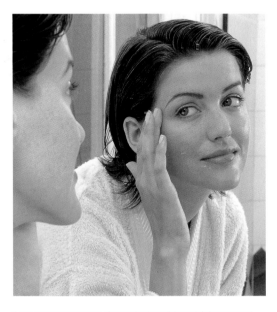

△ The single biggest cause of skin aging is sunlight. So it is important to choose a moisturizer that contains an effective sunscreen.

heard of, and undergo surgery to wipe the marks of time off our faces. But if the 20th century offered us quick fixes in abundance, it also taught us that there's a price to pay in the form of side effects, allergies and environmental damage. Our understanding of the natural world has been outstripped by our ability to manipulate it.

In the 21st century we are learning to evaluate new products and technologies more realistically. We are rediscovering the wisdom of our ancestors and learning to value what other cultures have to offer. Today, we can pick and mix from a treasure-trove of options: modern, traditional and worldwide.

This beautiful book is for anyone who wants to make the most of every stage of her life. "Natural" doesn't mean refusing the benefits of the world we

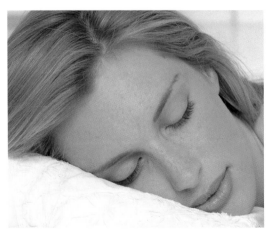

◁ It is important to get a good sleep every night if you truly want to help keep yourself looking young and carefree.

▷ Individual hair types need individual treatments: adopt a personal routine to keep your hair at its best. A massage with warm olive oil is ideal for a dry, tight scalp.

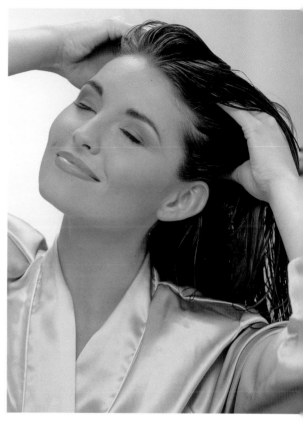

were born into. We're happy to use medicinal drugs or commercial make-up products for example, as long as they work without causing harm. If we don't need them, we'd rather try gentle remedies such as essential oils as the basis for relaxing footbath or an Ayurvedic massage to soothe away the strains and stresses of the day.

The rapidly growing popularity of complementary therapies has brought aromatherapy into the mainstream. But, as world-renowned pioneer Shirley Price explains, the reality is much less widely understood. Far from simply inspiring a range of nice-smelling toiletries, this therapy can relieve many ailments, both physical and psychological. A drop of lavender oil on a pillow has for generations offered gentler relief from insomnia than anything a doctor could prescribe.

This book covers every aspect of women's health and beauty, head to toe, inside and out. Beauty – looking good, feeling great and making the best of all your physical features – is an important part of improving every aspect of a woman's life.

▽ Keeping your fingernails filed regularly will minimize breakage. File them straight across with a soft emery board.

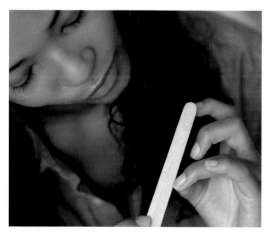

## skincare and make-up

While your actual skin type is determined by your genes, there is plenty you can do daily to ensure it always looks as good as possible. Understanding how your skin functions will help you to understand its special needs. In the skincare section, you can find out how to care for your own specific skin type. You can't neglect your complexion for months or years, then make up for it with expensive and intensive attention in the short term. Regularly spending time and care on your skin is a great investment – it's never too early or too late to follow a good skincare regime – and the results will last a lifetime.

Skincare is all about making sure your skin is in good shape – clear, soft and supple – and then keeping it that way through good habits, sensible cleansing and using skincare products in the right way. The bodycare section will also show you how to freshen, tone, pamper and maintain your whole

# introduction

body from top to toe – from bathroom essentials to natural pampering treats – to help you achieve natural, beautiful, hassle-free skin. The key to successful make-up is to understand how to enhance your features using the best cosmetic fomulations and colours around. If you research the best of the products available to you, brush up your application techniques and give yourself plenty of time to experiment, you can find the perfect look for you.

Every woman can use make-up to enhance her looks, but the secret is understanding your own beauty needs. This section provides fresh and inspiring ideas to help you find a look to suit you.

## haircare and styling

Beautiful, silky, shining hair makes you feel fantastic, it reflects well-being and has a natural beauty of its own. Hair can also be a versatile fashion accessory, and can be coloured, curled, dressed up or smoothed down – all in a matter of minutes. However, too much attention – washing, styling, dry-

▽ Choosing delicious, fresh fruit as an alternative to stodgy snacks is a simple way of beginning a healthier way of life.

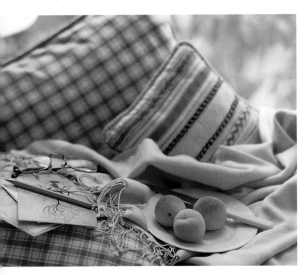

ing and colouring – can strip your hair of its vitality, and leave it looking lifeless. A daily haircare routine and prompt treatment when problems do arise are of vital importance in maintaining the natural beauty of healthy hair.

The haircare and styling section provides a complete guide to making the most of your hair. There are tips for establishing good haircare habits, and tricks and treatments to get your hair in great shape – from aromatic shampoos, herbal tonics and intensive conditioning treatments to colouring, bleaching and tinting – as well as a range of inspirational styling ideas for every season and occasion.

## exercise and healthy eating

It is particularly important that you make regular exercise and healthy eating a key part of your beauty routine. Walking, swimming, cycling, working out, yoga and Pilates are all great ways to stay fit, increase your stamina and keep your body toned and supple. Exercise boosts circulation, allowing the body to absorb nutrients and eliminate toxins and waste more efficiently. The exercise and healthy eating section provides a complete guide to health and fitness, from finding the right sports to relaxation and stress-reducing techniques. There are simple step-by-step sequences for general fitness to fit into your daily routine, as well as an introduction to the benefits of Pilates.

A healthy diet involves eating foods that provide all the nourishment your body requires for growth, tissue repair, energy to carry out vital internal processes and to make sure you are fit and active. The healthy eating chapter has a clear, comprehensive breakdown of foods and nutritional values to help you achieve a balance in your daily diet. There is advice on the best foods to eat to improve your skin, hair and nails, and hints on how to change your eating habits.

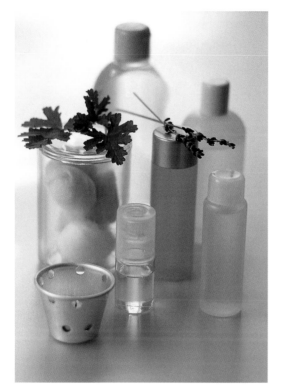

△ Many different plant extracts are used in beauty products. An extract is chosen not only for its fragrance, but also for its healing properties.

## healing aromatherapy

This section offers ideas for health and well-being at all stages of a woman's life. It describes what aromatic essential oils are, how they work and which oils and blends can be used to target specific problems and restore the mind–body harmony that is needed for good health.

## ayurvedic beauty

This is the ancient Indian system that covers all aspects of human life. Ayurveda's rules for healthy living, laid down 3,000 years ago, are still relevant today. Beauty shines through skin nourished by pure food, from a mind and body that work harmoniously — with stress relieved by meditation and a body tuned by yoga. This section is also packed with easy-to-make recipes for creams and scrubs, still widely used in India.

One great change from our ancestors' time is in our lifespans. Surviving longer than ever before, women in developed countries can now expect to live for nearly 30 years after the menopause. Time to relax and enjoy all the pleasures of a more leisurely life so long as we remain healthy.

## aging naturally

In this final section there is ample self-help information that can make this a long and rewarding period of any woman's life. Almonds and pumpkin seeds, for example, provide vital minerals to keep bones healthy. Adding a few flexibility exercises to your daily routine can release a grace of movement you never thought possible. So don't wait till you start slowing down — now's the time to start getting more out of life, the natural way.

▽ Fresh flowers bring beauty into our lives and stimulate feelings of happiness and well-being.

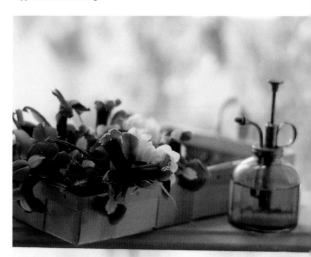

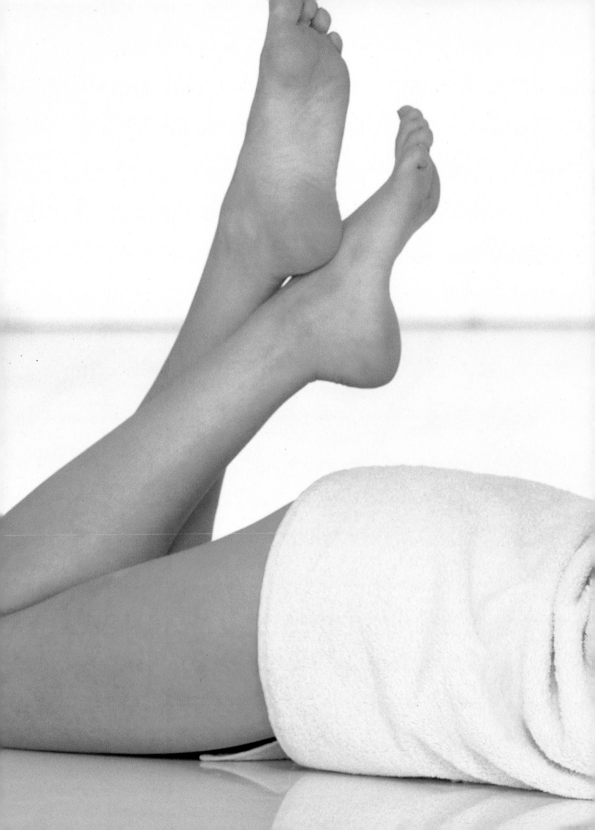

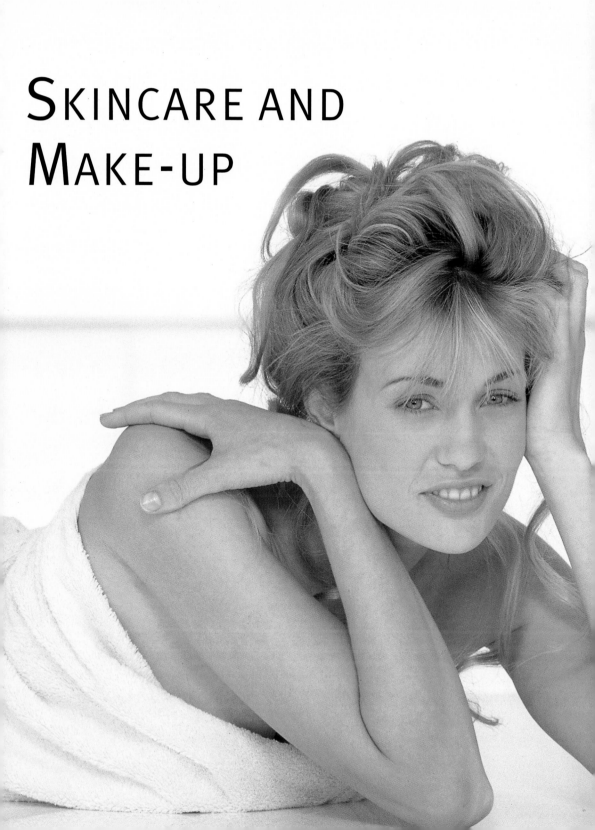

# Skincare and Make-up

# What is skin?

Skin is your body's largest organ, covering and protecting every single surface of your body. The secret of beautiful, healthy skin is to understand how your skin functions because this will help you to treat it correctly, keeping it strong and supple. Your skin is made up of two main layers, called the epidermis and the dermis.

## the epidermis

This is the top layer of skin and the one you can actually see. It protects your body from invasion and infection and helps to seal in moisture. It's built up of several layers of living cells which are then topped by sheets of dead cells. It's constantly growing, with new cells being produced at its base. They quickly die, and are pushed up to the surface by the arrival of new ones. These dead cells eventually flake away, which means that every new layer of skin is another chance to have a soft, glowing complexion.

The lower levels of living cells are fed by the blood supply from underneath, whereas the upper dead cells only require a supply of water to make sure that they are kept plump and smooth.

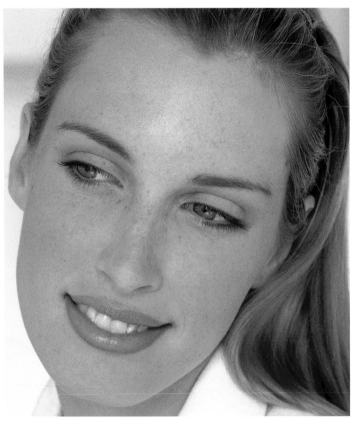

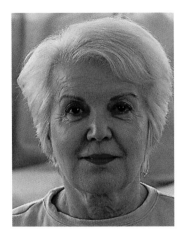

△ Every woman can have beautiful skin regardless of age, race or colouring.

The epidermis is responsible for your colouring, because it holds the skin's pigment. Its thickness varies from area to area. For instance, it's much thicker on the soles of your feet than on your eyelids.

## the dermis

The layer that lies underneath the epidermis is called the dermis, and it is composed entirely of living cells. It consists of bundles of tough fibres, which give your skin its elasticity, firmness and strength. There are also blood vessels, which feed vital nutrients to these areas.

The epidermis is usually able to repair and restore itself to make itself as good as

△ Understanding your skin the way a beauty therapist would allows you to give it the care it deserves and to appreciate why certain factors are good for it – and others are not.

new, but the dermis will be permanently damaged by injury. The dermis also contains the following specialized organs:

**Sebaceous glands:** These are tiny organs that usually open into hair follicles on the surface of your skin. They produce an oily secretion, called sebum, which is your skin's natural lubricant. The sebaceous glands are concentrated on the scalp and face, around the nose, cheeks, chin and forehead (the T-zone), which are usually the most oily areas.

▷ The condition of your skin is an overall sign of your health. It reveals stress, a poor diet and a lack of sleep. Taking care of your health will benefit your skin.

**Sweat glands**: These are located all over your body. There are millions of them and their main function is to control and regulate your body temperature. When sweat evaporates on the skin's surface, the temperature of your skin drops.

**Hairs**: Growing out of the hair follicles, these can help to keep your body warm by trapping air underneath them. There are no hairs on the soles of your feet or the palms of your hands.

**THE MAIN FUNCTIONS OF YOUR SKIN**
• It acts as a thermostat, retaining heat or cooling you down with sweat.
• It offers protection from potentially harmful things.
• It acts as a waste disposal system. Certain waste is expelled from your body 24 hours a day through your skin.
• It provides a sense of touch, which enables you to interact and communicate with other people and function in your environment.

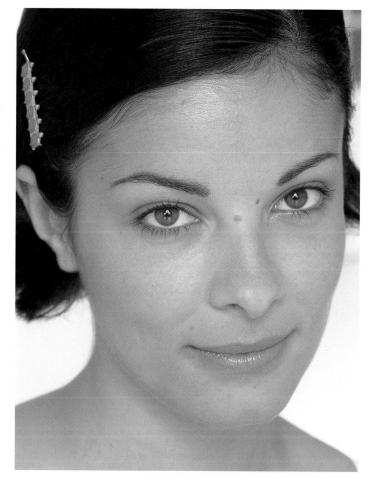

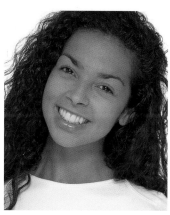

△ Skin is a barometer of your emotions. It becomes red when you're embarrassed and quickly shows the signs of stress.

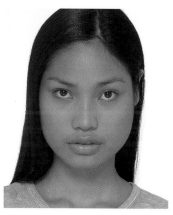

△ Your skin can cleanse, heal and even renew itself. How effectively it does these things is partly governed by you.

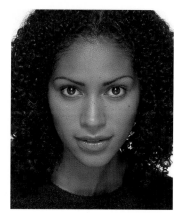

△ Your skin is a sensor of pain, touch and temperature, offering protection and a means of eliminating waste.

skincare and make-up

# What is your skin type?

There's no point spending a fortune on expensive skincare products if you buy the wrong ones for your skin type and make a collection of assorted once-used bottles. The key to developing a skincare regime that works for you is to analyse your skin-type first.

## skincare quiz

To develop a better understanding of your skin and what will suit it best, start by answering the questions here. Then add up your score and check the list at the end to discover which of the skin types you fit into.

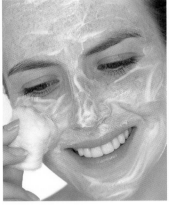

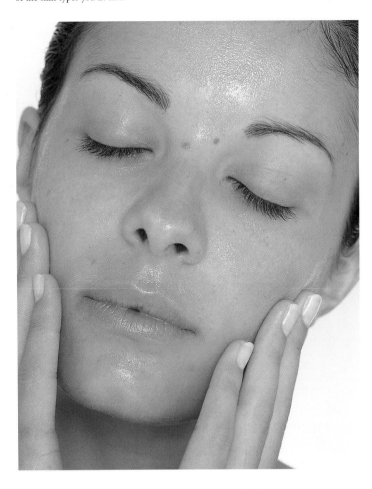

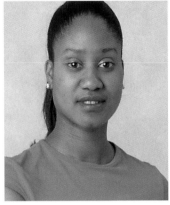

**2** How does your skin feel if you cleanse it with cream cleanser?

**A** Relatively comfortable.

**B** Smooth and comfortable.

**C** Sometimes comfortable, sometimes itchy.

**D** Quite oily.

**E** Oily in some areas and smooth in others.

**3** How does your skin usually look by the middle of the day?

**A** Flaky patches appearing.

**B** Fresh and clean.

**C** Flaky patches and some redness.

**D** Shiny.

**E** Shiny in the T-zone.

**1** How does your skin feel if you cleanse it with facial wash and water?

**A** Tight, as though it's too small for your face.

**B** Smooth and comfortable.

**C** Dry and itchy in places.

**D** Fine – quite comfortable.

**E** Dry in some areas and smooth in others.

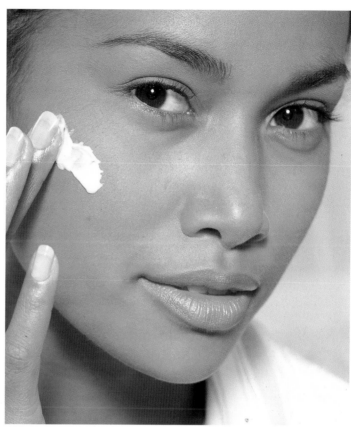

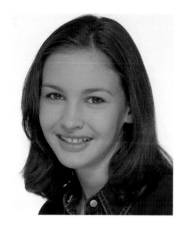

**4** How often do you break out in spots?

**A** Hardly ever.

**B** Occasionally, perhaps before or during your period.

**C** Occasionally.

**D** Often.

**E** Often – in the T-zone.

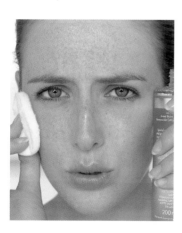
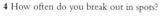

**5** How does your skin react when you use facial toner?

**A** It stings.

**B** No problems.

**C** Stings and itches.

**D** Feels fresher.

**E** Feels fresher in some areas but stings in others.

**6** How does your skin react when you have applied a rich night cream?

**A** It feels very comfortable.

**B** Comfortable.

**C** Sometimes feels comfortable, other times feels irritated.

**D** Makes your skin feel very oily.

**E** Oily in the T-zone, comfortable on the cheeks.

Now add up your A's, B's, C's, D's and E's. Your skin-type is the one that has the majority of answers.

**Mostly A's:** Your skin is DRY.

**Mostly B's:** Your skin is NORMAL.

**Mostly C's:** Your skin is SENSITIVE.

**Mostly D's:** Your skin is OILY.

**Mostly E's:** Your skin is COMBINATION.

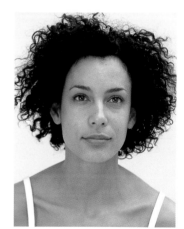

△ You know best how your skin reacts to different things so check your skin type before you buy lots of skincare products. Even if you've been told what your skin type is at some stage, it is a good idea to run through this quiz now as your skin will change over a period of time.

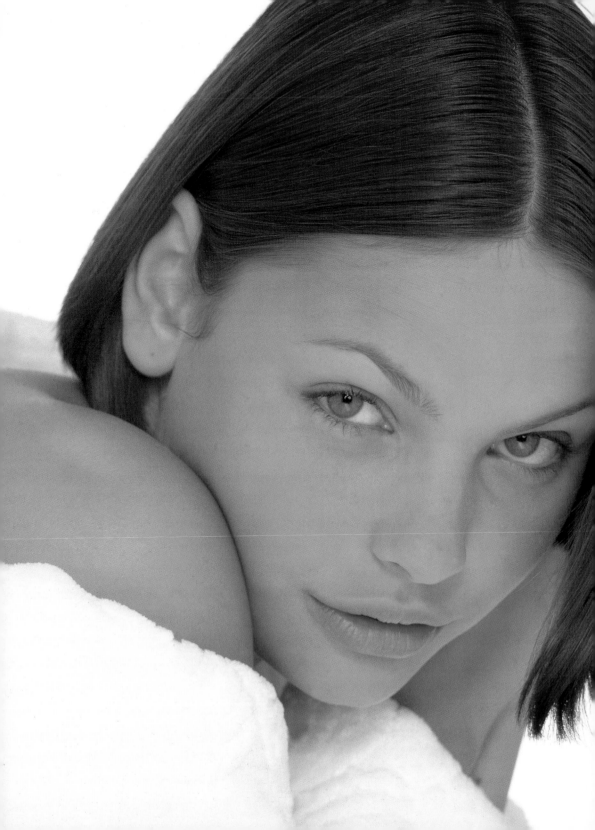

# Caring for your Skin

Clear, soft and supple skin is one of the greatest beauty assets, and there is plenty you can do every day to ensure that your skin always looks as good as possible. You'll soon realize the benefits of regularly spending time on your skin, and the results will last a lifetime.

Before you can devise the best regime for yourself and give your skin some special care, you need to understand what the main skincare products are designed to do.

## the key treatments

From the old soap and water cleansing routine, today's skincare has evolved into a modern range of products.

### facial washes

These liquids are designed to be lathered with water to dissolve grime, dirt and stale make-up from the skin's surface.

### cleansing bars

Ordinary soap is too drying for most skins. Now you can foam up with these special bars, which will cleanse your skin without stripping it of moisture. They're refreshing for oilier skin-types, and help keep pores clear and prevent pimples and blackheads.

### cream cleansers

A wonderful way to cleanse drier complexions, they generally have a light, fluid consistency that spreads more easily on to the skin. They contain oils to dissolve surface dirt and make-up, and can be quickly removed with cotton wool (cotton).

### toners and astringents

Refreshing and cooling your skin, they quickly evaporate after being applied with cotton wool. They can also remove excess oil from the surface layers of your skin. The word "astringent" means it has a higher alcohol content, and is suitable only for oily skins. The words "tonic" and "toner" mean that they're useful for normal or combination skins, as they are gentler. Those with dry and sensitive skins should avoid these products, as they can be too drying. Generally, if the product stings your face, move on to a gentler foundation or weaken it by adding a few drops of distilled water (available from a pharmacist).

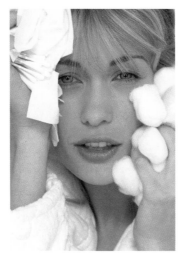

### moisturizers

The key function of a moisturizer is to form a barrier film on the skin's surface to prevent moisture loss. This makes the skin feel softer and smoother. Generally, the drier your skin the thicker the moisturizer you should choose. All skin types need a moisturizer, and one of the most valuable ingredients to look for is a UV filter. This ensures your moisturizer will give your skin year-round protection from the burning rays of the sun.

### eye make-up removers

Ordinary cleansers aren't usually sufficient to remove stubborn eye make-up, which is why these special products are so useful.

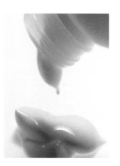

◁ Put some zing into your skincare regime with a refreshing toner or astringent.

If you wear waterproof mascara you will probably need to check that the cleanser you use is designed to remove it.

## special treatments

In addition to a basic wardrobe of skincare products, you can add a few extras.

### face masks

These intensive treatments deep-cleanse your skin or boost its moisture levels.

### facial scrubs and exfoliators

These creams or gels contain hundreds of tiny abrasive particles. When massaged into damp skin, the particles dislodge dead surface skin cells, revealing the younger, fresher cells underneath.

### eye creams

The delicate skin around your eyes is usually the first to show the signs of ageing. These gels and creams contain ingredients to plump out fine lines. They can also reduce puffiness and under-eye shadows.

### night creams

These intensive creams are designed to pamper your skin while you sleep. They can have a thicker consistency because you won't need to apply make-up over the top.

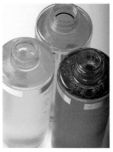

◁◁ Creamy cleansers should be a top priority for drier complexions, as they cleanse and nourish at the same time.

◁ Before you tailor-make a skincare regime for yourself, you need to know the key benefits of each product.

# A fresh approach to oily skin

This skin type usually has open pores and an oily surface, with a tendency towards pimples, blackheads and a sallow appearance. This is due to the over-production of the oily substance called sebum by the oil glands in the lower layers of the skin. Unfortunately, this skin-type is the one most prone to acne. The good news is that this oiliness will make your skin stay younger-looking for longer – so there are some benefits!

**ACNE ALERT**

This is a distressing condition that usually appears in our lives at a time when we're already feeling insecure – adolescence. A condition that often runs in families, it is thought to be triggered by a hormonal change which causes your skin to produce more sebum. It can be aggravated by stress and poor diet, and careful skincare helps keep acne under control. Avoid picking at pimples, as this can lead to scarring. Try over-the-counter blemish treatments, as today's formulations contain ingredients that are successful at treating this problem. Products containing tea tree oil can also be effective. If these aren't successful, consult your doctor who may provide treatment, or can refer you to a dermatologist.

## special care for oily skin

It's very important not to treat oily skin too rigorously, although you may well feel that you want to take drastic action when you are faced with a fresh outbreak of pimples. Remember that over-enthusiastic cleansing treatments can actually encourage the oil glands to produce even more sebum, and they will also leave the surface layers of your skin dry and dehydrated.

The best approach for oily skin is to use a range of products that gently cleanse away oils from the surface and unblock pores, without drying out and damaging the skin. The visible part of your skin actually requires water, not oil, in order to stay soft, healthy and supple.

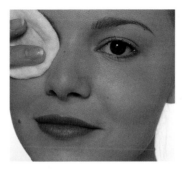

△ **1** Even though your skin is prone to oiliness, the skin around your eyes is delicate, so don't drag it when removing eye make-up. Soak a cotton wool (cotton) pad with a non-oily remover and hold over your eyes for a few seconds to dissolve the make-up, then lightly wipe it away from the eyelids and lashes.

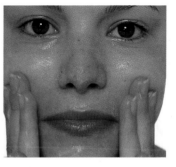

△ **2** Lather up with a gentle foaming facial wash. This is a better choice than ordinary soap, as it won't strip away moisture from your skin, but will remove grime, dirt and oil. Massage gently over damp skin with your fingertips, then rinse away the soapy suds with lots of warm water.

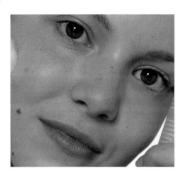

△ **3** Soak a cotton wool ball with astringent lotion, and sweep it over your skin to refresh it. This shouldn't irritate your skin – if it does, change to a gentler one. Continue until the cotton wool comes up clean.

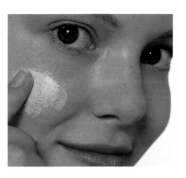

△ **4** Even oily skins need moisturizer, because it helps seal water into the top layers to keep the skin soft and supple. Don't load the skin down with a heavy formulation. Instead, choose a light, watery fluid.

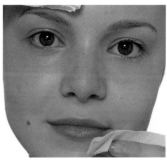

△ **5** Allow the moisturizer to sink in for a few minutes, then press a clean tissue over your face to absorb the excess, and to prevent a shiny complexion.

# Nourishing care for dry skin

If your skin tends to feel tight, as if it is one size too small, it's a fair bet you've got a dry complexion. This is caused by too little sebum in the lower levels of skin, and too little moisture in the upper levels. At its best, it can feel tight and itchy after washing. At its worst it can be flaky, with little patches of dandruff in your eyebrows, and a tendency to premature ageing with the emergence of fine lines and wrinkles. It requires a regular routine of soothing care to keep it looking its best.

## special care for dry skin

The condition of dry skin can be aggravated by over-use of soap, detergents and toners. It can also be adversely affected by exposure to hot sun, cold winds and central heating. For these reasons it is advisable to opt for a gentle, nourishing approach that concentrates on boosting the skin's moisture levels. This will plump out fine lines and keep the skin soft and supple.

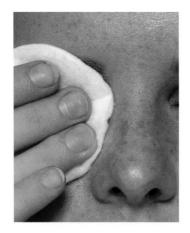

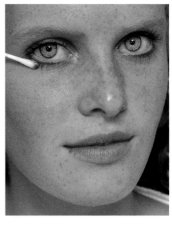

△ **1** Pour a little oil-based eye make-up remover on to a cotton wool (cotton) pad and sweep it over the eye area. This oily product will also help soothe away dryness in the delicate eye area, but a little goes a long way. If you overload the skin here with an oily product it can cause puffiness and irritation.

△ **2** If there are any stubborn flecks of mascara left behind, tackle them with a cotton bud (swab) dipped in the eye make-up remover. Take great care that the remover does not get in your eyes, but you will need to work as closely as you can to the eyelashes to remove all signs of make-up.

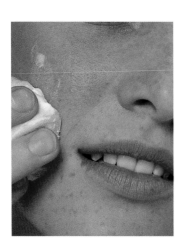

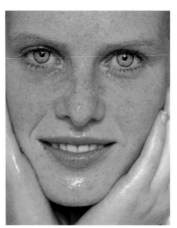

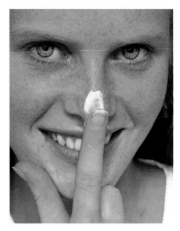

△ **3** Choose a creamy cleanser as it's vital that your skin is really clean. Leave the cleanser on for a few moments, before sweeping it away with a cotton wool pad. Use gentle upward movements to prevent stretching the skin and encouraging lines.

△ **4** Many women with dry skin complain that they miss the feeling of water on their skin. However, you can splash your face with cool water to remove excess cleanser and to refresh your skin. This also helps boost the circulation.

△ **5** Finally, apply a nourishing cream to seal in moisture. Opt for a thick cream, not a runny lotion, as this contains more oil than water, and helps seal in moisture. Give the moisturizer a few minutes to sink in before applying make-up.

# Balanced care for combination skin

Combination skin needs careful attention because it has a blend of oily and dry patches. The centre panel or T-zone, across the forehead and down the nose and chin, tends to be oily, and needs to be treated like oily skin. However, the other areas are prone to dryness and flakiness from lack of moisture, and need to be treated like dry skin.

Having said this, some combination skins don't follow the T-zone pattern and can have patches of dry and oily skin in other arrangements. If you're unsure of your skin's oily and dry areas, press a tissue to your face an hour after washing it. Any greasy patches on the tissue signify oily areas.

## special care for combination skin

Skin that has a combination of dry and oily patches requires a dual approach to skincare. Treating your entire complexion like oily skin will leave the dry areas even drier and tighter than before. In the same way, treating it only like dry skin can provoke excess oiliness and even an outbreak of blemishes. This means that you need to deal with the different areas of skin individually, with products to suit. This isn't as complicated and difficult as it sounds, and the result will be a softer, smoother and clearer complexion than before!

A dual approach to skincare will double the benefits for combination skin, and it needn't be terribly time-consuming.

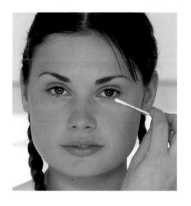

△ **1** Choose an oil-based eye make-up remover to clear away every trace of eye make-up from this delicate area which is prone to dryness. Use a cotton bud (swab) to remove any stubborn traces. Splash with cool water afterwards to rinse away any excess oil.

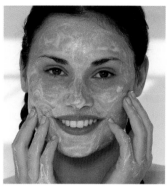

△ **2** Use a foaming facial wash in the morning. This ensures oily areas are clean, and clears pores to prevent blackheads. Massage a little on to damp skin, especially oily areas. Leave for a few seconds to dissolve the dirt, then splash clean with cool water.

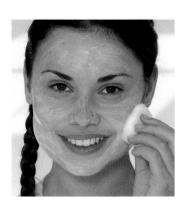

△ **3** In the evening, switch to a cream cleanser, to keep dry areas of skin clean and soothed. This will balance excess oiliness or dryness in your complexion. Massage well into your skin, concentrating on the drier areas, then gently remove with cotton wool (cotton) pads.

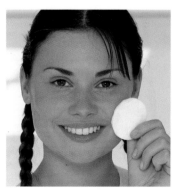

△ **4** To freshen your skin, you need two different strengths of toner to deal with the differing skin types. Choose a stronger astringent for oily areas, and a mild skin freshener for drier ones. This isn't as costly as you think, because you will use only a little of each. Sweep over your skin with cotton wool pads.

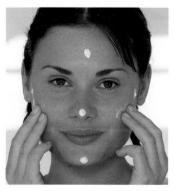

△ **5** Smooth moisturizer on to your entire face, concentrating on the drier areas. Then blot off any excess from the oily areas with a tissue. This will give all your skin the nourishment it needs.

# Maintaining normal skin

This is the perfect, balanced skin-type. It has a healthy glow, with a fine texture and no open pores. It rarely develops spots or shiny areas. The truth is that it is actually quite rare to find a perfectly normal skin, especially because all skins tend to become slightly drier as you get older.

## special care for normal skin

Your main concern is to maintain normal skin, to keep it functioning well, and as a result of this let it continue the good job it's already doing! It naturally has a good balance of oil and moisture levels. Your routine should include gently cleansing your skin to ensure surface grime and stale make-up are removed, and to prevent a build-up of sebum. Then you should boost moisture levels with moisturizer, to protect and pamper your skin.

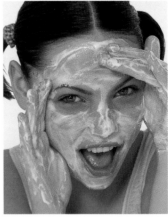

△ **1** Always remove eye make-up carefully. Going to bed with your mascara still on can lead to sore, puffy eyes. Applying new make-up on top of old, stale make-up is unhygienic, too! Choose your cleanser according to whether you're wearing ordinary or waterproof mascara.

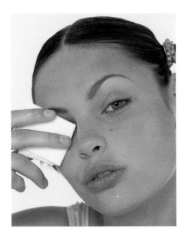

△ **2** Splash your face with water, then massage in a gentle facial wash and work it up to a lather for about 30 seconds. It is a good idea to massage your skin lightly, because this will boost the supply of blood to the surface of your skin – which means a rosier complexion.

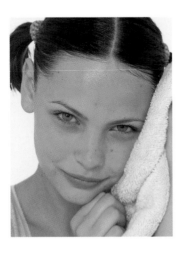

△ **3** Rinse with clear water until every soapy trace has been removed from your face. Then pat your face with a soft towel to absorb residual water from the surface of your skin. Don't rub at your skin, especially around the eyes, as this can encourage wrinkling.

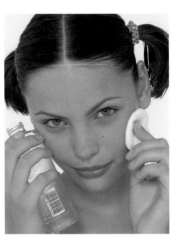

△ **4** Cool your skin with a freshening toner. Again, avoid the delicate eye area as this can become more prone to dryness.

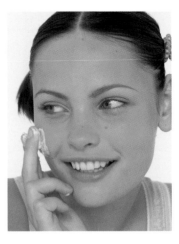

△ **5** Smooth your skin with moisturizing lotion. Dot on to your face, then massage in with your fingertips using light upward strokes. This leaves a protective film on the skin, so make-up can be easily applied and the moisture content is balanced.

# Soothing care for sensitive skin

Sensitive skin is usually quite fine in texture, with a tendency to be rosier than usual. Easily irritated by products and external factors, it's also prone to redness and allergy, and may have fine broken veins across the cheeks and nose. There are varying levels of sensitivity. If you feel you can't use any products on your skin without irritating it, cleanse with whole milk and moisturize with a solution of glycerin and rosewater. These should soothe it.

## special care for sensitive skin

**Your skin needs extra-gentle products to keep it supple and healthy. Choose from a wide range of hypo-allergenic products that are specially formulated to protect sensitive skin. These products are free of common irritants, such as fragrance, that can cause dryness, itchiness or even an allergic reaction.**

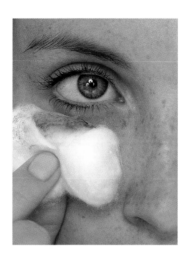

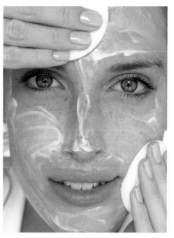

△ **1** Make sure the make-up you use is hypo-allergenic, too, and remove it thoroughly. First use a soothing eye make-up remover. Apply with a cotton wool (cotton) ball, then remove every last trace with a clean cotton bud (swab).

△ **2** It is advisable not to use facial washes and soaps, as these are likely to strip your skin of oil and moisture which can increase its sensitivity even more. So, instead, choose a light, hypo-allergenic cleansing lotion.

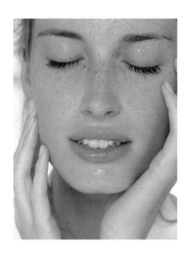

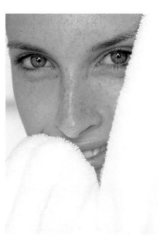

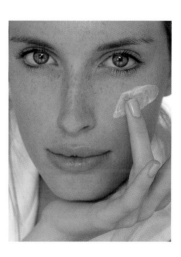

△ **3** Even mild skin fresheners can break down the natural protection your delicate skin needs against the elements. So freshen it by splashing with warm water instead. This also removes the final traces of cleanser and eye make-up remover from your skin.

△ **4** To dry your skin, lightly pat your face with a soft towel, taking care not to rub the skin because this could irritate it.

△ **5** It is vital to keep your skin moisturized to keep it strong and supple and provide a barrier against irritants that can lead to sensitivity. Dryness can make sensitive skin more uncomfortable, so it is a good idea to choose an unscented moisturizer.

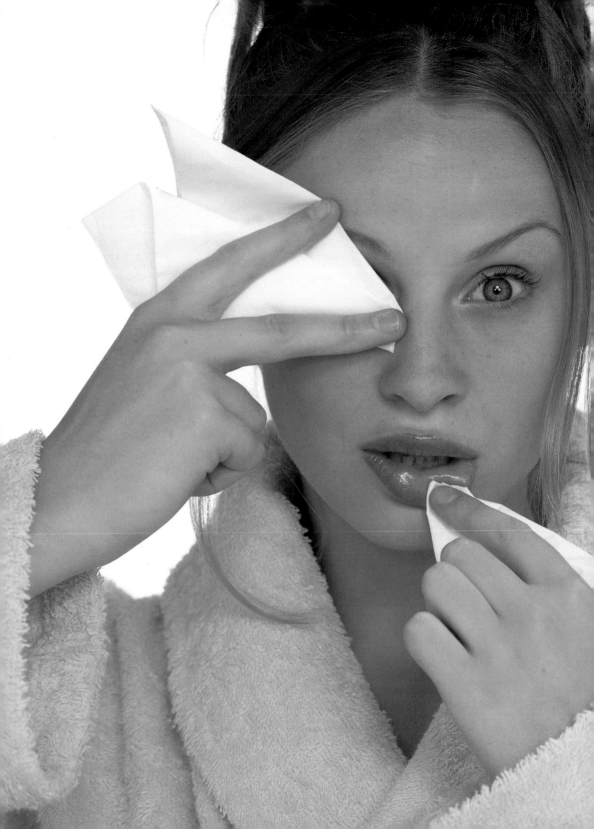

# Special Treatments

However well you care for your skin on a daily basis, from time to time a special treatment can make it feel even better. This chapter is packed with fabulous facials, healing masks, invigorating scrubs and soothing massages, as well as hints and tips on tackling particular problems.

# Miraculous masks

If there's one skincare item that can work miracles, it's a face mask. But, like any other skincare product, you should choose carefully to pick the right one for you.

## mask it!

Choose from the wonderful selection of face masks on the market to find one that is perfect for your skin.

### moisturizing masks

These are ideal for dry complexions because they boost the moisture levels of your skin. This means they can help banish dry patches, flakiness and even fine lines. They work quickly like an intensive moisturizer, and are usually left on the skin for 5–10 minutes before being removed with a tissue. The slight residue left on your skin will continue to work until you next cleanse your skin. They are a soothing treat, particularly after too much sun, or when your skin feels "tight".

### clay and mud masks

Ideal for oily skins, they absorb excess grease and impurities. They're an ideal way to "shrink" open pores, reduce shine and clear troublesome blemishes. They dry on your skin over a period of 5–15 minutes, then you simply wash them away with warm water, rinsing dead skin cells, dirt and grime away at the same time. They're a fantastic pick-me-up for skin.

### exfoliating masks

Masks with a light exfoliating action can keep your skin in tip-top condition. Even normal skins sometimes suffer from the build-up of dead skin cells, which can create a dull look and lead to future problems such as blackheads. Masks that cleanse and exfoliate are the perfect solution. They smooth on like a clay mask, and are left to dry. When you rinse them away, their tiny abrasive particles slough away the skin's surface debris.

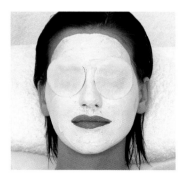

### peel-off masks

Ideal for all skin types, the gel is smoothed on, left to dry and peeled off. The light formulation refreshes oily areas, clears clogged pores and nourishes drier skins.

### gel masks

These are suitable for sensitive skins, as well as oily complexions, as they have a wonderfully soothing and cooling effect.

◁ **Clay and mud masks dry on your skin over a period of 5–15 minutes.**

Simply apply the gel, lie back, then wipe off excess after 5–10 minutes. Ideal after too much sun, or if your skin feels irritated.

## face mask tips

Your skin can change with the seasons. Skin that becomes oily in the hot summer months can become drier in winter and in central heating. So take your skin's quirks into account when choosing your mask.

• Cleanse your face before applying your chosen mask. Afterwards, rinse with warm water, than apply moisturizer.

• Most masks should be left on the skin for between 3 and 10 minutes. For the best results, read the instructions carefully.

• If you have combination skin, use two masks – one suitable for oily skin and one for dry skin. Just apply each one to the area that needs it.

---

**NATURAL NOURISHERS**
Making masks from natural ingredients is easy to do and can be very effective.

### avocado mash

Avocados make excellent face masks for dry skin. They boast 14 minerals as well as the antioxidant vitamins E and A. To prepare a face mask, mash up an avocado, add a touch of sweet almond oil and smooth the mixture over your face; keep it on for as long as possible to nourish and soften your skin.

### gentle oatmeal mask

A good face mask for oily skin, this recipe is sufficient for one treatment and must be applied as soon as it is mixed.

### ingredients

• 15ml/1 tbsp runny honey
• 1 egg yolk
• up to 60ml/4 tbsp fine oatmeal

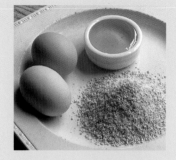

Mix honey and egg yolk together in a small bowl, then slowly stir in enough oatmeal to make a soft paste. Smooth the mask on to the skin of the face and neck and leave for 15 minutes. Rinse off with lukewarm water and pat your skin dry.

# Facial scrubs

Brighten up your complexion in an instant with this skincare treat – if you don't include a facial scrub in your weekly skincare regime, then you've been missing out! Technically known as exfoliation, it's a simple method that whisks away dead cells from the surface of your skin, revealing the plumper, younger ones underneath. It also encourages your skin to speed up cell production, which means that the cells that reach the surface are younger and better-looking. The result is a brighter, smoother complexion – no matter what your age or skin type.

## action tactics

Use an exfoliater on dry or normal skin once or twice a week. Oily or combination skins can be exfoliated every other day. As a rule, avoid this treatment on sensitive skin, or if you have bad acne. However, you can gently exfoliate pimple-prone skin once a week to help keep pores clear and prevent break-outs.

## getting to the nitty-gritty

Apply a blob of facial scrub cream to damp skin, massage gently, then rinse away with lots of cool water. Opt for an exfoliater that contains gentler, rounded beads, rather than scratchy ones such as crushed kernels.

You could also try a mini exfoliating pad, lathering up with soap or facial wash.

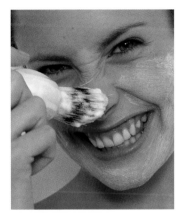

△ Instead of using a facial scrub, gently massage your skin with a soft flannel, facial brush or old, clean shaving brush and facial wash.

## applying a facial scrub
Using a facial scrub is a quick and invigorating way to cleanse and smooth your skin.

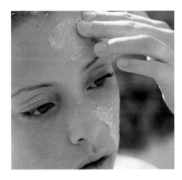

△ **1** With a light touch, gently rub the facial scrub into damp skin, using a circular motion and taking care to avoid the delicate area of skin around the eyes.

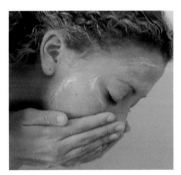

△ **2** Rinse the facial scrub off thoroughly and slowly with splashes of warm water and then gently pat your face dry with a soft towel.

### GENTLE FACE SCRUB

This is a luxurious blend of almonds, oatmeal, milk and rose petals. The rose petals should be bought from a herbalist or, if you want to use petals from your garden, be sure that they have not been sprayed with chemicals. The rose petals can be powdered in a pestle and mortar or in an electric coffee grinder. When mixed with almond oil, the scrub will cleanse the face and leave it silky soft.

### ingredients
Makes enough for 10 treatments.

- 45ml/3 tbsp ground almonds (without skin)
- 45ml/3 tbsp medium oatmeal
- 45ml/3 tbsp powdered milk
- 30ml/2 tbsp powdered rose petals
- almond oil
- mixing bowl
- spoon
- lidded glass jar

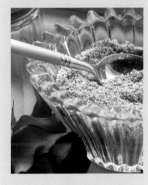

Put all the ingredients in a bowl and combine thoroughly. Then store the mixture in a sealed glass jar. When you are ready to use the facial scrub, take a handful of the mixture and blend it to make a soft paste with a little almond oil. Apply and remove as shown (left).

# Fabulous face pampering

For deep-down cleansing and a definite improvement in skin tone, try an at-home facial. If you apply this treatment just once a month you will notice an improvement in your complexion. Simply follow these step-by-step instructions for a fabulous facial to recreate the benefits of the beauty salon in the comfort and privacy of your own home.

**SKIN TONIC RECIPE**

This flower skin tonic is suitable for normal skin, and can be applied to soothe and freshen the skin.

**ingredients**
- 75ml/5 tbsp orangeflower water
- 25ml/1½ tbsp rosewater

Pour the ingredients into a glass bottle and shake to mix. Apply to skin with a cotton wool (cotton) pad.

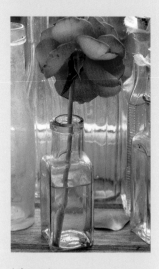

△ **If you make your own rosewater any fragrant roses are suitable for this recipe, as long as they have not been sprayed with pesticide. Pink or red ones are best.**

## freshening facial

**Facial skin is delicate and needs regular cleansing to keep the pores dirt-free so the skin can breathe.**

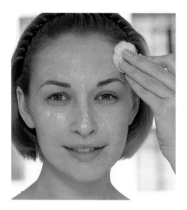

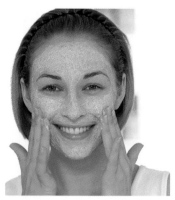

△ **1** Smooth your skin with cleansing cream. Leave on for 1–2 minutes to give it time to dissolve grime, oil and stale make-up. Then gently smooth away with a cotton wool (cotton) ball.

△ **2** Dampen your skin with warm water. Then gently massage with a blob of facial scrub, taking care to avoid the delicate eye area. This will loosen dead surface skin cells, and leave your skin softer and smoother. It will also prepare your complexion for the beneficial treatments to come. Rinse away with splashes of warm water.

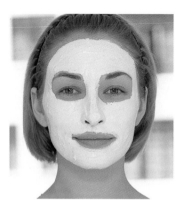

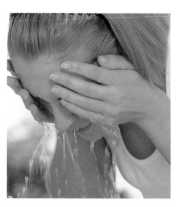

△ **4** Smooth on a face mask. Choose a clay-based one if you have oily skin, or a moisturizing one if you have dry or normal skin. Leave the mask on your skin for 5 minutes, or for as long as specified by the instructions on the product.

△ **5** Rinse away the face mask with warm water. Once all the mask is removed, finish off with a few splashes of cool water to close your pores and freshen your skin, then pat dry with a towel.

# face massage

**Dot your skin with moisturizer and smooth in. Following your facial, continue the pampering by taking the opportunity to massage your skin, as this encourages a brighter complexion and can help to reduce puffiness.**

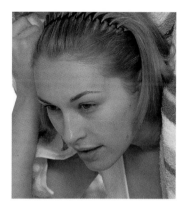

△ **3** Fill a bowl or washbasin with boiling water. Lean over it, capturing the steam with a towel placed over your head. Allow the steam to warm and soften your skin for 5 minutes. If you have blackheads, try to remove them gently with tissue-covered fingers after this treatment. If you suffer from sensitive skin, or are prone to broken veins, you should avoid this step.

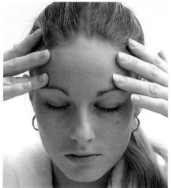

△ **1** Starting in the centre of your forehead, make small circular motions with your fingertips and work slowly out towards the temples. Repeat 3 times.

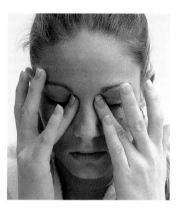

△ **2** Use your fingers to apply gentle pressure to the area where the eye socket meets your nose. Repeat at least 3 times.

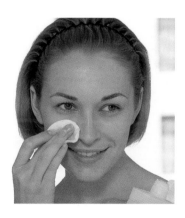

△ **6** Soak a cotton wool pad with a skin toner lotion or a homemade tonic, and smooth over oily areas, such as the nose, chin and forehead.

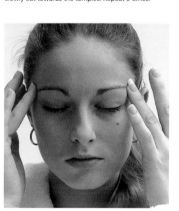

△ **3** Move your fingers outwards along the brow bone from the top of your nose. Repeat 5 times. The skin around the eyes is the most delicate on the face and the first to show signs of stress, so it is important that you treat this area very gently.

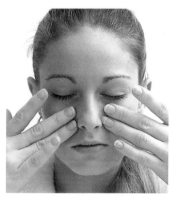

△ **4** Starting either side of your nose, move your fingers outwards using circular motions along the cheekbone to the jaw. Pay particular attention to the jaw area. Repeat 5 times. Finally, gently smooth your undereye area with a soothing eye cream to reduce fine lines and wrinkles, and make the skin ultra-soft.

# Care for eyes

The fine, delicate skin around your eyes is the first to show the signs of ageing. However, don't be tempted to deal with the problem by slapping on heavy oils and moisturizers because they are usually too heavy for the skin in the eye area. They can also block tear ducts, causing puffiness. The delicate skin around your eyes needs particularly special care because it is significantly thinner than the skin on the rest of your face, and this means that it is less able to hold in moisture. There are also fewer oil glands in this area, making it particularly susceptible to dryness, and also meaning that there is no fatty layer underneath to act as a shock absorber. Consequently this area of skin quickly loses its suppleness and elasticity.

## choosing an eye treatment

There is a huge range of products to choose from, and it is important to find the right one for you. Gel-based ones are suitable for young or oily skins, and are refreshing to use. However, most women find light eye creams and balms more effective.

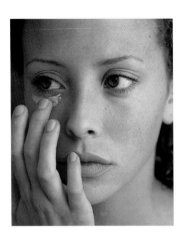

△ The skin around the eyes is soft and delicate so it is important to apply moisturizer to this area very gently.

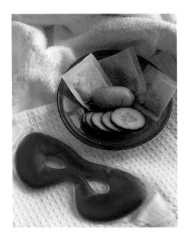

△ There is a range of remedies for eyes, from special pads to home-made therapies. Experiment to find out which works best for you.

Use a tiny amount of the eye treatment, as it's better to apply it regularly in small quantities than apply lots occasionally. Apply with your middle finger, as this is the weakest one and won't stretch the delicate skin. This will help keep your skin more supple and prevent premature wrinkling in this area.

## preventing puffy eyes

This is one of the most common beauty problems. These ideas can help:
• Gently tap your skin with your ring finger when you're applying eye cream to encourage the excess fluid to drain away.
• Store creams in the refrigerator, as the coldness will also help reduce puffiness.
• Place thin strips of potato underneath your eyes to reduce swelling. The starch in the potato seems to tighten the skin.
• Fill a small bowl with iced water or ice-cold milk. Soak two cotton wool (cotton) pads and lie down with the pads over your eyes. Replace the pads as soon as they become warm. Continue for 15 minutes. This treatment reduces puffiness and brightens the whites of your eyes.

## cooling cucumber

This is a super-quick and simple treatment. Place a slice of cucumber over each eye, then just lie back and relax for 15 minutes. Cucumber will gently tone and soothe the skin around the eyes.

## herbal eyepads

A compress over your eyes will refresh them, reduce puffiness and relieve itchiness.

### fennel decoction

Make a decoction by boiling 10ml/2 tsp fennel seeds in 300ml/$^1$/$_2$ pint/1$^1$/$_4$ cups purified water for 30 minutes. Strain and cool, then use to soak cotton wool pads.

### teabag treatments

Use a teabag to make tea then apply to the eyes when cool. Chamomile is good for tired eyes. The tannin in Indian tea is an astringent and will firm the skin.

### rosewater

Soak cotton wool pads in an infusion of rose petals and purified water.

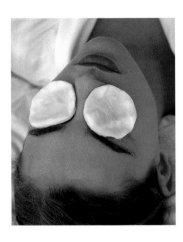

△ Whichever eye treatment you decide to use, it is vital that you take time to lie down and relax for at least 10 minutes.

# Goodnight creams

Going to bed with night cream on your face can benefit your skin while you are sleeping. The main difference between night creams and ordinary daily moisturizers is that most night creams have special added ingredients such as vitamins and anti-ageing components. They can also be thicker and more intensive than creams you apply during the day because you won't need to apply make-up on top of them.

Your skin's cell renewal is more active during the night, and night creams are designed to make the most of these hours. Using a night cream gives your skin the chance to repair the daily wear and tear caused by pollution, make-up and ultra-violet light.

## who needs night creams?

While very young skins do not generally require the extra nourishing properties of night creams, most women will benefit from using one regularly. Dry and very dry skins will respond particularly well to this treatment. Remember that you don't have to choose very rich formulations, as there

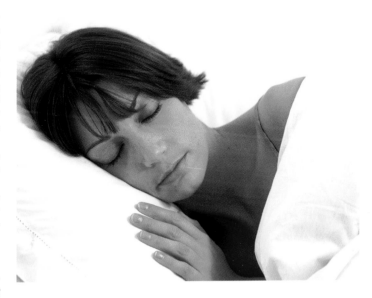

are lighter alternatives that contain the same special ingredients. Choose the formulation carefully on the basis of how dry your skin is – it is important that your skin shouldn't feel overloaded.

△ Applying night cream before you go to bed means waking up to a softer, smoother complexion. If you apply cream to slightly damp skin this can really boost its performance, as it seals in extra moisture.

▽ Dab a little night cream in your palm, then gently rub your hands together. The heat will liquefy the cream so that it is more easily absorbed as you massage it into your skin.

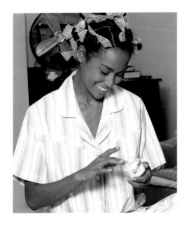

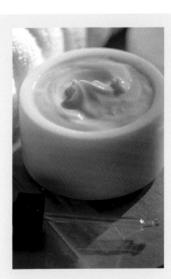

### NOURISHING NIGHT CREAM

As we get older, our skin becomes drier and more in need of regular care. Jasmine and rose oils help to rehydrate the skin, while frankincense helps to reduce wrinkles and restore tone to slack muscles.

### ingredients

- 50g/2oz jar of unperfumed base cream with a close-fitting lid
- 3 drops of rose essential oil
- 2 drops of frankincense essential oil
- 1 drop of jasmine essential oil

Add the oils to the cream, and mix well together. Apply a little of the cream just before going to bed.

# Special skin treatments

As well as basic moisturizers, there is a vast range of special treatments, serums and gels that have been carefully formulated to treat specific problems.

## key treatments

Special skin treatments come in all shapes and sizes, and in various formulations:

### serums and gels

These have an ultraviolet formulation, a non-greasy texture and a high concentration of active ingredients. They're not usually designed to be used on their own, except on oily skins. They're generally applied under a moisturizer to enhance its benefits and boost the anti-ageing process.

### skin firmers

You can lift your skin instantly with creams that are designed to tighten, firm and smooth. They work by forming an ultra-fine film on the skin, which tightens your complexion and reduces the appearance of fine lines. The effects last for a few hours, and make-up can easily be applied on top. These products are a wonderful treat for a special night out or when you're feeling particularly tired.

### skin energizers

These creams contain special ingredients designed to accelerate the natural production and repair of skin cells. As well as producing a fresher, younger-looking skin, they are also thought to help combat the signs of ageing.

### ampule treatments

These concentrated active ingredients are contained in sealed glass phials or ampules, to ensure that they're fresh. Typical extracts include herbs, wheatgerm, vitamins and collagen – used for their intensive and fast-acting results. Vitamin E is another great skin saver. Break open a capsule and smooth the oil on to your face for a fast skin treat.

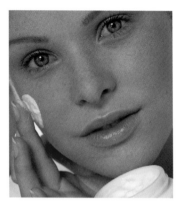

△ Choose a cream that contains specialized ingredients to improve your skin.

### liposomes creams

These are tiny spheres in the cream which carry special ingredients into the skin. Their shells break down as they're absorbed into your skin, releasing the active ingredients.

---

**AHA KNOW-HOW**

Alpha-hydroxy acids, also commonly known as fruit acids, are found in natural products. These include citric acid from citrus fruit, lactic acid from sour milk, tartaric acid from wine, and malic acid from apples and other fruits. Incorporated in small amounts, AHAs are often a key ingredient in specialized skincare products.

They work by breaking down the protein bonds that hold together the dead cells on the surface of your skin. They then lift them away to reveal brighter, plumper cells underneath. This gentle process cleans and clears blocked pores, improves your skintone and softens the look of fine lines. Basically, they're the ideal solution to most minor skincare problems. You should see results within a couple of weeks, although many women report an improvement after only a few days.

Without even realizing it, women have used AHAs for centuries and have reaped the benefits for their skins. For example, Cleopatra is said to

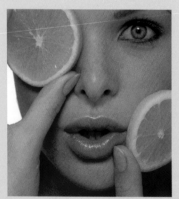

◁ AHAs (also known as fruit acids) are an effective way to replace the zing in your skin.

have bathed in sour asses' milk, and ladies of the French court applied wine to their faces to keep their skin smooth and blemish-free – both these ancient beauty aids contain AHAs.

AHA products are best used under your ordinary everyday moisturizer as a treatment cream. You should avoid applying them to the delicate eye and lip areas. If you have sensitive skin, you may find they're not suitable for you, but some women do experience a slight tingling sensation as the product gets to work. The great news is that AHA products are now becoming more affordable, and not just the preserve of more expensive skincare companies. Many mid-market companies are including the benefits of AHAs in their products, so everyone can give their skin the treatment it deserves. You can also find AHA products for the hands and body, so you can reap the benefits from top to toe.

# 10 ways to beat wrinkles

Fine lines and wrinkles aren't inevitable. In fact, skin experts believe that most skin damage can be prevented with some special care. Here are the 10 main points to bear in mind, no matter what your age.

## 1 sun protection

The single biggest cause of skin ageing is sunlight. You should use a sunscreen every day because the aging effects of the sun are as prevalent in the cold winter months as in the hot summer ones. This will help prevent your skin from aging prematurely, and will guard against burning.

## 2 stop smoking

Cigarette smoke speeds up the ageing process as it strips your skin of oxygen and slows down the regeneration of new cells. It can give the skin a grey, sluggish look, and cause fine lines around the mouth because heavy smokers are constantly pursing their lips to draw on a cigarette.

## 3 deep cleanse

Many older women don't cleanse their skin as thoroughly as they should, believing this can lead to dryness and lines. However, it's essential to ensure your skin is clear of dead skin cells, dirt and make-up to give it a youthful, fresh glow.

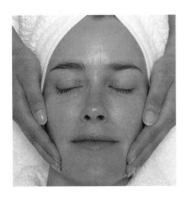

△ Relax and enjoy a beneficial facial!

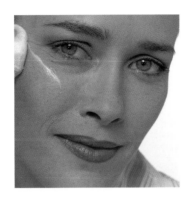

△ **Whatever you are applying to your skin, always use gentle strokes and an upward motion.**

Don't use harsh products – a creamy cleanser removed with cotton wool (cotton) is effective for most women. If your skin is very dry, massage with an oily cleanser. Leave on your skin for a few minutes, then rinse away the excess with warm water.

## 4 deep moisturize

As well as using a daily moisturizer, you can also boost your skin's water levels weekly. Either use a nourishing face mask, or apply a thick layer of your usual moisturizer or night cream. Whichever you choose, leave on the skin for 5–10 minutes, then remove the excess with tissues. Apply to damp skin for greater effect.

## 5 boost the circulation

Buy a gentle facial scrub or exfoliater, and use once a week to keep the surface of your skin soft and smooth. This increases the blood-flow to the top layers of skin, and encourages cell renewal. You can get the same effect by lathering a facial wash on your skin using a clean shaving brush.

## 6 disguise lines

Existing lines can be minimized to the naked eye by opting for the latest light-reflecting foundations, concealers and powders. These contain luminescent particles to bounce light away from your skin, making lines less noticeable and giving your skin a wonderful luminosity.

## 7 pamper regularly

As well as daily skincare, remember to treat your skin from time to time with special treatments such as facials, serums and anti-ageing creams.

## 8 be weather vain

Extremes of cold and hot weather can strip your skin of essential moisture, leaving it dry and more prone to damage. Central heating can have the same effect. For this reason, ensure you moisturize regularly, changing your products according to the seasons.

For instance, in the winter you may need a more oily product, which will keep the cold out and won't freeze on the skin's surface. In hot weather, lighter formulations are more comfortable on the skin, and you can boost their activity by using a few drops of special treatment serum underneath.

## 9 be gentle

Be careful not to drag at your skin when applying skincare products or make-up. The skin around your eyes is particularly likely to show signs of ageing. A heavy touch can cause the skin to stretch. So, always use a light touch, and take your strokes upwards, rather than drag the skin down. Also, avoid any products that make your skin itch, sting or feel sensitive. If any product causes this sort of reaction, stop using it at once and switch to a gentler formulation.

## 10 clever make-up

Skincare benefits aren't limited to skincare products. In fact, many make-up products now contain UV filters and skin-nourishing ingredients to treat your skin as well as superficially improve its appearance. So investigate the latest products – it's well worth making use of them.

# Eating for beautiful skin

While lotions and potions can improve your skin from the outside, a healthy diet works from the inside out. A nutritious, balanced diet isn't only a delicious way to eat – it can work wonders for your skin.

## you are what you eat

A diet for a healthy body is the same one as for a healthy, clear complexion. That is, one that contains lots of fresh fruit and vegetables, is high in fibre, low in fat and low in added sugar and salt. This should provide your body and skin with all the vitamins and minerals they need to function at their very best.

## healthy skin checklist

These are the essentials your body needs to keep your skin in tip-top condition.
• The most essential element is water. Although there's water in the foods you eat, you should drink at least two litres (quarts) of water a day to keep your body healthy and your skin clear.
• Cellulose carbohydrates, better known as fibre foods, have another less direct effect on the skin. Their action in keeping you

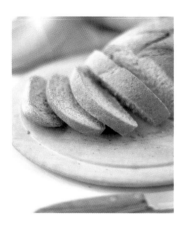

△ Wholegrain cereals, such as bread, are an excellent source of B vitamins and also provide the fibre that your body needs to stay healthy.

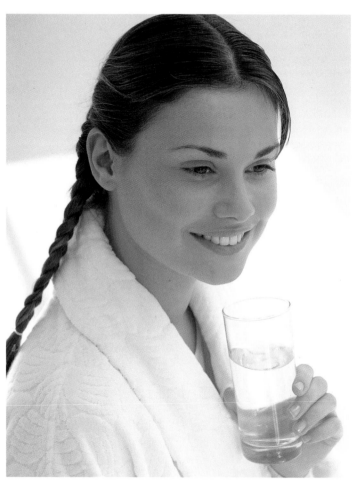

regular can help to give you a brighter, clearer complexion.
• Vitamin A is essential for growth and repair of certain skin tissues. Lack of it causes dryness, itching and loss of skin elasticity. It's found in foods such as carrots, spinach, broccoli and apricots.
• Vitamin C is needed for collagen production, to help keep your skin firm. It's found in foods such as strawberries, citrus fruits, cabbage, tomatoes and watercress.
• Vitamin E is an antioxidant vitamin that

△ Drinking plenty of water during the day helps rehydrate and purify your body.

neutralizes free radicals – highly reactive molecules that can cause ageing. It occurs in foods such as almonds, hazelnuts and wheat germ.
• Zinc works with vitamin A in the making of collagen and elastin, the fibres that give your skin its strength, elasticity and firmness. It occurs in shellfish, wholegrains, milk, cheese and yoghurt.

▷ Eating a selection of fresh fruit every day
provides your body with the minerals and
vitamins it needs.

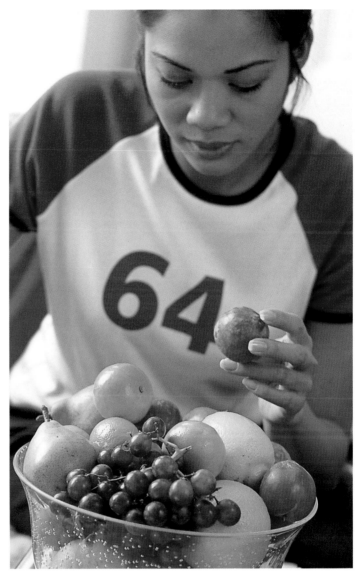

## diet Q & A

A healthy diet and a beautiful complexion
go hand in hand. Check you know the facts.

### yo-yo dieting

**Q** *"Is it true that if you are constantly losing
and then gaining weight it can have a bad effect
on your skin?"*

**A** Yes. Eating too much and becoming
overweight thickens the layer of fat under
your skin and consequently stretches it.
Crash dieting can then result in your skin
collapsing, leading to the appearance of lines
and wrinkles. What's more, a crash diet will
deprive your skin and body of the essential
nutrients they need to stay healthy and look
good. If you need to lose weight, do it
slowly, sensibly and steadily, to give your skin
time to acclimatize. Consult your doctor
before starting any weight-loss programme.

### daily diet

**Q** *"What would be a good typical day's diet for
a clearer complexion?"*

**A** One that follows the rules already
outlined. For example, here's a typical day
you could follow:

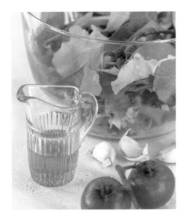

△ Fresh raw vegetables and salads provide your
body and your skin with valuable nutrients. Aim
to eat five portions of fruit and vegetables a day.

**Breakfast:** Glass of unsweetened fruit juice;
bowl of unsweetened muesli (granola), with
a chopped banana and semi-skimmed (low-
fat) milk; two slices of wholewheat toast
with a scraping of low-fat spread.

**Lunch:** Baked potato filled with low-fat
cottage cheese and plenty of fresh, raw salad;
one low-fat yogurt, any flavour.

**Evening meal:** Grilled fish or chicken with
boiled brown rice and plenty of steamed
vegetables. Fresh fruit salad, topped with
natural yogurt and nuts.

### on the spot

**Q** *"I love eating chocolate but have heard that it
cause pimples. Is this true?"*

**A** There isn't any scientific evidence that
links eating chocolate to having break-outs
of spots, but as a healthy low-fat, high-fibre
diet is known to be good for the skin, keep
snacks such as chocolate to a minimum
and eat them only as an occasional treat. If
you find yourself craving sweet snacks, try
eating a low-fat yoghurt or a delicious bowl
of strawberries.

# Your top 20 skincare questions answered

Here are quick and simple remedies, and sound advice, for a range of common skincare problems.

## 1 night watch

**Q** *"My dry skin needs night cream, but I seem to lose most of it on my pillow."*

**A** Try placing the cream in a teaspoon, and heating it gently over a low heat on the cooker until just warm, before applying. It sounds strange, but it really works!

## 2 polished perfection

**Q** *"I spend a fortune on skincare, but resent paying for exfoliators. Are there alternatives?"*

**A** Yes. After washing your skin, gently massage with a soft facecloth or natural sponge to ease away the dead surface skin cells. If you have dry skin, massage cream cleanser on to damp skin, then rub over the top with your flannel. Rinse afterwards, then apply moisturizer in the normal way. It is essential to wash the facecloth after every couple of uses, and to hang it up to dry in between to prevent the build-up of bacteria.

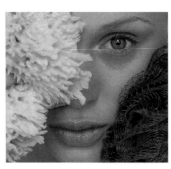

△ The soft touch of a natural sponge is a cheap and effective alternative to a facial scrub.

## 3 lip tricks

**Q** *"How can I stop my lips getting so chapped and flaky in winter?"*

**A** This three-step action plan will help:

• Massage dry lips with petroleum jelly. Leave for a couple of minutes to soften the skin, then gently rub your lips with a warm, damp facecloth. As the petroleum jelly is removed, the flakes of skin will come with it!

• Smooth your lips morning and night with a lip balm.

• Switch to a moisturizing lipstick to prevent lips from drying out during the daytime.

## 4 red nose day

**Q** *"How can I cover my red winter nose?"*

**A** Try smoothing a little green foundation or concealer over the red area before applying foundation and powder. The green works by cancelling out the redness.

## 5 winter sun

**Q** *"Is it true that you should still wear a sunscreen in winter?"*

**A** Yes. Exposure to sunlight is thought to be the main cause of wrinkling, and the ultraviolet A rays that are responsible for this process are around all year, so choose a moisturizer that contains sunscreens.

## 6 lighten up

**Q** *"My skin feels as though it needs a richer cream in the winter months, but I find most of them too heavy"*

**A** A heavier moisturizer doesn't necessarily mean it's more effective, so choose one that feels right for you. Help seal moisture into your skin by spritzing your face with water before applying it. Also, choose a nourishing foundation or tinted moisturizer to ensure your skin stays smooth and soft all day long.

## 7 water factor

**Q** *"I like the feeling of water on my face, but I find soap too drying. Should I switch to a cream cleanser instead?"*

**A** For dry skin, it's generally better to use a creamy cleanser – applied with your fingertips and removed with cotton wool (cotton) or soft tissues. This prevents too much moisture from being lost from the skin's surface. Normal and oily skins should

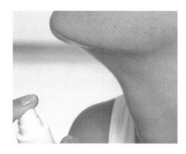

△ Boost the moisture in your skin with a refreshing spritz.

be fine with water but a facial wash or wash-off cleanser is formulated to be non-drying, while still cleaning your skin.

## 8 age spots

**Q** *"I've noticed 'liver spots' on the back of my hands. How are they caused – and how can I get rid of them?"*

**A** Many people find these light-to-dark-brown patches on the back of their hands as they grow older. They can also appear on the forehead and temples. They're caused by an uneven production of the melanin tanning pigment in the skin. This can be caused by excess sun exposure, or merely highlighted by it.

You can use a cream containing hydroquinone, which penetrates the skin tissue to 'dissolve' the melanin. In six to eight weeks, your skin should be back to normal. However, you must use a safe level of hydroquinone – the recommended amount in a cream is two per cent. Using a sunscreen on a daily basis can prevent these patches from appearing again.

## 9 sensitive issue

**Q** *"Why does my skin feel more sensitive in winter than in summer?"*

**A** Eighty per cent of women claim to have sensitive skin – which tingles, itches and is prone to dryness. It can be aggravated by harsh winter winds and cold, because this breaks down the natural protective oily layer. Moisturizing regularly with a hypo-allergenic cream formulated for sensitive skin should help.

## 10 pregnant pause

**Q** *"I'm pregnant and have patches of darker colour on my face, particularly under my eyes and around my mouth. What is this?"*

**A** This is called chloasma, or "the mask of pregnancy". It's triggered by a change in hormones, and is made more obvious by sunbathing. Cover up in the sun and use sunblock to stop patches becoming denser. It usually fades within a few months of having your baby. Chloasma can also be triggered by birth-control pills, but disappears once you stop taking them.

## 11 on the spot

**Q** *"I suffer from oily skin, but find blemish creams too drying. What can you suggest?"*

**A** Choose an antibacterial cream to kill off the cause of your blemishes while soothing the skin around them.

## 12 treatment sprays

**Q** *"I find body lotions too hot and sticky to wear after bathing. What else can I try?"*

**A** There are body treatment sprays, combining moisturizer, toner and fragrance. Your skin will be lightly moisturized and smell fantastic.

## 13 the throat vote

**Q** *"The skin on my neck looks grey and dull. Are there any special treats to use?"*

**A** Necks show the signs of ageing, mainly because they lack sebaceous glands. Using a creamy cleanser can help. Massage in, leave

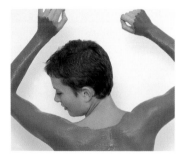

△ **Back to basics with a clay mask for the body.**

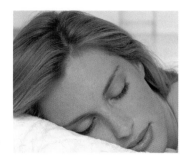

△ **Don't forget your beauty sleep.**

to dissolve dirt, and remove with cotton wool (cotton) pads. Dull grey skin benefits from regular exfoliation – scrub briskly with a facecloth or soft shaving brush. Boost softness by smoothing on moisturizer.

## 14 beautiful back

**Q** *"What can I do for pimples on my back?"*

**A** Backs are hard to reach, so they're prone to break-outs. Keep your back blemish-free by exfoliating daily with a loofah or back brush to remove dead skin. For stubborn pimples, try a clay mask to draw out deep-seated impurities.

## 15 mole watch

**Q** *"I understand you need to keep an eye on moles on your skin to monitor the risk of skin cancer. What should I look for?"*

**A** Moles are clumps of clustered pigment cells, usually darker than freckles. All changes in existing moles should be checked by your doctor. Any that cause concern will be removed and sent off for analysis. You should also check moles yourself once a month. Try the following A.B.C.D. code: check for A (asymmetry); B (border irregularity); C (colour change); D (change in diameter).

## 16 shadow sense

**Q** *"What's best for shadows under my eyes?"*

**A** Dark shadows can have a variety of causes, including fatigue, anaemia, lack of fresh air and poor digestion. They can also be hereditary. If in doubt, consult your doctor. Take steps to cut out causes such as getting a good night's sleep and keeping to a low-fat, high-fibre diet. Try bathing the eyes with pads soaked in ice-cold water for 15 minutes, to lessen the shadow effect temporarily. Or cover by dotting on concealer.

## 17 brown baby

**Q** *"Is there any way to prolong my tan?"*

**A** Your skin is dried by sunbathing, and so sheds old cells more quickly. Prolong colour by applying lots of body lotion. Use while your skin is damp to make it extra effective. Apply a little fake tan every few days to keep your colour topped up. Better still, protect your skin by using fake tan all the time.

## 18 sticky situation

**Q** *"I exercise a lot, and find body odour a problem. How can I prevent it?"*

**A** Sweating is your body's natural cooling device. Sweat itself has no odour, but smells when it comes into contact with bacteria on the skin. So, opt for an antiperspirant deodorant. Antiperspirants prevent sweating, while deodorant helps prevent odour. Also wear fresh, natural fibres next to your skin.

## 19 massage magic

**Q** *"Can I give myself a facial massage?"*

**A** A massage is the ideal way to give your complexion a workout. Pour a few drops of vegetable oil into the palms of your hands and smooth it on to your face and neck. Then follow these steps:
• Use finger pads to stroke upwards from the base of your neck to your chin.
• Continue with long strokes up one side of your face, then the other. Then go around your nose and up towards your forehead.
• When you get to your forehead, stroke it across from left to right using one hand. Finish off by gently drawing a circle around each eye using one finger.

## 20 stretch marks

**Q** *"Can I get rid of the stretch marks on my stomach, breasts and thighs?"*

**A** Stretch marks are a sign of your skin's inability to cope with the rapid expansion of flesh underneath. The collagen and elastin fibres underneath actually tear with the strain. They usually appear in times of rapid weight gain, such as puberty and pregnancy. They look quite red at first, although with time, they fade away to a pale silvery shade. There's nothing you can do once you've got them, except wait until they start to fade. However, moisturizing well can help guard against them. Apply body lotion after a bath or shower, and give it time to sink in.

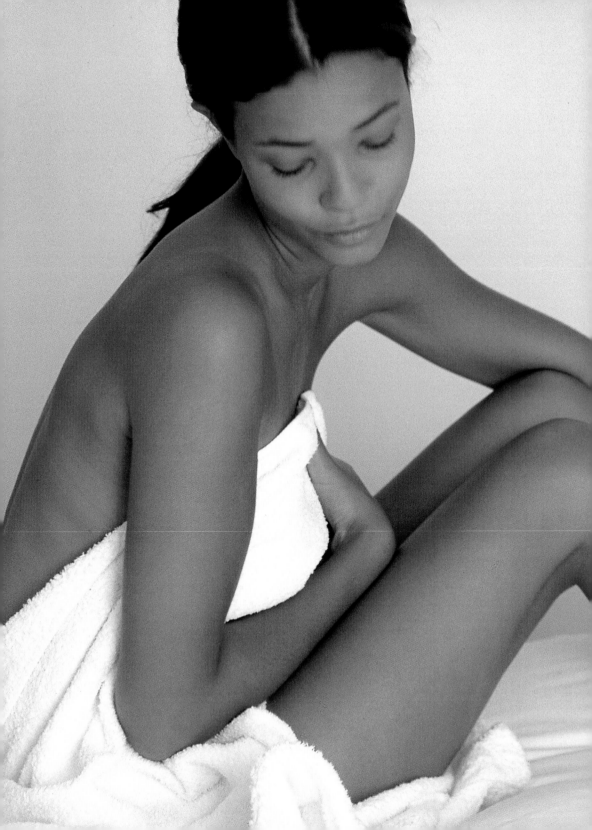

# Complete Bodycare

The secret to a beautifully maintained
body is to lavish the same care on it as
you do on your complexion and make-up.
You need to take into account both
general maintenance and any special needs
it may have. Whatever beauty boosts your
body needs, you'll find the help you
need in this section of the book.

# Caring for your body

One of the most effective ways to care for your body is to build bodycare treatments into your everyday bathroom routine. Hands and feet, elbows and necks can be forgotten and neglected because we are not in the habit of focusing our attention on them. Regular pampering may seem like an indulgence but in fact taking care of your whole body is vital to keeping it healthy. The power of touch to identify problem areas and notice changes, as you moisturize, scrub and massage, should not be underestimated.

## throat
• Does skincare stop at your neck?
• Is the skin rough and grey?
• Do you indulge yourself with special treats to keep your skin in tip-top condition?

## chest
• Do you give your breasts the care they need?
• Is your chest prone to break-outs?
• Do you protect this area of your skin from the harmful rays of the sun?

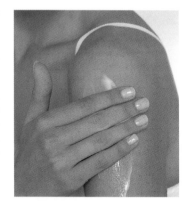

△ **Tops and especially the backs of arms need care too, so that they stay soft, smooth and firm.**

## arms
• Are your elbows grey and dull in tone?
• Is the skin soft and supple, or rough and dry?
• Do darker hairs on your lower arms need bleaching?
• If you remove hair from your underarms, have you found the best method, the one that suits you for convenience and results?
• Have you found the solution to underarm freshness?

## hands
• Do they suffer from too much housework?
• Do they need some moisturizing care?
• Are your nails neatly filed and shaped?
• Would a lick of polish or a French manicure give them a helping hand?

## legs
• Are they free from stubbly hairs?
• Is the skin as smooth as it could be?
• Would they benefit from a light touch of fake tan?
• Are they prone to cellulite?
• Would bathtime treats improve the look of your skin?

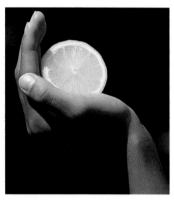

△ **The juice of a lemon is a good natural bleach for nails stained by dark nail polish.**

## bikini line
• If you remove hair from this area, have you found the best method for you?

## feet
• Are they free from hard skin, corns and calluses?
• Are your nails neatly trimmed?
• Do you smooth a foot cream on them regularly to ensure that the skin stays soft?

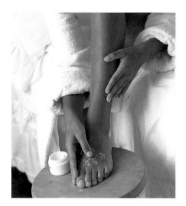

△ **As you massage your feet, take care to apply cream to the soles of your feet, as the skin on the heels can often become dry and cracked.**

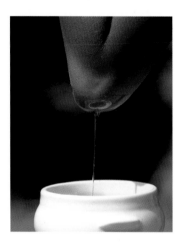

△ **The skin on your elbows can miss out on moisturizing and become very dry. Evening primrose oil is especially nourishing for dry skin.**

# Bathroom essentials

A pleasing, well-stocked bathroom can make all the difference at the start of a busy day and can be transformed into a sensual haven to help you unwind at the end of it.

The skin is the body's largest organ and forms a protective barrier against bacteria and other invaders. Although it continually sheds and renews itself, the skin has a lot to cope with and it deserves special attention. Scrubbing our skin removes dead skin cells and stimulates the blood supply, leaving skin tingling and toned. So keeping clean is vital for the overall health of the skin and body.

## sponges and facecloths

These are useful for lathering soaps and gels on your skin, and dislodging dirt and grime from your body. Wash your facecloth regularly, and allow it to dry between uses. Natural sponges are a more expensive but long-lasting alternative. Squeeze out afterwards in warm clear water and allow to dry naturally.

## pumice stone

These are made from very porous volcanic rock, and work best if you lather up with soap before rubbing at hardened areas of skin in a circular motion. Don't rub too fiercely or you'll make the skin sore. Little and often is best.

## loofah or back brush

Try using a loofah as an exfoliator as its length makes it useful for scrubbing difficult-to-reach areas such as the back. Loofahs are actually the pod of an Egyptian plant and need a bit of care if they're going to last. Rinse and drain them thoroughly after use to prevent them going black and mouldy. Avoid rinsing them in vinegar and lemon juice as this can be too harsh for these once-living things.

Back brushes are also useful for areas of skin that are hard to reach, and are easier to care for: you simply rinse them in cool water after use and leave them to dry.

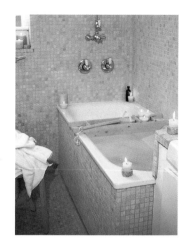

△ **A well-organized bathroom can be transformed into a haven to help you unwind.**

## soaps and cleansing bars

These are a cheap and effective way of cleansing your body. If you find them too drying, choose ones that contain moisturizing ingredients to minimize these effects. Most people can use ordinary soaps and cleansers without any problem. However, if you have particularly dry or sensitive skin, it is advisable to opt for the pH-balanced variety.

---

### BATHROOM BASICS

From cleaning your teeth to preventing underarm odour, there are a few basics that are essential for a well-stocked bathroom:

• **Toothbrush:** It is vital to choose the right toothbrush. A nylon brush is best, as bristle tends to split and lose its shape quickly. Choose one with a small head so you can easily clean your back teeth. A soft or medium brush is best as harder brushes may damage the tooth enamel and gums. Change your toothbrush approximately every month.

• **Dental floss:** Use floss at least once a day to clean between the teeth where the toothbrush can't reach. Waxed floss is best as it's less likely to catch on fillings or uneven edges. To floss, wind a short length around the second finger of each hand. Slide it gently down between two of the teeth, taking care to press it against the side of the tooth. Then gently slide it upwards out of the teeth, removing any food particles with it. Repeat between all of the teeth.

• **Antiperspirant deodorant:** Deodorants do not prevent perspiration – they only stop the bacteria from decomposing the sweat. If you perspire heavily, it is advisable to use an antiperspirant or even better an antiperspirant deodorant. The antiperspirant element prevents the production of sweat. Remember, though, not to use it on inflamed or broken skin or immediately after shaving.

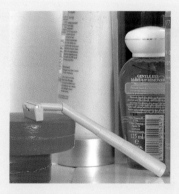

◁ **Stock your bathroom with bodycare products and bathtime treats for top-to-toe health and freshness.**

• **Talcum powder:** This white powder is made from finely ground magnesium silicate and is usually perfumed. It is considered to be rather old-fashioned, which is a shame because a good talcum powder makes you smell fresh and helps you slide into your clothes after bathing or swimming. However, there is no substitute for a thorough drying with a towel, especially between the toes, for keeping your skin healthy.

# Fresh ideas for the bath and shower

As well as a chance to cleanse your body, bath- or shower-time is the perfect opportunity to pamper and polish your skin, and indulge in some refreshing and energizing beauty treats.

## bathing beauty

The time of day and even the time of year will affect what you like using, so why not take the opportunity to try different products, adding any you particularly like to those you already know well.

### shower gels and bubble baths

These are mild detergents that help cleanse your body while you soak in the water. There are hundreds of varieties to choose from, including those containing a host of additives, ranging from herbs to essential oils. If you find them too harsh for your skin, look for the ones that offer 2-in-1 benefits – these also contain moisturizers, to soothe your skin.

### bath oils

These are a wonderful beauty boon for those with dry skins. They float on the top of the water, and your entire body becomes covered with a fine film when you step out

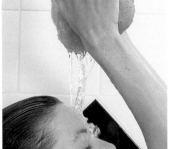
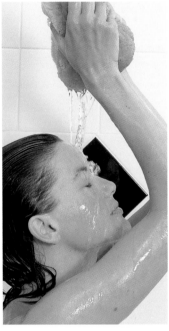

of the bath. Most cosmetic houses produce a bath oil, but if you're not worried about the fragrance, you can use a few drops of any vegetable oil, such as olive, corn or peanut.

◁ Just splashing water on your face will refresh and revive you. Take time to relax and enjoy your bath or shower.

### bath salts

Made from sodium carbonate, these are particularly useful for softening hard water, and for preventing your skin from becoming too dry. Combined with warm water, they are a popular way to soothe away aches and pains.

## bath-time treats

Once you've armed yourself with some bathroom treats and luxuries, try these water-baby bath treats to boost your body, beauty and mood.

### sleepy "sitz" bath

The combination of hot and cold temperatures is an effective way of helping you get to sleep. Try a "sitz" bath, which helps you relax by drawing energy away from your head and stopping your mind from racing. Here's how to create your own "sitz" bath:
• Ensure the bathroom is warm, then run approximately 7.5–10cm (3–4in) of cold water into the bath.
• Wrap the top half of your body in a warm sweater or towel, then immerse your hips and bottom in the cold water for 30 seconds.
• Get out of the bath, pat yourself dry, then climb into bed and fall asleep.

### learning to relax

Turn bathtime into an aromatherapy treat by adding relaxing essential oils such as chamomile and lavender to the water. Just add a few drops once you've run the bath, then lie back, inhale the vapours and relax completely. Salts and bubble baths that

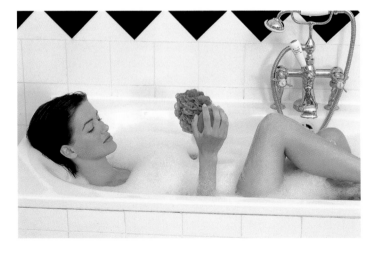

◁ Soaking in a warm bubble bath is a great opportunity to pamper and polish your skin, and has to be one of the most popular ways to relax.

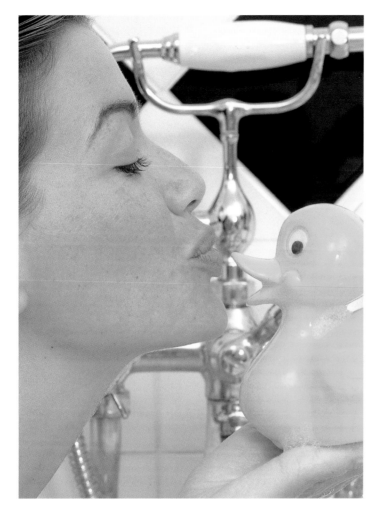

◁ There is nothing like a leisurely soak to melt away tension and to lift your spirits.

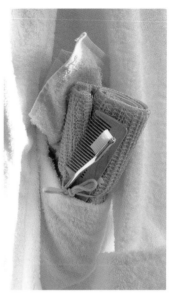

△ Make sure all the bath products you plan to use are close to hand, so you won't have to disturb your relaxing soak to fetch them.

contain sea minerals and kelp also have a relaxing effect, and purify your skin too. Bathing by candlelight and listening to calming music will make it even more of a treat. Put on soothing eye pads and relax for 10 minutes.

### be a natural beauty

You don't have to splash out on expensive bath additives – try adding some simple, natural remedies:

• Soothe irritated skin by adding a cup of cider vinegar to the running water.

• A cup of powdered milk will soothe rough skin.

• Sprinkle a cupful of oatmeal or bran to the water to cleanse, whiten and soothe your skin.

### sleek skin

Smooth your body with body oil before getting into the bath. After soaking for 10 minutes, rub your skin with a soft facecloth – you'll be amazed at how much dead skin you remove!

## shower-time treats

Showers are a wonderful opportunity to cleanse your body quickly and cheaply, and to wake yourself up. Here are some of the other benefits.

### circulation booster

Switch on the cold water before finishing your shower to help boost your circulation. It will also make you feel warmer once you get out of the shower! It also works well if

you concentrate the blasts of cold water on cellulite-prone areas, as this stimulates the sluggish circulation in these spots.

### boosting benefits

If you pat yourself dry after a bath, it'll help you to unwind, whereas briskly rubbing your skin with a towel will help to invigorate you.

### shower sensation

Add a few drops of essential oils to the floor of the shower itself. As they evaporate you will find that you're surrounded by a sensuous-smelling mist while you wash your body. Rosemary, peppermint and basil are classic refreshers, while grapefruit blended with geranium makes a stimulating mix.

# Natural bathing treats

Enjoyed in the evening, a warm bath helps the body to relax and can pave the way for a good night's sleep. Although you may be tempted, especially in cold weather, to have a steaming hot bath, a short soak in body-temperature water is far more effective at helping you unwind. Bathing in water that is too hot can cause thread veins and may make you feel unwell. The skin is also better able to release impurities at body temperature and to absorb the healing properties of any herbs and minerals that are added to the bathwater.

## essential oils

To make bathing a real indulgence you can create your own aromatic bath products. Lavender, chamomile, clary sage, neroli and rose all have a relaxing, soporific effect.

Add 5–10 drops of your chosen oil blend to your bath, then sink in and relax. Inhaling the wonderful aromas will soothe your mind, and the oils will also have a beneficial effect on your skin and body.

▽ **A good supply of clean, fluffy towels and beautiful candles can make taking a bath a glorious indulgence.**

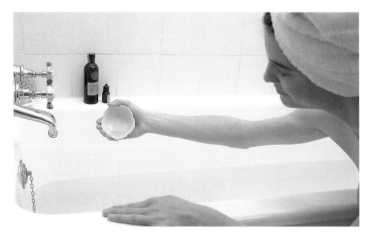

△ **Essential oils evaporate very quickly in hot water so the oils will be much more effective if you pour them into the bath water just before you climb in.**

## orange and grapefruit bath oil

At the end of the day, a scented bath is a therapeutic treat. Choose the oils depending on whether you want to be relaxed or invigorated. An orange and grapefruit bath will gently refresh you. Add one teaspoon once you have run the bath, otherwise the oils will evaporate before you get in.

### ingredients
- 45ml/3 tbsp sweet almond oil
- 5 drops grapefruit oil
- 5 drops orange oil

Pour the oils into a bottle and shake so that they are well combined before you add one teaspoon to the bathwater.

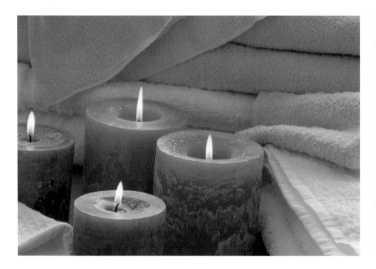

**THERAPEUTIC BATH OIL BLENDS**

Mix two or three essential oils in a base of sweet almond oil or jojoba oil. These quantities are for a 50ml/1/4 cup bottle of base oil. Add 20 drops of the mixed oil to the bathwater.

Alternatively, you can mix the oils with milk or honey because this will help to disperse them in the water.

- **Anti-stress mix:** 10 drops each marjoram, lavender and sandalwood.
- **Invigorating mix:** 5 drops rosemary, 5 drops camphor, 20 drops peppermint.
- **Healing mix for colds and flu:** 10 drops each eucalyptus, thyme and lavender.
- **Soothing arthritis:** 30 drops eucalyptus.

▷ Lavender is a versatile and widely used essential oil, well known for its fabulous scent and its soothing, relaxing and healing properties.

## lavender and olive oil soap

Use a good-quality pure olive oil soap to make this home-made soap. Enrich it with other oils and scent it with lavender to produce a gently rejuvenating cleanser.

### ingredients

- 175g/6oz good-quality olive oil soap
- 25ml/1¹/₂ tbsp coconut oil
- 25ml/1¹/₂ tbsp almond oil
- 30ml/2 tbsp ground almonds
- 10 drops lavender essential oil
- lavender buds for decorating

Grate the soap and place in a double boiler. Leave the soap to soften over a low heat. When soft, add all the other ingredients and mix evenly. Press the mixture into oiled moulds and leave to set overnight. Unmould, and decorate by pressing the top of each block of soap into a shallow tray of lavender buds.

## goodnight bath salts

Chamomile is a widely recognized sedative; for these bath salts it has been combined with sweet marjoram, which is an effective treatment for insomnia.

### ingredients

- 450g/1lb/2¹/₄ cups coarse sea salt
- 10 drops chamomile essential oil
- 10 drops sweet marjoram essential oil
- 1–3 drops green food colouring (optional)

Combine all the ingredients and pour into a glass storage jar with a close-fitting lid. Put the lid on firmly. Just before bedtime, light a scented candle, add a handful of the salts to your bath, immerse yourself in the warm water and relax.

## herbal bath mix

All the ingredients for this mix are easily available to buy, or they can be grown in a herb garden or window box. They are associated with purification and cleansing.

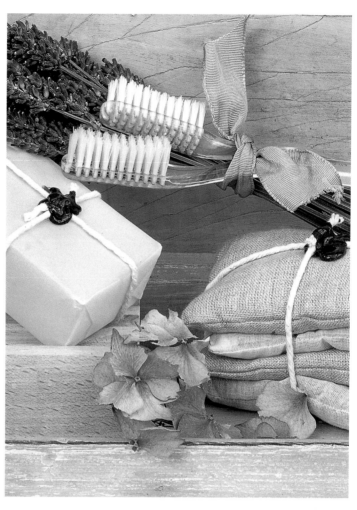

### ingredients

- 7 basil leaves
- 3 bay leaves
- 3 sprigs oregano
- 1 sprig tarragon
- small square of cotton muslin
- 10ml/2 tsp organic oats
- pinch rock or sea salt
- thread to tie up muslin

Use fresh herbs for this recipe if possible. Pile the herbs in the centre of the muslin square, then sprinkle the oats on top. Top with the rock or sea salt, pick up the corners of the muslin and tie with thread. Hang the sachet from the bath tap so that as the water runs over the bag it is infused with the essence of the mixture.

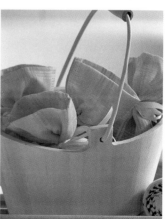

△ Fragrant bath bags will lightly scent the bath.

# Be a smoothie

Most women aspire to smooth, healthy skin free of dry patches, superfluous hair, and blemishes. And the chances are, even if your skin isn't prone to spottiness or flaky patches, it will suffer from dullness and poor condition from time to time. This is where body scrubs and exfoliators come into their own. They work by shifting dead cells from the skin surface, revealing the younger, fresher ones underneath. This process also stimulates the circulation of blood in the skin tissues, giving it a rosy glow.

Hair on a woman's body is completely natural, but fashion and cultural practices mean that it is usually removed. There are a number of ways of removing hair for smooth, soft skin and it is simply a matter of finding the method that suits you best.

## exfoliation methods

There are lots of different ways you can exfoliate your body – so there's one to suit every budget and preference.

• Your first option is to buy an exfoliating scrub, which is a cream- or gel-based product containing tiny abrasive particles.

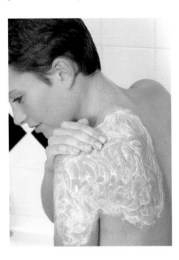

△ **A body scrub is a quick and easy way to keep your skin sleek and smooth.**

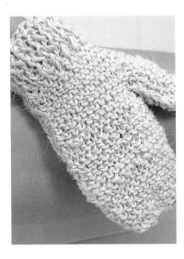

△ **Keep a sisal mitt to hand for super-soft skin.**

Look for the type with rounded particles which won't irritate delicate skin. Simply massage the scrub into damp skin, then rinse away with lots of warm water.

• Bath mitts, loofahs and sisal mitts are a cinch to use, and cost-effective too. They can be quite harsh on the skin if you press too hard, so go easily at first. Rinse them well after use, and allow them to dry naturally. Simply sweep over your body when you're in the shower or bath.

• Your ordinary facecloth or bath sponge can also double up as an exfoliator. Lather up with plenty of soap or shower gel, and massage over damp skin before rinsing away with clear water.

• Copy what health spas do, and keep a large tub of natural sea salt by the shower. Scoop up a handful when you get in, and massage over your skin. Rinse away thoroughly afterwards.

• You can also make your own body scrub at home by mixing sea salt with body oil or olive oil. Allow the mixture to soak into your skin for a few minutes to allow the edges of the salt crystals to dissolve before massaging in, then rinsing away.

• Body brushes are also useful. The best way to use them is on dry skin before you get in the bath or shower, as this is particularly good for loosening dead skin cells. You can also use them in the water, lathering them up with soap or gel.

## perfecting your exfoliation technique

Whichever method you use, the best thing to do is concentrate on problem areas such as upper arms, thighs, bottom, heels and elbows. Also sweep over the rest of your body. However, go gently on delicate areas of skin, such as the inner arms, stomach and inner thighs. Work in large strokes, in the direction of your heart.

Oilier skin types will benefit from exfoliation 2–3 times a week, while once a week is sufficient for others. Never exfoliate broken, inflamed or acne-prone skins.

After exfoliating, always apply body lotion to seal moisture into the fresh new skin you've exposed.

> **BEAUTY TIP**
> For speedy super-soft skin, you should massage your body with oil before climbing into the bath or shower. Then proceed as usual with your preferred exfoliating method.

## hair removal

These are the main removal methods for superfluous hair. Each method has advantages and disadvantages, and these have been outlined here:

### shaving

Using a razorblade, shaving works by cutting the hair at the skin surface. Shaving is most effective for legs and underarms.

**Pros:** Cheap, quick and painless.

**Cons:** Regrowth (stubble) appears very quickly, usually within a couple of days.

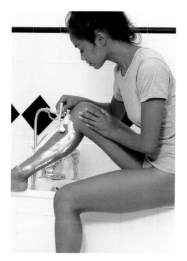

◁ **For many women, shaving is the no-fuss option for silky smooth legs.**

### SHAVING TIPS

• Use with a moisturizing shave foam or gel for a close shave. Moisturize afterwards to soothe your skin.
• A closer shave means you will have to shave your legs less frequently.
• Let the shaving cream get to work and soften the hair for a few moments before using your razor.

### tweezing

This rather time-consuming method involves plucking out hairs one at a time so it is most effective for small areas such as eyebrows, or for removing the odd stray hair missed by waxing.

**Pros:** Good control for shaping.

**Cons:** Can be painful and may make skin slightly reddened for a while afterwards. You also need to remember to check the area regularly in a mirror to see that you don't need to re-tweeze.

### TWEEZER TIP

Before you begin, hold a warm facecloth over the area of skin you are going to work on. This will dampen and soften the skin, and open the pores, making tweezing easier. Or you could try pressing an ice cube over the area to numb the skin first if you find it really painful.

### waxing

This method uproots the hair from below the skin's surface. Either wax is smoothed on to the skin and removed with strips, or pre-prepared wax strips are used. This is a form of hair removal that can be safely used on any part of the body.

**Pros:** The results last for 2–6 weeks.

**Cons:** This method can be extremely painful and there is also the risk of sore, red and blotchy legs and of ingrowing hairs. Also, hair has to be left to grow until it is long enough to wax effectively, so you have to put up with regrowth to give the hairs time to grow back sufficiently. If the hair is too short, it won't come out, or it will be removed patchily.

### WAXING TIPS

• After waxing the bikini area, apply an antibacterial cream to prevent infection or a rash.
• Wear loose clothing after waxing.
• Never wax a sore area.

### depilatory creams

These creams contain chemicals that weaken the hair at the skin's surface, so hair can be wiped away. Simply apply, leave for 5–10 minutes, then rinse away. (Check the packaging for exact instructions.) You can use a depilatory cream anywhere, especially as some companies produce different formulations for specific areas. Do a patch test 24 hours before use to make sure it won't cause irritation or an allergy.

**Pros:** It is cheap, and the results last a bit longer than a razor – up to a week.

**Cons:** Can be messy, and takes time. The smell of some products can be off-putting although formulations have improved.

### bleaching

This is not technically hair removal, but it's a good way to make hair less noticeable. A hydrogen peroxide solution is used to lighten the hair. Bleaching is best for arms, upper lip and face.

**Pros:** Results last between 2 and 6 weeks, and there's no regrowth.

**Cons:** Not suitable for coarse hair.

### BLEACHING TIP

It is a good idea to carry out a patch test on your skin first to ensure you don't react to the product's bleaching agents.

### sugaring

This works in a similar way to waxing, but uses a paste made from sugar, lemon and water. It's well known in the Middle East, and is growing in popularity elsewhere.

**Pros:** Has the same benefits as waxing and can be used anywhere on the body.

**Cons:** Can be fairly painful and there is a risk of ingrowing hairs.

### electrolysis

A needlelike probe conducts an electric current into the hair follicle, inactivating it. This method is best for small areas such as breasts and face. Go to a qualified practitioner (and ask to see proof of their qualifications).

**Pros:** A permanent solution.

**Cons:** Expensive, and more painful for some people than others, depending upon the pain threshold. You may find that you are more sensitive to the pain just before or during your period.

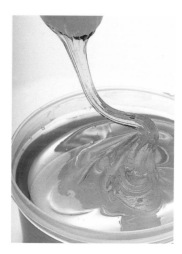

△ **Sugaring – the sweeter way to removing superfluous hair.**

# Simple steps to softer skin

Slick on a body moisturizer to create a wonderfully silky body. Add a moisturizing body treat to your daily beauty regime, and you'll soon reap the benefits.

## moisturizing matters

Just as you choose a moisturizer for your face with care, you should opt for the best formulation that is suited to the skin type on your body.

• Gels are the lightest formulation and are perfect for very hot days or oilier skin types. They contain many nourishing ingredients even though they're very easy to wear.

• Lotions and oils are good for most skin types, and easy to apply, as they're not sticky. Creams give better results for those with dry skins, especially on very dry areas.

## make the most of body moisturizer

• Apply using firm strokes to boost your circulation as you massage in the product. Apply the moisturizer straight on to clean, damp skin – after a bath or shower is the ideal time. This helps seal extra moisture into the upper layers of your skin, making it softer than ever.

• Soften cracked feet by rubbing them with rich body lotion, pulling on a pair of cotton socks and heading for bed. They'll be beautifully soft by the next morning!

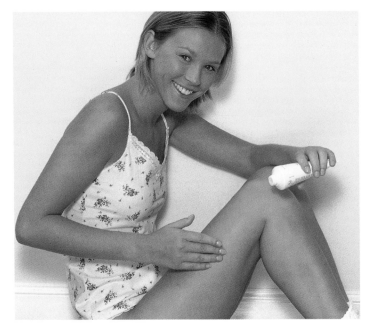

△ Take the time before dressing to moisturize your skin. Why not apply body lotion and then allow your skin to absorb it while you clean your teeth or dry your hair?

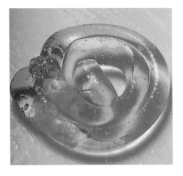

△ Opt for the light touch with a moisturizing gel.

• Concentrate on rubbing moisturizer into particularly dry areas such as heels, knees and elbows. The calves are also very prone to dryness because there aren't many oil glands present there.

• If you don't have time to apply moisturizer after your bath, simply add a few drops of body oil to the water. When you step out of the bath, your skin will be coated with a fine film of nourishing oil. Always remember to rinse the bath well afterwards to prevent you from slipping the next time you climb into the bath.

• Your breasts don't have any supportive muscle from the nipple to the collarbone and skin is very fine here. Firming creams won't work miracles, but can help maintain the elasticity and suppleness of this delicate area. Regular application of body lotion can have similar effects.

### SMELLING SENSATIONAL

Opt for a scented body lotion as a treat. They can often be longer-lasting than the fragrances themselves. Alternatively, use them as part of "fragrance layering". This simply means taking advantage of the various scent formulations available. Start with a scented bath oil and soap, move on to the matching body lotion and powder, and leave the house wearing the fragrance itself sprayed on to pulse points.

However, be careful you don't clash fragrances. Choose unscented products if you're also wearing perfume, unless you're going to be wearing a matching scented body lotion. You don't want cheaper products to compete with your more expensive perfume.

▷ For super-soft skin apply moisturizer immediately after showering or bathing. Cream is better absorbed by warm, damp skin and this will help to seal in extra moisture.

## home-made lotions

For pure pampering pleasure nothing beats a tailor-made beauty preparation, and you can choose the ingredients specially to suit your own skincare needs. Mixing oils or adding your favourite essential oil to a ready-made unscented cream is easy to do and very rewarding.

## geranium body lotion

This is a spicy, fragrant lotion. Geranium oil is derived from a relative of the scented geranium leaf and the fragrance is pleasantly sharp and aromatic.

### ingredients
- 175ml/6 fl oz unscented body lotion
- 15 drops geranium essential oil

Add the geranium oil to the body lotion, mix them well and pour into a bottle with a tight lid.

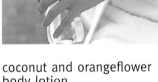

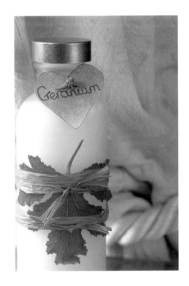

△ It is a good idea to label and date home-made lotion. It should keep for a month or so if it is stored in a sealed bottle in a cool place, but will not keep indefinitely.

## coconut and orangeflower body lotion

This creamy preparation is soothing and nourishing for dry skin. Wheatgerm oil is rich in vitamin E, an antioxidant that protects skin cells against premature aging.

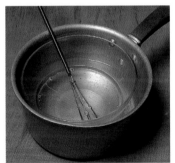

△ **1** Melt the coconut oil in a heatproof bowl over gently simmering water. Stir in the sunflower and wheatgerm oils. Leave to cool, then add the fragrance and pour into a jar.

### ingredients
- 50g/2oz coconut oil
- 60ml/4 tbsp sunflower oil
- 10ml/2 tsp wheatgerm oil
- 10 drops orangeflower essence or 5 drops neroli essential oil

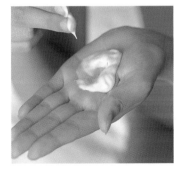

△ **2** The lotion will solidify after several hours. For the best results warm the cream on your hands briefly before applying to dry areas of skin.

# Simple aromatherapy recipes

Many more of us are waking up to the benefits of aromatherapy and natural beauty products these days, and for very good reasons. Natural therapies are wonderful to use, easily available and can give immediate results.

Aromatherapy uses essential oils, which are the distilled essences of herbs, plants, flowers and trees. These oils smell wonderful and are a pleasure to use. It's this smell that usually attracts people to them for treating a variety of physical and mental conditions, from skin infections to stress.

## aromatherapy massage

Mix 3–4 drops of essential oil into 10ml/ 2 tsp of a neutral carrier oil such as sweet almond oil, and use to massage your body – or ask someone else to massage you.

### tips for using essential oils

• Essential oils are natural products but their effects can be powerful, so they must be used with care.
• If you don't want to buy individual essential oils, buy them ready-blended, or treat yourself to bath and body products that contain them.
• Some oils are thought to carry some risk during pregnancy. For this reason, consult a qualified aromatherapist for advice if you are pregnant and want to use essential oils.
• Don't try to treat medical conditions with them – always consult your doctor.
• Essential oils can be expensive, but a little goes a long way.
• Do not apply essential oils to the skin undiluted as they're far too concentrated in this form, and can result in inflammation. The only exception is lavender, which can be used directly on the skin for insect bites and stings. Otherwise, essential oils should be mixed with a carrier oil.
• Don't take essential oils internally. Essential oils are approximately 50 to 100 times more powerful than the plant from which they were extracted.

• Don't apply oils to areas of broken, inflamed or recently scarred skin.
• Whichever method of aromatherapy you use, shut the door to the room to prevent the aroma from escaping!
• For immediate results add about 4 drops of your chosen oil to a bowl of hot water, lean over it and cover your head with a towel. Inhale deeply for about 5 minutes.
• Place a few drops of your favourite oil on a tissue, so you can inhale it whenever you like. Eucalyptus is great for blocked sinuses or if you have a cold. Alternatively, sprinkle a few drops of chamomile or lavender on your pillow to help you sleep.
• If you have sensitive skin it is a good idea to carry out a patch test before you use an oil. Apply diluted oil to a small patch of skin and leave it for a few hours to make sure you do not have an adverse reaction to it.

## hand and foot creams

These creams are made by adding suitable essential oils to an unscented cream, which means that you can easily adapt the recipe

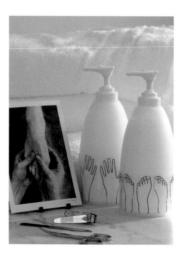

△ **Plastic pump-action bottles such as these make lotions easier to use so that you are much more likely to apply them regularly.**

to suit you. Look out for a lanolin-rich cream or one that includes cocoa butter, as both hands and feet benefit from something with a richer formulation. Although most creams and lotions are best stored in glass or ceramic containers, in this case it is practical to keep the lotion in a pump-action plastic bottle, which makes it much easier to use, and more likely that you will apply it regularly.

## tea tree foot cream

Well-cared-for feet look and feel so much better. Tea tree is one of the best essential oils to add to a foot cream. It has healing, antiseptic properties and an effective fungicidal action.

### ingredients
• 120ml/4fl oz unscented cream
• 15 drops tea tree essential oil
• bowl and spoon for mixing
• pump-action plastic bottle
• funnel

Blend the essential oils thoroughly into the unscented cream and pour into the plastic bottle through a funnel.

## healing hand cream

The oils in this cream are good for the hands: the chamomile soothes, the geranium helps heal cuts and grazes and the lemon softens the skin.

### ingredients
• 120ml/4fl oz unscented hand cream
• 10 drops chamomile essential oil
• 5 drops geranium essential oil
• 5 drops lemon essential oil
• bowl and spoon for mixing
• pump-action plastic bottle
• funnel

Blend the essential oils thoroughly into the unscented hand cream and pour into the plastic bottle through a funnel.

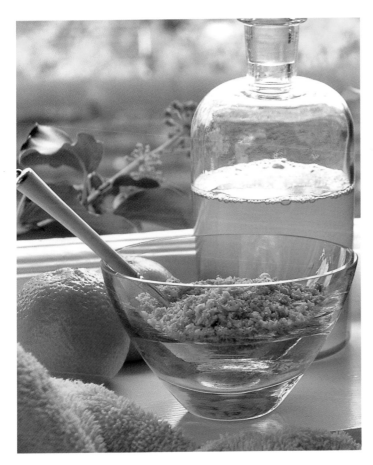

◁ The combination of aromatic orange peel and refreshing grapefruit oil in this body scrub gives it a stimulating, clean scent.

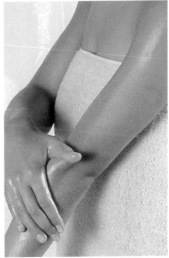

△ For a soothing and moisturizing massage on a problem area, mix 15ml/1 tbsp almond oil with a suitable essential oil and massage gently. Breathe deeply as you massage to maximize the therapeutic effect.

## citrus body scrub

Orange peel is mixed with the slightly gritty texture of ground sunflower seeds, oatmeal and sea salt in this reviving scrub, helping to remove dead skin cells and stimulate the blood supply to the skin, leaving it feeling tingling and toned.

### ingredients

- 45ml/3 tbsp freshly ground sunflower seeds
- 45ml/3 tbsp medium oatmeal
- 45ml/3 tbsp flaked sea salt
- 45ml/3 tbsp finely grated orange peel
- 3 drops grapefruit essential oil
- almond oil

Mix together all the ingredients except the almond oil and store in a sealed glass jar. Using just a little at a time, mix with some almond oil to make a thick paste, then rub over damp skin.

**APPLYING A BODY SCRUB**

For smoother, softer skin, mix the scrub with water or oil to make a paste.

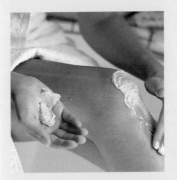

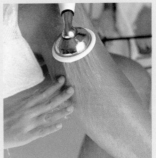

△ **1** Work the scrub into damp skin using a firm pressure and paying particular attention to areas of dry skin such as the elbows, knees and ankles.

△ **2** Use a dry flannel to remove most of the scrub and then gently rinse the rest away with warm water.

# Fabulous foot pampering

Setting aside time for a regular treatment will help you to care for your feet and keep them healthy all year round. A pamper session once a month will greatly improve their appearance, and will also soften the skin and help boost the circulation. You can also do it to pep up your feet at the start of the summer or before going on holiday.

You'll need at least an hour to do the treatment properly – or you can really indulge yourself and take two hours for the session. Use this as a time to relax – you will find that focusing on your feet is a great way to forget about day-to-day worries.

## foot pamper routine

This routine uses the luxury foot scrub (opposite). If you don't have time to make this, buy one that includes essential oils so that you can benefit from their soothing properties. You also need foaming bath or foot gel, a large foot bowl, one large towel and two smaller ones, two plastic bags that are large enough to slip your feet into, a pumice stone and pedicure tools.

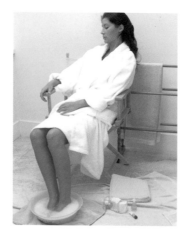

△ **1** Half fill a large bowl with warm water. Place the bowl on a large towel on the floor. Add a little foaming gel, and perhaps a couple of drops of essential oil which have been diluted first in a carrier oil. Swish the water around with your hand to create plenty of bubbles and to release the aroma of the essential oil. Put both feet into the water, then sit back and relax as you soak them for a good five minutes. Remove your feet from the bowl and rub on the floor towel to remove most of the water.

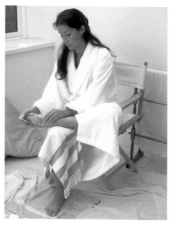

△ **2** Put a towel on your right knee and rest the left foot on top. Massage the foot scrub all over the sole, paying extra attention to any rough skin, and rub into cuticles. Place your foot in a plastic bag and secure.

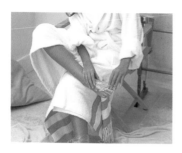

△ **3** Repeat on the right foot. Wait ten minutes, then remove the bag from the left foot, sliding it firmly down the foot to remove the foot scrub. Do the same for the right foot. Dip both feet into the water. This will have cooled down, so it will stimulate the circulation.

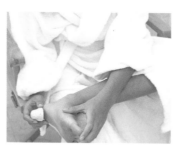

△ **4** Remove your feet from the bowl. Place your left foot on the right knee. Take the pumice stone and rub over the sole. Use firm pressure on the heel and ball, and light pressure on the arch. Now rub the pumice all over the top of the foot, using light pressure. This helps to improve the skin texture and bring nutrient-rich blood to the surface, which will help improve the appearance. Repeat on the left foot.

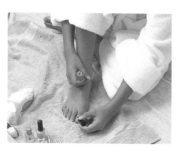

△ **5** Trim the nails straight across, then smooth the edges with an emery board. Use a cotton bud (swab) to apply cuticle remover, wait a few minutes, then gently push the cuticle back with a hoof stick. Soak the feet again, then carefully clean under the nail. Dry the feet, then apply base coat, polish and top coat, using cotton wool (cotton) to separate the toes and allowing each layer to dry before applying the next.

## luxury foot scrub

The following recipe is an excellent cleanser and softener for the feet. It can be used whenever you feel they need a boost. For the best results, though, set aside enough time for a long pamper session.

### ingredients

• 5ml/1 tsp each almond oil, jojoba oil and glycerine – to nourish and soften the skin

• 5ml/1 tsp each Fullers earth and rock salt – to soften and cleanse

• 10ml/2 tsp foaming foot or bath wash – to cleanse the skin and soften the cuticles

• 3 drops essential oil – for aromatic feel-good factor. Choose whichever oil you like best, or use a blend: mandarin and geranium, or lavender and lemon are relaxing, cleansing combinations

In a small clean bottle, mix the foaming wash, essential oil and glycerine. Shake and set aside while you prepare the other ingredients. Put the Fullers earth and rock salt into a medium-sized dish and mix together. Mix in the almond and jojoba oils. Add the glycerine mixture to the bowl, and mix all the ingredients together with a metal spoon. You should now have a runny paste.

## lemon verbena and lavender foot bath

### ingredients

• 15g/¹/₂oz dried lemon verbena

• 30ml/2 tbsp dried lavender

• 5 drops lavender essential oil

• 30ml/2 tbsp cider vinegar

Put the lemon verbena and lavender into a basin and pour in enough hot water to cover the feet. When it has cooled add the lavender oil and cider vinegar. Sit down and immerse your feet in the bath for 15 minutes. Dry your feet thoroughly afterwards.

**CARING FOR YOUR FEET**

A pedicure will help to keep your feet attractive and healthy. You will need a few special items, but because they will last a long time they are definitely a worthwhile investment.

• **Nail-polish remover**: It's a good idea to choose a conditioning one.

• **Cotton wool (cotton)**: Ideal for removing nail polish and also useful for separating toes while you paint them.

• **Nail brush or orange stick** (tip covered with cotton wool): Useful for cleaning under the nail.

• **Hoof stick or cotton buds (swabs)**: Vital for pushing back the cuticles.

• **Toenail clippers**: These are often easier to use than scissors.

• **Emery board:** Toenails are harder than fingernails so you'll need a strong one.

• **Cuticle remover**: Invaluable for softening and loosening the cuticle.

• **Nail polish and a clear top coat**: Great for sealing polish and preventing chipping.

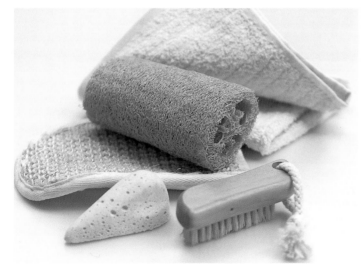

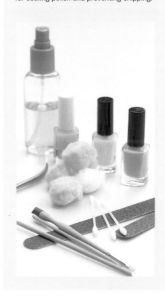

△ After soaking your feet in a footbath for ten minutes, use a loofah or nail brush to scrub and deep-cleanse, then use a pumice on the dead skin all over the soles of the feet. Pat them dry, then give your feet a quick massage using a blend of neroli and lemon essential oils well diluted in almond oil.

# Beating cellulite

It's not just plumper, older women who suffer from "orange-peel skin" on their thighs, hips, bottom and even tummy – many slim, young women suffer too. Sadly, there is no miracle cure for cellulite, but there are some practical things you can do to see great results.

## facts on cellulite

Experts disagree about what causes cellulite. It seems likely that it's an accumulation of fat, fluid and toxins trapped in the hardened network of elastin and collagen fibres in the deeper levels of your skin. This causes the dimpled effect and feel of cellulite areas. These areas also tend to feel cold to the touch because the flow of blood is constricted and the lymphatic system, which is responsible for eliminating toxins, can't work properly. This can worsen the problem and make the cellulite feel puffy and spongy.

## testing for cellulite

Try squeezing the skin of your upper thigh between your thumb and index finger. If the flesh feels lumpy and looks bumpy, you have cellulite. Further clues may be that these areas look whiter and feel colder than elsewhere on your legs.

## common causes

Cellulite can be caused and/or aggravated by the following:
• A poor diet is full of toxins and puts the body under great strain to get rid of vast quantities of waste. Also, an unhealthy low-fibre, high-fat diet means that the body's digestive system can't work effectively to expel toxins from the body.
• Stress and lack of exercise make your body sluggish and can slow down blood circulation and the lymphatic system.
• Hereditary factors – if your mother has cellulite, it's a fair bet you will have, too.
• Hormones, such as the contraceptive pill or hormone replacement therapy, may contribute.

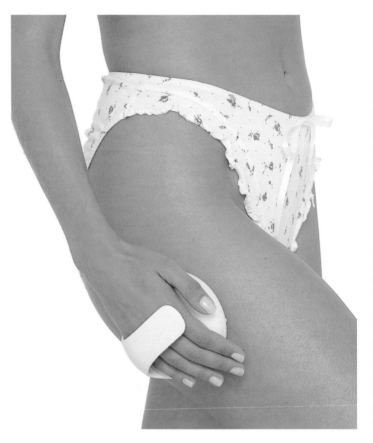

## tackling cellulite

There are dozens of products around designed to deal with cellulite, but it is debatable how effective they really are. To actually tackle the problem effectively you should attempt to follow a three-pronged approach, combining:
• Circulation-boosting tactics
• Diet
• Exercise

## boost your circulation

Here are several ways to boost your circulation and your lymphatic system. Whichever one you choose, aim to follow it for at least 5 minutes a day.

△ Pep up your circulation and lymphatic system to help beat that cellulite.

• Use a soft body brush on damp or dry skin. Brush the skin in long sweeping movements over the affected area, and make sure you are working in the direction of the heart.
• Use a massage glove or rough sisal mitt in the same way as above.
• Use a cellulite cream. These usually contain natural ingredients such as horse chestnut, ivy and caffeine to boost your circulation. However, you can make them doubly effective by massaging them thoroughly into the skin with your

## step up your exercise

Exercise will boost your sluggish circulation and lymphatic system, and encourage your body to get rid of the toxins causing your cellulite. Do a regular aerobic workout, exercising for 20–40 minutes, 3–5 times a week, and choose from these: brisk walking, swimming, cycling, tennis, badminton, aerobic classes or running. (It is always wise to consult your doctor before embarking on a new form of exercise.)

**tone it up!**

You can also try these exercises to increase circulation, firm up your legs and give them a better shape. Carried out daily, they will help you win the cellulite battle.

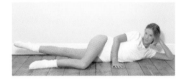

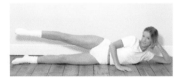

△ **Inner thigh toner**: Lie on your side on the floor, supporting your head with your arm. With your top leg resting on the floor in front, raise the lower leg off the floor as far as you can without straining, then gently lower it again. Repeat 10 times, then turn over and work the other leg.

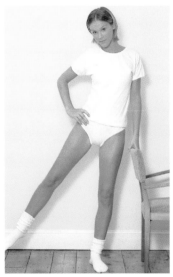

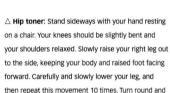

**MAKE YOUR OWN CELLULITE CREAM**
Aromatherapy has been found to be very effective for treating cellulite. There are a number of ready-blended oils on the market, but you can easily make your own. Simply add two drops each of rosemary and fennel essential oils to 15ml/1 tbsp of carrier oil, such as almond oil. Massage this mixture thoroughly into the affected areas and try to do this every day.

fingertips. Some cellulite creams even come with their own plastic or rubber hand-held mitts to help boost the circulation.

## anti-cellulite diet

To cleanse your body you need to follow a healthy low-fat, high-fibre diet – one that contains plenty of fresh fruit and vegetables. The great news is, if you have any excess weight to lose it will naturally fall away by following these rules.

• Eat at least five servings of fresh fruit and vegetables every day.

• Cut down on the amount of fat you eat. For instance, grill rather than fry foods, and cut off visible fat from meat. For many foods you buy, look out for a low-fat alternative. Water cleanses your system and flushes toxins from body cells, so drink at least 2 litres (quarts) of pure water every day.

• Change from caffeine-laden tea and coffee to herbal teas and decaffeinated coffee. Sip pure fruit juices rather than fizzy drinks.

• Steer clear of alcohol as much as possible as it adversely affects your liver – your body's main de-toxifier.

• Drink a glass of hot water containing the juice of a fresh lemon when you get up in the morning – it's a wonderful way to detoxify your body.

• Avoid eating sugary snacks between meals – eat a piece of fruit, raw vegetables or rice cakes instead.

△ **Hip toner**: Stand sideways with your hand resting on a chair. Your knees should be slightly bent and your shoulders relaxed. Slowly raise your right leg out to the side, keeping your body and raised foot facing forward. Carefully and slowly lower your leg, and then repeat this movement 10 times. Turn round and repeat with the other leg.

△ **Outer thigh toner**: Lie on your side, supporting your head with your hand. Bend your lower leg behind you and tilt your hips slightly forward. Place your other hand on the floor in front of you for balance. Slowly lift your upper leg, then bring it down to touch the lower one, and repeat this action 6 times. Repeat on the other side.

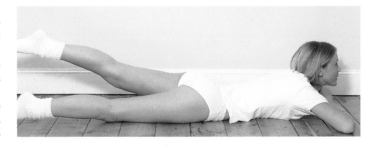

△ **Bottom toner**: Lie on your front with your hands on top of one another, resting your chin on them if you wish. Raise one leg about 13cm/5in off the floor and hold for a count of 10. Bring your leg back to the floor, and repeat 15–20 times with each leg.

# Holiday skincare

There's nothing that lifts your spirits like spending time in the sunshine and a certain amount of exposure to the sun is actually good for our bodies. However, it is important that you take special care of your skin against the dangers of suntanning. The secret is to give your skin the protection it needs, while you gradually develop a light attractive colour.

## the right product

There is a wide range of sun creams, lotions and blocks available, and it is vital to use the right one because burning ages your skin and increases your chances of skin cancer. Play safe by following our two-step plan:

### step 1: know your SPFs

SPF stands for Sun Protection Factor. The higher the number of the SPF, the more protection the product will give you from the burning ultraviolet B (UVB) rays. For instance, an SPF 2 will let you stay out in the sun for twice as long as you usually could before burning, whereas an SPF 8 will let you stay out eight times as long.

### step 2: go by skin type

To choose an SPF, you need to know how vulnerable your skin is to the sun's UVB rays. Dermatologists divide skins into six types, each needing a different level of protection, so you can ensure your skin is always well protected, wherever you travel.

**Skin-type 1:** Always burns, never tans. Fair-skinned, usually with freckles. Red or blonde hair. Typical Irish or Anglo-Saxon skin type.
UK/North Europe: Use total sunblock, or keep out of the sun.
USA/Tropics/Africa: Use total sunblock.
Mediterranean: Use total sunblock.

**Skin-type 2:** Burns easily and tans with difficulty. Fair hair and pale skin. Typical North European skin type.
UK/North Europe: Start with SPF 20 and use sunblock on delicate areas. Progress gradually to SPF 15.
USA/Tropics/Africa: Start with sunblock and progress gradually to SPF 20.
Mediterranean: Start with SPF 20, use sunblock on delicate areas, and progress gradually to SPF 15.

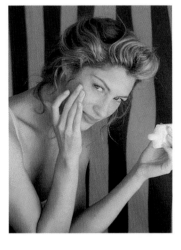

△ If your skin is going to be exposed to the sun, make sure you apply plenty of sunscreen to protect it.

**Skin-type 3:** Sometimes burns but tans well. Light brown hair and medium skin tone. Again, a typical North European skin type.
UK/North Europe: Start with SPF 10 and progress to SPF 8.
USA/Tropics/Africa: Start with SPF 20, moving to SPF 15, then SPF 10.
Mediterranean: Start with SPF 15, moving to SPF 10.

**Skin-type 4:** Occasionally burns but tans easily. Usually with brown hair and eyes, and olive skin. This is the typical Mediterranean skin type.
UK/North Europe: Start with SPF 8, moving to SPF 6.
USA/Tropics/Africa: Start with SPF 15, moving to SPF 8.
Mediterranean: Start with SPF 10, moving to SPF 6.

**Skin-type 5:** Hardly ever burns and tans very easily. Dark eyes, dark hair and olive skin. A

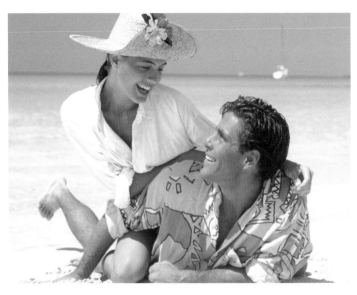

◁ If you are out in the sun during the hottest part of the day, make sure you cover up with a shirt and a hat.

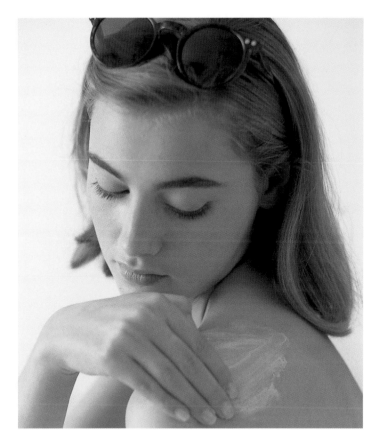

### wash-off tanners

A quick way to create an instant tan on your face and body. Simply smooth on the cream, then wash it away at the end of the day.

### self-tanners

If you haven't tried these formulations for years because you remember the awful smell, colour and streaky results, then you'll be pleasantly surprised at the improvements that have been made. In fact, choose carefully and you'll create an acceptable alternative to the real thing. These products contain an active ingredient called dihydroxyacetone (DHA), which is absorbed by surface skin cells and turns brown in the presence of oxygen, creating the "tan". This process usually takes 3–4 hours, and the effects last until these skin cells are naturally shed – which can be from a few days right up to a week.

### self-tanning tips

• Use a body scrub first to rub away the dead flaky skin that can create a patchy finish.

• Massage plenty of body lotion into the area to be treated. This will combat any remaining dry areas, and give a smooth surface on which to apply the tanning lotion.

• If there's a shade choice, go with the lighter one, because you can always apply more to get a darker colour.

• Use a small amount of the product at a time – you can apply a second layer later.

• Work the product firmly into the skin until it feels completely dry. Any excess left on the surface is likely to go patchy.

• If you've applied self-tan to your body, wipe areas that don't normally tan with damp cotton wool (cotton) – armpits, nipples, soles of feet and fingers. On the face, work the cotton wool around eyebrows, hairline and jawline.

• While there are self-tanning products that offer some protection from the sun until you wash your skin, it's best to use them in conjunction with the best sunscreen for your skin type.

---

typical Middle Eastern or Asian skin type.
UK/North Europe: Use SPF 6 throughout.
USA/Tropics/Africa: Start with SPF 8 and move to SPF 6.
Mediterranean: Start with SPF 8 and move to SPF 6.

**Skin-type 6:** Almost never burns. Has dark hair, eyes and skin. Typical African or Afro-Caribbean skin type.
UK/North Europe: No sunscreen needed.
USA/Tropics/Africa: Start with SPF 8, moving to SPF 6.
Mediterranean: Use SPF 6 throughout.

### safe tan plan

• Apply suntan lotion before you go into the sun, and before you dress, to ensure that you don't miss any areas.

• Gradually build up the time you spend in the sun. Never be tempted to stay in the sun so long that your skin burns – it's a sign of skin damage.

• Stay out of the sun between 12 noon and 3 o'clock when the sun is at its hottest. Move into the shade or cover up with a t-shirt and broad-brimmed hat.

• If you're playing a lot of sport or swimming, choose a special sports formula or waterproof formulation.

• Lips need a good lip screen to protect them from burning and chapping.

• If you have sensitive skin, there are hypo-allergenic products around, so ask your pharmacist.

### fake tan plan

The safest tan of all is one that comes out of a bottle! There are three main ways to fake a tan.

### bronzing powders

These are designed to be used on your face, and they act in the same way as a blusher. Make sure that the one you use is not too pearlized, or you'll shimmer a little too much in the sunshine.

# Skincare glossary

If you are confused about the various claims and ingredients in your skincare products, check out what they mean here in our guide to the most commonly found skincare terms on bottles and jars.

**Allergy-screened:** This means that the individual ingredients in the product have gone through exacting tests to ensure that they're safe to use and that there's just the minimum risk of causing allergy.

**Aloe vera:** The juice from the leaves of this succulent plant is often used in skincare ingredients because of its soothing, protecting and moisturizing qualities.

**Antioxidants:** These work by mopping up and absorbing 'free radicals' from your skin. These highly reactive molecules can damage your skin and cause premature aging. Good antioxidants are the ACE vitamins, that is vitamins A, C and E.

**Benzoyl peroxide:** This is an ingredient commonly used in over-the-counter spot and acne treatments because it gently peels surface skin and unclogs blocked follicles, which can cause spots.

**Cocoa butter:** This comes from the seeds of the cacao tree in tropical climates. Cocoa butter is an excellent moisturizer, especially for dry skin on the body.

**Collagen:** Collagen is an elastic substance in the underlying tissues of your skin that provides support and springiness. Old collagen fibres are less elastic than young collagen, which is one of the main reasons why skin can become less springy as it ages. Collagen is a popular ingredient in skincare treatments, although it's doubtful if a molecule this size can penetrate the skin.

**Dermatologically tested:** This means the product has been patch-tested on a panel of human volunteers to monitor it for any tendency to cause irritation. This means it's usually suitable for sensitive skins.

**Elastin:** These are fibres in the underlying layer of your skin, rather like collagen, which help give it strength and elasticity.

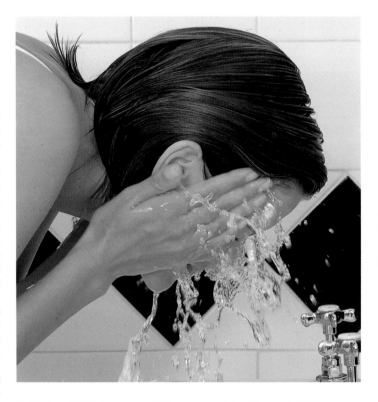

**Exfoliation:** Exfoliating means whisking away the top surface layers of dead cells from your skin. This has the effect of making it look brighter and feeling smoother. To exfoliate, you massage a gritty exfoliating scrub over damp skin, then rinse it away with warm water.

**Fruit acids:** Also known as AHAs or alpha-hydroxy acids. They're commonly found in natural products such as fruit, sour milk and wine. AHAs are included in many face creams because they work by breaking down the protein bonds that hold together the dead cells on the skin's surface, to reveal newer, fresher skin underneath.

**Humectants:** These ingredients are often found in moisturizers, as they work by attracting moisture to themselves, and so keep the surface layers of your skin well hydrated.

△ A pH-balanced facial wash will help prevent your skin from feeling tight.

**Hypo-allergenic:** These products are usually fragrance-free and contain the minimum of colouring agents and no known irritants or sensitizers. This is not a total guarantee that no one will have an allergic reaction to them. Some people are even allergic to water.

**Jojoba oil:** Jojoba is a liquid wax obtained from the seeds of a Mexican shrub. It was used for centuries by American Indians. It's a gentle, non-irritant oil that makes an excellent moisturizer as it is easily absorbed into the skin and helps improve the condition of the hair and scalp.

**Lanolin-free:** This means a product doesn't contain the ingredient lanolin – the fat stripped from sheep's wool. At one time it

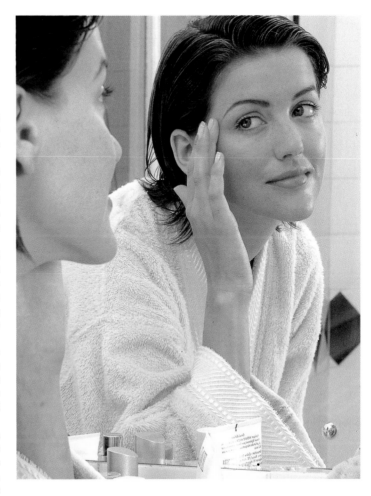

was thought that lanolin was a common skin allergen, although evidence does now seem to show that lanolin is even suitable for sensitive skins.

**Liposomes:** These are tiny fluid-filled spheres made of the same material that forms cell membranes. Their very small size is said to let them penetrate into the skin's living cells, where they act as delivery parcels and release their active ingredients.

**Milia:** Another word for whiteheads – small pimples on the skin. Oil produced from the sebaceous glands gathers to form a white plug, which is trapped under the skin. You can try to remove these by gentle squeezing with tissue-covered fingers or treat them with an antibacterial cream.

**Non-comedogenic**: A comedo is a blackhead, so this means the product has been screened to eliminate ingredients that can clog the follicles and encourage blackheads and spots. It's particularly useful for oily skins.

**Oil of evening primrose:** The oil taken from the seeds of the evening primrose plant is very useful for helping your skin retain its moisture. It's a wonderful moisturizer, particularly for dry or very dry skins, as it hydrates, protects and soothes. It also improves the skin's overall softness and suppleness. Many sufferers of eczema find it useful.

**pH-balanced:** The pH scale measures the acidity or alkalinity of a solution, with 7 meaning that it is neutral. Any number below that is acidic, and numbers above are alkaline. Healthy skin has a slightly acidic reading, so pH-balanced skincare products are slightly acidic to maintain this natural optimum level.

**Retin A:** Also known as Retinoic Acid, this is a derivative of vitamin A that has been used for years to treat acne. Now it's available on prescription, to be used under medical supervision, to help reverse the visible signs of ageing on the skin.

**SPF:** This stands for Sun Protection Factor. It will tell you how long the sun cream or moisturizer will protect you from the sun's burning ultraviolet B rays. The higher the number, the more protection it will give.

**T-zone:** This is the area across the forehead and down the centre of the face where the oil glands and sweat glands of the face are most concentrated.

**Ultraviolet (UV) rays:** Ultraviolet light damages your skin. UVB rays will burn your skin if you sunbathe for too long. UVA rays are strong all year round and cause ageing and wrinkling of the skin. Guard against this with a broad-spectrum sun cream, which contains both UVA and UVB filters.

**Vitamin E:** This is often used in moisturizers because it can help combat dryness and the signs of ageing. It's also useful for helping to heal scars and burns.

**Water-soluble:** When they contain oils to dissolve grime and make-up from your skin, cleansers are described as water-soluble, with the bonus that they can be quickly and easily rinsed away.

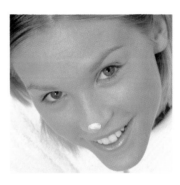

△ Discover the healing properties of vitamin E on your skin.

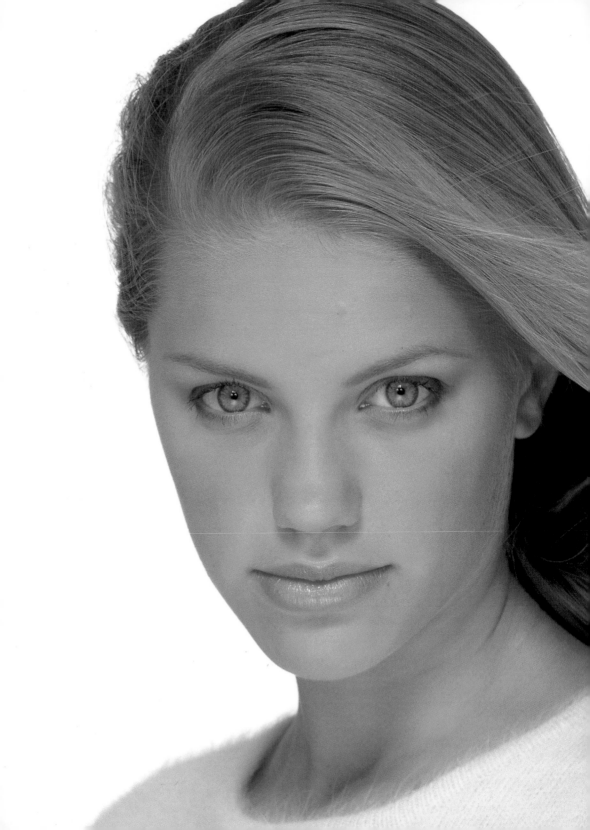

# Make-up Magic

The key to making-up successfully is to
understand how to enhance your
features using the best cosmetic
formulations and colours. Buy the best
products, brush up your techniques and
experiment to find the perfect look.

# Make-up basics

Being considered beautiful today no longer means conforming to one accepted ideal. The contemporary approach to beauty places the emphasis firmly on the individual and her own particular needs, aspirations and lifestyle. For although every woman is concerned to some extent about how she looks, everyone is very different. For instance, the make-up needs of a blue-eyed blonde are not the same as those of a dark-eyed woman with an Oriental skin-tone.

The great news is that make-up can be used to enhance everyone's features. Applied with a sensitive touch it should create a subtle emphasis, rather than a mask disguising the features.

Many women are wary of cosmetics because they are not sure which colours suit them or which make-up methods and textures are the most flattering. Good make-up hinges on experience: you learn what suits you by trial and error. Nobody wants to waste money on a lipstick that turns out to be the wrong colour when you try it at home; but it's easy to get stuck in a rut – so be brave and experiment a little.

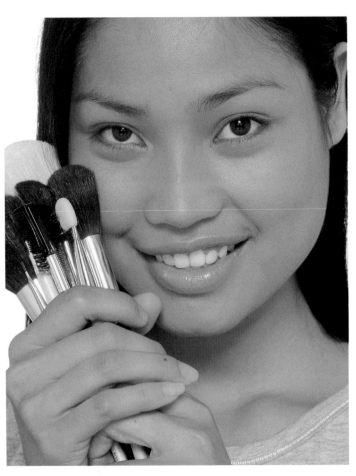

◁ **Every woman can use make-up to emphasize her best features.**

## product know-how

No two women are alike. When we're buying a pair of jeans, we don't just pick the same size, colour and pair as our sister, because we have different requirements. Make-up is the same. We need to choose carefully from the vast array of products and formulations around to create a look that's made-to-measure for our own complexions and features. Simply buying the most expensive product on the shelves is no guarantee of success, as it may not be the most suitable for your colouring or skin type.

These pages will take you through the myriad bottles, compacts and colours, and show you how to find the ones that work best for you, and how to apply them.

## tailor-made make-up

The perfect make-up for you will be effortless once you choose the correct shades for your skin tone and hair colour. It'll also work wonderfully, because you'll still look like you, only better! Checking your hair colour is easy – whether it's natural or comes out of a bottle. Deciding whether your skin is "warm" or "cool" seems slightly more difficult – however, there is an easy way to check. Simply look in a mirror and hold a piece of gold and a piece of silver in front of your face. These can just as easily be pieces of foil or costume jewellery as the real thing. The right metal will bring a healthy glow to your skin, whereas the wrong will make it look grey. If gold suits your skin, then it's "warm" toned. If silver suits it, it's "cool" toned. A further clue is how well you tan in the sun – cool skin tones tend to colour less easily.

## inspirational ideas

Sometimes make-up should be used just for the sheer fun of it. Try out a different look for a special occasion, bringing out the

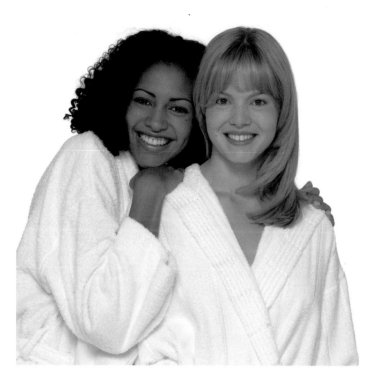

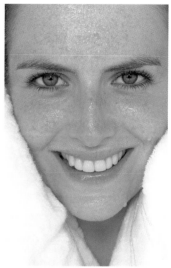

make-up artist in you. Whether you want to create an impact in the office or turn heads at a party, there are lots of ideas to help you put on the perfect face.

## how to reassess your image

Take a careful look at your make-up bag or drawer. How old are the cosmetics? Six months, a year or more? Now study your face when you are wearing your usual make-up, and ask yourself what your make-up does for you: does it widen or narrow your eyes or mouth, enhance the shape of your face, make you look younger or older? If it does not produce the effect you require and your cosmetics are more than a year old, it is time for a complete change. Bear these points in mind:

**Your age:** Make-up that suited you when you were 25 is not going to look right 10 years down the line. Changes in skin tone and texture, as well as in hair colour, require different make-up shades and textures: the right make-up can take years off your face.

**Your face shape and skin tone:** Make-up can improve face shape by illusion; it can also improve skin tone and texture.

**Your eye colour and size:** Deftly applied make-up can make small eyes look bigger, blue eyes look bluer and round eyes look longer; can your current make-up do this for you?

**Your hair colour:** Make-up should complement hair; if your hair is jet black and your skin is pale, deep red lipstick and black eye make-up (mascara and kohl) look stunning. If you are blonde, earthy tones look best (the bright colours can be a bit brassy). If you have brown or black hair, you will have almost limitless colour freedom.

**Your lifestyle:** Make make-up easy; there is no point choosing make-up that requires a great deal of time to apply properly if you have a very busy lifestyle.

## brush up your techniques

Don't just read about them but actually put new ideas into practice! Brush up on tips and tricks to help you maximize your looks, and deal with your own particular beauty needs. Perhaps you need a new look on a budget, speedy ideas or some expert help. The main thing is to spend a little time on making the most of yourself.

△ Take a close look at your face while you are washing or getting ready for bed. Which features would you like to enhance? Which would you like to play down?

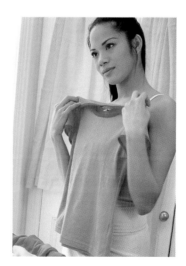

△ We already have a pretty good idea of colours that suit us, and it is important to work out what make-up colours and styles work best for you.

# Foundation that fits

Many women avoid foundation because they're scared of an unnatural, mask-like effect. In fact, finding the right product for your skin is simpler than you might think. There are two keys to success: the first is to pick the right formulation, and the second is to choose the perfect shade for your skin.

## find your formulation

Long gone are the days when you could only buy heavy pancake foundation. Now you can choose from many formulations, so you can get the best coverage for your particular skin type. Here are the products on offer, and who they're best for.

### tinted moisturizers

These are a cross between a moisturizer and a foundation, as they'll soothe your skin while giving a little coverage. They're ideal for young or clear skins. They're also great in the summer, when you want a sheer effect or to even out a fading tan. Unlike other foundations, you can blend tinted moisturizers on with your fingertips.

### liquid foundations

These are the most popular and versatile of all foundation types, because they smooth

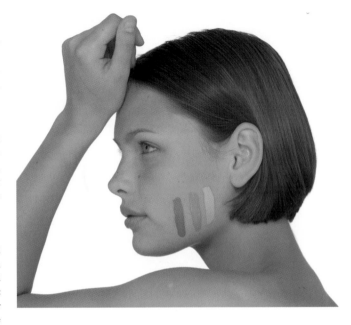

on easily and offer natural-looking coverage. They suit all but the driest skins. If you have oily skin or suffer from occasional spot break-outs, look for an oil-free liquid foundation, to cover the affected areas without aggravating them.

### cream foundations

These are thick, rich and moisturizing, making them ideal for dry or mature skins. As they have a fairly heavy texture, make sure you blend them well into your skin with a damp cosmetic sponge.

### mousse foundations

Again these are quite moisturizing and ideal for drier skins. The best way is to dab a little of the product on to the back of your hand, then dot on to your skin with a sponge.

### compact foundations

These are all-in-one formulations, which already contain powder. They come in a compact, usually with their own sponge for

△ **Before buying, check different foundation colours on your jawline for the perfect match.**

application. However, they actually give a lighter finish than you'd expect. They're great on all but dry skin types.

### stick foundations

These are the original foundation. They have a heavy texture, and so are best confined for use on badly blemished or scarred skin. Dot a little foundation directly on to the affected area, then blend gently with a damp sponge.

## shade selection

Once you've chosen the ideal formulation for you, you're ready to choose the perfect matching shade to your skin. At last cosmetic companies have woken up to the fact that not everyone has an "American tan" complexion! Now, there is a good selection of foundation shades from a pink-toned English rose to a yellow-hued, olive

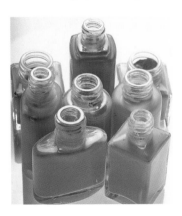

△ **It is well worth spending time to find the right foundation colour for you.**

▷ Blend, blend, blend for a professional finish. And don't forget to give all angles of your face a final check in the mirror to make sure you haven't got any unnatural lines where your foundation finishes.

▽ Liquid foundations are popular because they provide natural-looking coverage.

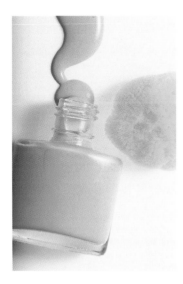

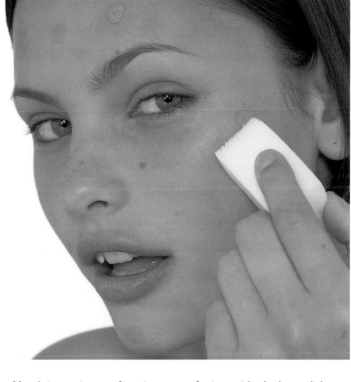

skin, as well as from the palest skin to the darkest one. There are some tried-and-tested methods for choosing the perfect one for your skin tone:

• Ensure you're in natural daylight when trying out foundation colours, so you can see exactly how your skin will look once you leave the shop or counter.

• Select a couple of shades to try that look as though they'll match your skin.

• Don't try foundation on your hand or on your wrist – they're a different colour to your face.

• Stroke a little colour on to your jawline to ensure you get a tone that will blend with your neck as well as your face. The shade that seems to "disappear" into your skin is the right one for you.

## application know-how

Apply foundation to freshly moisturized skin to ensure you have a perfect base on which to work.

• Use a cosmetic sponge to apply most types of foundation – using your fingertips can result in an uneven, greasy finish.

• Apply foundation in dots, then blend each one with your sponge.

• Dampen the sponge first of all, then squeeze out the excess moisture – this will prevent the sponge from soaking up too much costly foundation.

• Check for tell-tale "tidemarks" on your jawline, nose, forehead and chin.

## high performance foundation

Companies these days have made great improvements to their foundations. Here are some benefits to look out for:

• Many companies have added sunscreens to their foundations, so they'll protect you from the ageing effects of the sun while you wear them. Look out for the words UV Protection and Sun Protection Factor (SPF) numbers on the tube or bottle.

• Look for the new "light-diffusing" foundations, which are great for older skins. They contain hundreds of tiny light-reflective particles that bounce light away from your skin – making fine lines, wrinkles and blemishes less noticeable.

## correct colour

You can wear a colour corrective foundation under your normal foundation to alter your skin-tone. They can seem quite strange at first glance but are, in fact, highly effective at toning down a high colour or boosting the colour of your complexion. Use them sparingly at first until you feel confident that you have achieved an effective, but subtle, result.

• Green foundation cools down rosiness and is great for those who blush easily.

• Lavender foundation will brighten up a sallow complexion, and is great for when you're feeling tired.

• Apricot foundation will give a subtle glow to dull skin, and is a great beauty booster in the winter.

• White foundation gives a wonderful glow to all complexions, and is perfect for a special night out.

# Clever concealer

Concealers are a fast and effective way to disguise blemishes, shadows, scars and red veins, so your skin looks perfect.

## find your formulation

Concealers are concentrated foundation with a high pigment content, giving complete coverage to problem areas. Make-up artists argue as to whether concealer should be applied before or after foundation. Applying it after foundation is often best, as it's applied to specific areas which would be disturbed when the foundation was applied. If you're after a light effect, apply concealer to clean skin, then apply powder or all-in-one foundation/powder on top.

### stick concealers

These are easy to apply as you can simply stroke them straight on to the skin. Some have quite a thick consistency, so it's worth trying samples before buying.

### cream concealers

These usually come in a tube, with a sponge-tipped applicator. The coverage isn't as thick as the stick type, but the finished effect is natural.

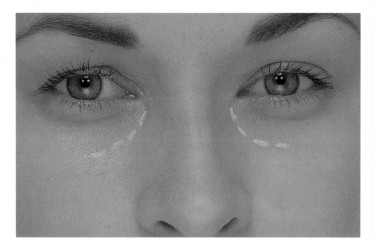

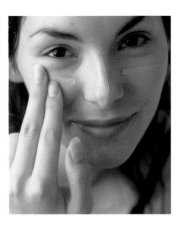

△ Cream concealer is easier to apply smoothly on larger areas.

### liquid concealers

Again, these come in a tube. Just squeeze a tiny amount on to your finger and smooth over the affected area. Look for the cream-to-powder formulations, which slick on like a cream and dry to a velvety powder finish.

## taking cover

Here's how to conceal all your beauty problems effectively.

### spots and blemishes

The ideal solution is to use a medicated stick concealer as this contains ingredients to deal with the pimple or blemish as well as cover it. Only apply the concealer on the pimple or blemish, as it can be quite drying, and then smooth away the edges with a clean cotton bud (swab). Applying concealer all around the area will make the spot more noticeable.

> **CONCEALER TIP**
> When choosing a concealer look for the colour that is nearest your own skin tone rather than a lighter one. Covering a problem area with a paler shade will simply accentuate it.

△ **If you have noticeable shadows under your eyes, you can tone them down very effectively with a few dots of concealer.**

### under-eye shadows

Opt for a creamy stick concealer or a liquid one, as dry formulations emphasize fine lines around your eyes. If you're blending with your fingertips, use your ring finger, as this is the weakest finger and less likely to drag at the delicate skin around your eyes.

### scars

Scars, including old acne or chickenpox marks, can be effectively covered using a concealer but it can be a time-consuming process. Begin by building the indentation up to skin level by dotting on layers of concealer. This is best applied using a fine brush. Take your time and allow each layer to settle into the skin properly.

### red veins

Stick or liquid concealer is ideal for tackling this problem. Apply a layer of concealer over the area with a fine eyeliner brush or clean cotton bud, then carefully feather and soften the edges to blend them in and make them less noticeable.

# The power of powder

Face powder is the make-up artist's best friend, as it can make your skin look really wonderful and is very versatile in its uses.

## why use powder

Here are four good reasons for putting on that powder!
• Powder gives a super-smooth sheen to your skin – with or without foundation.
• It "sets" your foundation, so it stays put and looks good for longer.
• Powder absorbs oils from your skin, and helps prevent shiny patches appearing.
• It helps conceal open pores.

## choose your powder

You'll need two types of powder – a loose form at home, and a powder compact for your handbag.

### loose powder

This gives the best and longest-lasting finish and is the choice of professional make-up artists and models. The best way to apply loose powder is to dust it lightly on to your skin using a large, soft powder brush. Then lightly brush over your face again to dust off the excess.

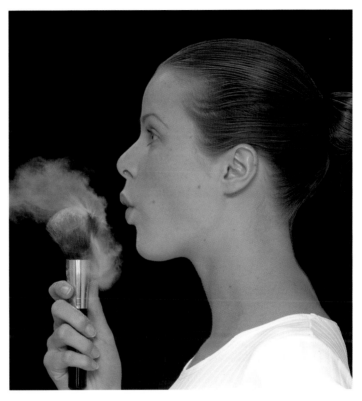

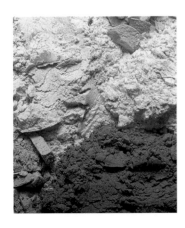

△ Take time to experiment so you choose the shade that best suits your colouring.

### pressed powder

Compacts containing pressed powder are ideal for carrying in your make-up bag as they're very quick to use and lightweight. Most come with their own application sponges, but you'll find you get a better result if you apply them with a brush. Look for brushes with retractable heads to carry in your make-up bag.

If you do use the sponge, use a light touch and wash it regularly, or you'll transfer the oils in your skin on to the powder and get a build-up.

### shade away

Don't make the mistake of thinking that one shade of powder suits all. Instead, choose one that closely matches your skin-

△ Careful application of the right powder as the final finishing and fixing touch should give your skin a soft, glowing and natural feel.

> **POWDER TIP**
> When dusting excess powder away from your skin, use your brush in light, downward strokes to help prevent the powder from getting caught in the fine hairs on your skin. Pay particular attention to the sides of the face and jawline which aren't so easy for you to see.

tone for a natural effect. Do this by dusting a little on your jawline, in the same way as you would with foundation.

# Beautiful blusher

Give your complexion a bloom of colour with this indispensable beauty aid.

## blush baby

Blusher is an instant way to give your looks a lift. It's old-fashioned to use blusher to sculpt your face, as it looks so unnatural. Instead, it should be applied in the way it was first intended to be used – to recreate a youthful flush.

### powder blusher

This should be applied over the top of your foundation and face powder. To apply powder blusher, dust over the compact with a large soft brush. If you've taken too much on to your brush, tap the handle on the back of your hand to remove the excess. It's better to waste a little blusher than to apply too much! A good guide is to use half as much blusher and twice as much blending as you first think you need.

Start applying the colour on the fullest parts of your cheeks, directly below the centre of your eyes. Then smile and dust the blusher over your cheekbones and up towards your temples. Blend the colour well towards the hairline, so you avoid harsh edges. This will effectively place colour where you would naturally blush.

### cream blusher

Breaking all the traditional beauty rules, cream blusher is applied with your fingertips. It's put on after foundation and before face powder. It drops out of fashion from time to time, but it's never long before it makes a comeback. This is for good reason, as it can give a lovely fresh glow to every skin type.

To apply, dab a few dots of cream blusher over your cheeks, from the plump part up towards your cheekbone. Using your fingertips, blend well. Build up the effect gradually, adding more blusher to create just the look you want. Or, if you prefer, you can use a foundation wedge to blend in cream blusher.

## colour choice

There is a kaleidoscope of blusher shades to choose from. However, as a rule, it's best to opt for a shade that tones well with your skin colouring, and co-ordinates with the rest of your make-up. You can opt for lighter or darker shades, depending on the season.

## Blusher colour guide

| COLOURING | CHOOSE |
|---|---|
| Blonde hair, cool skin | Baby pink |
| Blonde hair, warm skin | Tawny pink |
| Dark hair, cool skin | Cool rose |
| Dark hair, warm skin | Rosy brown |
| Red hair, cool skin | Soft peach |
| Red hair, warm skin | Warm peach |
| Dark hair, olive skin | Warm brown |
| Black hair, dark skin | Terracotta |

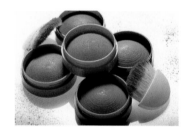

△ **Powder blusher is a quick and easy option.**

▽ **Be a blushing beauty with a light touch of powder blusher (left). Or go for more of a glow with cream blusher (right).**

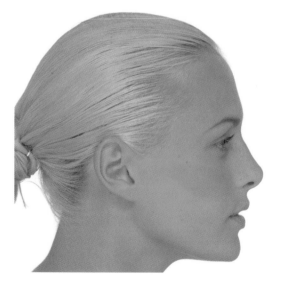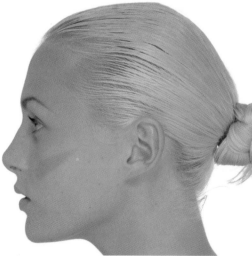

# Brush up your make-up

Even the most expensive make-up in the world won't look particularly great if it's applied carelessly and using your fingertips.

## basic tools

For a professional finish you need the right tools. This means investing in a set of good brushes and applicators.

### make-up sponge

Have a wedge-shaped one, so you can use the finer edges to help blend in foundation round your nose and jawline, and the flatter edges for the cheeks, forehead and chin. However, if you prefer not to use a synthetic sponge try the small, natural ones instead. Remember to use it damp, not dry.

### powder brush

Get used to using a powder brush each time you put make-up on. To prevent a caked or clogged finish to your face powder, use a large, soft brush to dust away any excess.

### blusher brush

Use to add a pretty glow to your skin with a light dusting of powder blusher. A blusher brush is slightly smaller than a powder brush to make it easier to control.

### eyeshadow brush

Smooth on any shade of eyeshadow with this brush.

### eyeshadow sponge

A sponge applicator is great for applying a sweep of pale eyeshadow that doesn't need much blending, or for applying highlighter to your brow bones.

### all-in-one eyelash brush/comb

Great for combing through your lashes between coats of mascara for a clump-free finish. Flip the comb over and use the brush side to sweep your eyebrows into shape, or soften pencilled-in brows.

### lip brush

Create a perfect outline and then use it to fill in the shape with your lipstick.

### eyebrow tweezers

It is essential to have a good pair of tweezers for regularly tidying up the eyebrows.

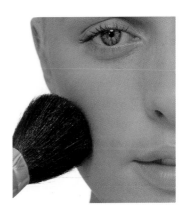

△ Use a big soft brush to blend the colour on to your cheeks.

### eyelash curlers

Once used, they'll soon become a beauty essential! Curlier eyelashes make a huge difference to the way your lashes look and help open up the eyes.

▽ Bring out the creative make-up artist in you with a good-quality set of brushes and a basic make-up tool kit.

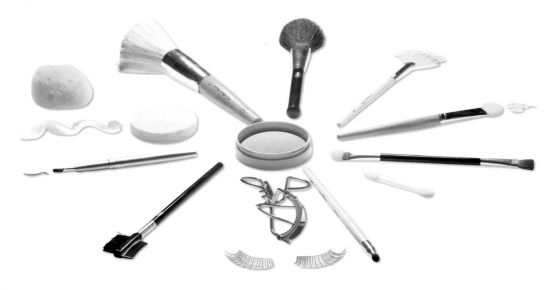

# Eye-catching make-up

Eye make-up is the most popular type of cosmetic, and for good reason. Just the simplest touch of mascara can open up your eyes, while a splash of colour can transform them instantly. Whatever your eye shape and colour, you can take steps to ensure that they always look stunning.

## mastering the basics

Many women hesitate to experiment with eye make-up, because it seems too time-consuming and complicated. The sheer quantity of products on the shelves and make-up counters can make it even more intimidating. However, you can create a huge variety of looks – from the simplest to the most extreme – by opening your eyes to the basic techniques.

## eyebrow know-how

Many women tend to ignore their eyebrows completely. Or sometimes, which is usually even worse, they will overpluck them. When it comes to eye make-up, the eyebrows make a very important impression. They can provide a balanced look to your face so it's well worth making the effort to master the techniques and to get them looking right.

**natural brows**

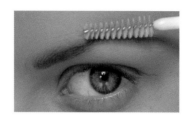

△ For perfectly groomed brows in an instant, try combing through them with a brush to flick away any powder or foundation. Comb the hairs upwards and outwards. This will also help give you a wide-eyed look. Then lightly slick them with clear gel to hold the shape in place.

## lining up liner

Eyeliner can be applied to flatter all eye shapes and sizes. If you have never applied eyeliner before, try this straightforward technique. Sit down in front of a mirror in a good light. Take your eyeliner in your hand and rest your elbow on the table to keep your arm and hand steady. You might want to give yourself extra support by resting your little finger on your cheek. Eyeliner should be applied after eyeshadow and before mascara.

**liquid liners**

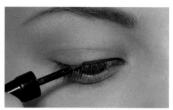

△ These have a fluid consistency, and usually come with a brush attached to the cap. To apply, look down into a mirror to prevent smudging. Stay like this for a few seconds after applying to give it time to dry.

**pencil liners**

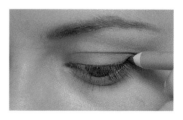

△ This is the easiest way, and one of the most effective, to add extra emphasis to your eyes. Using a pencil, carefully draw a soft line, keeping close to your upper lashes, then repeat under your lower lashes.

## define your eyebrows with powder or pencil colour

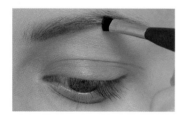

△ **1** To define your brows you can use eyebrow powder or pencil. Apply powder with an eyebrow brush, dusting it through your brows and taking care not to sweep it on to the surrounding skin. This gives a natural effect, and requires little blending.

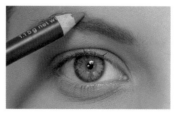

△ **2** Alternatively, use a well-sharpened pencil to draw on tiny strokes, taking care not to press too hard or the finished effect will be unnatural.

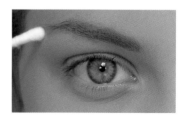

△ **3** Then soften the lines you've made with the eye pencil by lightly stroking a clean cotton bud (swab) through your brows.

## false eyelashes

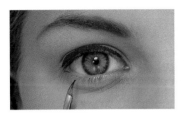

△ These luscious lashes are great for party looks but they can be tricky to apply. The strip lashes can look too obvious unless you apply them perfectly. It's a better idea to use the individual lashes on the outer corners of your eyes. Dot the roots with a little glue, then use a pair of tweezers to position them exactly.

## magic mascara

Mascara creates a flattering fringe to your eyes – particularly if your lashes are fair. Most mascaras are applied with spiral wands that are quick and easy to use. Some contain fibres to add length and thickness. Opt for a waterproof variety to withstand tears, showers and swimming – but remember you'll need a special eye make-up remover as it clings more fiercely to your lashes.

**EYEING UP EYESHADOWS**
Choose neutral colours to enhance your looks subtly, or play with a kaleidoscope of different shades.

• **powder eyeshadows**: The most popular type, these come in pressed cakes of powder either with a small brush or a sponge applicator. You can build up their density from barely-there to dramatic. Apply using a damp brush or sponge if you want a deep colour for an evening look.

• **cream shadows**: These are oil-based and come in little pots or compacts. They're applied with either a brush or fingertips. They're a good choice for dry or older skins that need extra moisturizing.

• **stick shadows**: These are wax-based and smoothed on to eyelids from the stick. Ensure they have a creamy texture before you buy, so they won't drag at your skin.

• **liquid shadows**: Usually these come in a slim bottle with a sponge applicator. Look out for the cream-to-powder ones that smooth on as a liquid and then blend to a velvety powder finish.

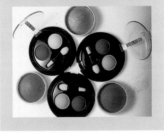

## eyeshadow as eyeliner

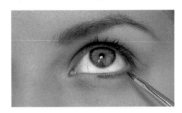

△ **1** Make-up artists often use eyeshadow to outline the eyes, and it's a trick worth stealing! It looks very effective because it gives a soft smoky effect. Use a small brush to apply shadow under your lower lashes and to make an impact over the top of the eyelid, taking care to keep the shadow close to the eyelashes.

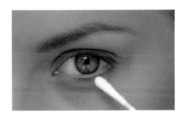

△ **2** To create an even softer effect, simply sweep over the eyeshadow liner with a cotton bud.

## simple steps for creating perfect lashes

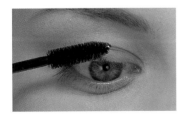

△ **1** Start by applying mascara to your upper lashes. Brush them downwards to start with, then brush them upwards from underneath. Use a tiny zig-zag movement to prevent mascara from clogging on your lashes.

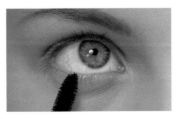

△ **2** Next, use the tip of the mascara wand to brush your lower lashes, using a gentle side-to-side technique. Take care to keep your hand steady while you are applying the mascara, and don't blink while the mascara is still wet.

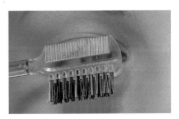

△ **3** Comb through your lashes with an eyelash comb to remove any excess, and to prevent your lashes from clumping. For a more defined effect, repeat the two previous steps twice more, allowing each layer of mascara to dry before applying the next.

# Eye make-up masterclass

Now that you know where to start and have mastered the basic techniques, you can begin to experiment with more sophisticated eye make-up methods to create a variety of stunning looks.

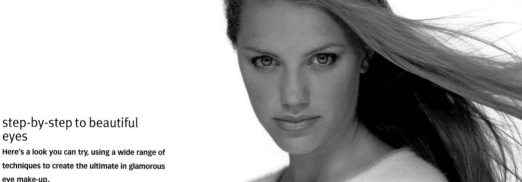

## step-by-step to beautiful eyes

Here's a look you can try, using a wide range of techniques to create the ultimate in glamorous eye make-up.

△ For our main look here, we used a palette of ivory and blue eyeshadow, combined with black eyeliner and mascara. Take time to experiment with different colours to find a look that suits you and your colouring.

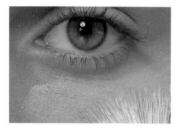

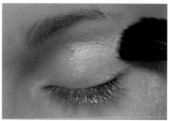

△ **1** Smooth over your eyelids with foundation to create an even base on which to work, and to give your eye make-up something to cling to.

△ **2** Sweep over your eyelids with a brush loaded with translucent face powder.

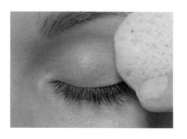

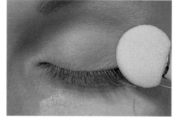

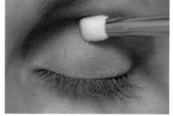

△ **3** Dust a little translucent powder under your eyes to catch any flecks of fallen eyeshadow. Use a very soft brush for this.

△ **4** Use a sponge applicator to sweep a neutral ivory shade over your eyelids. Work it right up towards your eyebrows for a balanced overall effect.

△ **5** Smudge a brown eyeshadow into the socket line of your eyes, using a sponge applicator. A slightly shimmery powder is easier to blend on.

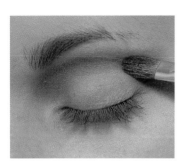

△ **6** Use a brush to sweep over the top of the brown shadow as this will remove any harsh edges.

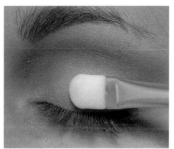

△ **7** To create a perfectly blended finish, sweep some more ivory shadow over the edges of the brown eyeshadow using a sponge applicator.

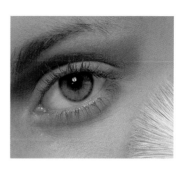

△ **8** Now that you've completed your eyeshadow, flick away the powder from under your eyes.

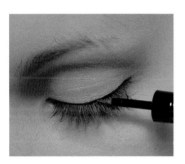

△ **9** Looking down into a mirror and keeping your hand as steady as possible, apply liquid eyeliner along your eyelid.

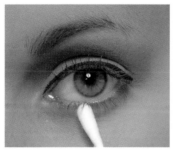

△ **10** Use a clean cotton bud (swab) to work some brown eyeshadow under your lower lashes to add some subtle definition.

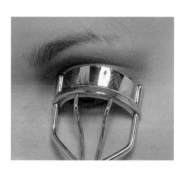

△ **11** Squeeze your lashes with eyelash curlers to make them bend, before applying mascara. This will "open up" the eye area.

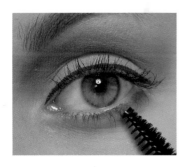

△ **12** Apply mascara to your upper lashes and then use the tip of the mascara wand to coat your lower lashes.

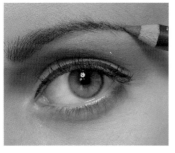

△ **13** Stroke your eyebrows with pencil to shape them and fill in any patches.

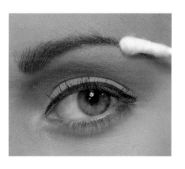

△ **14** Smooth over the top with a cotton bud to soften the eyebrow pencil line.

# Lipstick colour

Lipstick has been around for about 5,000 years, and women have always loved using it. It is the easiest and quickest way to give your face a focus and an instant splash of colour.

## a lick of colour

Lipsticks in a bullet form are the most popular way to use lip colour. The more pigment a lipstick has, the longer it'll last on your lips. The best way to apply lipstick is with a lip brush.

Another way of applying a touch of colour is with a lip gloss. This can be used alone to give your lips an attractive sheen, or applied over the top of lipstick to catch the light.

Lip liners are used to provide an outline to your lips before applying lipstick. You can also use them over your entire lip for a dark, matte effect. However, you may need to add a touch of lipsalve (balm) over the top to prevent drying out this delicate area of skin. It is particularly important because this area of skin is prone to developing fine lines.

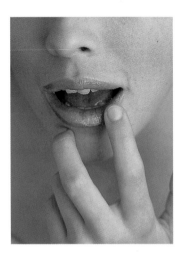

△ **Tinted lip gloss helps to keep lips soft and supple and gives your lips a hint of colour. Use it on its own, or under or over your lipstick.**

## step-by-step to perfect lips

**Follow this simple guide to apply a perfect layer of luscious colour to your lips.**

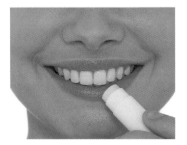

△ **1** Ensure your lips are soft and supple by smoothing over some lipsalve before you start.

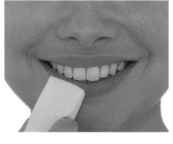

△ **2** Prime your lips with foundation, using a make-up sponge so you reach every crevice on the surface.

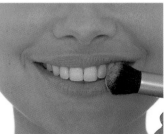

△ **3** Lightly dust over the top of the foundation with your usual face powder, to ensure your lipstick will stay put for longer.

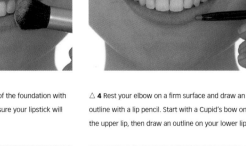

△ **4** Rest your elbow on a firm surface and draw an outline with a lip pencil. Start with a Cupid's bow on the upper lip, then draw an outline on your lower lip.

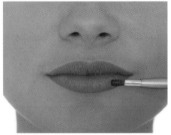

△ **5** Use a lip brush to fill the outline with lipstick; this helps get a more precise definition. Open your mouth to brush the colour into the corners of your lips.

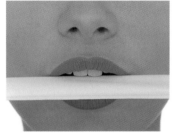

△ **6** You'll make your lipstick last longer if you blot over the surface with a tissue. It'll also give an attractive, semi-matte finish to your lips.

## SPECIAL INGREDIENTS

Today's lipsticks offer more than just a pigment to add colour to your lips. In just the same way as technology has been used in skincare products, lipsticks often contain other specially developed ingredients so that they provide optimum care for the delicate skin on your lips. Here are some of the extra ingredients that may be included in your lipstick:

• Vegetable wax to make your lipstick easier to apply smoothly, and to give your lips a natural soft sheen.

• Liposomes containing active moisturizing ingredients, to keep your lips soft.

• Chamomile to soothe and heal the skin on your lips.

• Shea butter to deep-moisturize your lips, especially in extremes of weather and wind, which can have drastic effects.

• Silicas to help give your lipstick a slightly matte effect.

• UV filters to protect your lips from the aging effects of the sun's rays.

• Vitamin E to help heal any cuts, and protect your lips against the fine lines associated with aging.

## lavender lip balm

### ingredients

- 5ml/1 tsp beeswax
- 5ml/1 tsp cocoa butter
- 5ml/1 tsp wheatgerm oil
- 5ml/1 tsp almond oil
- 3 drops lavender essential oil

Put all the ingredients, except the lavender oil, in a small bowl. Then set the bowl over a pan of simmering water and keep stirring the mixture until the wax has melted. Remember that beeswax has a high melting point so you will need to be patient. Remove from the heat and allow the mixture to cool for a few minutes before adding the lavender oil. Pour into a small jar and leave to set.

▷ **This sweet-scented lavender lip balm is a natural way to soothe and condition your lips.**

## Lipstick colour coding

Believe it or not, everyone can wear red lipstick. The key to success is to choose just the right shade for your colouring.

| COLOURING | CHOOSE |
|---|---|
| **Blonde hair, cool skin** | If you're daring enough you can wear any bright red shade, such as crimson or fire-engine red. Any bold shade will look really effective and striking on you. |
| **Blonde hair, warm skin** | Lovely pink-reds look great with your colouring. They're delicate enough not to look too harsh, while the pinky undertones complement the warmth of your skin. |
| **Dark hair, cool skin** | Rich blue reds, such as wine, burgundy and blood-red, look wonderful on your China-doll features. The contrast of dark hair, pale skin and red lips is really stunning! |
| **Dark hair, warm skin** | Rich brick reds and ruby jewel-like shades suit you. Their warmth is very flattering to your complexion, while the intensity of colour looks great against your hair. |
| **Red hair, cool skin** | A delicate orange-red, a paler version of the one mentioned above, will add a splash of colour without overpowering you. |
| **Red hair, warm skin** | Warm, fiery reds with brown undertones will complement your rich hair colour and rosy skin. |
| **Dark hair, olive skin** | Rich red with orange undertones will flatter your skin. Go for a bold colour, as you can carry it off. |
| **Black hair, brown skin** | Berry reds and burgundy reds look wonderful on your skin. |

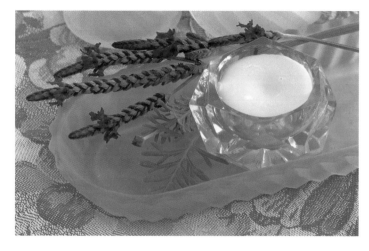

# Beautiful nails

Regular care and a little manual labour is all it takes to have nails that you will want to show off, rather than ones you want to hide away.

## laying the foundations for healthy nails

There's no point in slicking your nails with colour if they're not in good condition to start with. Following this advice will ensure that they're ultra-tough.

### filing know-how

Keep your nails slightly square or oval – not pointed – to prevent them from breaking. Filing low into the corners and sides can weaken nails. File gently in one long stroke, from the side to the centre of the nail. The classic length that suits most hands is just over the fingertip.

### condition-plus

Smooth your nails every evening with a nourishing oil or conditioning cream. This helps seal moisture into your nails to prevent flaking and splitting. A tiny drop of olive oil is a great cheap alternative.

### cuticle care

Go carefully with tough or overgrown cuticles. Most manicurists are against cutting them with scissors, as this can lead to infection. Instead, soak your nails in warm soapy water to soften the cuticles. Then

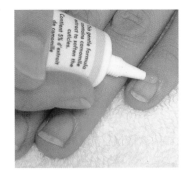

△ Soften cuticles with a cream or gel before pushing them back.

smooth them with a little cuticle softening cream or gel, before gently pushing them back with a manicure hoof stick or clean cotton bud (swab). You can then gently scrub away the flakes of dead skin that are still clinging to the nail bed.

## colour coding

• If you have long, elegant fingers you can carry off any shade, including the dramatic deep reds, russets and burgundies. Short nails look best with pale or beige-toned polish.

• Pale colours also suit broad nails, but you can make them look narrower by leaving a little space at the sides of each nail unpainted.

• If you love barely-there shades for the daytime, but prefer something more exotic at night, try a pale pearlized polish – the shimmer will be caught by the evening light.

• If you find strong colours too bold on your fingers, try painting your toenails instead. A glimpse of colour in open-toed shoes or on bare feet can look sophisticated. You can create a great look by mixing a little dark red and black nail polish before applying.

• Coral polish and pearlized formulations work very well against a tanned skin.

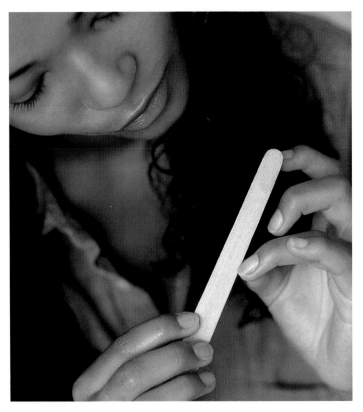

◁ **Fingernails should be filed regularly. To minimize breakage, file them straight across with a soft emery board.**

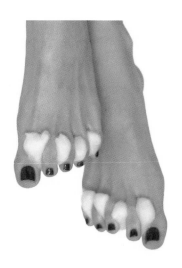

◁ **Use pieces of cotton wool (cotton) between your toes, to keep them apart while you are painting them.**

## the French manicure

**This is a popular look because it makes all lengths of nail look clean and healthy. It combines white tips with a pink polish over the entire nail. It is suitable for all occasions, from an ultra-natural to a glamorous look. It does take a little practice at first, but it's worth persevering. There are also special kits that contain all you need to get it right.**

### BEAUTIFUL NAIL TIP

The key to this look is to be very patient! It is important that you wait for each coat to dry thoroughly before applying the next one. If you rush the stages and apply the coats too quickly, the manicure will not be perfect because you are sure to end up with smudges and a rather messy finish.

## top 10 nail tips

**1** Avoid using acetone nail polish removers, as these can strip your nails of essential moisture. Choose the conditioning variety of nail polish remover instead.

**2** Apply hand cream every time you wash your hands. The oils in the cream will seal moisture into your skin.

**3** The most common cause of soft nails is exposure to water, so wear rubber gloves when doing the dishes.

**4** If you have very weak nails, try painting your base coat and nail polish under the tip of your nails to give them extra strength.

**5** Dry wet nails in an instant by plunging them into ice-cold water.

**6** To repair a split nail, tear a little paper from a teabag or coffee filter paper and glue it over the tear with nail glue. Once it's dry, buff until smooth, and then apply your polish on top.

**7** If you're planning to do some gardening or messy work, drag your nails over a bar of soap. The undersides of your nails will fill up with soap, and dirt won't be able to get in.

**8** Clean ink and stains from your fingertips by using a toothbrush and toothpaste on the affected areas.

**9** Never file your nails immediately after a bath, as this is when they're at their weakest and most likely to split.

**10** Use a cotton bud with a pointed end to clean under your nails – it's gentler than scrubbing with a nail brush.

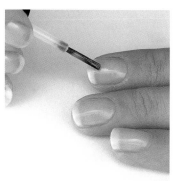

△ **1** Apply a clear base coat to protect your nails and help to prevent chipping.

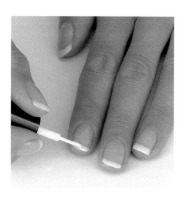

△ **2** Apply two thin coats of white polish to the tips of your nails. Try to apply it in one long stroke, working from one side of your nail to the other.

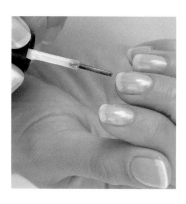

△ **3** Allow the white polish to dry completely, then apply a coat of pink polish over the entire nail. If you like a very natural finish, apply just one coat of pink polish; if you prefer a bolder effect, apply two coats.

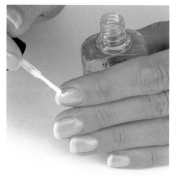

△ **4** Apply a clear top coat over the entire nail for added protection.

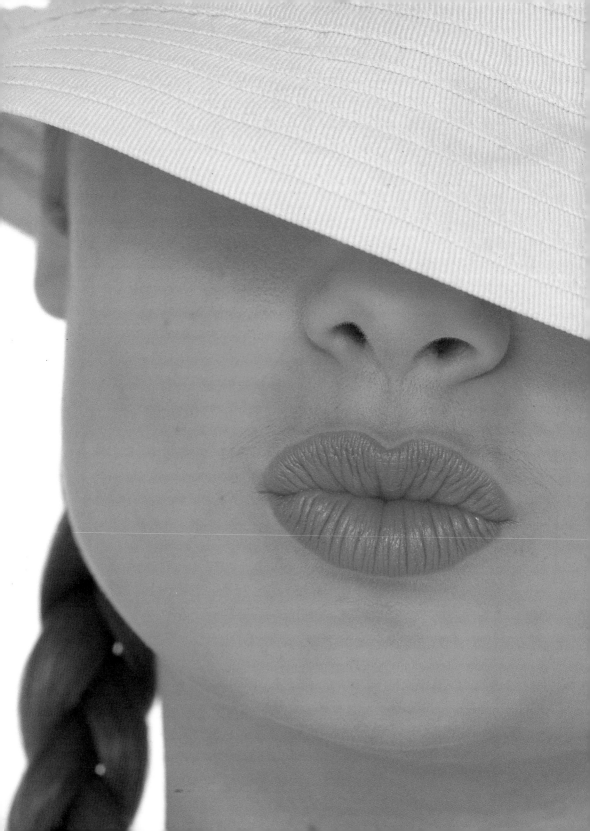

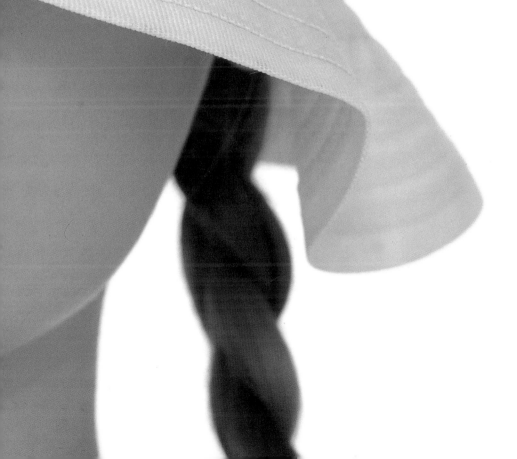

# Choosing Styles and Colours

Every woman can use make-up to enhance her looks, but individual make-up needs will differ from woman to woman. This chapter offers fresh and inspiring ideas to help you find a look to suit you.

# Cool skin, blonde hair

With your porcelain complexion and pale hair, you should opt for baby pastel tones with sheer formulations and a hint of shimmer. This flatters your colouring with a light, fresh make-up look, without overpowering it.

## this look suits you if ...

• You have pale blonde to mousey or mid-blonde hair. It also suits women with white or steel-grey hair.

• Your eyes are blue, grey, hazel or green.

• You have pale skin, including whiter-than-white, ivory or a pinky "English rose" style of complexion.

▷ These subtle pastels and shimmering shades flatter your cool, pale colouring for a soft yet vibrant look.

**EYESHADOW TIPS**

• If you're over 35 or unsure about wearing blue eyeshadow, swap it for a cool grey shade. This will create the same soft effect, but it's slightly more subtle.

• Shimmery eyeshadow can highlight crêpey eyelids, so you may prefer to use a matte ivory shadow instead.

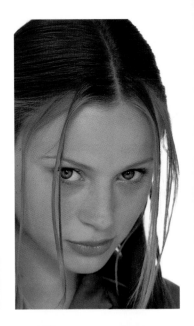

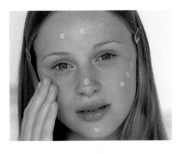

△**1** Your delicate skin doesn't need heavy coverage, so use a light tinted moisturizer. Dot it on to your nose, cheeks, forehead and chin, then blend it in with your fingertips.

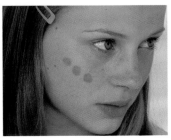

△ **2** Cool pink cream blusher will give your skin a soft glow. Dot on to your cheeks, then blend in with your fingertips. You can either skip powder to leave your skin with a dewy glow, or dust a little over your face. However, use a gentle touch, as you want to let your natural skin tone shine through.

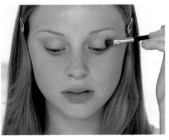

△**3** Take some baby blue eyeshadow on to an eyeshadow brush and sweep it evenly over your entire eyelid. Stroke the brush gently over your eyelid a few times until you've swept away any obvious edges to the colour. Also work a little eyeshadow under your lower lashes.

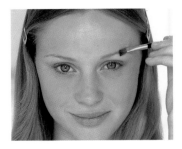

△ **4** Sweep a shimmery ivory shadow from the crease of your eyelid up towards the brow bone. Finish with two coats of brown/black mascara.

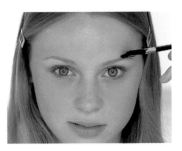

△ **5** Stroke your eyebrows into shape with an eyebrow brush. This will also flick away any powder that's got caught in the hairs.

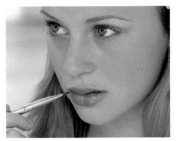

△ **6** Cool pink lipstick should be applied with a lip brush. If you like, you can slick a little lipgloss or lip balm on top for a sexy shimmer.

# Warm skin, blonde hair

Although you have a warm skin tone, your overall look is quite delicate. This means you should opt for tawny, neutral shades of make-up, and apply them with a light touch so you enhance your basic colouring.

## this look suits you if ...

• You have golden, warm blonde or dark blonde hair. This look also suits women with greying hair that has warm or yellow undertones.

• Your eyes are brown, blue, hazel or green.

• You have a warm skin tone that can develop a light, golden tan.

• Your skin tone and blonde hair mean your colouring is quite delicate. If so, you need to choose make-up shades that are not too intense, such as those shown here.

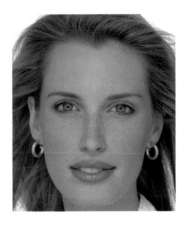

△ **Light neutral shades enhance the warmth of the skin while retaining the delicate tones.**

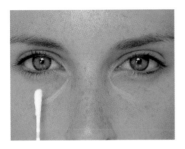

△ **1** After applying a light tinted moisturizer, stroke concealer on to problem areas. Blondes tend to have fine skin, often prone to surface thread veins. Cover these effectively with concealer, applied with a clean cotton bud (swab).

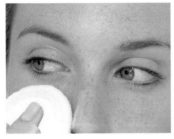

△ **2** Dip a powder puff into loose powder and lightly press over the areas of your face that are prone to oiliness. This will absorb excess oil throughout the day, and leave your skin beautifully matte. Dust off any excess powder with a clean powder brush.

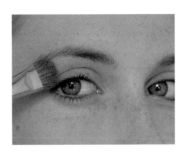

△ **3** Sweep peach eyeshadow over your entire eyelid. It will blend with your natural skin tone, but give a clean, wide-eyed look to your make-up.

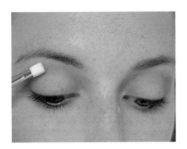

△ **4** Use an eyeshadow brush to work a tiny amount of soft brown eyeshadow into the crease of your eyelid to give depth and definition to your eyes. Sweep it towards the outer corner of your eyes too.

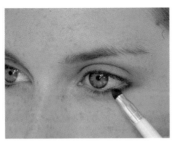

△ **5** Using the same brown eyeshadow, work a little underneath your lower lashes. This gives a softer effect than traditional kohl pencil or eyeliner, and is particularly suitable for those with pale or blonde hair who often can't carry off very strong eye make-up. Finish with two coats of brown/black mascara.

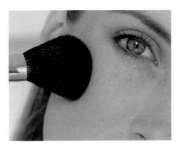

△ **6** Apply a barely-there shade of nude lipstick with a lipbrush. Then apply a tawny blusher, sweeping it a little at a time over your cheeks, forehead and chin. You can even dust a little over the tip of your nose! The advantage of applying blusher after you've completed your make-up is that you can assess exactly how much you need.

# Cool skin, dark hair

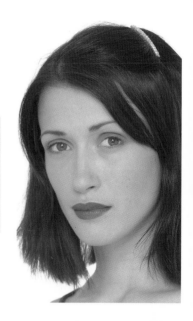

If you are a pale-skinned brunette you will look fabulous with strong, cool shades of cosmetics. The density of colour provides a striking contrast to your ivory skin tone, while the coolness blends beautifully with your natural look.

## this look suits you if ...

• Your hair is mid-brown to dark brown in colour.
• Your eyes are brown, blue, hazel, grey or green.
• You have a cool, China-doll skin tone that tans slowly in the sun.

**MAKE-UP TIPS**
• To stop your mascara from clogging, wiggle the mascara wand slightly from side to side as you pull it through your lashes.
• If you find cream blusher hard to apply, you can opt for the powder variety, applying it after face powder.

▷ **Strong, dense shades enhance dark hair and cool skin tones.**

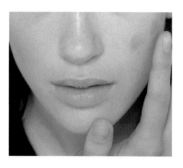

△ **1** Apply foundation or tinted moisturizer. If using foundation, it's likely you'll need the palest of shades. Blend in a few dots of tawny cream blusher, and finish with a dusting of loose powder.

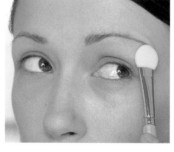

△ **2** Smudge a cool ivory shadow over your eyelids, right up to your eyebrows. Stroke over it with a cotton bud (swab) to blend it if you find it gathers in creases close to your upper eyelashes.

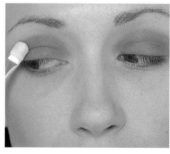

△ **3** Add extra definition with a touch of taupe or khaki eyeshadow on your eyelids. This shade works beautifully on your cool colouring, and emphasizes the colour of your eyes.

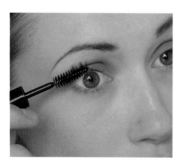

△ **4** Now move on to your eyelashes. You need to apply two thin coats of black mascara to create an effective frame to your eyes.

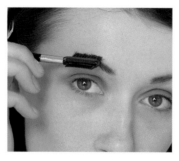

△ **5** Slick your eyebrows into place with an eyebrow brush. If they tend to look untidy, hold them in place by spritzing the brush with a little hairspray first.

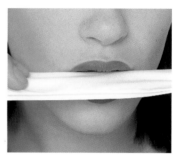

△ **6** Choose a clear shade of berry lipstick to give your look a polished finish. Blot after one coat with a tissue, then re-apply for a longer-lasting finish.

# Warm skin, dark hair

Your skin tone can carry off burnished browns, warm reds and earthy shades beautifully. They'll complement your complexion and emphasize your features.

## this look suits you if ...

• You have mid- to dark brown hair.
• Your eyes are brown, dark blue, grey, hazel or green.
• You have a warm skin tone that usually tans quite well. Even if it is pale in winter, your skin still has a yellow undertone.

▷ A flaming red lipstick combines powerfully with the burnished browns to create a warm, sophisticated look.

**POWDER TIP**
Carry a powder compact with you during the day to blot break-through shine on nose, forehead and chin.

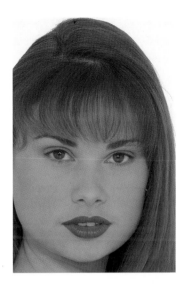

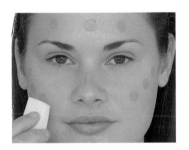

△ **1** Dot liquid foundation on to your skin and blend in with a damp cosmetic sponge. Blend the colour into your neckline for a natural effect. Then apply concealer to any blemishes that need it.

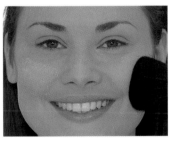

△ **2** Pat your face with translucent loose powder, then brush off the excess with a large, soft brush.

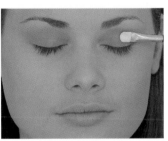

△ **3** Use a sponge-tipped eyeshadow applicator to sweep a red-brown shadow over your entire eyelid. The advantage of the sponge over a brush is that it doesn't tend to flick colour around. Complete your eyes with two thin coats of mascara.

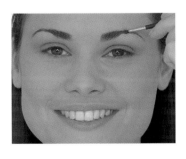

△ **4** Your eyebrows need subtle emphasis for this look. Either pencil them in with soft strokes of brown eyebrow pencil, or use a brown eyeshadow for a softer effect. Whichever method you use, brush them with an eyebrow brush to blend the strokes and slick the hairs in place.

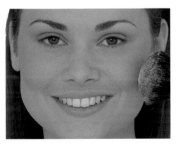

△ **5** Opt for a warm, tawny brown shade of powder blusher, dusted over your cheeks and up towards your temples. As this colour is quite strong, you may need to tone it down a little afterwards by dusting lightly over the top with translucent loose powder.

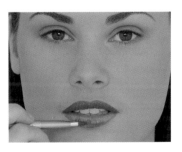

△ **6** A fiery red lipstick balances the overall look. Take care to use a lip brush to ensure you fill in every tiny crease and crevice on the lip surface – this will help your lipstick colour stay put for longer as well as creating a perfect finish.

# Cool skin, red hair

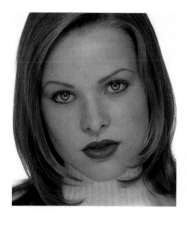

Redheads with cool skin tones often stick to soft colours, but you can experiment with brighter colours to contrast with your wonderful colouring. Greens give an exciting dimension to your eyes, and strong earthy shades supercharge your lips.

## this look suits you if ...

• You have strawberry blonde or pale red hair, and these rules apply even if the colour has faded.

• Your eyes are blue, grey, hazel or green.

• You have pale skin, ranging from ivory to a pink-toned complexion.

**FRECKLE TIP**
If you have freckles, don't fall into the trap of trying to cover them with dark-toned foundation. Instead, match your foundation to your skin tone to avoid a mask-like effect.

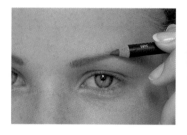

△ A rich burnished red lipstick adds a touch of drama to this look while soft greens enhance the striking colour of the eyes.

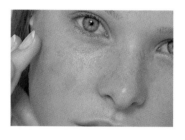

△ **1** Apply foundation and concealer, then dot a peachy shade of cream blusher on to your cheekbones. Unlike powder blusher, you can blend the cream variety with your fingertips, as the warmth from your skin will help smooth it in evenly. Apply a little cream blusher at a time. Finish with a dusting of translucent powder.

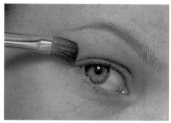

△ **2** A neutral, peach-toned eyeshadow swept over your eyelids will emphasize your eye colour without fighting with it. Ensure you take care to work it close to your eyelashes, to create a balanced effect.

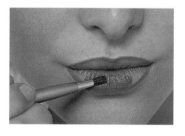

△ **3** Redheads usually have fair eyebrows, so don't forget to emphasize them to create a frame to your eyes. Otherwise the rest of your make-up will look unbalanced as the focus will be placed on your forehead. Opt for a very pale eyebrow pencil, in a subtle grey-brown tone. Stroke it through your eyebrows, taking care to fill any bald spots. Then soften the lines by brushing through with an eyebrow comb.

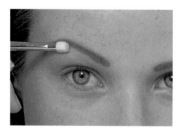

△ **4** Brush a hint of gold, shimmery eyeshadow into the arch under your eyebrows to give your eyes an extra dimension and bring them subtly into focus. This is a particularly good way to bring out gold flecks or warmth in the iris of your irises.

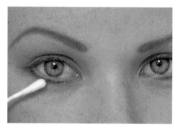

△ **5** Green eyeliner looks great but don't smudge it under your lower lashes as this will drag your features down. Work it along the upper lashes and into the eye corners. Then smudge with a cotton bud (swab) to give a soft finish. Brush with translucent powder to ensure it stays put. Finish with two coats of brown mascara.

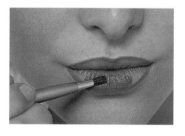

△ **6** Burnished orange lipstick complements this look. Begin by outlining your lips with a toning lip liner to prevent the colour from bleeding. Then use a lipbrush to fill in with the lipstick.

# Warm skin, red hair

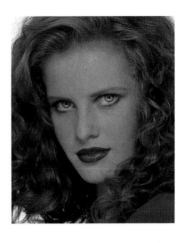

Your vibrant Pre-Raphaelite colouring is suited to bold shades of wine, purple and brown. These deep, blue-toned colours look fabulous with your warm skin and hair tones, and can make you look truly stunning.

## this look suits you if ...

• You have medium to dark red hair. This look may also suit brunettes who have a lot of red tones to their hair.
• Your eyes are blue, grey, hazel, brown or green.
• You have a medium to warm skin tone.
• Your skin takes on a golden colour in the summer, although you're unlikely to get a deep tan. It's quite likely that you have freckles.

△ Fiery hair and warm skin tones gain added vibrancy from purples, plums and browns.

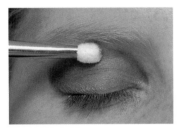

△ **1** After applying foundation, concealer and powder, smooth a wine shade of shadow over your entire eyelid. Using a sponge-tipped eyeshadow applicator will give you more control when applying this colour. You may find it easier to blend in if you sweep some translucent powder over your eyelids first, to create a smooth base on which to work.

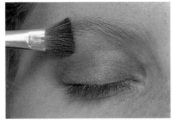

△ **2** Use a pale mauve eyeshadow over your brow bone to balance your eye make-up. Blend it into the crease, to soften any harsh edges of the wine-toned eyeshadow. Take time at this stage for a professional-looking finish.

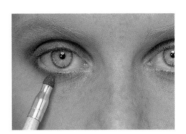

△ **3** Smudge a little of the wine-toned eyeshadow under your lower lashes as well. This will give a modern look to your eye make-up, and give a softer effect than kohl pencil. Ensure you also work it into the outer corners of your eyes, sweeping it slightly upwards to give your eyes a lift. Then finish with two coats of brown mascara. Take care to take the mascara right to the roots of your lashes, especially if they're pale.

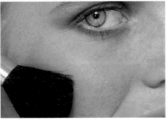

△ **4** Use a soft brown eyeshadow to give your eyebrows subtle emphasis, using either a small brush or a cotton bud (swab). Brush the eyebrows through afterwards with an eyebrow comb for a soft finish.

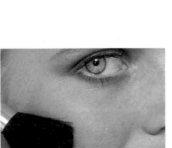

△ **5** Choose a brown-toned blusher or bronzing powder to give your skin warmth. Dust it on with a large blusher brush, blending it towards your hairline for a natural glow. The key is to use a little at a time, increasing the intensity of colour as you go. Avoid shimmery blushers, as these can give your skin an unnatural-looking sheen.

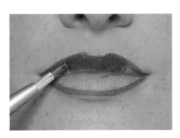

△ **6** You can carry off a deep plum shade of lipstick, outlined with a toning lip pencil. This strong colour needs perfect application to look good, so apply two coats, blotting the first with a tissue. This will also ensure your lipstick stays put for ages, and avoids the need for constant retouching.

# Olive skin, dark hair

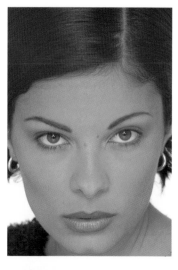

Your skin tones are easy to complement with rich browns, oranges and a hint of gold or bronze. These shades define your features and work well on your wonderful skin tones.

## this look suits you if...

- You have dark brown to black hair.
- Your eyes are brown, hazel or green.
- Your olive skin tans beautifully, or you have Asian or Indian colouring.

▷ **Shimmery soft orange lipstick and rich golds and browns complement your warm skin-tones.**

**LIPSTICK TIP**
To create a perfect lip line, stretch your mouth into an "O" shape and fill in the corners with your lip pencil.

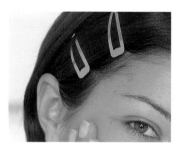

△ **1** Even out minor skin blemishes with a tinted moisturizer, blending it in smoothly with fingertips. If you need more coverage, opt for a liquid or cream foundation. Now apply a concealer and a light dusting of face powder.

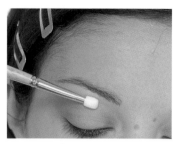

△ **2** After sweeping a golden shadow across your entire eyelid, apply a darker bronze shade into the crease and then apply some carefully under the lower lashes. This gives a wonderfully sultry look to your eyes.

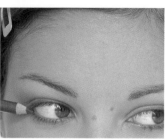

△ **3** Take a warm brown eyeliner and work it along your upper and lower lashes for a strong look that you can carry off beautifully. If you find the effect too harsh, smudge with a clean cotton bud (swab). Apply two coats of black mascara.

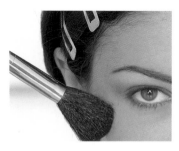

△ **4** A peach-brown powder blusher adds a sunkissed warmth to your cheeks. Apply just a little at a time, increasing the effect as you go.

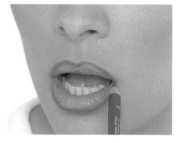

△ **5** Outline your lips with an orange-brown lip pencil. Start at the Cupid's bow on the upper lip, and move outwards. Then complete the other side, and finish with the lower lip.

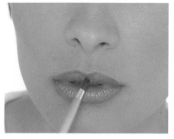

△ **6** To complete the look fill in with a sunny orange shade of lipstick. If you prefer a glamorous, glossy finish, don't blot your lips with a tissue. You can even add a dab of lip balm for extra shine if you wish. But if you prefer a semi-matte look, blot after one coat with a tissue, then re-apply your lipstick for a longer-lasting finish.

# Oriental colouring, dark hair

Your black hair and pale – but yellow-toned – skin are best complemented by soft, warm colours. These will define your looks and counteract any sallowness in your complexion.

## this look suits you if ...

• You have very dark brown to blue-black hair. It also works if you have grey flecks in your hair.

• Your eyes are hazel or brown.

• You have a pale to medium skin tone. It does tan, although it has a tendency to look quite yellow.

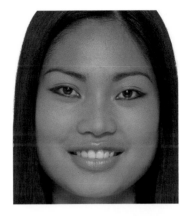

◁ Baby pink gives your lips a cool, soft look and blue-black eyeliner emphasizes the beautiful shape of your eyes.

**EYELASH TIP**

Oriental eyelashes are often poker-straight and so you can really benefit from the use of eyelash curlers.

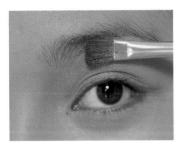

△ **1** After applying foundation, concealer and powder, sweep some lilac eyeshadow over your eyelid. This pale colour is a better option than using darker eyeshadows near the eyes, which have a tendency to make them look deep-set, particularly as your eyelids tend to be quite small.

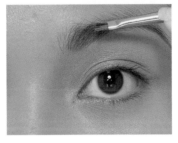

△ **2** Lightly fill in your eyebrows with a dark brown eyeshadow or eyebrow pencil to provide a strong frame to your eyes. This will help balance the eyeliner, which is going to be applied next.

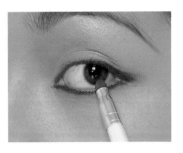

△ **3** A lick of blue-black eyeliner will emphasize your beautifully shaped eyes, and help correct any droopiness. Slick it under the lower lashes and into the outer corners of your eyes to create balance. To prevent the overall look from seeming too harsh, use a cotton bud (swab) to soften the eyeliner slightly.

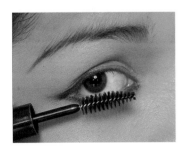

△ **4** Place your eyelashes between the pads of a curler, and gently squeeze for a few seconds. Then apply two coats of black mascara.

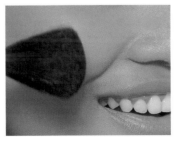

△ **5** A warm pink blusher gives a wonderful boost to your complexion, and brings out its natural glow. Dust it over the plumpest part of your cheeks.

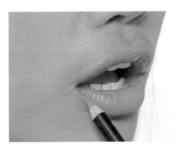

△ **6** A baby pink lipliner and lipstick bring your lips fashionably into focus. The cool blue tone to this shade works very well on your colouring.

# Pale black skin, black hair

This make-up combination emphasizes your looks with earthy shades. Your pale black, or brown skin works well with beige, brown and copper colours.

## this look suits you if...

• You have black hair with golden or reddish highlights. It also works if you have grey flecks in your hair.
• You have hazel or brown eyes.
• You have a black skin.

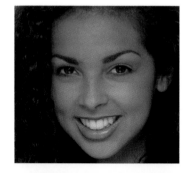

◁ **Ivory-toned eyeshadow and pearly pink-brown lipstick create a pretty contrast with your warm skin tone.**

**DARK SKIN TIP**
Look at cosmetic ranges especially designed for darker skins for your foundation and powder.

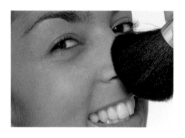

△ **1** After applying foundation, dust on a translucent face powder, ensuring it perfectly matches your skin tone to avoid a chalky-looking complexion. Dust off the excess with a large powder brush, using downward strokes.

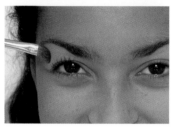

△ **2** Use an eyeshadow brush to dust an ivory-toned shadow over your entire eyelid, creating a contrast with your warm skin tone.

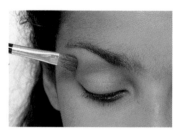

△ **3** Smudge a deep-toned brown eyeshadow into the crease of your eyelid, blending it thoroughly. Also work a little of this colour into the outer corners and underneath your lower lashes, to make your eyes look really striking.

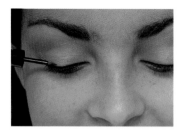

△ **4** Black liquid eyeliner swept along your upper lashes will give a supermodel look to your eyes. A sponge-tipped applicator is easier to use than a brush. Apply the eyeliner while looking down into a mirror, as this stretches any creases out of your eyelids. Rest your elbow on a firm surface. Complete your eyes with two coats of black mascara.

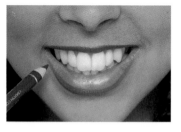

△ **5** Use a brown lipliner pencil to outline your lips. You can use an ordinary brown eyeliner pencil if this is the only thing you have to hand. Blend the line lightly into your lips, using a cotton bud (swab) for a softer effect.

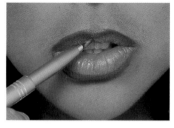

△ **6** A neutral pink-brown lipstick gives a natural-looking sheen to your lips, and instantly updates your look. Apply it with a lip brush for an even finish.

# Black skin, black hair

You can experiment with endless colour possibilities as your dark eyes, hair and skin provide the perfect canvas on which to work. The key to success is to choose bold, deep colours as your skin demands these to achieve a wonderful glow.

## this look suits you if ...

- You have deep black hair, even if it has flecks of grey.
- You have dark hazel or brown eyes.
- You have a dark black skin.

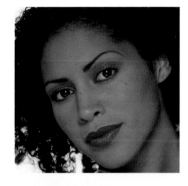

◁ Soft red lipstick, blackcurrant eyeshadow and tawny blusher combine dramatically with your dark hair and skin.

**MAKE-UP TIP**

While dramatic colours suit your skin tone and colouring perfectly, be sure to apply them with a light touch to get a fresh and vibrant look.

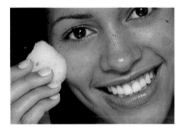

△ **1** Take care to find a foundation that matches your skin tone exactly. Apply it with a sponge so it blends in perfectly. Dampen the sponge with water first to give it extra "slip", and to prevent the sponge from absorbing too much expensive foundation. Blend in thoroughly along your jaw and hairline to avoid tidemarks. Finally, set with a light dusting of translucent loose powder.

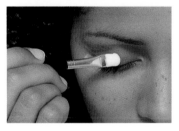

△ **2** Next, sweep a dark blackcurrant eyeshadow over your eyelids. Dust a little loose powder under your eyes first to catch any falling specks of this dark shade, and prevent it from ruining your completed foundation.

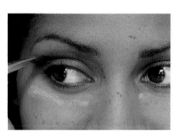

△ **3** Apply a dark charcoal eyeshadow into the crease of your eyelid using an eyeshadow brush. Only take a little colour at a time on to the brush to prevent it from spilling on to your eyelid. If necessary, tap the brush on the back of your hand first to shake away any excess.

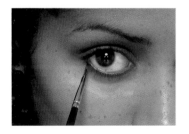

△ **4** Use an eyeliner brush to work some of this charcoal shade under your lower lashes, as this is the ideal colour with which to outline your eyes. Hold the mirror slightly above your eyeliner so that you can achieve an accurate liner effect. Finish with two coats of black mascara.

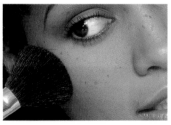

△ **5** A tawny-brown shade of blusher complements your skin beautifully. With a large round brush, dust it over the apples of your cheeks, working it lightly out towards your hairline.

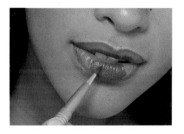

△ **6** After outlining your lips with a toning lip pencil, fill in with a dark plum shade of lipstick, using a lip brush for extra definition.

# Look younger in six steps

It is best to avoid fashion extremes and bright colours when you're over 40. Younger skins can get away with garish make-up, but it emphasizes fine lines and wrinkles on most women. Flatter your looks with subtle colours and throw away bright eyeshadows and neon lipsticks. If you don't know where to start, make an appointment for a free makeover. You'll be able to see which shades suit you, before you buy.

▷ **The latest foundations and concealers contain hundreds of light-reflective particles and these bounce light away from your skin. This gives it the illusion of added vitality, and helps disguise problem areas such as fine lines and under-eye shadows.**

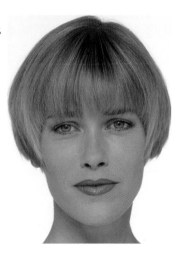

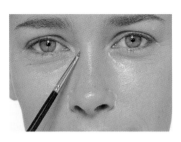

△ **1** Apply your foundation with a damp sponge, blending away any harsh edges to avoid tell-tale tidemarks. This is the stage at which to apply concealer, dotting it on to under-eye shadows, blemishes and thread veins with a brush. Apply a tiny amount at a time, and blend it in thoroughly.

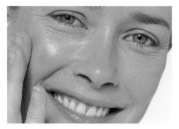

△ **2** Use half as much blusher and twice as much blending. Cream blusher gives your skin a soft glow. Dot the blusher on and blend with your fingertips. Set foundation and blusher with translucent powder, but remember that too much powder will settle into fine lines and wrinkles, and emphasize them. The best way to apply powder is only to blot the areas that need it, then brush away the excess with a large powder brush, stroking downwards.

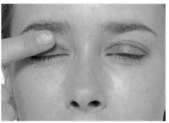

△ **3** Many women don't feel confident about applying eyeshadow properly. One of the most effective is an eyeshadow formulation that is easy to apply – cream-to-powder eyeshadow. It applies as a smooth cream, and dries quickly to a super-soft powder finish. Opt for a subtle shade such as mid-brown, grey or taupe.

A good tip if your eyes look rather droopy is to blend eyeshadow upwards and outwards at the outer corners. Remember to blend it in well.

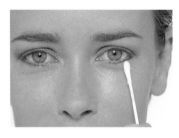

△ **4** Harsh lines of colour close to your eyes can be hard and unflattering. You'll emphasize your eyes much better if you smudge a little neutral-toned powder eyeshadow under your lower lashes with a clean cotton bud (swab).

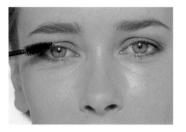

△ **5** Most women's colouring fades slightly over the years. This means that the black mascara you're used to wearing can now look too obvious and harsh. Try switching to a lighter shade for a more flattering effect. Apply two thin coats, allowing time for the first to dry thoroughly before you apply the second.

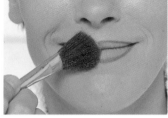

△ **6** If lipstick tends to "bleed" into the lines around your mouth, use a toning lipliner first. Keep it firm to give a precise line, yet soft so as not to drag the skin. Outline your top lip first, working outwards from the centre. Dust your lips with loose powder to set the lipliner, before applying a glossy, moisturizing lipstick.

# Classic chic

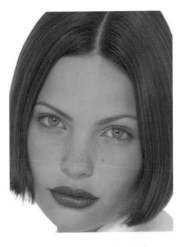

Whatever your age or colouring, this cool, sophisticated, classic look is very easy to apply and will always make a pleasing impact. Whether you are going to an important meeting or getting ready for an interview for a dream job, this simple but striking make-up combination will ensure that you feel completely confident about the way you look.

▷ Red is a lipstick classic, but the range of reds available is truly astonishing. It is simply a matter of experimenting with different tones and shades to find the perfect red for you.

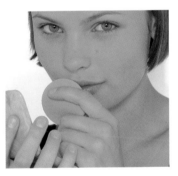

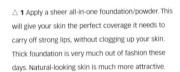

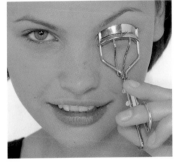

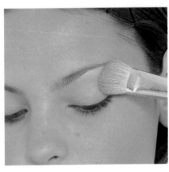

△ **1** Apply a sheer all-in-one foundation/powder. This will give your skin the perfect coverage it needs to carry off strong lips, without clogging up your skin. Thick foundation is very much out of fashion these days. Natural-looking skin is much more attractive.

△ **2** The eye make-up for this look is very understated. So, use an eyelash curler to open up your eyes and give them a fresh look.

△ **3** Sweep pale ivory eyeshadow across your entire eyelid using a blender brush. Then complete your eyes with two thin coats of brown/black or black mascara.

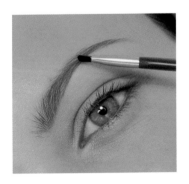

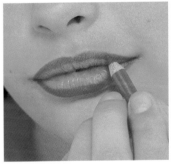

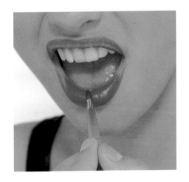

△ **4** Well-groomed eyebrows are essential. Brush them against the growth to remove any stray flecks of powder or foundation. Then lightly fill in any gaps with a toning eyeshadow. This gives a softer, more natural effect than a pencil.

△ **5** Your lips are the focus of this chic look. To ensure that you create a perfect outline, use a toning red lip pencil. Rest your elbow on a hard surface when using the pencil to prevent your hand from wobbling.

△ **6** Use a lip brush to fill in with a bold shade of red lipstick. Apply one coat, blot with a tissue, then reapply for a long-lasting finish.

# Country girl

Having fun with your make-up and experimenting with different styles is the best way to discover what is right for you. Why not try a sunkissed, outdoor look – a summery make-up combination that creates a muted, natural look, complete with fake freckles!

▷ Natural lipstick, light touches of mascara and eyeshadow and a hint of shimmery blusher will give you a glowing, wholesome look that is perfect for the outdoor days of summer.

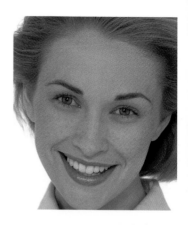

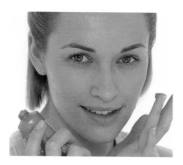

△ **1** You need to avoid heavy foundations when you're outside, so tinted moisturizer is the perfect solution. It'll both nourish your skin and lightly cover any minor blemishes. Apply with your fingertips for ease.

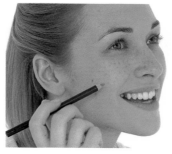

△ **2** If you already have freckles, don't try to hide them – they're perfect for a fresh-air look. If you don't have them, then fake them! Use an eyebrow pencil rather than an eyeliner pencil as it has a harder consistency and is less likely to melt on the skin. Use a mid-brown shade, and dot on the freckles, concentrating them on the nose and cheeks. Be extra creative and apply different sizes of freckles for a realistic look.

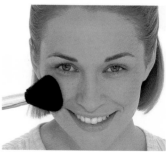

△ **3** A bronzing powder rather than a blusher will give your skin a sunkissed outdoor look. Choose one with minimum pearl or shimmer. Apply it to the plumpest part of your cheeks, where the sun would naturally catch your face. Dust the bronzing powder over your temples, too.

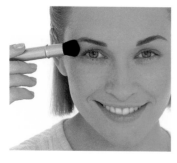

△ **4** Swap to an eyeshadow blending brush to gently sweep some of the bronzing powder over your eyelids. Natural colours like brown work best for this look. Remove any harsh edges with a clean cotton bud (swab).

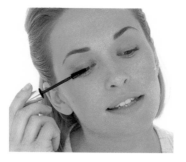

△ **5** Keep mascara to a minimum. Choose a natural-looking brown or brown/black shade, and apply just one coat. The waterproof type is great for hot days and sudden downpours but remember you'll need a suitable eye make-up remover, too.

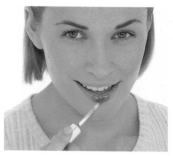

△ **6** Don't overpower this subtle look with bold lipstick. Opt for a muted brown-pink shade that's close to your natural lip colour, or use a softly tinted lipgloss for a natural sheen.

# City chic

This super-successful look is perfect for work and in the city. Simple, immaculately applied colours can help you put together a polished working image. This stylish, balanced look will help you to feel super-confident, whatever the day at the office brings.

▷ **These clever make-up moves create a simple, stylish look to keep you feeling super-cool throughout the working day.**

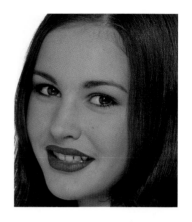

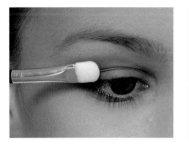

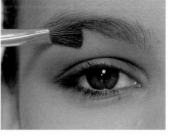

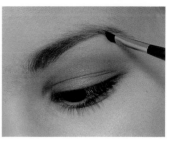

△ **1** After applying a light foundation and dusting your skin with powder to blot out shine, sweep your eyelids with a mid-grey eyeshadow. Use a matte powder formulation as this tends not to crease as much during the day. Use a sponge-tipped applicator to make the eyeshadow easier to apply.

△ **2** Use a beige highlighting eyeshadow over your brow bone to soften the edges of the grey shadow and to bring your eyes into focus. Take care not to leave flecks of powder in your eyebrow hairs – if necessary, flick them away with an eyebrow brush. Finish with two coats of mascara – blondes should use brown or brown/black mascara, while other colourings can opt for black.

△ **3** Brush your eyebrows with brown eyeshadow to fill in any gaps. This helps to create a strong frame to your make-up look.

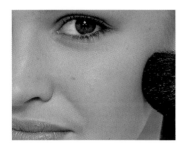

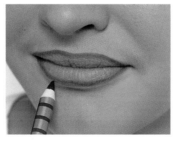

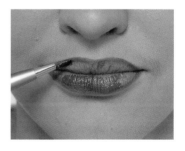

△ **4** A soft pink shade of blusher will give your skin a rosy glow, and neatly co-ordinate the rest of your make-up. It will also give pale work-a-day faces an immediate lift!

△ **5** Try soft blackcurrant shades as these can work beautifully on your lips, and make a welcome alternative to red. Start by using a lipliner to outline, ensuring you take it well into the outer corners. If you create any wobbly edges, whisk over the top with a clean cotton bud (swab) dipped in a little cleansing lotion. Then powder and try again!

△ **6** Fill in your lips with a matching shade of blackcurrant lipstick. Blot your lips with a tissue afterwards for a semi-matte finish that's perfect for a day at the office.

# Quick-fix evening make-up

Follow these six quick steps to achieve a striking, elegant look in just five minutes. When you are in a hurry, there is no time to experiment with new ideas, so the key to a successful quick-fix is to choose simple styles, applied with the minimum of fuss ... so here you have straightforward steps to a stunning look!

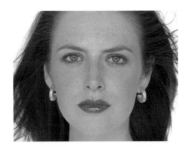

◁ When you don't have much spare time, but want to look presentable fast, try this quick and simple make-up combination for evening sophistication.

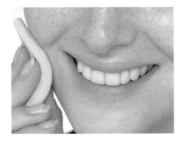

△ **five minutes to go ...**

**1** The all-in-one foundation/powder formulations give your skin the medium coverage it needs for this look in half the normal time. Also, take it over your lips and eyelids as this will make the rest of your make-up easier to apply and ensure it lasts the whole evening.

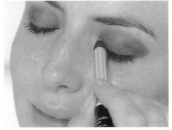

△ **four minutes to go ...**

**2** Cream eyeshadow applied straight from the stick is quick and easy to apply. Opt for a brown shade as it'll bring out the colour of your eyes, and give them a sexy, sultry finish. Slick it over your entire eyelid, right up to the crease of the eye socket.

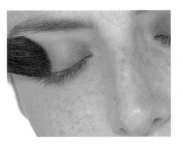

△ **three and a half minutes to go ...**

**3** A swift way to blend in your eyeshadow is to brush over the top with a layer of translucent loose powder. This will tone down the colour and blend away any harsh edges.

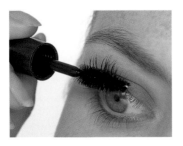

△ **two and a half minutes to go ...**

**4** Apply a coat of mascara to your lashes, taking care to colour your lower lashes as well as your upper ones. Use the tip of the mascara wand to coat the lower lashes, as this will prevent it from clogging on the hairs – and prevent you from spending valuable time having to use an eyelash comb.

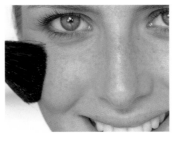

△ **one and a half minutes to go ...**

**5** A warm berry red blusher will give your skin a fabulous flush. Apply it with a blusher brush, sweeping it from your cheeks up towards your eyes to give your face a lift.

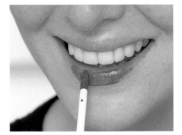

△ **thirty seconds to go ...**

**6** Choose a berry shade of lip gloss to add instant bold colour to your lips, sweeping it straight on with the sponge-tipped applicator. Cover your lower lip first, then press your lips together to transfer some of the colour on to your upper lip. Touch up any areas you've missed with the applicator, and you're ready to go!

# Go for glamour

There's usually one time when you want to make a special effort with your make-up and pull out all the stops, and that is the big night out!

Here's how to create this stunning look in six simple steps. Just follow the step-by-step instructions to create a sultry mixture of dark and light tones.

▷ **Smoky dark-brown eyeshadow, black eyeliner to make sure the focus is on the eyes, and a soft, neutral shade on the lips combine to create a fabulously sultry effect.**

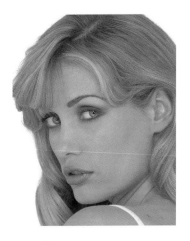

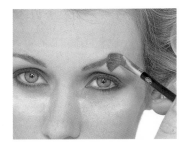

△ **1** This is a sophisticated look, with the focus very much on the eyes. Once you've applied foundation, concealer and powder, you're ready to start work on your eye make-up. Sweep a smoky dark brown eyeshadow over your entire eyelid and blend it carefully into the crease. A simple sponge applicator is less likely to flick colour away than a brush, but still take the precaution of sweeping a line of loose powder under your eyes to catch any falling specks of dark shadow.

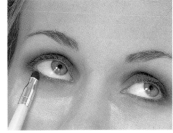

△ **2** Apply a little of the same eyeshadow under your lower lashes to accentuate the shape of your eyes. This will give a balanced look to your eye make-up, and provide a smooth base on which to apply your eyeliner at the next stage. The emphasis is on glamour and impact!

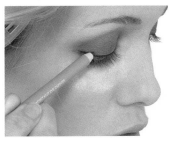

△ **3** Although black eyeliner is usually too severe for harsh daylight, it's perfect for this look, which is designed to be seen in softer, sexier light! Using a pencil, carefully draw a fine line above and below your eyelashes. If you find it hard to create a steady line, try drawing a series of tiny dots, then blend them together with a clean cotton bud (swab).

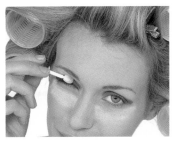

△ **4** To contrast with the dark, smoky look on your eyelids, sweep a pearly ivory shadow over your brow bones for a wide-eyed look. Apply a little at a time, building up the effect gradually. Complete the look with two coats of black mascara.

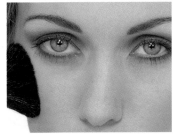

△ **5** Tawny blusher or a bronzing powder is ideal for this look, as the natural colour won't compete with the rest of your make-up. Sweep it smoothly over your cheekbones, taking care to blend away the edges into your hairline.

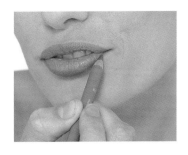

△ **6** Keeping the lips neutral gives this look its real impact, and updates it. Opt for a pinkish-beige shade of lip pencil and smudge it over your entire mouth for a matte, understated effect.

# 20 make-up problem-solvers

Whether you've made a mistake, have run out of a vital product or are simply stuck for inspiration, the following problem solvers will give you all the help you need.

## 1 polish remover has run out

If you want to re-paint your nails, but have run out of remover, try coating one nail at a time with a clear base coat. Leave to dry for a few seconds, then press a tissue over the nail and remove it quickly – the base coat and coloured polish will come off in one quick move, and you are ready for a fresh coat of colour.

## 2 poker-straight eyelashes

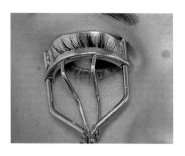

△ A set of eyelash curlers can make a significant difference to the way your eyes look. Gently squeeze your upper lashes between the cushioned pads to curl your lashes beautifully.

## 3 patchy powder

If you apply powder with a light touch to freshly moisturized skin, or on top of foundation that is applied with a clean sponge, it should look perfect. If it doesn't, check you're not making the common mistake of using the wrong colour powder for your skin. It needs to be matched closely to your natural skin tone, as closely as your foundation. So, try dusting a sample of powder on to your skin in natural daylight before buying it, to check you've found the perfect match.

## 4 yellow nails

Yellow nails are usually caused by wearing dark-coloured nail polish without using a protective clear base coat, so wear one in future to prevent this from happening. You can also try switching to paler coloured polishes that contain lower levels of pigment so are less likely to stain your nails.

To cure yellow nails, rub with lemon juice to remove stains, then massage your hands and nails with moisturizer. Try going polish-free one day a week. If your problem recurs, consult your doctor to check that there's no underlying cause.

## 5 flaky mascara

This usually means the mascara is too old and the oils that give it a creamy consistency have dried out. This can be made worse by pumping air into the dispenser when replacing the cap – so go gently. Replace your mascara every few months.

Revive an old mascara by dropping it into a glass of warm water for a few minutes before applying it. If mascara flakes on your lashes, the only solution is to remove it thoroughly and make a clean start.

## 6 a blemish appears

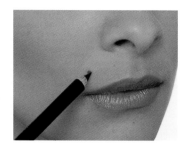

△ The immediate solution is to transform the blemish into a beauty mark! First, soothe the blemish by dabbing it with a gentle astringent on a clean cotton bud (swab). This will dry out excess oils from the skin and help the beauty mark last longer.

To create your beauty mark, dot over the top with an eyebrow pencil – this is better than using an eyeliner pencil as it has a drier texture and so is less likely to melt and smudge. Finally, set your beauty mark in place with a light dusting of loose powder.

## 7 melting lipstick

If you're out and about, and your lipstick is starting to melt, dust over the top with a little loose powder. This will give a slightly drier texture and help the lipstick stay put for longer. Loose powder will also create a lovely matte finish.

## 8 smudged eyeliner

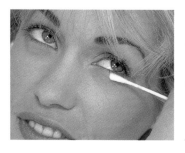

△ Tidy under-eye areas by dipping a cotton bud in eye make-up remover. Whisk it over the problem area to remove smudges, then re-powder. A little loose powder over eyeliner will combat the smudging that occurs as the wax in the pencil melts.

## 9 red skin

A red skin colour can be toned down by smoothing your skin with a specialized green-tinted foundation. Apply with a light touch to the areas that really need it. The green pigment in the cream has the effect of cancelling out the red in your skin.

To avoid a ghostly glow, you'll need to apply a light coating of your ordinary foundation on top, set with a dusting of loose powder. This tip is also good for covering an angry spot or blemish.

## 10 foundation turns orange

Mix 5g/1 tsp of bicarbonate of soda into your loose face powder, then dust the powder mixture lightly over your skin before applying your foundation. The bicarbonate of soda will give your skin a slightly acid pH to prevent it from turning orange.

## 11 bleeding lipstick

A lipliner can prevent lipstick from bleeding into the fine lines around your mouth. Trace the lip outline, then apply lip colour with a brush. A drier-textured matte lipstick is less prone to bleed than the moisturizing variety. Also, lightly powder over and around your lips before you start.

## 12 disappearing foundation

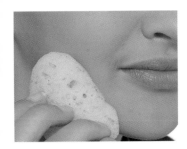

△ If your foundation seems to sink into your skin on hot or damp days, the trick is to apply it to cool skin. Do this by holding a damp facecloth on to your skin for a few moments, then apply your foundation.

Storing your foundation in the refrigerator will ensure it's cool when it goes on. Apply the foundation with a damp sponge, not your fingers, as the natural oils from your skin will leave a streaky finish. Set with a light dusting of loose powder.

## 13 yellow teeth

First of all, visit your dentist or dental hygienist for regular check-ups and thorough cleaning to ensure your teeth are as white as possible, and also bear in mind that yellow teeth tend to be stronger than whiter ones. To make them look whiter, avoid coral or brown-based lipsticks as the warm colours will emphasize the yellow ones in your teeth. Clear pink or red shades will make them appear whiter.

## 14 bloodshot eyes

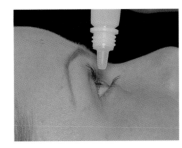

△ Red eyes are caused by the swelling of tiny blood vessels on the eye surface, from lack of sleep, excessive time in front of a computer, a smoky atmosphere or an infection. If it's an ongoing problem, consult your doctor, or visit an optician for an eyesight examination to ensure there's no underlying cause.

For a quick temporary fix, use eye drops to bring the sparkle back to your eyes. These contain ingredients that will reduce the swelling in the blood vessels, decrease redness and cut down on dryness and itching.

## 15 tidemarks of foundation

If you can see edges to the foundation on your chin, jawline or hairline, blend and soften them away with a damp cosmetic sponge. Do this in natural daylight so you can check the finished effect. Powder as usual afterwards.

## 16 unhealthy nails

However strong nails are, their overall effect can be spoilt by clear or yellowing tips. A quick way to improve them is to run a white manicure pencil under the edges of the nails to give them a cleaner appearance. Combine with a coat of clear polish for a fresh, natural look.

## 17 droopy eyes

To help lift droopy eyes, sweep a light-toned eyeshadow all over your eyelid. Then apply a little eyeshadow with a clean cotton bud under your eyes, sweeping it slightly upwards. Apply extra coats of mascara on the lashes just above the iris of the eye to draw attention to the centre of your eye rather than the outer corners.

## 18 straggly eyebrows

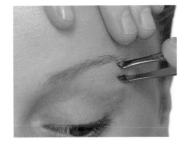

△ Women often don't take much notice of their eyebrows until they look messy! The best plan is to tidy them with regular tweezing sessions. The ideal time is after a bath when your skin is warm and soft, the pores will be open from the heat and the hairs are easier to remove. Before bedtime is also good, so you don't have to face the day with blotchy skin.

First of all, use an eyebrow brush to sweep your brows into place, so that you can see their natural shape. Then pluck one hair at a time, always pulling in the direction of growth. First remove the hairs between your brows, and then thin out overall – generally, don't pluck above the eyebrow or you'll risk distorting the shape of your brows. The only exception is if there are hairs growing well above the natural browline. Finally, tweeze any stray hairs at the outer sides.

## 19 over-applied blusher

If you've forgotten to build up your blusher slowly and gradually, you may need to tone down an over-enthusiastic application of colour. The quickest and easiest way is to dust a little loose powder over the top of the problem area, until you've reached a softer blusher shade.

## 20 sore ears from cheap earrings

If you don't want to throw away cheap earrings that make your ears react, try coating the posts and back of the earrings with hypo-allergenic clear nail polish. This should make them less likely to react with your sensitive skin. If your ears are sore, always give the skin plenty of time to heal up before wearing troublesome earrings again.

# 50 effective beauty tips

When you don't have time for trial and error, you need beauty tips that really work. Here are 50 of the most effective.

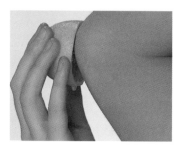

△ **1** Brighten grey elbows by rubbing them with half a fresh lemon – it has a natural bleaching effect. Moisturize afterwards to counteract the drying effects of the juice.

**2** Turn foundation into a tinted moisturizer by mixing a few drops of it with a little moisturizer on the back of your hand before applying. It's perfect for summer.

**3** Carry a spray of mineral water in your handbag to freshen up your foundation while you're out and about.

**4** Sleeping on your back helps stop wrinkles, according to recent research. It's certainly worth a try!

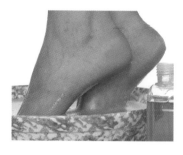

△ **5** Dunk feet into a bowl containing warm water and 45ml/3 tbsp Epsom salts to help ease swollen ankles.

**6** If you have very soft nails, file them while the polish is still on, which will prevent them from cracking.

**7** If you find eyebrow tweezing painful, hold an ice cube over the area first to numb it before you start.

**8** Warm up your looks by dusting a little blusher over your temples, chin and the tip of your nose as well as your cheeks.

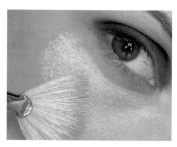

△ **9** Sweep a little loose powder under your eyes when applying dark eye-shadow to catch falling specks and prevent them from staining your skin.

**10** Make your lips appear larger by wearing a bright, light lipstick. Make them appear smaller by wearing a dark or muted coloured lipstick.

**11** Soak nails in a bowl of olive oil once a week to strengthen them.

**12** If you haven't got time for a full make-up, but want to look great, paint on a bright red lipstick – it's a happy, glamorous colour that can immediately brighten your face.

**13** If you don't have a different coloured blusher for your cheeks, simply use an ordinary face powder a couple of shades darker than your usual one to slim round cheeks.

**14** Add a drop of witch hazel – available from all good pharmacists – to turn ordinary foundation into a medicated one – it's great for oily or blemish-prone skins.

**15** Mascara your lashes before applying false ones to help them stick properly.

**16** If you look tired, blend a little concealer just away from the outer corner of your eye – it makes you look as though you had a good night's sleep!

**17** Go lightly with powder on wrinkles around the eyes – too much will settle into them and emphasize them.

**18** When plucking your eyebrows, coat the hairs you want to remove with concealer – it'll help you visualize exactly the shape of brow you're after.

**19** Never apply your make-up before blow-drying your hair – the heat from the dryer can make you perspire and cause your make-up to smudge.

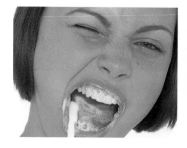

△ **20** Keep your smile looking its best by changing your toothbrush once the bristles begin to splay. This means at least every three months. You should brush for at least two minutes, both morning and evening.

**21** Powder eyeshadow can be made to look more intense by dipping your eyeshadow brush in water first.

22 Keep lashes supple by brushing them with petroleum jelly before going to bed.

23 Apply cream blusher in light downward movements, to prevent it from creasing and specks of colour from catching in the fine hairs on your face.

24 If mascara tends to clog on your lower lashes, try using a small thin brush to paint colour on to individual lashes.

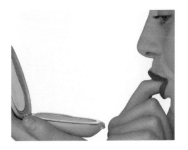

△ 25 To prevent lipstick getting on your teeth, after applying it put your finger in your mouth, purse your lips and pull it out.

26 Give moisturizer time to sink in before you start applying your make-up – it'll help your make-up go on more easily.

27 To make your eyes sparkle, try outlining them just inside your lower eyelashes with a soft white cosmetic pencil.

28 Apply a dot of lipgloss in the centre of your lower lip for a sophisticated look.

29 Hide cracked or chipped nails under stick-on false ones.

30 If your eyeliner is too hard and drags your skin, hold it next to a light bulb for a few seconds before applying.

31 If you find your lashes clog with mascara, try rolling the brush in a tissue first to blot off the excess, leaving a light, manageable film on the bristles.

32 If you're unsure where to apply blusher, gently pinch your cheeks, and if you like the effect, apply blusher in the same area for a natural look.

33 If you're near-sighted, glasses make your eyes look smaller. So, opt for bolder shadows and lots of mascara to enhance them. If you're far-sighted, lenses make your eyes look bigger and make-up more prominent. So, opt for more muted colours.

34 A little foundation lightly rubbed in your eyebrows and brushed with an old toothbrush will instantly lighten them.

35 Coloured mascara can look super-effective if applied with a light hand. Start by coating your lashes with two coats of black mascara. Once the lashes are dry, slick a little coloured mascara – try blue, violet or green – on the underside of your upper lashes. Each time you blink, your eyelashes will reveal a dash of unexpected colour.

36 If you use hypo-allergenic make-up for your sensitive skin, remember to use hypo-allergenic nail polish, too – you constantly touch your face with your hands and can easily trigger a reaction.

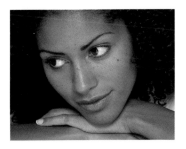

△ 37 For a longer-lasting blusher on hot days, apply cream and powder. Apply the cream formulation, set it with translucent powder then dust with powder blush.

38 Let nails breathe when applying polish by leaving a tiny gap at the base of the nail where the cuticle meets the nail – this is where the new nail cells are growing.

39 Make over-prominent eyes appear smaller with a wide coat of liquid liner.

40 Calm an angry red blemish by holding an ice cube over it for a few seconds to cool and soothe the skin. Then apply your medicated concealer.

41 If you've run out of loose powder it is just as effective to use a dusting of unperfumed talcum powder.

42 Use a little green eyeshadow on red eyelids to mask the ruddiness.

43 If you've run out of liquid eyeliner, dip a thin brush into your mascara.

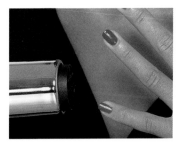

△ 44 If you need to dry your nail polish extra quickly, you can blast your nails with a cold jet of air from your hairdryer to speed up the process.

45 Use a toothpick or dental floss regularly to clean between your teeth. This ensures your teeth are completely clean and cuts down the risk of cavities.

46 Apply foundation/powder with a damp sponge for thicker opaque coverage.

47 Run your freshly sharpened eyeliner pencil across a tissue before you use it. This will round off any sharp edges and remove small particles of wood.

48 If you have obvious under-eye shadows, cover them with a light coat of blue cream eyeshadow before applying your concealer.

49 Remove any excess mascara by placing a folded tissue between your upper and lower lashes and then blinking two or three times.

50 Get together friends and take turns to make each other up – it's good fun, you'll get feedback from your friends, and it's a fantastic way to experiment and find yourself a new look.

# 50 budget beauty tips

If you can't afford top-of-the-range, expensive beauty products, here are 50 fabulous tips to help you follow a successful beauty regime on a tight budget.

**1** Cotton wool (cotton) balls soak up liquids such as toner, so dampen them with water first. Squeeze out the excess, then use as usual.

**2** A drop of remover added to a bottle of dried-up nail polish will revive it in a few seconds. Shake well to encourage it to mix in thoroughly.

**3** Stand a dried-up mascara in a glass of warm water to bring it back to life.

**4** Keep new soaps from getting soft by storing them in a warm cupboard. This helps dry the moisture out, which makes them harder and longer-lasting.

**5** To get the last drop from almost-empty bottles, store them upside-down overnight. You'll reap the rewards!

**6** Don't rip the cellophane off translucent powder – prick a few holes in it instead – it'll stop you spilling and wasting it.

**7** Keep perfume strips from magazines in case you need an instant freshen-up.

**8** Sachets in magazines make ideal travel packs for weekends away.

**9** Look out for "3 for the price of 2" offers on your favourite products.

**10** Turn ordinary mascara into the lash-lengthening variety by dusting eyelashes with a little translucent powder first.

**11** Rub a dab of petroleum jelly around the neck of a new nail-polish bottle, and it should be easy to open for the entire life of the product.

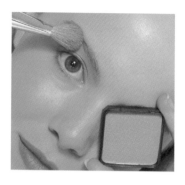

△ **12** Dust blusher over your eyelids as an instant subtle eyeshadow. It's quick to apply, and will give a balanced look to your make-up.

**13** One-length hair with no layers is the easiest and cheapest hairstyle to maintain as it doesn't require as many visits to the hairdresser to keep it looking good.

**14** Swap commercial face scrubs for a handful of oatmeal massaged directly on to your skin – smooth soft skin naturally.

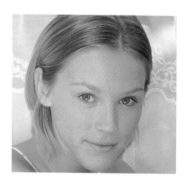

△ **15** If you've run out of blusher, dot a little pink lipstick on to your cheeks and blend well with your fingertips.

**16** Don't use too much toothpaste – it's the brushing action that gets teeth really clean. A pea-sized blob is enough.

**17** Pick the largest-sized products you can afford – it's much cheaper that way.

**18** Don't shop for beauty goodies just in glitzy department stores and fancy pharmacies. These days, your local supermarket can offer a good range.

**19** If you're happy to forgo a fancy label, look out for great value own-label product ranges at drug store chains.

**20** Sometimes you're just as well off with cheap alternatives. Indulge yourself with the products that are really worth it! For instance, buy cheap and cheerful lip liners, then show off with a fancy lipstick. As well as looking good, expensive lipsticks tend to contain more pigment than cheaper ones – which means they look better and last even longer.

**21** Buy cheap but effective moisturizers instead of expensive fragranced ones. This will mean you can save your money to splash out on your favourite perfume.

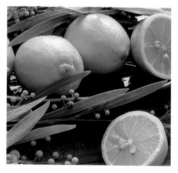

△ **22** A cheap way to boost the shine of dark hair is to rinse it with diluted vinegar. Blonde hair benefits from lemon juice being applied in the same way. Both act by sealing down the outer cuticles of the hair, which helps it to reflect the light more effectively.

23 It used to be that only the pricier ranges offered hi-tech products. However, these days more companies are offering state-of-the-art products – at budget prices. This means you'll get all the benefits without spending a fortune. For instance, there are now affordable skin creams that contain the anti-ageing alpha-hydroxy ingredients at a third or quarter of the price of prestige brands.

24 Many of the more expensive prestige make-up, skincare and fragrance companies offer sample products at their counters. It's always worth asking, especially if you're already buying something from them.

25 There's a great trend at the moment for 2-in-1 products. They're worth trying out, because they can save you money – as you buy only one product that does two jobs. The types of products included are shower gels that are also body scrubs and hair shampoos with built-in conditioners.

26 If you want to indulge in some new make-up, then ask for a makeover at a cosmetic counter. It can be the best way to see how the colours and formulations look on your skin before you buy anything – and can also mean you'll look great for an evening out!

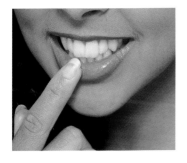

△ 27 Turn lipstick into lip gloss with a coat of lip balm after applying colour.

28 De-fuzz using a razor with replaceable blades – it works out much cheaper in the end than buying disposable razors.

29 Don't throw away an item of make-up just because the colour's not in fashion at the moment – you might like it again in a few months, or be able to blend it with something.

30 Make cheap nail polish last longer by sealing it with a clear top coat.

31 Pure glycerine is an extremely cheap and effective moisturizer when you don't have much to spend.

32 Store your make-up and fragrance in a cool dark place to extend their life span.

33 Double up your lip liner to fill in your lips as well as outline them.

34 Prise eyeshadows out of their cases, and stick into an old paint-box or lid to create a make-up artist's colour palette. It ensures you use the products you've got because you can see them all at a glance.

35 Add a few drops of your favourite *eau de toilette* to some olive oil, and use as a scented bath oil as a cheap treat.

36 Neutral make-up colours are a better investment because they are more versatile.

37 Eyeshadow doubles up as eyeliner, if applied with a cotton bud (swab). Dampen the end of the bud first to get a cleaner line under the eye.

38 If you're choosing a new fragrance, buy the weaker and cheaper *eau de toilette* before splashing out on stronger and more expensive perfume.

39 Check out model nights at your local hairdressers when trainees will style your hair for a fraction of the normal price.

40 Mix different colour lipsticks on the back of your hand with a brush, to create new shades for free!

41 When you're out of toothpaste, brush with bicarbonate of soda – it'll make them extra white, too.

42 Put your lip and eye pencils in the refrigerator before sharpening, as this means they're less likely to break.

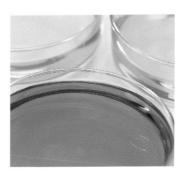

△ 43 A drop of olive oil rubbed nightly into your nails will help them grow long and strong, and is cheaper than shop-bought manicure oils.

44 Make powder eyeshadows last and stay crease-free by dusting eyelids with translucent powder. This keeps make-up looking fresher for longer.

45 Sharpen dull eyebrow tweezers by rubbing sandpaper along the tips.

46 Add a drop of water to the remains of a foundation to use every last dot.

47 Keep the plastic seals or paper discs that come with products and replace after use. It helps prevent air from getting into the products and bacteria from breeding – so your product stays fresher for longer.

48 Spritz your hair lightly with water and blow dry again to revive products already in the hair and revitalize your style.

49 A cup of bicarbonate of soda in your bath is a cheap and cheerful water softener.

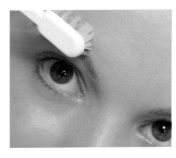

△ 50 Use an old clean toothbrush to slick unruly eyebrows into shape.

# Your top 10 make-up questions answered

## 1 blush baby

**Q** *"Can I reshape my face using blusher?"*

**A** The best way to apply blusher is to smile, find the apples of your cheeks, and blend the colour upwards. For special occasions, try using your normal blusher, combined with a barely-there highlighter colour and a colour that is slightly darker than your usual blusher, to reshape your face. Check your face shape and try the following techniques:

• Slim a round face by blending your usual blusher upwards from your cheeks into your hairline. Then highlight along your cheekbones, and use the shader in the hollows of your cheeks.

• Soften a square face by concentrating your blusher in a circle on the rounded parts of your cheeks. Apply shader into the hollows of your cheeks, and also lightly on the square edges of your chin. Lightly dust highlighter on to the bridge of your nose and across the tip of your chin.

• Balance a heart-shaped face by dusting your blusher slightly lower than your cheekbones into the actual hollows of your cheeks. Dust some highlighter on to the tip of your chin, and apply shader to your temples, making sure that you blend it well into your hairline.

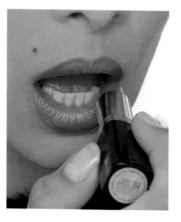

◁ A good quality lipstick will keep your lips feeling and looking good all day long.

## 2 long-lasting lipstick

**Q** *"Is there any way to make my lipstick stay put all day?"*

**A** Unfortunately there's no such thing as a 24-hour lipstick, no matter what some cosmetic manufacturers claim. The longest-lasting lipsticks are those with the thickest, driest textures, although this can mean they leave your lips feeling quite dry, especially if you use them day in, day out. However, you can look for lipstick sealers, which are clear gels that you paint over your lips after you've applied your lipstick. Once they're dry, these lipstick sealers help your lipstick stay put at least past your first coffee of the day.

## 3 over-plucked brows

**Q** *"I plucked my eyebrows very thin last year. Now I'd like to grow them back. How can I do it successfully?"*

**A** Choose a natural-looking brown eyeshadow. Apply it lightly and evenly with a firm-bristled eyebrow brush, using short sharp strokes across the brow. As the hairs that grow back are often unruly, a light coat of clear mascara can be applied to help keep them in place.

Try to ignore the periodic fashions for highly plucked eyebrows. The fashions don't last for long – but eyebrows can take ages to grow back! It's better to stick with your natural eyebrow shape, just removing stray hairs from underneath the arch and between the brows.

## 4 covering birthmarks

**Q** *"Can you recommend something that will cover my birthmark, even when I go swimming?"*

**A** You need a specialized foundation that will give ultimate coverage, look opaque and be waterproof. Look for a specialized range of camouflage creams tailor-made to

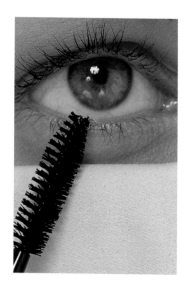

△ Avoid mascara smudges by holding a piece of tissue underneath your lower lashes while you are applying your mascara.

cover skin imperfections, such as scars and port wine stains, as well as birthmarks. The formulation means they are applied differently to ordinary foundation. They're applied with fingertips using a "dab, pat" motion. They're available from make-up suppliers and some dermatologists.

## 5 spider veins

**Q** *"What can I do about facial spider veins?"*

**A** Spider or thread veins, known as "telangiectases", are a common beauty problem. An electrolysist qualified in diathermy, or a dermatologist, can treat them by inserting a fine needle into the vein. The heat from the needle coagulates the blood in the vein, rendering it inactive. The number of treatments depends on the size of the area to be treated, and the number of spider veins.

You can also cover the veins with a light covering of concealer, applied with a fine brush and set with a dusting of powder.

▷ Generally most women can wear any colour, but the important thing is to find the shade that suits your colouring.

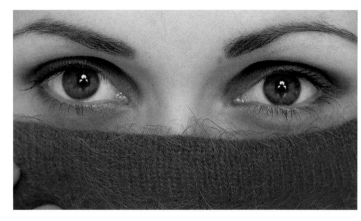

## 6 mascara matters

**Q** *"My mascara always seems to run on to my skin and leaves me with 'panda eyes'. What can I do?"*

**A** Using a waterproof variety of mascara should help if you're prone to this problem, or you can "seal" your normal mascara with a coat of clear mascara.

Alternatively, dip a cotton bud (swab) in eye make-up remover for fast touch-ups before the mascara can dry on your skin. Another, more long-term, solution is to have your eyelashes permanently dyed regularly at a reputable beauty salon.

## 7 smoother lips

**Q** *"Lipstick always looks awful on my mouth because my lips are so flaky, and it's impossible to create a smooth finish. Is there a solution?"*

**A** Slick your lips with a thick coat of petroleum jelly, and leave for 10 minutes to give it a chance to soften any hard flakes of skin. Then cover your index finger with a damp flannel and gently massage your lips. This removes the petroleum jelly and the flakes of dead skin should come off with it, leaving your lips supple and smooth.

▽ Applying your lipstick with a brush will make it much easier to achieve a perfectly smooth finish.

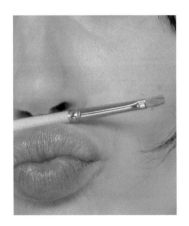

## 8 colour coding

**Q** *"Are there colours that some people can never wear?"*

**A** As a general rule, everyone can wear every colour. However, if you want to wear a particular colour, you should choose the particular shade of it very carefully. For instance, everyone can wear red lipstick, but in different shades. A pale-skinned blonde will suit a soft pink-red, whereas a warm-toned redhead will be able to carry off an orange-based fiery shade of the colour.

In the same way, a blue-eyed, cool-skinned blonde can carry off a pale pastel, baby-blue eyeshadow, whereas her brunette colleague will look much better wearing a darker version to complement her skin tone.

▽ Rolling a nail varnish bottle between your hands to mix it up ensures it is smooth to apply.

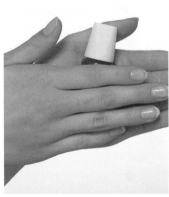

## 9 problem polish

**Q** *"I always have bottles of nail varnish that I can't use because they're either dried up, or full of bubbles so they don't go on smoothly. What can I do?"*

**A** There are some simple solutions to your problem. Dried-up polish can be revived by stirring in a few drops of polish remover before using. You can help prevent it from thickening in the first place by storing it in the refrigerator, as the cold temperature will stem evaporation and stop it changing in texture.

Bubbles of air in the polish will ruin its finish, as it won't create an even surface. You can prevent this by rolling the bottle between the palms of your hands to mix it up before using, rather than shaking it vigorously – as it is this that creates the bubbles in the first place.

## 10 the changing face of foundation

**Q** *"I have difficulty keeping up with the changing colour of my skin in the summer, as I gradually get a tan. It's so expensive constantly buying new foundations!"*

**A** Stick with the colour that suits you when you're at your palest in the middle of winter. Then, also buy a small tube of dark foundation designed for black skins. Blend just a drop or two into your ordinary foundation on the back of your hand before applying, to darken it so that it matches your tan. This means you can change your foundation as often as you need to, without having to spend a fortune on different shades.

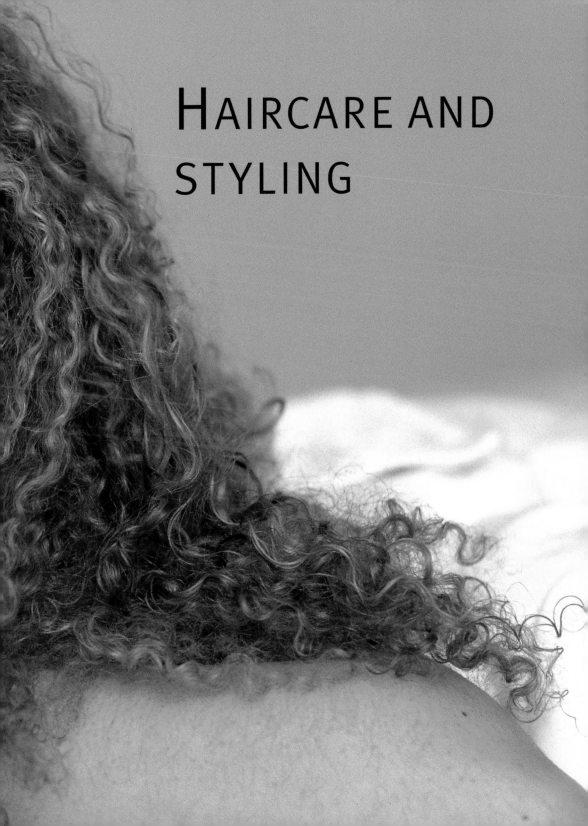

# Haircare and styling

# The structure of hair

A human hair consists mainly of a protein called keratin. It also contains some moisture and the trace metals and minerals found in the rest of the body. The visible part of the hair, called the shaft, is composed of dead tissue: the only living part of the hair is its root, the dermal papilla, which lies snugly below the surface of the scalp in a tube-like depression known as the follicle. The dermal papilla is made up of cells that are fed by the bloodstream.

Each hair consists of three layers. The outer layer, or cuticle, is the hair's protective shield and has tiny overlapping scales, rather like tiles on a roof. When the cuticle scales lie flat and neatly overlap, the hair feels silky-soft and looks glossy. If, however, the cuticle scales have been physically or chemically damaged or broken, the hair will be dull and brittle and will tangle easily.

Under the cuticle lies the cortex, which is made up of fibre-like cells that give hair its strength and elasticity. The cortex also contains the pigment called melanin, which gives hair its natural colour. At the centre of each hair is the medulla, consisting of very soft keratin cells interspersed with spaces. The actual function of the medulla is not known, but some authorities believe that it carries nutrients and other substances to the cortex and cuticle. This could explain why hair is affected so rapidly by changes in health.

Hair's natural shine is supplied by its own conditioner, sebum, an oil composed of waxes and fats and also containing a natural antiseptic that helps fight infection. Sebum is produced by the sebaceous glands present in the dermis. The glands are linked to the hair follicles and release sebum into them. As a lubricant, sebum gives an excellent protective coating to the hair shaft, smoothing the cuticle scales and helping hair retain its natural moisture and elasticity. The smoother the surface of the cuticle, the more light will be reflected from the hair, and therefore the higher will be the gloss. This is why it is more difficult to obtain a sheen on curly hair than on straight hair.

**HAIR STRUCTURE**

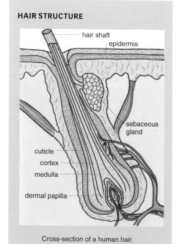

hair shaft
epidermis
sebaceous gland
cuticle
cortex
medulla
dermal papilla

Cross-section of a human hair.

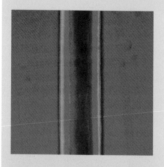

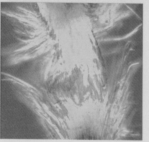

△ Pictures of a human hair magnified 200 times. A strand of hair in good condition is smooth, but if it has been damaged the outer layer is frayed and broken.

Under some circumstances, for example excessive hormonal activity, the sebaceous glands produce too much sebum, and the result is oily hair. Conversely, if too little sebum is produced, the hair will be dry.

## the growth cycle

The only living part of hair is underneath the scalp – when the hair has grown through the scalp it is dead tissue. Hair has three stages of growth: the anagen phase when it actively grows; the catagen, or transitional, phase when the hair stops growing but cellular activity continues in the papilla; and the telogen, or resting, phase when growth stops completely. During the telogen phase there is no further growth or activity at the papilla; eventually the old hair is pushed out by the new growth and the cycle begins again. The anagen phase continues for a period of two to four years, the catagen phase for only about 15-20 days, and the telogen phase for 90-120 days. At any given time, about 93 per cent of an individual's hair is in the anagen phase, 1 per cent is in the catagen phase and 6 per cent is in the telogen phase. Scalp hair, which reacts to hormonal stimuli like the hair on the rest of the body, is genetically programmed to repeat its growth cycle 24–25 times in the average person's lifetime.

**FACT FILE**

• Hair grows an average of 12mm/½ in per month.

• A single strand lives for up to seven years.

• If a person never had their hair cut it would grow to a length of about 107cm/42 in before falling out.

• Women have more hair than men.

• Hair grows faster in the summer and during sleep.

• Hair grows fastest between the ages of 16 and 24.

• Between the ages of 40 and 50 women tend to lose about 20 per cent of their hair.

• Hair becomes drier with age.

# the importance of diet

What you eat is soon reflected in the health of your hair. Like the rest of the body, the hair depends on a good diet to ensure it is supplied with all the necessary nutrients for sustained growth and health. Regular exercise is also important as it promotes good blood circulation, which in turn ensures that vital oxygen and nutrients are transported to the hair root via the blood. Poor eating habits and lack of exercise are soon reflected in the state of the hair; even a minor case of ill-health will usually make it look limp and lacklustre.

An adequate supply of protein in the diet is essential. Good sources include lean meat, poultry, fish, cheese and eggs as well as nuts, seeds and pulses. Fish, seaweed, almonds, brazil nuts, yoghurt and cottage cheese all help to give hair strength and a natural shine.

Wholegrain foods and those with natural oils are highly recommended for the formation of keratin, the major component of hair. Seeds are a rich source of vitamins and minerals as well as protein. Try to eat at least three pieces of fruit a day – it is packed with fibre, vitamins and minerals. Avoid saturated fat, which is found in red meat, fried foods and dairy products. Choose skimmed or semi-skimmed (low-fat) milk rather than the whole varieties, and low-fat cheese and yogurt instead of whole cheese and cream. Use vegetable oils such as sunflower, safflower and olive oil instead of animal fats. These foods all provide nutrients that are essential for luxuriant hair.

If you eat a balanced diet with plenty of fresh ingredients you shouldn't need to take any supplementary vitamins to promote healthy hair growth.

## colour

Hair colour is closely related to skin colour, which is governed by the same type of pigment, melanin. The number of melanin granules in the cortex of the hair, and the shape of the granules, determines a person's natural hair colour. In the majority of cases the melanin granules are elongated in shape. People who have a large number of elongated melanin granules in the cortex have black hair, those with slightly fewer elongated granules have brown hair, and people with even fewer will be blonde. In

**PROMOTING HEALTHY HAIR**

• Cut down on tea and coffee – they are powerful stimulants that act on the nervous, respiratory and cardiovascular systems, increasing the excretion of water and important nutrients. They also hamper the absorption of minerals crucial for hair health. Drink mineral water (between six and eight glasses a day), herbal teas and unsweetened fruit juice.

• Alcohol dilates blood vessels and so helps increase blood flow to the tissues. However, it is antagonistic to several minerals and vitamins that are vital for healthy hair. Limit yourself to an occasional drink.

• Regular exercise stimulates the circulatory system, encouraging a healthy blood supply to all cells and nourishing and helping to regenerate and repair.

• Some contraceptive pills deplete the B-complex vitamins and zinc. If you notice a change in your hair after starting to take the Pill, or changing brands, ask your doctor or nutritionist for advice.

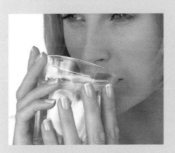

△ **Drink plenty of water every day to keep your hair healthy.**

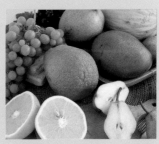

△ **Eating 2 or 3 pieces of fruit a day provides your hair with vital vitamins and minerals.**

other people the melanin granules are spherical or oval in shape rather than elongated, and this makes the hair appear red.

Spherical or oval granules sometimes appear in combination with a moderate amount of the elongated ones, and then the person will have rich, reddish-brown tinges. If, however, spherical granules occur in combination with a large number of elongated granules then the blackness of the hair will almost mask the redness, although it will still be present to give a subtle tinge to the hair and differentiate it from pure black.

Hair darkens with age, but at some stage in the middle years of life the pigment formation slows down and silvery-grey hairs begin to appear. Gradually, the production of melanin ceases, and all the hair becomes colourless – or what is generally termed grey.

When melanin granules are completely lacking from birth, as in albinos, the hair has no colour and is pure white.

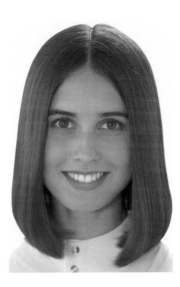

◁ The colour of your hair is determined by the amount of pigment in the hair and also by the shape of the pigment granules. People with dark hair have larger quantities of pigment than people with blonde hair. In both brunettes and blondes the pigment granules are elongated in shape; red hair results from the presence of oval granules.

# Hair analysis – texture and type

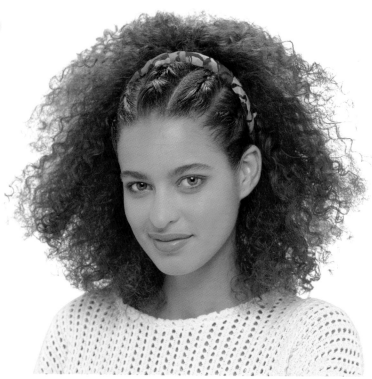

◁ Hair with a very curly texture needs intensive moisturizing treatments to keep the spring in the curl. On this type of hair always use a wide-toothed comb, never a brush, which will make the hair frizz. Leave-in conditioners are good for curly hair as they help to give curl separation. To revitalize curls, mist with water and scrunch with the hands.

## HAIR FACT FILE
• Healthy hair is highly elastic and can stretch 20 or 30 per cent before snapping.
• Chinese circus acrobats have been known to perform tricks while suspended by their hair.
• A human hair is stronger than copper wire of the same thickness.
• The combined strength of a headful of human hair is capable of supporting a weight equivalent to that of 99 people.

The texture of your hair is determined by the size and shape of the hair follicle, which is a genetic trait controlled by hormones and related to age and racial characteristics.

Whether hair is curly, wavy or straight depends on two things: its shape as it grows out of the follicle, and the distribution of keratin-producing cells at the roots. When viewed in cross section, straight hair tends to be round, wavy hair tends to be oval, and curly hair kidney-shaped. Straight hair is formed by roots that produce the same number of keratin cells all around the follicle. In wavy and curly hair, the production of keratin cells is uneven, so that at any given time there are more cells on one side of the oval-shaped follicle than on the other. Furthermore, the production of excess cells alternates between the sides. This causes the developing hair to grow first in one direction and then in the other. The result is wavy or curly hair.

The natural colour of the hair also affects the texture. Natural blondes have finer hair than brunettes, while redheads have the thickest hair.

Generally speaking, hair can be divided into three categories: fine, medium, and coarse and thick. Fine hair can be strong or weak; however, because of its texture, all fine hair has the same characteristic – it lacks volume. As the name suggests, medium hair is neither too thick nor too thin, and is strong and elastic. Thick and coarse hair is abundant and heavy, with a tendency to grow outwards from the scalp as well as downwards. It often lacks elasticity and is frizzy.

A single head of hair may consist of several different textures. For example, fine hair is often found on the temples, the hairline at the front and on the nape of the head, while the texture over the rest of the head may be medium or even coarse.

## ETHNIC DIFFERENCES
Generally, people from Scandinavia have thin, straight, baby-fine hair, and mid-European populations have hair that is neither too fine nor too coarse. People native to the Indian subcontinent have thick-textured tresses while Middle-Eastern populations have strong hair. In very general terms, the further east you travel the coarser hair becomes. The hair of Chinese and Japanese people is usually extremely straight; and that of Latin-speaking and North African peoples can be very frizzy and thick.

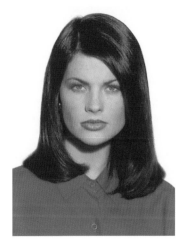

△ Thick straight hair can be made sleeker if you remember always to blow-dry downwards. This encourages the cuticles to lie flat and reflect the light.

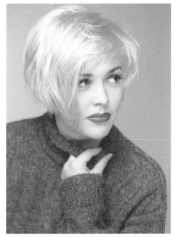

△ Fine hair needs regular expert cutting to maximize the volume. Here, gel spray was used to give lift at the roots and the hair was then blow-dried.

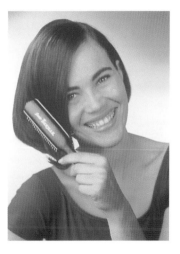

△ Normal hair generally holds a style well. It is usually very easy to look after and responds well to regular brushing, smoothing and polishing.

## normal, dry or oily?

Hair type is determined by the hair's natural condition – that is, the amount of sebum the body produces. Treatments such as perming, colouring and heat styling will also have an effect on hair type. Natural hair types and those produced by applying treatments are described here, with advice on haircare where appropriate.

### dry hair

It can look dull, feels dry and tangles easily. It is difficult to brush, particularly when it is wet. It is often quite thick at the roots but thinner, and sometimes split, at the ends.

*Causes* Excessive shampooing, over-use of heat-styling equipment, misuse of colour or perms, damage from the sun, or harsh weather conditions. Each of these factors depletes the moisture content of hair, so that it loses its elasticity, bounce and suppleness. Dryness can also be the result of a sebum deficiency on the hair's surface, caused by a decrease in or absence of sebaceous gland secretions.

*Solutions* Use a nourishing shampoo and an intensive conditioner. Dry hair naturally.

### normal hair

It is neither oily nor dry, has not been permed or coloured, holds its style, and looks good most of the time. Normal hair is suited to the daily use of two-in-one conditioning shampoos. These are formulated to provide a two-stage process in one application. When the product is lathered into wet hair the shampoo removes dirt, grease and styling products. At this stage the conditioner remains in the lather. As the hair is rinsed with more water, the grease and dirt are washed away, and the micro-fine conditioning droplets are released on to the hair, leaving it shiny and easy to comb.

### oily hair

It looks lank and greasy and needs frequent washing to look good.

*Causes* Overproduction of sebum as a result of hormone disturbances, stress, hot and humid atmosphere, excessive brushing, or constantly running hands through the hair, perspiration, or a diet rich in saturated fat. The hair becomes oily, sticky and unmanageable in just a few days, or sometimes within hours.

*Solutions* Use a gentle, non-aggressive shampoo that also gives the hair volume. A light perm will lift the hair at the roots and limit the dispersal of sebum. Rethink your diet: cut out as many dairy fats and greasy foods as you can. Try to eat plenty of fresh food, and drink six to eight glasses of water every day.

### combination hair

It is oily at the roots but dry and sometimes split at the ends.

*Causes* Chemical treatments, using detergent-based shampoos too frequently, overexposure to sunlight, and over-use of heat-styling equipment. Such repeated abuse often provokes a reaction in sebum secretion at the roots and a partial alteration in the scales, which can no longer fulfil their protective role. The hair ends therefore become dry.

*Solutions* Use products that have only a gentle action on the hair. Excessive use of formulations for oily hair and those for dry hair may contribute to the problem. Ideally, use a product specially designed for combination hair. If this is not possible try using a shampoo for oily hair and finish by applying a conditioner from the middle lengths to the ends of the hair only.

### coloured or permed hair

It is very often more porous than untreated hair, so it needs to be treated with gentle cleansers and good conditioners. Colour-care products will help prevent fading by protecting the hair from the damaging rays of sunlight. Products specially designed for permed hair can also help maintain elasticity, giving longer-lasting results.

# Times of change

Hair goes through many different stages during a lifetime. Each stage brings with it different requirements in haircare. The most significant stages are described below, together with recommendations for promoting hair health during each phase.

## beginnings: the baby and child

A baby's hair characteristics are determined from the very moment of conception. By the 16th week of pregnancy the foetus will be covered with lanugo, a downy body hair that is usually shed before birth. The first hair appears on the head at around 20 weeks' gestation and it is at this time that the pigment melanin, which will determine the colour of the hair, is first produced.

A few weeks after birth, the baby's original hair begins to fall out or is rubbed off. The new hair is quite different from the initial downy mass, so a baby born with blonde wispy curls might have dark straight hair by the age of six months.

Cradle cap, which appears as thick, yellow scales in patches over the scalp, causes many mothers concern. Cradle cap is the result of a natural build-up of skin cells. It is nothing to worry about and can be gently loosened by rubbing a little baby oil on to the scalp at night and washing it off in the morning. This may need to be repeated for several days until all the loose scales have been lifted and washed away.

Mothers often carefully trim their baby's hair when necessary, and it is not until the child is about two years of age that a visit to a hairdressing salon may be necessary. Children's hair is normally in beautiful condition and is best cut and styled simply.

At the onset of puberty young adults suddenly become much more interested in experimenting with their hair. This is when they may experience oily hair and skin for the first time. A re-evaluation of the shampoos and conditioners currently in use is often necessary to keep hair looking good.

## haircare during pregnancy

During pregnancy the hair often looks its best. However after the birth, or after breast-feeding ceases, about 50 per cent of new mothers experience what appears to be excessive hair loss. This is related to the three stages of hair growth (see page 104). During pregnancy and breast-feeding, hormones keep the hair at the growing stage for longer than usual, so it appears thicker and fuller. Some time after the birth – usually about 12 weeks later – this hair enters the resting stage, at the end of which all the hair that has been in the resting phase is shed. What appears to be excessive hair loss is therefore simply a postponement of a natural occurrence, a condition that is known as post-partum alopecia.

A more significant problem that may occur during pregnancy is caused by a depletion in the protein content of the hair. As a result the hair becomes drier and more brittle. Combat this by frequent use of an intensive conditioning treatment.

**GROWING UP**

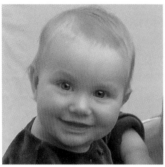

△ A baby's hair is soft and downy at first but it takes on its individual characteristics within six months of birth.

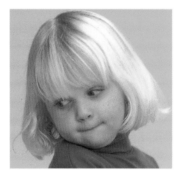

△ The toddler's hair requires a simple cut. At this stage the child is usually taken for her first visit to a salon.

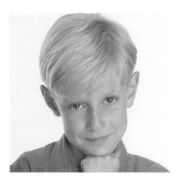

△ Young boys need a hair cut that is easily straight hair, but need regular trims.

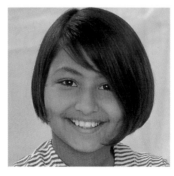

△ Bobs suit most girls and are perfect for straight hair, but need regular trims.

smoke and natural gas from cookers discolour white hair and make it look yellow. Mineral deposits from chlorinated water can give white hair a greenish tinge. Chelating, clarifying or purifying shampoos will help to strip this build-up from the hair.

To counteract dryness associated with aging, use richer shampoos and conditioning products. As well as regular conditioning, weekly intensive treatments are essential to counteract moisture loss.

Avoid perming during pregnancy because the hair is in an altered state and the result can be unpredictable. Try a herbal rinse to give your hair and your spirits a lift.

## growing older

With aging the whole body slows down, including the hair follicles, which become less efficient and produce hairs that are finer in diameter and shorter in length. Such shrinkage is gradual and the hair begins to feel slightly thinner, with less volume and density. At the same time the sebaceous glands start to produce less sebum and the hair begins to lose its colour as the production of melanin decreases.

Blonde hair fades, brunettes lose natural highlights, and redheads tone down to brown shades. When melanin production stops altogether the new hair that grows is white, not grey as is commonly perceived. The production of melanin is governed by genetic factors, and the best indication of when an individual's hair will become white is the age at which their parents' hair did. Pigment, apart from giving hair its colour, also helps to soften and make each strand more flexible. This is why white hair tends to become wirier and coarser in texture.

As the texture of the hair changes, it is inclined to pick up dust and smoke from the atmosphere, so that it soon appears to be discoloured and dirty. This is particularly true for those who live in a town or spend time in smoky atmospheres. Cigarette

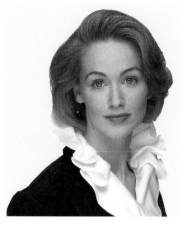

△ As women grow older the hair becomes thinner. A mid-length to short cut makes the hair less prone to droop.

### AS THE YEARS GO BY

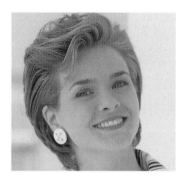

△ Medium-textured hair that has gone flat and needs a lift can be given height on the crown with a root perm.

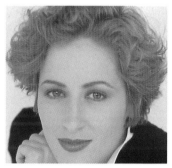

△ The hair has been cut to create more movement and softness. It was then scrunch-dried and finished with wax.

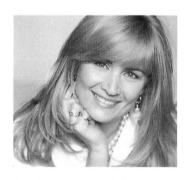

△ Long hair was softened by feathering the sides and cutting a full fringe (bangs). A semi-permanent colour added gloss.

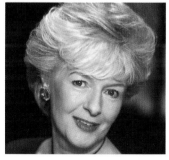

△ This fine grey hair was highlighted and then toned using a rinse before blow-drying with a round brush.

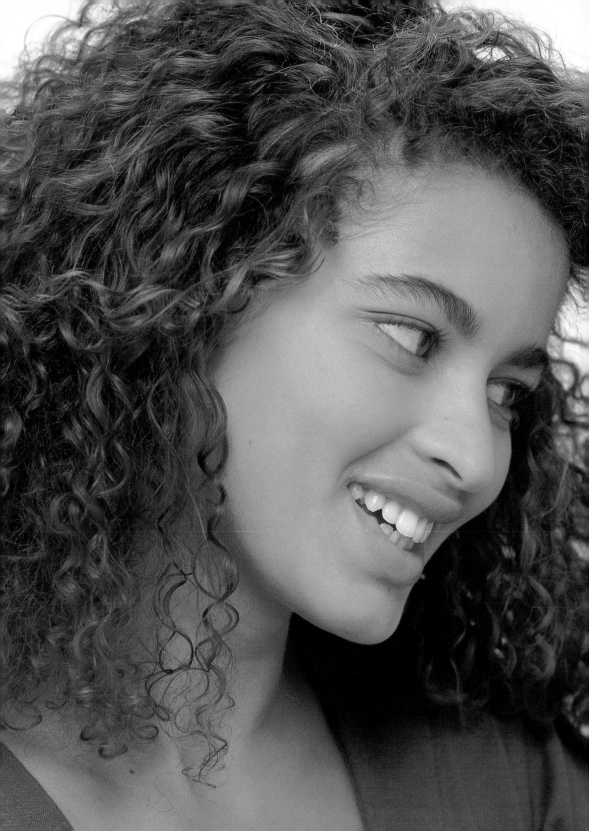

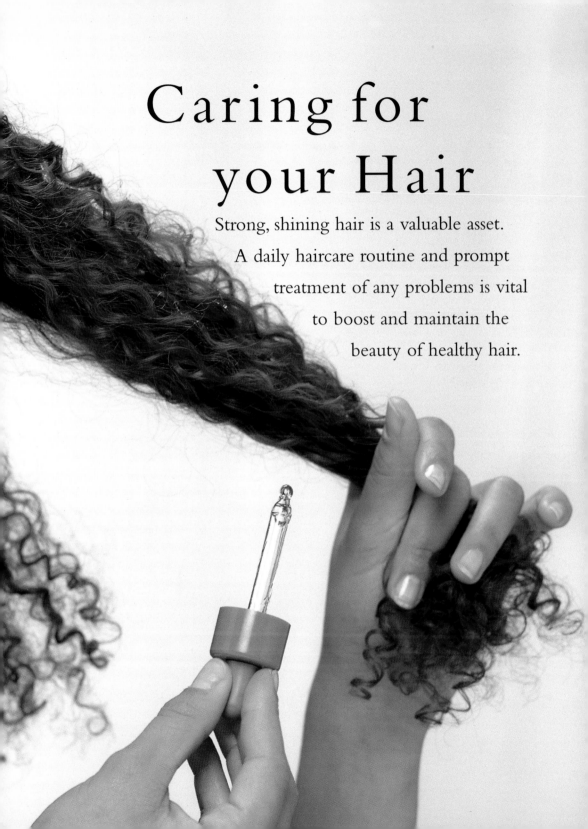

# Caring for your Hair

Strong, shining hair is a valuable asset.
A daily haircare routine and prompt
treatment of any problems is vital
to boost and maintain the
beauty of healthy hair.

# The cut

Hair growth varies over different parts of the head. This is why your cut can appear to be out of shape very quickly. As a general rule, a short precision cut needs trimming every four weeks, a longer style every six to eight weeks. Even if you want to grow your hair long it is essential to have it trimmed regularly – at least every three months – to prevent splitting and keep the ends even.

Hairdressers use a variety of techniques and tools to make hair appear thicker, fuller, straighter or curlier, whatever the desired effect. These techniques and tools are explained below.

Blunt cutting, in which the ends are cut straight across, is often used for hair of one length. The weight and fullness of the hair is distributed around the perimeter of the shape.

**Clippers:** Used for close-cut styles and sometimes to finish off a cut. Shaved clipper cuts are popular with teenagers.

**Graduated hair:** This is cut at an angle to give fullness on top and blend the top hair into shorter lengths at the nape.

**Layering the hair:** This technique evenly distributes the weight and fullness, giving a round appearance to the style.

**Slide cutting:** (also called slithering or feathering) This thins the hair. Scissors are used in a sliding action, backwards and forwards along the hair length. This technique is often done when the hair is dry.

**Razor cutting:** Used to create softness, tapering and internal movement so that the hair moves more freely. It can also be used to shorten hair.

**Thinning:** Either with thinning scissors or a razor, removes bulk and weight without affecting the overall length of the hair.

## clever cuts

Fine, thin, flyaway hair can be given volume, bounce and movement by blunt cutting. Mid-length hair can benefit from being lightly layered to give extra volume, while short, thin hair can be blunt cut and the edges graduated to give movement.

Some hairdressers razor cut fine hair to give a thicker and more voluminous effect. It is best not to let fine hair grow too long. As soon as it reaches the shoulders it tends to look wispy and out of control.

Thick and coarse hair can be controlled by reducing the weight to give more style

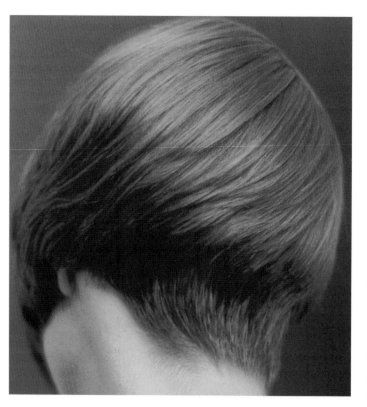

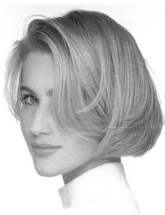

△ For this style the model's straight hair was cut so that it would swing back into shape with every movement of the head. The shine was improved by using a longer-lasting semi-permanent colour.

◁ This heavily layered, graduated bob was cut close into the nape, and then the shape of the hair was emphasized by using a vegetable colour to give tone and shine. The hair was styled by blow-drying.

# cutting to add volume and shape

A good stylist can, with technical expertise, make the most of any type of hair, so take time to discuss what you like and dislike about your hair. A good haircut should need the minimum of styling products and drying to achieve the desired result.

and direction. Avoid very short styles because the hair will tend to stick out. Try a layered cut with movement.

Layering also helps achieve height and eliminate weight. On shorter styles the weight can be reduced with thinning scissors expertly used on the ends only.

Sometimes hair grows in different directions, which may cause styling problems. For example, a cowlick is normally found on the front hairline and occurs when the hair grows in a swirl, backwards and then forwards. Clever cutting can redistribute the weight and go some way to solving this problem. A double crown occurs when there are two pivots for natural hair at the top of the head, rather than the usual one. Styles with height at the crown are most suitable here.

To maximize the effect of a widow's peak the hair should be taken in the reverse direction to the growth. This gives the impression of a natural wave.

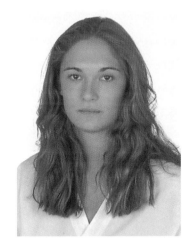

△ **1** Before she had her hair cut, our model's long hair had natural movement but the weight was pulling the hair down and spoiling the shape. For her new style she wanted a shorter, more sophisticated look, and one that would be easy to maintain.

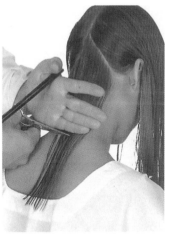

△ **2** First the model's hair was shampooed, conditioned and then combed through to remove any tangles. The stylist was then ready to start cutting. He began by sectioning off the front hair so that the hair at the back could be cut to the required length.

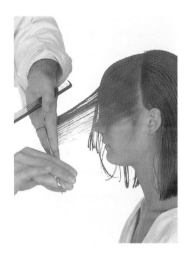

△ **3** Next the front hair was combed forward and cut straight across at an angle. This ensured that when the model's hair was dry it would fall easily into shape.

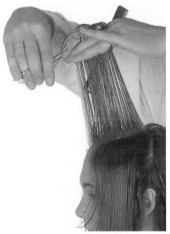

△ **4** The top hair was graduated to help build volume and lift into the style. This versatile cut makes it possible for the hair to be styled either towards the face or towards the back of the head.

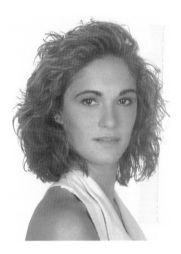

△ **5** To finish, the stylist scrunched the hair, using a blow-dryer and some mousse to encourage the formation of curls. On this type of style a diffuser fitted to the dryer will spread the airflow and give added movement to the hair.

# Shampoos

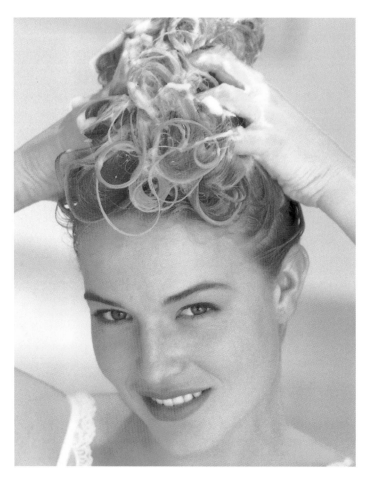

Shampoos are designed to cleanse the hair and scalp thoroughly, removing dirt, grease and grime without stripping away too much of the protective natural sebum. They contain cleansing agents, perfume and preservatives, and some have conditioning properties that can coat the hair shaft to make the hair appear thicker. The conditioning agents also smooth the cuticle scales so the hair doesn't tangle, and help eliminate static electricity from the hair when it dries.

## the pH factor

The letters pH relate to the acid/alkaline level of a substance. This level is calculated on a scale of 1 to 14. Numbers below 7 denote acidity, those over 7 indicate alkalinity. The majority of shampoos range between a pH factor of 5 and 7; medicated varieties have a pH of about 7.3, which is near neutral.

Sebum has a pH factor of between 4.5 and 5.5, which is mildly acidic. Bacteria cannot survive in this pH, so it is very important to maintain this protective layer in order to keep the skin, scalp and hair in optimum condition.

◁ Shampoos are available in different formulas to suit all hair types and conditions. Make sure you choose one that is right for your hair and use it as often as necessary to keep your hair clean. Rinse out the shampoo thoroughly.

**SHAMPOO TIPS**
- Use the correct shampoo (and not too much) for your hair type. If in doubt use the mildest shampoo you can buy.
- Don't wash your hair in washing-up liquid, soap or other detergents; they are highly alkaline and will upset your hair's natural pH balance by stripping out the natural oils.
- Read the instructions first. Some shampoos need to be left on the scalp for a few minutes before rinsing.

- If you can, buy small packets of shampoo to test which brand is most suitable for your hair.
- Never wash your hair in the bath; dirty bath water is not conducive to clean hair, and it is difficult to rinse properly without a shower attachment or separate pourer.

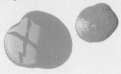

- Always wash your brush and comb when you shampoo your hair.
- Change your shampoo every now and then; hair seems to develop a resistance to certain ingredients after a period of time.
- Don't throw away a shampoo that doesn't lather. The amount of suds is determined by the active level of detergent. Some shampoos have less suds than others but this has no effect on their cleansing ability. In fact, quite often, the more effective the product, the fewer the bubbles.

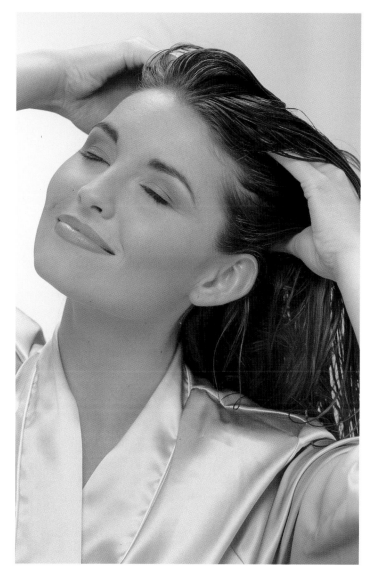

▷ **A head massage reduces scalp tension as well as promoting healthy hair growth.** It is also a relaxing and pampering treatment that you can do yourself at home.

Many shampoos are labelled "pH balanced", and this means they have the same acidity level as hair. Individuals with fragile, permed or coloured hair should use a shampoo of this type. However, for strong hair in good condition, a pH balanced shampoo is unnecessary, provided shampooing is followed by conditioning.

## shampoo success

Always use a product formulated for your hair type – dry, normal, oily or chemically treated – and before shampooing brush your hair to free any tangles and loosen dirt and dead skin cells. Use lukewarm water, as hot water can be uncomfortable.

Wet the hair, then apply a small amount of shampoo and gently massage into the roots using the pads of your fingertips; never use your nails. Pay special attention to the hairline area, where make-up and dirt can become trapped. Allow the lather to work its way to the ends of the hair. Don't rub vigorously or you will stretch the hair.

When you have finished shampooing, rinse thoroughly until the water runs clean and clear. Repeat the process only if you think your hair needs it, again using only a small amount of shampoo. Finally, blot the hair with a towel to remove excess water before applying conditioner.

## massaging the scalp

Massage helps maintain a healthy scalp. It brings extra blood to the tissues, which enhances the delivery of nutrients and oxygen to the hair follicle. It also reduces scalp tension, which can contribute to hair loss, loosens dead skin cells and helps redress the overproduction of sebum, which makes hair oily.

You can give yourself a scalp massage at home. Use warm olive oil if the scalp is dry or tight. Try equal parts of witch hazel and mineral water if you have an oily scalp. For a normal scalp, use equal parts rose and mineral waters.

Begin the massage by gently rotating your scalp using the tips of your fingers. Start at the forehead, move to the sides, and work over the crown to the nape of the neck. Then place your fingertips firmly on the scalp without exerting too much pressure. Push the fingers together then pull them apart through the hair in a kneading motion, without lifting or moving them. When you have massaged for about a minute, move to the next section. Continue until your entire scalp and upper neck have been treated.

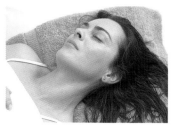

△ **For a really deep conditioning treatment,** oils can be left on overnight to continue working while you recharge with a restful sleep.

# Getting into condition

In an ideal world a regular shampoo would be sufficient to guarantee a glossy head of hair. Unfortunately very few people are able to wash their hair and let the matter rest at that; most need some sort of help just to overcome the effects of modern living, not to mention the occasional problem that needs treatment. Here is a guide to the vast array of products available to get the hair in excellent condition.

## the conditioners

Glossy hair has cuticle scales that lie flat and neatly overlap, thus reflecting the light. Perming and colouring, rough handling and heat styling all conspire to lift the cuticles, allowing moisture to be lost from the cortex and making hair dry, lacklustre and prone to knotting and tangling. Severely damaged cuticles break off completely, resulting in thinner hair which eventually breaks.

To put the shine back into hair and restore its natural lustre it may be necessary to use a specific conditioner that meets the hair's requirements. Conditioners, with the exception of hot oils, should be applied to freshly shampooed hair that has been blotted dry with a towel to remove excess moisture.

Today there is a large, and sometimes confusing, number of conditioners on the market. The following list describes those that are widely available:

**Basic conditioners:** These coat the hair with a fine film, temporarily smoothing down the cuticle and making hair glossier and easier to manage. Leave for a few minutes before rinsing thoroughly.

**Conditioning sprays:** These are used prior to styling and form a protective barrier against the harmful effects of heat. They are also good for reducing static electricity on flyaway hair.

**Hot oils:** Used to give an intensive, deep nourishing treatment. To use, place the unopened tube in a cup of hot tap water and leave to heat for one minute. Next, wet the hair and towel it dry before twisting off the

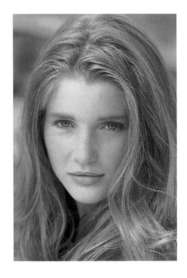

△ **Long hair needs a regular conditioning regime to keep it healthy and shiny.**

tube top. Massage the hot oil evenly into the scalp and through the hair for one to three minutes. For a more intensive treatment cover the head with a shower cap. To finish, rinse the hair and shampoo.

**Intensive conditioners:** These can help hair to retain its natural moisture balance, replenishing it where necessary. Use this type if the hair is split, dry, frizzy or difficult to manage. Distribute the conditioner evenly through the hair and then allow it to penetrate for two to five minutes, or longer if required. Rinse very thoroughly with lots of fresh, warm water, lifting your hair from the scalp to ensure any residue is washed away.

**Leave-in conditioners:** Designed to help retain moisture, reduce static and add shine, they are especially good for fine hair as they avoid conditioner overload, which can cause lankness. Convenient and easy to use, they also provide a protective barrier against the effects of heat styling. Apply after shampooing but don't rinse off. These products are ideal for daily use.

**Restructants:** These penetrate the cortex, helping to repair and strengthen the inner part of damaged hair. They are helpful if the hair is lank and limp and has lost its natural elasticity as a result of chemical treatments or physical damage.

**Split end treatments/serums:** Used to condition damaged hair. The best course of action for split ends is to have the ends trimmed, but this does not always solve the whole problem because the hair tends to break off and split at different levels. As an intermediate solution, split ends can be temporarily sealed using these specialized conditioners. They should be worked into the ends of newly washed hair so that they surround the hair with a microscopic film that leaves the hair shaft smoother.

**Colour/perm conditioners:** These are designed for chemically treated hair. After-colour products add a protective film around porous areas of the hair, preventing colour loss. After-perm products help stabilize the hair, thus keeping the bounce in the curl.

## problems and solutions

Split ends, dandruff and a dry, itchy scalp are common problems that can detract from otherwise healthy hair. In most cases such problems can be overcome by giving the appropriate treatment.

**Dandruff:** This consists of scaly particles with an oily sheen that lie close to the hair root. This condition should not be confused with a flaky scalp (see below).

*Causes* Poor diet, sluggish metabolism, stress, a hormonal imbalance, and sometimes infection. These conditions usually produce increased cell renewal on the scalp, which is often associated with an increase in sebum. The scales will absorb the excess oil, however if the problem remains untreated it will become worse.

*Solutions* Rethink your diet and lifestyle. Learn relaxation techniques if the problem appears to be caused by stress. Brush the hair

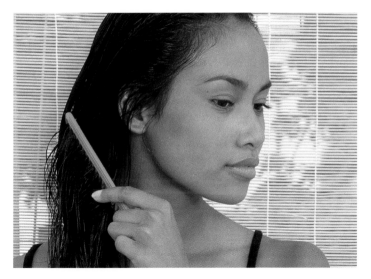

conditioner. The hair is often best styled with a gel, and it is most effective if it is applied when the hair is wet. Alternatively, allow the hair to dry naturally and then style it using a wax or pomade. Serums can also help. These are silicone-based products that work by surrounding the cuticle with a transparent microscopic film, which leaves the hair shaft smoother. Serums effectively prevent moisture loss and inhibit the absorption of dampness from the surrounding air.

**Split ends:** These occur when the cuticle is damaged and the fibres of the cortex unravel. The hair is dry, brittle and prone to tangling, and can split at the end or anywhere along the shaft.

*Causes* Over-perming or colouring, insufficient conditioning, or too much brushing or backcombing, especially with poor-quality combs or brushes. Careless use of spiky rollers and hair pins, excessive heat styling and not having the hair trimmed regularly can also cause the problem.

*Solutions* Split ends cannot be repaired; the only long-term solution is to have them snipped off regularly. What is lost in the length will be gained in quality. It may help if you reduce the frequency with which you shampoo, as this in itself is stressful to hair and causes split ends to extend up the hair shaft. Never use a dryer too near the hair, or set it on too high a temperature. Minimize the use of heated appliances. Try conditioners and serums that are designed to seal split ends temporarily and give resistance to further splitting.

**Product build-up:** This is caused by the residue of styling products and two-in-one shampoo formulation left on the hair shaft.

*Causes* When these residues combine with mineral deposits in the water a build-up occurs, preventing thorough cleansing and conditioning. The result is hair that is dull and lack lustre; it is often difficult to perm or colour successfully because there is a barrier preventing the chemicals from penetrating the hair shaft. The colour can be patchy and the perm uneven.

*Solutions* Use one of the stripping, chelating or clarifying shampoos, which are specially designed to strip out product build-up. This is particularly important prior to perming or colouring.

before shampooing and scrupulously wash combs and brushes. Always choose a mild shampoo with an antidandruff action that gently loosens scales and helps prevent new ones. Follow with a treatment lotion, massaged into the scalp using the fingertips. The treatment must be used regularly if it is to be effective. Avoid excessive use of heat stylers. If the dandruff persists, consult your doctor or trichologist.

**Flaky/itchy scalp:** This condition produces tiny white pieces of dead skin that flake off the scalp and are usually first noticed on the shoulders. This condition can often be confused with dandruff but the two are not related. Sometimes the scalp is red or itchy and feels tight. The hair usually has a dull appearance.

*Causes* Hereditary traits, stress, insufficient rinsing of shampoo, lack of sebum, using a harsh shampoo, vitamin imbalance, pollution, air conditioning and central heating.

*Solutions* Choose a moisturizing shampoo and a conditioner with herbal extracts to help soothe and remoisturize the scalp.

**Fine hair:** This tends to look flat, and is hard to style because it does not hold a shape.

*Causes* The texture is hereditary, but the problem is often made worse by using too heavy a conditioner, which weighs the hair down. Excessive use of styling products can have the same effect.

*Solutions* Wash hair frequently with a mild shampoo and use a light conditioner.

△ **Leaving the oils in your hair after an oil massage is a holistic treatment and helps leave your hair and scalp in excellent condition.**

Volumizing shampoos can help give body, and soft perms will make hair appear thicker.

**Frizzy hair:** This can result from the merest hint of rain or other air moisture being absorbed into the hair. It looks dry, lacks lustre, and is difficult to control.

*Causes* It can be inherited or it can be caused by rough treatment, such as too much harsh brushing or regularly pulling the hair into rubber bands.

*Solutions* When washing the hair, massage the shampoo into the roots and allow the lather to work its way to the ends. Apply a conditioner from the mid-lengths of the hair to the ends, or use a leave-in

# Natural hair treatments

For thousands of years, herbs and plants have been mixed and blended and then used to heal, freshen, pamper and beautify hair. The following are a few age-old haircare recipes that you might like to try at home. Remember to use these treatments immediately after you have made them because they won't keep well.

## natural dandruff treatment

Mix a few drops of oil of rosemary with 30ml/2 tbsp olive oil and rub well into the scalp at bedtime. Shampoo and rinse thoroughly in the morning.

## easy egg shampoo

In a blender mix together two small (US medium) eggs with 50ml/2fl oz/¼ cup still mineral water and 15ml/1 tbsp cider vinegar or lemon juice. Blend for 30 seconds at low speed. Massage well into the scalp and rinse very thoroughly using lukewarm water (if the water is any hotter the egg will begin to set).

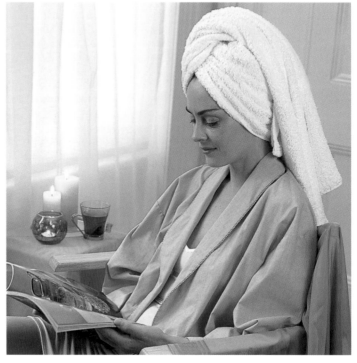

△ Once you have applied a conditioning treatment to your hair, wrap your hair in a warm towel. Then lie back and relax for 20 minutes or so, to allow the treatment plenty of time to work.

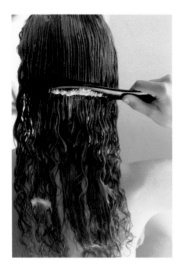

△ Treatments can be applied more thoroughly to the hair by using a wide-toothed comb. This ensures it is applied from root to tip.

## herbal shampoo

Crush a few dried bay leaves with a rolling pin, or with a pestle and mortar, and mix with a handful of dried chamomile flowers and one of rosemary. Place in a large jug and pour over 900ml/3½ cups boiling water. Strain after 2–3 minutes and mix in 5ml/ 1 tsp soft or liquid soap. Apply to the hair, massaging well. Rinse thoroughly.

## zesty hair cream

Beat 150ml/⅔ cup natural yoghurt with an egg; add 5ml/1 tsp sea kelp powder and 5ml/1 tsp finely grated lemon rind. Mix thoroughly and work into the hair. Cover your hair with a plastic shower cap and leave in place for 40 minutes. Shampoo and rinse.

## hair rescuer

For dry, damaged hair, apply this mixture after shampooing. Leave for 5 minutes, then rinse.

**ingredients**

- 30ml/2 tbsp olive oil
- 30ml/2 tbsp light sesame oil
- 2 eggs
- 30ml/2 tbsp coconut milk
- 30ml/2 tbsp runny honey
- 5ml/1 tsp coconut oil
- blender or food processor
- bottle

Process the ingredients until smooth. Transfer to a bottle. Keep in the fridge and use within 3 days.

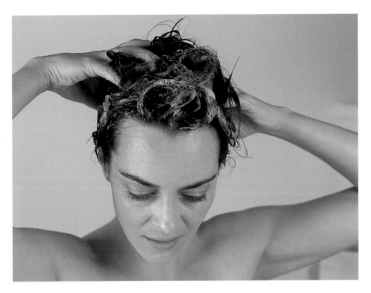

◁ As you apply the treatments, gently massage your scalp for a few minutes to improve circulation and allow the treatment to have the most beneficial effect.

## rosemary hair tonic

This hair tonic made from fresh-smelling rosemary can be used as a substitute for mildly medicated shampoos. It is also effective in controlling greasy hair and enhances the shine and natural colour, especially of dark hair. Use this tonic as a final finishing rinse after shampooing, catching it in a bowl and pouring it repeatedly through the hair.

### ingredients

- 250ml/8 fl oz/1 cup fresh rosemary tips
- 1.2 litres/2 pints/5 cups bottled water
- pan
- strainer
- funnel
- bottle

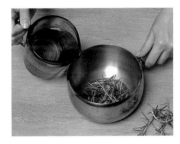

△ 1 Place the rosemary and water in a saucepan and bring to the boil. Simmer for approximately 20 minutes, then allow to cool in the pan.

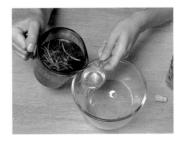

△ 2 Strain the liquid and use a funnel to pour it into a clean bottle. Store in a cool place. Apply as a soothing and invigorating rinse after shampooing.

## parsley hair paste

This hair paste stimulates circulation, aids hair growth and leaves hair healthy and glossy.

### ingredients

- 1 large handful parsley sprigs
- blender or food processor
- 30ml/2 tbsp water

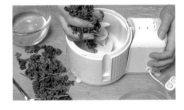

△ 1 Place the parsley in a blender or food processor with the water.

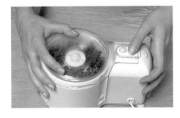

△ 2 Process until the parsley is ground to a smooth green purée. Apply the lotion to your scalp, then wrap a warm towel around your head. Leave for about an hour before washing your hair as usual.

### BENEFITS OF NATURAL HAIR TREATMENTS

Commercial haircare products may work to a certain extent; however, a more holistic approach is required if we are to achieve the strong, lustrous hair that most of us long for. Strong hair growth is closely related to our general state of health and also to diet and fitness.

In some cultures people do not shampoo their hair but use other treatments such as oiling or just washing with water. It is true that when left alone the hair reaches a point of homeostasis where it is protected by its natural oils and there is no need for soap. Frequent hair-washing is actually damaging to the hair. It strips it of all its natural oils and dries out the scalp. This stimulates the sebaceous glands to produce more oil to compensate, which then leads to greasy hair and more hair washing.

Hairdryers and heated styling devices also have a damaging and drying-out effect on the hair so it is best to leave it to dry naturally.

Research suggests that there may be some risks associated with using chemical dyes or other products on the hair, as they can be absorbed into the bloodstream through the scalp and could be toxic for the body. There are many plant- or vegetable-based dyes and natural treatments available that do not pose this risk.

## hot oil treatment

Any vegetable oil is suitable for conditioning. Just heat the oil until slightly warm. Rub a little into your scalp and then through every part of your hair, massaging gently as you go. Cover your head with a plastic shower cap for 20 minutes; the heat from your head will help the oil penetrate the hair shaft. Shampoo and rinse thoroughly.

## intensive conditioning

Warm 15ml/1 tbsp each wheatgerm and olive oil and massage gently into the scalp. Wrap a warm towel around the head and leave for 10 minutes. Then rinse with a basin of water to which you have added the juice of a lemon.

## using essential oils

Pure aromatherapy oils can be used for hair-care. The following recipes come from world-famous aromatherapist Robert Tisserand. The number of drops of oil, as listed, should be diluted in 30ml/2 tbsp vegetable oil, which will act as a carrier oil.

**Dry hair:** rosewood 9, sandalwood 6.
**Oily hair:** bergamot 9, lavender 6.
**Dandruff:** eucalyptus 9, rosemary 6.

Mix the required treatment and apply to dry or wet hair. Massage the scalp using the fingertips. Leave for two to five minutes. Shampoo your hair as usual and then rinse thoroughly.

## warm oil treatment

These treatments feel better and are more easily absorbed by the scalp. If you apply this treatment once a month, it should improve the texture of your hair and the condition of your scalp.

### ingredients
- 90ml/6 tbsp coconut oil
- 3 drops rosemary essential oil
- 2 drops tea tree essential oil
- 2 drops lavender essential oil
- dark-coloured glass bottle with stopper

**1** Pour all the ingredients into the bottle and shake gently to mix. Use the oil sparingly on dry hair; the head should not be soaked.
**2** Massage the oil in, then cover your head with a warm towel for 20 minutes. Shampoo as normal.

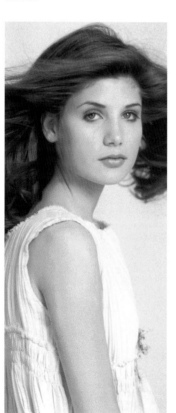

◁ **Natural ingredients such as herbs and essential oils can help you achieve beautifully conditioned hair. Here a hot oil treatment was applied to the model's hair to enhance its shine and condition. Natural oils that are suitable for applying to the hair and scalp include vegetable oils, but rosemary, ylang ylang and lavender essential oils are fragrant alternatives. Use according to the manufacturer's directions.**

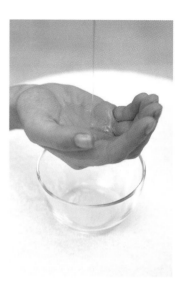

△ **Warm the oil in the palm of your hand or on a radiator before applying it. Heated oil is more easily absorbed by the hair and scalp and is more pleasant to apply**

### HEAD MASSAGE FOR COMMON HAIR PROBLEMS

For a therapeutic head massage, warm the oil in the palm of your hand and apply it to the top of your head. Using the pads of your fingers make circular strokes across your scalp with medium pressure. Work methodically from the front to the back, covering the whole head. When you have finished, cover your head and leave the oils for as long as possible to sink into your hair and scalp.

• **Greasy hair:** Massage stimulates the sebaceous glands to work properly and help prevent the hair follicles from clogging up with sebum. Jojoba oil helps to regulate over-productive sebaceous glands. For hair washing, use mild shampoos and avoid washing too often.

• **Dry hair:** Massage, combined with regular hot-oil treatments, is ideal for conditioning and moisturizing dry hair. Ideally leave the oil in overnight. Avoid hair products that contain isopropyl or ethyl alcohol, which dry the hair.

• **Hair loss:** Massage will have a stimulating effect, speeding up the delivery of nutrients to the roots and hair shaft and encouraging new hair growth.

▷ Many natural hair treatments can be made safely, economically and simply at home. Fresh herbs are most effective and a wide range of beautifully scented herbs are easy to grow in pots and window boxes.

## natural hair rinses

Hair rinses are simple to make, use fresh, natural ingredients, and are a pleasantly sweet-scented finishing treatment after you have shampooed your hair.

### lemon verbena rinse

This rinse fragrances your hair and stimulates the pores and circulation of the scalp. Lemon verbena is easy to grow in the garden.

Put a handful of lemon verbena leaves in a bowl and pour 250ml/8fl oz/1 cup boiling water over them. Infuse for an hour. Strain and discard the leaves. Pour over your hair after conditioning.

### geranium and chamomile condition rinse

Chamomile flowers will not affect the colour of medium to dark hair, but they will help to brighten naturally fair hair. The geranium flowers add a delightful scent.

▽ Use a natural hair rinse after shampooing to treat and gently fragrance your hair.

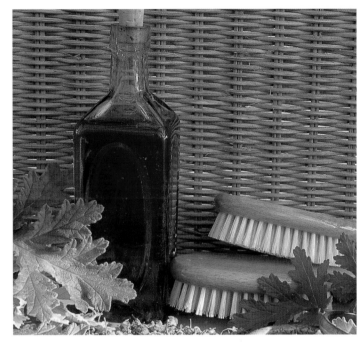

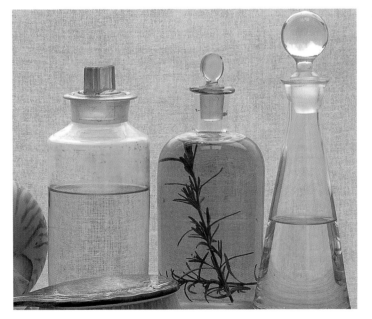

Put 25g/1 oz/$^1$/4 cup of chamomile flowers in a pan with 600ml/1 pint/2$^1$/2 cups water. Boil and then simmer for 15 minutes. Strain the hot liquid over scented geranium leaves and leave to soak for 30-40 minutes. Strain into a bottle.

### cider vinegar rinse

This traditional country treatment will invigorate your scalp and give your hair a deep, natural shine. This recipe makes enough for one treatment. Mix 250ml/8fl oz/1 cup cider with 1 litre/3$^3$/4 pints/4 cups warm water, and use as a final rinse for your hair. Towel dry, gently comb through and leave to dry naturally.

Other rinses (to use as a finishing treatment after shampooing) can be made up to treat various hair problems. First, make an infusion by placing 30ml/2 tbsp of the fresh herb (see below) in a china or glass bowl. Fresh herbs are best, but if you use dried herbs remember they are stronger so you will need to halve the amount required. Add 475ml/16fl oz/2 cups boiling water, cover and leave to steep for three hours. Strain before using.

**HAIR INFUSIONS**

Make infusions with the following herbs for the specific uses as listed:
- Southernwood to combat grease.
- Nettle to stimulate hair growth.
- Rosemary to prevent static.
- Lavender to soothe a tight scalp.

# Holiday haircare

More damage can be done to the hair during a two-week holiday in the sun than is accrued during the rest of the year. The ultraviolet rays or radiation (UVRs) from sunlight that can cause damage to the skin can also have an adverse effect on the hair, depleting the natural oils and removing moisture. Strong winds whip unprotected hair into a tangle, causing breakage and split ends. Chlorinated and salt water cause colour fading and result in drooping perms.

Hair that is permed or coloured is weakened by chemicals and loses moisture at a faster rate than untreated hair. White hair is particularly susceptible to the effects of the sun because it has lost its natural pigmentation (melanin), which to some degree helps to filter out harmful UVRs.

## out in the midday sun

Protecting the hair from the sun's harmful rays makes as much sense as protecting the skin. Wear a hat or scarf on the beach or use a sun-protective spray to shield the hair from the sun's harmful rays. After a swim, rinse the salt or chlorinated water thoroughly from the hair using plenty of fresh, clean water. If fresh water is not available take some with you in an empty soft drinks bottle or use bottled water.

Sunscreen gels are available for the hair and these offer a good deal of protection. Comb the gel through your hair and leave on all day. Remember to reapply the gel after swimming. Alternatively, use a leave-in conditioner, choosing one that protects the hair against UVRs.

On windy or blustery days keep long hair tied back to prevent tangles. Long hair can also be braided when it is wet and the braid left in all day. When evening comes and you undo the braids you will have a cascade of rippling, pre-Raphaelite curls.

If your hair does get tangled by the wind, untangle it gently by using a wide-toothed comb and work from the ends of the hair up towards the roots.

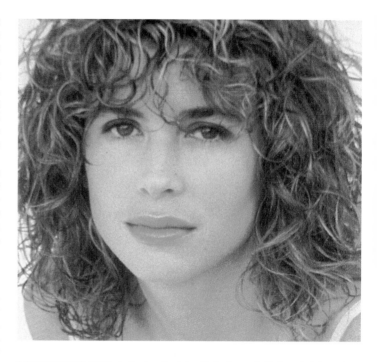

△ Permed hair needs extra protection from the drying effects of sun, salt, chlorine and wind. Use plenty of conditioner and always rinse your hair after swimming. Curl revitalizers help by putting moisture back and keeping curls bouncy.

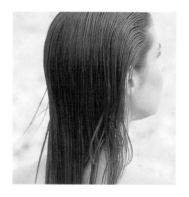

△ After swimming rinse the hair in clean, clear water and comb through with a wide-toothed comb. Use a sun-protection gel with a UVR filter for maximum care.

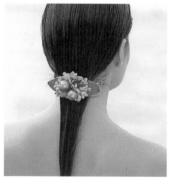

△ To keep the hair in place, clasp it into a pretty clip (barrette). Colourful accessories are great for the beach; take a selection to mix and match with your swimwear.

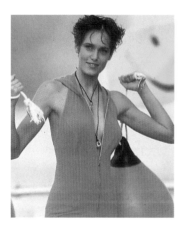

△ Slick short hair back with gel to keep it under control. Leave the gel in all day, then rinse out and style your hair in the evening.

▷ It is often a good idea to plait or braid your hair when you are out in the sea and sun all day. Pinning fresh or silk flowers in the braids will soften and add allure to this practical style.

Keep your head and hair protected even when you are away from the beach. Wear a sun hat when shopping or sightseeing, especially in the middle of the day. When the sun sets, shampoo and condition your hair and, if possible, let it dry naturally. Leave heat styling for those special nights out.

## winter haircare

During the winter, and particularly on a winter break, your hair will be exposed to damaging conditions such as harsh biting winds and the drying effects of low temperatures and central heating. Central heating draws moisture from the hair and scalp, causing static. Extreme cold makes the hair brittle and dry, and wet weather spells disaster for a style, making curly hair frizzy and straight hair limp.

These effects can be counteracted with a few simple measures. To reduce the drying effects of central heating, place large bowls of water near the radiators or use humidifiers. Use a more intensive conditioner on your hair in the winter to combat dryness caused by cold. In damp weather apply a mousse, gel or hairspray; they are invaluable for keeping a style in place and giving some degree of protection.

**BEFORE YOU GO**

• Any hair colouring you are planning should be done at least one week prior to your holiday. This will allow the colour to "soften" and allow time for some intensive conditioning on any dry ends.

• If you want to have a perm before your holiday, book the appointment at least three weeks before departure to allow your hair to settle. You will also have the opportunity to learn how best to manage your new style and help overcome any dryness.

• Remember to pack all your holiday hair needs – your favourite shampoos, conditioners and styling products. And pack a selection of scarves and hair accessories. You will have more time to experiment on holiday.

• If possible take a travel dryer with dual voltage, and remember to pack an adaptor.

• Battery-powered stylers are convenient for holidays but remember to buy several replacements and to carry all the batteries separately from the styler. Airlines do not permit operational electric or battery-powered accessories.

• Soft, bendy rollers are a good alternative to heated ones – they are also kinder to the hair.

• Have a trim before you go, but not a new style, as you won't want to worry about coping with a new look. Whatever you do, don't be tempted to have your hair cut abroad. Wait until you are back home and can visit your regular stylist.

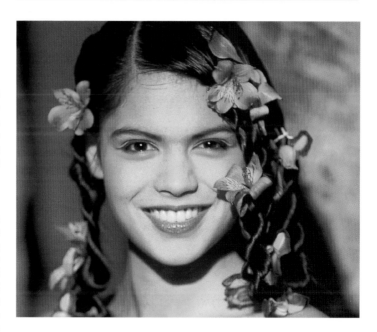

**ON THE PISTE**

• The sun's rays are intensified by reflection from the snow, so hair needs extra protection in the form of a hair sunscreen.

• Wind, blasts of snow, and sunshine are a damaging combination for hair, so wear a hat whenever possible.

• In freezing temperatures hair picks up static electricity, making it flyaway and unmanageable. Calm the static by spraying your brush with hairspray before brushing your hair.

• With sudden temperature changes – from icy-cold slopes to a warm hotel – and constantly changing headgear your hair may need daily shampooing. Use a mild shampoo and light conditioner.

# Colouring and bleaching

Hair colourants have never been technically better; nowadays it is a simple matter to add a temporary tone and gloss to the hair or make a more permanent change. And there is a wide variety of home colouring products from which to choose.

## the choice

Temporary colours are usually water-based and are applied to pre-shampooed, wet hair. They work by coating the outside, or cuticle layer, of the hair. The colour washes away in the next shampoo. Temporary colours are

**COLOUR FACT FILE**
• Colouring swells the hair shaft, making fine hair appear thicker.
• Because colour changes the porosity of the hair it can help combat oiliness.
• Rich tones reflect more light and give hair a thicker appearance.
• Highlights give fine hair extra texture and break up the heaviness of very thick hair.
• Too light a hair colour can make the hair appear thinner.

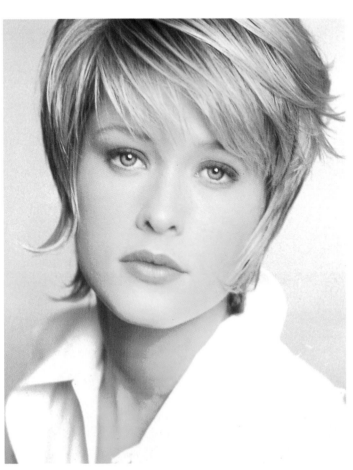

good for a quick, but fleeting, change or for counteracting discolouration in blonde or white hair. Colour-enhanced shampoos combine a wash-out colour with a shampoo. They are similar to temporary colours, are easy to use at home, and are perfect for adding tone to grey, white or bleached hair.

Semi-permanent colours give a more noticeable effect that lasts for six to eight shampoos. They can only add to, enrich, or darken hair colour, they cannot make it any lighter. Semi-permanent colours penetrate the cuticle and coat the outer edge of the cortex (the inner layer of the hair). The colour fades gradually and is ideal for those who want to experiment with colour but don't want to commit themselves to a more permanent change.

Longer-lasting semi-permanent colours remain in the hair for 12-20 shampoos and are perfect for blending in the first grey hairs. The colour penetrates even deeper into the cortex than in semi-permanent colours. This type is perfect for a more lasting change.

Permanent colours lighten or darken, and effectively cover white. The colour enters the cortex during the development time (around 30 minutes) after which oxygen in the developer swells the pigments in the colourant, and holds them in. The roots may need retouching every six weeks. When retouching it is important to colour only the new hair growth. If the new colour overlaps previously treated hair there will be a build-up of colour from the mid-lengths to the ends, which will make the hair more porous.

◁ The model's fine hair was made to look thicker by working fine highlights of different tonal values throughout the hair. The feather cut was then styled forward and blow-dried into shape. A little wax was rubbed between the palms of the hands and applied to the hair with the fingertips to give further definition.

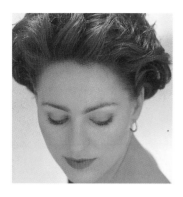

△ These copper tones were achieved by applying a permanent tint; the volume of hair was then increased by using a hot air brush to style the hair away from the face. You can get the same effect by working on one section of the hair at a time. Finish with firm-hold hairspray.

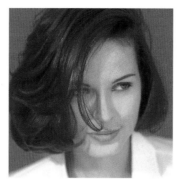

△ Here, reddish hues were created with a longer-lasting semi-permanent colour that added deep tones and luminosity. The hair was blow-dried straight, pointing the nozzle of the dryer downwards in order to polish and encourage the shine.

It is always wise to test the henna you intend to use on a few loose hairs (the ones in your hairbrush will do), noting the length of time it takes to produce the result you want.

Neutral henna can be used to add gloss and lustre to the hair without changing the colour. Mix the henna with water to a stiff paste. Stir in an egg yolk for extra conditioning, plus a little milk to help keep the paste pliable. Apply to the hair and leave for an hour before rinsing. Repeat every two to three months.

## natural colouring – chamomile

Chamomile has a gentle lightening effect on hair and is good for sun-streaking blonde and light brown hair. However, it takes several applications and a good deal of time to produce the desired effect. The advantage of chamomile over chemical bleach is that it never gives a brassy or yellow tone. Best for blonde hair, it will also gently lighten red.

To make a chamomile rinse to use after shampooing, add 30m/2 tbsp dried chamomile flowers to 600ml/1 pint/2$\frac{1}{2}$ cups boiling water. Simmer for 15 minutes, strain and cool before use. For more positive results add 50g/2oz/1 cup dried chamomile flowers to 250ml/8fl oz/1 cup boiling water and leave to steep for 15 minutes. Cool, simmer and strain. Stir in the juice of a fresh lemon along with 30ml/2 tbsp of a rich conditioner. Comb through the hair and leave to dry – in the sun, if possible. Finally, shampoo and condition your hair as usual.

## natural colouring – henna

Vegetable colourants such as henna and chamomile have been used since ancient times to colour hair, and henna was particularly popular with the Ancient Egyptians. Although henna is the most widely used natural dye, others can be extracted from a wide variety of plants, including marigold petals, cloves, rhubarb stalks and even tea leaves. Natural dyes work in much the same way as semi-permanent colourants by staining the outside of the hair. However, results are variable and a residue is often left behind, making further colouring with permanent tints or bleaches inadvisable.

Henna enhances natural highlights, making colour appear richer. It is available today as a powder, which is mixed with water to form a paste. The colour fades gradually but frequent applications will give a stronger, longer-lasting effect. The result that is achieved when using henna depends on the natural colour of the hair. On brunette or black hair it produces a lovely reddish glow, while lighter hair becomes a beautiful titian. Henna will not lighten, and it is not suitable for use on blonde hair. On hair that is more than 20 per cent grey, white, tinted, bleached or highlighted, the resultant colour will be orange.

The longer the henna is left on the hair, the more intense the result. Timings vary from one to two hours, but some Indian women leave henna on the hair for 24 hours, anointing their heads with oil to keep the paste supple.

The condition of the hair being treated is another factor that effects the intensity. The ends of long hair are always slightly lighter than the roots because they are more exposed to the sun, and henna will emphasize this effect. The resulting colour will be darker on the roots to the mid-lengths and more vibrant from the mid-lengths to the ends.

---

**DO'S AND DON'TS**

• Do rinse henna paste thoroughly, or the hair and scalp will feel gritty.

• Don't expose hennaed hair to strong sunlight and always rinse salt and chlorine from the hair immediately after swimming.

• Do use a henna shampoo between colour applications to enhance the tone.

• Don't use shampoos and conditioners containing henna on blonde hair, grey hair or hair that has been chemically treated.

• Do use the same henna product each time you apply henna.

• Don't use compound henna (one that has had metallic salts added); it can cause long-term hair-colouring problems.

---

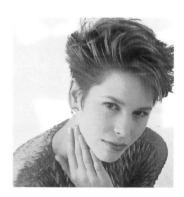

△ Russet tones were further emphasized by weaving a few lighter colours into the front hair. The hair was blow-dried with styling gel to get lift at the roots.

## choosing a new colour

When choosing a colour a basic rule is to keep to one or two shades at each side of your original tone. It is probably best to try a temporary colourant first; if you like the result you can choose a semi-permanent or permanent colourant next time. If you want to be a platinum blonde and you are a natural brunette, you should seek the advice of a professional hairdresser.

There are two important points to remember when considering a change of colour. First, only have a colour change if your hair is in a healthy condition; dry, porous hair absorbs colour too rapidly, and this will lead to a patchy result. Second, your make-up may need changing to suit your new colour.

## special techniques

Hairdressers have devised an array of colouring methods to create different effects. These include:

**Hair painting:** (flying colours) This is where a combination of colours is applied with combs and brushes to the middle lengths and tips of the hair.

**Highlights/lowlights:** Fine strands of hair are bleached or tinted lighter or darker, or colour is added just to give varying tones throughout the hair. This technique is sometimes called frosting or shimmering, particularly when bleach is used to give an overall lighter effect.

▷ There is a wide range of natural tones to choose from when you are looking for a new hair colour. The alternative is to opt for more vibrant fashion shades.

**Slices:** This is a technique where assorted colours are applied through the hair to emphasize a cut and show movement.

## covering white hair

If you just want to cover a few white hairs use a temporary or semi-permanent colour that will last for six to eight weeks. Choose one that is similar to your natural colour. If the hair is brown, applying a warm brown colour will pick out the white areas and give lighter chestnut highlights. Alternatively, henna will give a glossy finish, and at the same time produce stunning red highlights. For salt and pepper hair – hair with a mixed amount of white with the natural colour – try a longer lasting semi-permanent colour. These last for up to 20 shampoos and also add shine.

When hair is completely white it can be covered with a permanent tint, but with this type of colourant it is necessary to update the colour every four to six weeks, a fact that should be taken into consideration before choosing this option. Those who prefer to stay with their natural shade of white can improve on the colour by using toning shampoos, conditioners and styling products, which will remove any brassiness and add beautiful silvery tones.

## caring for coloured hair

Chlorinated and salt water, perspiration and the weather all conspire to fade coloured hair, particularly red hair. However, certain special products are available that will help counteract fading, such as those containing ultraviolet filters that protect coloured hair from the effects of the sun. Other protective measures include always rinsing the hair after you have been swimming, and using a shampoo that is specially designed for coloured hair, followed by a separate conditioner. Gently blot the hair with a towel after shampooing – never rub it vigorously as this ruffles the cuticle and can result in colour "escaping". Finally, use an intensive conditioning treatment at least once a month.

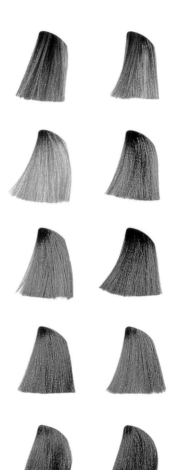

## bleaching

Anything that lightens the hair bleaches it, but here bleaching refers to any treatment that removes colour from the hair – rather than adding colour, which is the purpose of permanent colourants. There are several different types of bleach on the market and they range from the mild brighteners that lift hair colour a couple of shades to the more powerful mixes that completely strip hair of its natural colour.

Bleaching is difficult to do and is best left to a professional hairdresser. To get the best results make sure that your hair is in optimum condition. Once the hair has been bleached, regular intensive conditioning treatments are essential.

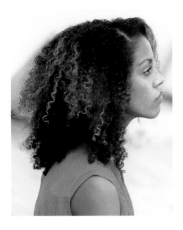

△ Fine strands of tinted or highlighted hair look particularly striking against dark hair.

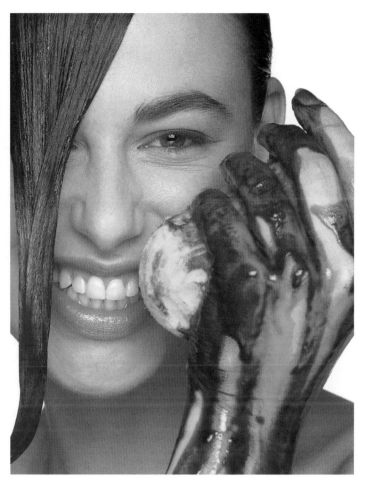

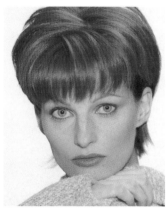

◁ A variety of herbs and other plants have been used in the past to colour hair, and many of them have remained popular to this day. The natural dyes provide a semi-permanent colour, although the results that can be achieved will vary. They depend on the quality of the raw ingredients combined with the natural colour of the hair and how porous it is. Many top hairdressers mix their own vegetable dyes using a wide range of ingredients, as well as using commercial colours.

△ Burnished Titian red tones give one of the most effective results when applied to natural brown hair. However reddish hues are particularly prone to fading so protect coloured hair from the sun. Specialized shampoos and conditioners should be used to help maintain colour.

**FACT FILE**

In the Middle Ages saffron and a mixture of sulphur, alum and honey were used for bleaching and colouring hair. These concoctions were not always safe however, and in 1562 a certain Dr Marinello from Moderna, Italy, wrote a treatise warning of the possible and extremely undesirable consequences of bleaching the hair in this way. He warned: "The scalp could be seriously damaged and the hair be destroyed at the roots and fall out."

## colour correction

If you have been colouring your hair for some time and want to go back to your natural colour and tone, consult a professional hairdresser. Hair that has been tinted darker than its normal shade will have to be colour-stripped with a bleach bath until the desired colour is achieved. Hair that has been bleached or highlighted will need to be re-pigmented and then tinted to match the original colour. For best results, all these processes must be carried out in a salon where the technicians have access to a variety of special products, and the expertise to use them properly.

## helpful hints for home hair-colouring

Always read the directions supplied with the product before you start your treatment, and follow them precisely. Make sure you do a strand and skin sensitivity test, as detailed in the directions.

If you are retouching the roots of tinted or bleached hair, apply new colour only to the regrowth area. Any overlap results in uneven colour and porosity, which may adversely affect the condition of your hair.

Don't colour your hair at home if the hair is split or visibly damaged, or if you have used bleach or any type of henna; you must allow previously treated hair to grow out before applying new colour. Avoid colouring your hair if you are taking prescribed drugs, as the chemical balance of your hair can alter. Check with your doctor first.

If your hair has been permed it is advisable to consult a hairdresser before using a hair colourant. And if you are in any doubt about using a colour, always check with the manufacturer or consult a professional hair colourist.

# Permanent solutions

Making straight hair curly is not a new idea. Women in Ancient Egypt coated their hair in mud, wound it around wooden rods and then used the heat from the sun to create the curls.

Waves that won't wash out are a more recent innovation. Modern perms were pioneered by A. F. Willat, who invented the "cold permanent wave" technique in 1934. Since then, improved formulations and evermore sophisticated techniques have made perms the most versatile styling option in hairdressing.

## how perms work

Perms work by breaking down inner structures (links) in your hair and re-forming them around a curler to give a new shape. Hair should be washed prior to perming as this causes the scales on the cuticles to rise gently, allowing the perming lotion to enter the hair shaft more quickly. The perming lotion alters the keratin and breaks down the sulphur bonds that link the fibre-like cells together in the inner layers of each hair. When these fibres have become loose, they can be formed into a new shape when the hair is stretched over a curler or perming rod.

Once the curlers or rods are in place, more lotion is applied and the perm is left to develop to fix the new shape. The development time varies according to the condition and texture of the hair. When the development is complete, the changed links in the hair are re-formed into their new shape by the application of a second chemical known as the neutralizer. The neutralizer contains an oxidizing agent that is effectively responsible for closing up the broken links and producing the wave or curl – permanently.

The type of curl that is produced depends on a number of factors. The size of the curler is perhaps the most important as this determines the size of the curl. Generally speaking the smaller the curler the smaller and therefore tighter the curl, whereas medium to large curlers tend to give a much

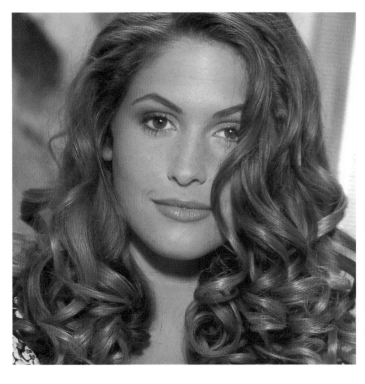

△ **Specialist formulations enable your hairdresser to perm long hair while maintaining it in optimum condition. Here the hair was wound on to large rods to achieve soft curls.**

looser effect. The strength of lotion can also make a difference, as can the texture and type of hair. Hair in good condition takes a perm much better than hair in poor condition, and fine hair curls more easily than coarse hair.

After a perm it takes 48 hours for the keratin in the hair to harden naturally. At this time the hair is vulnerable to damage and must be treated with care. Resist shampooing, brushing or combing, blow-drying or setting, which may cause the perm to drop.

Once hair has been permed it remains curly and shaped the way it has been formed, although new growth will be straight. As time goes by the curl can soften, and if the hair is long its weight may make the curl and the wave appear much looser.

## home versus salon

Perming is such a delicate, and potentially hazardous operation that the majority of women prefer to leave it in the hands of experienced professional hairdressers. The advantages of having hair permed in a salon are several. The hair is first analysed to find out whether it is in good enough condition to take a perm; coloured, out-of-condition or over-processed hair may well be damaged even more by a perm. With a perm carried out by a professional there is also a greater variety in the type of curl and texture you can choose – different strengths of lotion and different winding techniques all give a range of curls that are not generally available in home perms.

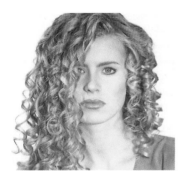

△ Spiral perming gives a ringlet effect on long hair. It is important with hair of this length to re-perm only at the roots when the hair grows, or you may cause damage to previously permed hair.

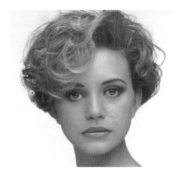

△ A soft perm gives volume to short hair. Set the hair on rollers to achieve the maximum amount of lift, and to give extra height and body to short hair.

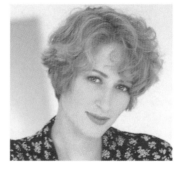

△ Tinted hair can also be permed if the correct formulation is chosen. Your stylist will be able to advise you on the formulation that is most suitable for you.

## home rules

If you do use a perm at home, it is essential that you read the instructions that are supplied with the product and that you follow them very carefully. Remember to do a test curl to check whether your hair is suitable, and check to make certain you have enough curlers. You will probably want to enlist the help of a friend, as it is impossible to curl the back sections of your own hair properly, so you will definitely need a helping hand.

Timing is crucial – don't be tempted to remove the lotion before the time given or leave it on longer than directed.

## salon perms – the choices

Professional hairdressers can offer a number of different types of perm that are not available for home use:

**Acid perms:** These produce highly conditioned, flexible curls. Ideally suited to hair that is fine, sensitive, fragile, damaged or tinted, they have a mildly acidic action that minimizes the risk of hair damage.

**Alkaline perms:** These give strong, firm curl results on normal and resistant hair.

**Exothermic perms:** For bouncy, resilient curls, "exothermic" refers to the gentle heat that is produced by the chemical reaction that occurs when the lotion is mixed. The heat allows the lotion to penetrate the hair cuticle, which will have the effect of conditioning and strengthening the hair from inside as the lotion moulds the hair into its new shape.

## perming techniques

Any of the above types of perm can be used with different techniques to produce a number of results.

**Body perms:** These are soft, loose perms created using large curlers, or sometimes rollers. They add volume with a hint of wave and movement rather than curls.

**Root perms:** These add lift and volume to the root area only. They will add height and fullness, and are therefore ideal for short hair that tends to go flat.

**POST-PERM TIPS**

- Don't wash newly permed hair for 48 hours after processing as any stress can cause curls to relax.
- Use shampoos and conditioners formulated for permed hair. They help retain the correct moisture balance and prolong the perm.
- Always use a wide-toothed comb and work from the ends upwards. Never brush the hair.
- Blot wet hair dry before it is styled to help prevent stretching.
- Avoid using too much heat on permed hair. If possible, wash, condition and then leave it to dry naturally.
- If your perm has lost its bounce, mist with water or try a curl reviver. These are designed to put instant volume and bounce into permed hair. They are also ideal for eliminating frizziness on naturally curly hair.
- Expect your perm to last three to six months, depending on the technique and lotion used.

**Pin curl perms:** These give soft, natural waves and curls, achieved by perming small sections of hair that have been pinned into pre-formed curls.

**Stack perms:** This perm gives curl and volume to one-length hair by means of different-sized curlers. The hair on top of the head is left unpermed while the middle and ends have curl and movement.

**Spiral perms:** These create romantic spiral curls, an effect produced by winding the hair around special long curlers. The mass of curls makes long hair look much thicker.

**Spot perms:** These give support on the area to which they are applied. For example, if the hair needs lift, the perm is applied just on the crown. They can also be used on the fringe (bangs) or side areas around the face.

**Weave perms:** These involve perming sections of hair and leaving the rest straight to give a mixture of texture and natural-looking body and bounce, particularly on areas around the face such as the fringe.

## regrowth problem

When a perm is growing out, the areas of new growth can be permed if a barrier is created between old and new growth. The barrier can be a special cream or a plastic protector, both of which effectively prevent the perming lotion and neutralizer from touching previously permed areas.

There are also products that facilitate re-perming the length of hair without damaging the structure. These complex solutions are available only from salons.

# Black hair

Black hair is fragile yet difficult to control, therefore it needs specialist care and pampering if it is to look its best.

This type of hair is almost always curly, although the degree of wave varies enormously. As a general rule, it is brittle and has a tendency to split and break. This is because the sebaceous glands produce insufficient sebum to moisturize the hair. In addition, because the hair is tightly curled, the sebum is unable to travel downwards to condition it naturally. If the curl forms kinks, this makes the hair thinner, and therefore weaker, at each bend.

Other types of black hair (such as Asian, Indian and Native American) can be very fine, making it difficult to style and set.

To treat excessive dryness choose a specialist formulation that replaces the natural oils lacking in black hair. If the product is massaged in daily, or whenever necessary, the hair will become more manageable with improved condition and shine. It is also important to deep-condition the hair regularly.

## hair straightening

Straightening, or relaxing, is in fact perming in reverse. A hair straightener, also known as a chemical relaxer, is combed or worked through the hair to change the structure and to straighten it. The result is permanent, only disappearing as the hair grows. Chemical relaxers come in different strengths to suit different hair textures and styles. They are particularly effective on longer styles as the weight of the hair helps to maintain the straightened look. If you do this at home get advice first, and make sure you use high-quality branded products and follow the instructions precisely to achieve the best results.

> **PROFESSIONAL TIP**
> Hair needs to be strong and healthy to take any type of chemical treatment. To check hair strength and natural elasticity, pluck out a hair and hold it firmly between the fingers of both hands, then pull gently. If the hair breaks with hardly any stretching, it is weak and in poor condition, in which case all chemical treatments should be avoided.

## demi perming

Extremely curly hair can also be tamed by perming. This enables tight curls to be transformed into larger, looser ones. Demi-perms are particularly good for short hair, giving a more controlled, manageable shape; on long hair they produce a softer, bouncier effect. The more advanced perms involve softening the hair by weaving it on

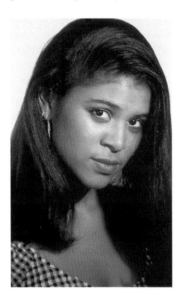

△ Hair that has been straightened is blow-dried using a vent brush to make it smooth. Hair straighteners could also be used to achieve a similarly smooth effect.

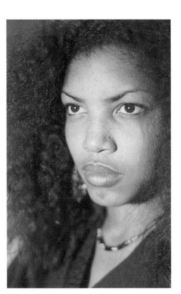

△ Before: Long, thick natural hair can be totally transformed with the technique known as weaving. The hair is corn-row braided and then weaves are sewn on to the braided base.

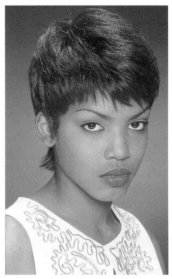

△ After: Once the weave has been sewn into place, the new hair is cut and styled as desired. The result of all this work is a completely different look.

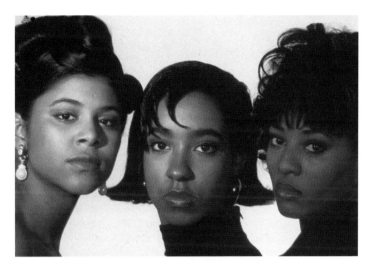

to rollers and then neutralizing it so that the curls are permanently set into their new shape.

To prevent frizziness and maintain the shape and definition of curls, special lotions called curl activators and moisturizing sprays can be used to revive and preserve the formation of curls.

As with all chemical treatments, relaxing and perming can be harmful and damaging to the hair. This is because it removes natural moisture and leaves the hair in a weakened state. For this reason it is always advisable to obtain skilled professional help and advice.

## hot combs

Before chemical relaxers became available the most popular hair-straightening method was "hot pressing". This involved putting a pre-heated iron comb through the hair to loosen the curls. Up-to-date versions, known as thermal texturizers, are electric pressing combs, which work in a similar way to loosen and soften very curly hair.

## colour options

Because of its natural dryness and porosity, black hair should be coloured with caution. If you still want to colour your hair it should be carried out by a professional hairdresser who will be able to advise you properly. If the hair has been straightened, relaxed or permed it may simply be too weak to colour successfully. Techniques such as highlighting, lowlighting or tipping the ends are best for this type of hair.

△ **After straightening or relaxing, black hair can be styled smooth using blow-drying techniques.**
*Left:* **The hair has been smoothed into curls.**
*Centre:* **Here it has been flicked up at the ends and the fringe curved.**
*Right:* **For this style it was piled into soft curls and given a fuller fringe (bangs).**

## special problems

Traction hair loss is caused by braiding or weaving the hair too tightly. If the hair is pulled too forcibly too often, it disrupts the hair follicles, causes scar tissue to form and, ultimately, could result in hair loss. If you are thinking of having your hair straightened it is important to go to a reputable salon.

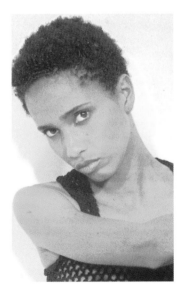

△ **One of the most effective ways of styling very curly hair is to crop it close and short. With this type of cut you just need to shampoo, condition and finish with soft wax.**

**KEEPING BLACK HAIR BEAUTIFUL**
• Use a wide-toothed afro comb for curly hair and a natural bristle brush for relaxed hair. Combing will help spread the natural oils through the hair, making it look shinier and healthier. Use intensive pre-shampoo treatments.
• Massage the scalp regularly to encourage oil production.
• Shampoo as often as you feel necessary but only lather once, using a small amount of shampoo. Rinse thoroughly. Towel-blot, don't rub hair.
• Once a month try a hot oil treatment, which will lubricate dry scalp conditions as well as moisturize brittle hair.
• If you have delicate baby-fine hair around the hairline (sometimes from breakage, sometimes an inherited trait), use a tiny round brush and a hairdryer to blend in this hair.
• Gels are good for moulding black hair into shape: choose non-oily formulas that give hair a healthy sheen.
• If you use hot combs or curling tongs, make sure you shield the hair by using a protective product.
• For extra hold and added shine use a finishing spray.
• Braided hair needs a softening shampoo that maintains the moisture balance and helps to treat and even eliminate a dry scalp.

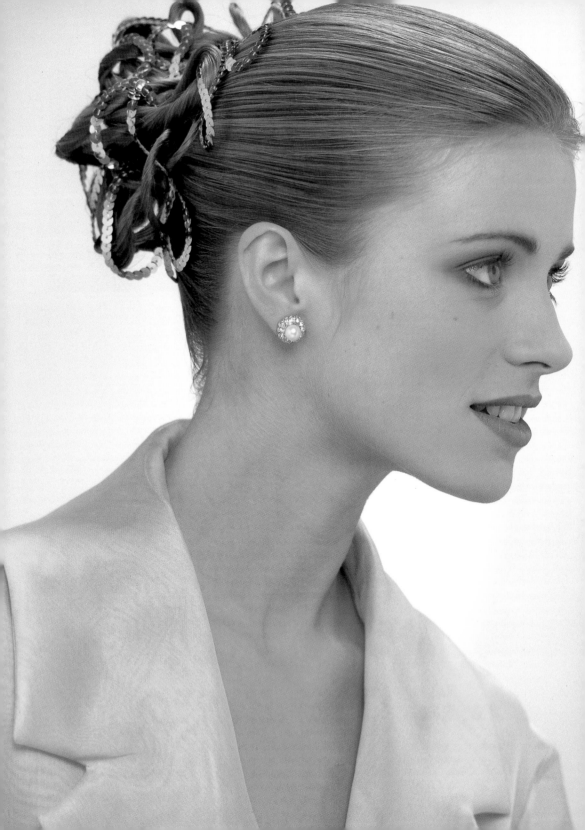

# Choosing a Style

Successful styling means choosing a hairstyle that suits your looks and lifestyle, and then learning the techniques that will ensure a perfect finish. There is an enormous range of gadgets, hair products and heated styling equipment available, all of which, if used properly, can effect wonderful transformations. The trick is to know what to use and when in order to achieve the desired results. Here we show you how.

# Choosing a style to suit your face

Make the most of your looks by choosing a style that maximizes your best features. The first feature you should consider is the shape of your face – is it round, oval, square or long? If you are not sure what shape your face is, the easiest way to find out is to scrape your hair away from your face so that you can see all your features clearly. Stand squarely in front of a mirror and use a lipstick to trace around the outline of your face so that the shape is transferred to the mirror. When you stand back you should be able to see into which of the following categories your face shape falls.

## the square face

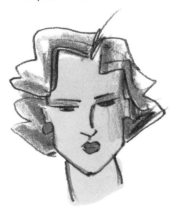

The square face is angular with a broad forehead and a square jawline. To make the best of this shape, choose a hairstyle with long layers, preferably one that features soft waves or curls. This will create a softness that detracts from the hard lines particularly around the jaw. The hair should be parted at the side of the head and any fringe (bangs) combed away from the face.
**Styles to avoid:** Very severe geometric cuts – they will only have the effect of emphasizing the squareness of your face; long bobs with a heavy fringe; severe styles in which the hair is scraped off the face and with a parting down the centre.

## the round face

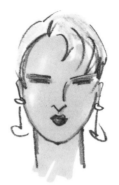

On the round face the distance between the forehead and the chin is about equal to the distance between the cheeks. Choose a style with a short fringe, which lengthens the face, and a short cut, which makes the face look thinner.
**Styles to avoid:** Curly, because they will draw attention to the roundness; very full, long hair; styles that are pulled right back off the face.

## the oval face

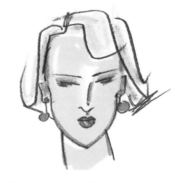

The oval face has wide cheekbones that taper down into a small, often pointed, chin and up to a fairly narrow forehead. This is regarded by many experts as the perfect face shape. If your face is oval in shape then you have the advantage of being able to wear any hairstyle you choose.

## the long face

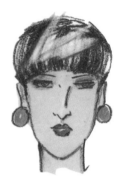

A long face is characterized by a high forehead and long chin, and needs to be given the illusion of width. Soften the effect with short layers, or go for a bob with a fringe to create horizontal lines. Scrunch-dried or curly bobs balance a long face.
**Styles to avoid:** Styles without a fringe; long, straight, blunt cuts.

## the complete you

When choosing a new style you should also take into account your overall body shape. If you are a traditional pear-shape don't go for elfin styles; they will draw attention to the lower half of your body, making your hips look even wider. Petite women should avoid masses of very curly hair as this makes the head appear large and out of proportion with the body.

**IF YOU WEAR GLASSES . . .**
Try to choose frames and a hairstyle that complement each other. Large spectacles could spoil a neat, feathery cut, and very fine frames could be overpowered by a large, voluminous style. Remember to take your glasses to the salon when having your hair restyled, so that your stylist can take their shape into consideration when deciding on the overall effect.

## SPECIFIC PROBLEMS

- Prominent nose: incorporate softness into your style.
- Pointed chin: style hair with width at the jawline.
- Low forehead: choose a style with a wispy fringe, rather than one with a full fringe.
- High forehead: disguise with a fringe.
- Receding chin: select a style that comes to just below chin level, with waves or curls.
- Uneven hairline: fringes should conceal this problem.

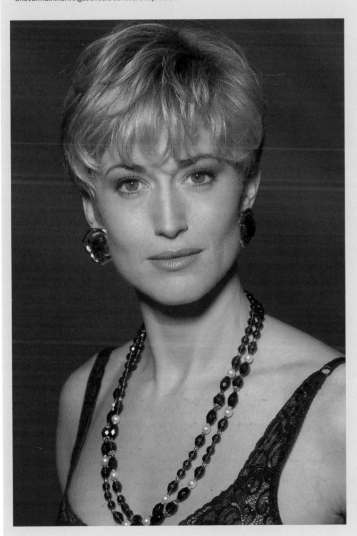

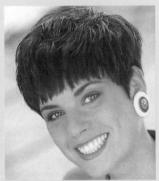

△ A high forehead or uneven hairline can be hidden under a fringe.

◁ A wispy fringe stylishly disguises a low forehead.

▽ Strong features benefit from a soft, full hairstyle.

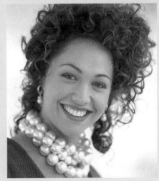

# Style gallery, short hair

Short hair is usually easier to maintain but it does need more regular cutting. It can be cut close to the shape of the head, cropped or layered in a variety of styles. Generally a short cut will make the face look thinner.

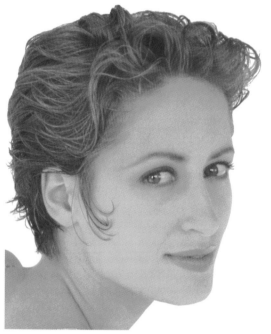

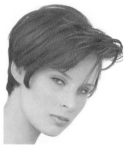

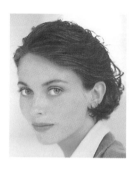

△ Fine, straight hair was lightly layered and cut close into the nape. A root perm provided extra volume at the crown of the head. The hair was then finger-dried using a styling mousse.

△ Naturally wavy hair was cut into a one-length bob and taken behind the ears, using wet-look gel to give definition and accentuate the waves.

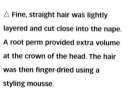

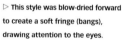

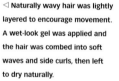

▷ This style was blow-dried forward to create a soft fringe (bangs), drawing attention to the eyes.

◁ Naturally wavy hair was lightly layered to encourage movement. A wet-look gel was applied and the hair was combed into soft waves and side curls, then left to dry naturally.

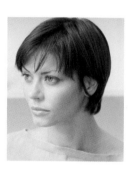

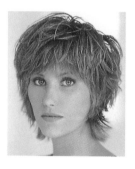

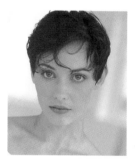

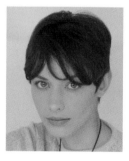

△ Thick hair was feather-cut into layers, with slightly longer lengths left at the nape. The hair was highlighted and then blow-dried into shape using a styling brush.

△ For a different look the hair was combed down over the ears.

△ Fine hair was softly layered and given an application of mousse, then ruffle-dried with the fingers to create just a little lift at the roots.

△ The same haircut was blow-dried forwards using a styling brush.

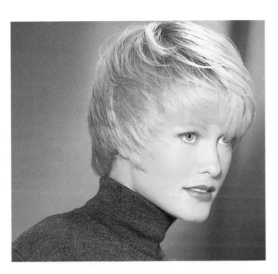

◁ Medium-textured hair was cut into layers of the same length, then blow-dried using a strong-hold mousse to get lift, and finished with a mist of firm-hold hairspray.

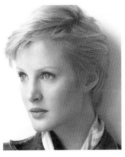

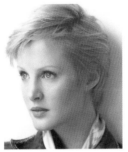

△ Choppy layers give an uneven texture to this thick hair. The hair was blow-dried using mousse and a styling brush to create lift.

△ A root perm helped to give lift at the crown on this short, layered look. Mousse was applied to give extra lift and the hair was blow-dried forwards from the crown.

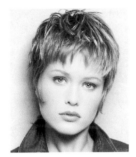

△ A short cut was given extra interest by bleaching the hair honey-blonde. It was then blow-dried into shape and finished using wax to create separation.

△ A short, urchin cut is good for all hair textures. Highlights give extra interest and add thickness to finer hair.

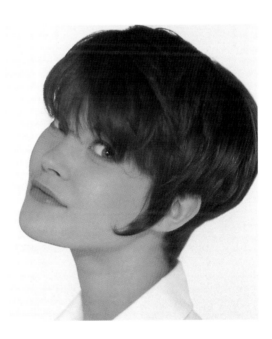

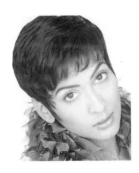

△ Very curly, wiry hair was cropped close to the head, then dressed using just a little wax to give definition and separation.

△ Very straight hair was cut into a neat, face-framing shape, then blow-dried forwards. It was finished with a mist of shine spray for added gloss.

△ Medium-textured hair was graduated to give this head-hugging cut. Mousse was applied from the roots to the ends, then the hair was blow-dried forwards from the crown.

# Style gallery, mid-length hair

Hair of medium length has the advantage of being a little more versatile, because it can be worn in a smooth, sleek bob or lightly layered to allow for more variety in styling.

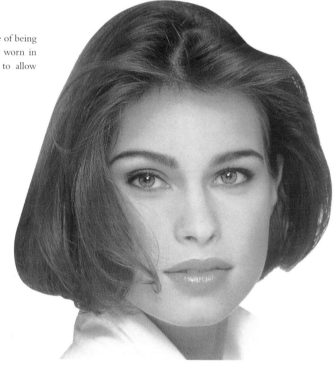

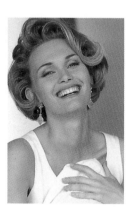

△ Medium-textured hair was cut into a one-length bob. Styling spray was applied to partially dried hair, which was then wound on large rollers and heat set. After the rollers were removed the hair was brushed into shape.

△ Fine mid-length hair can be made to look thicker by blunt cutting just below ear level. This style can be roller-set and brushed through with a bristle brush to smooth, or simply blow-dried with a round brush.

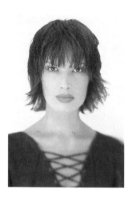

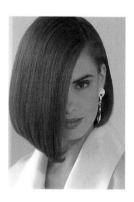

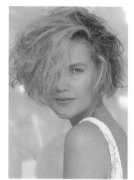

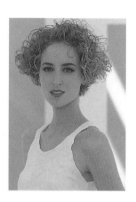

△ Layering gives this 70s-inspired style a fresh look. The hair was misted with styling spray and rough-dried before finishing with a little gloss.

△ This longer, one-length, graduated bob is perfect for thick, straight hair. Add extra shine by using a longer-lasting semi-permanent colour.

△ A mid-length bleached bob was scrunch-dried with mousse to give a tousled look. Use a diffuser to encourage more volume.

△ This layered cut was permed to give plenty of movement. The hair was scrunch-dried and styled, with the head held forward to give maximum volume.

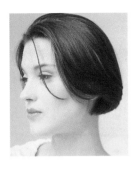

△ A soft body perm gives volume to this one-length bob. The hair was gently dried using mousse for additional lift.

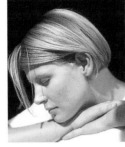

△ Thick, straight hair was heavily highlighted and cut into a blunt, short bob. Either blow-dry or leave to dry naturally.

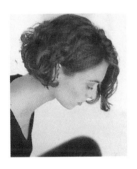

△ Natural movement was encouraged by blunt cutting and leaving the hair to dry naturally. Alternatively, the hair could be dried using a flat diffuser attachment on the dryer.

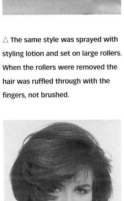

△ The same style was sprayed with styling lotion and set on large rollers. When the rollers were removed the hair was ruffled through with the fingers, not brushed.

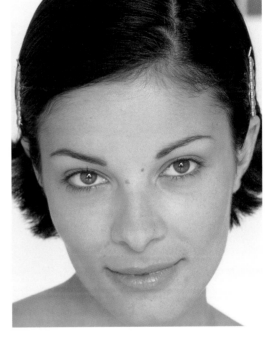

△ This fine straight hair has been cut in a simple short bob that is easy to style but can also be left to dry naturally.

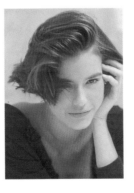

△ A bob was highlighted using a light, golden-blonde colour to give natural, warm lights, then styled and blow-dried using a soft sculpting spray.

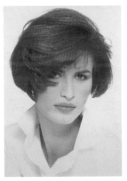

△ A razor-cut bob gives graduation so the hair moves freely. The hair was coloured with a shade of mahogany to give more depth, and then blow-dried using mousse.

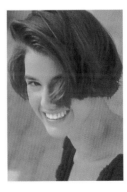

△ Thick hair was cut into a bob, then sprayed with styling lotion before setting on large rollers. After drying, the hair was brushed through to give a smooth style.

△ The same cut was blow-dried smooth using a styling brush.

# Style gallery, long hair

Long locks are particularly versatile and can be transformed into a fabulous range of styles using different techniques. They can be waved, curled, straightened or left to fall free.

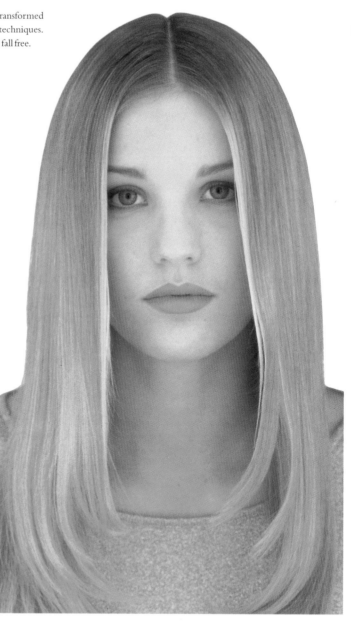

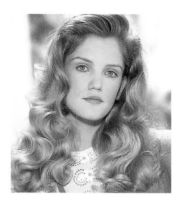

△ Naturally wavy hair was roller-set and heat-dried, then brushed through lightly. A similar look could be achieved with a soft perm.

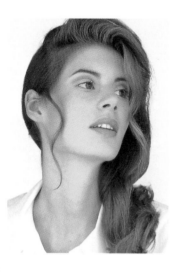

△ After an application of styling spray the hair was set on large rollers. When dry the hair was combed to one side and allowed to fall into soft waves, with a tiny tendril pulled in front of one ear.

△ Straight hair was graduated at the sides to give interest. It was then shampooed and conditioned, and left to dry naturally.

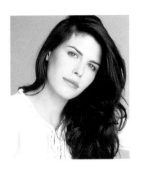

△ A vegetable colour adds depth and makes hair appear even thicker. The hair was then simply styled by blow-drying.

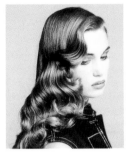

△ Soft, undulating waves were achieved by tonging the hair, then lightly combing it through. Spray shine was applied to the finish.

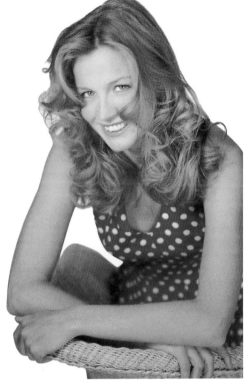

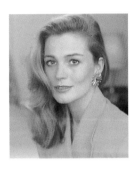

△ Mousse was applied to rough-dried hair, which was then set on heated rollers. The hair was then brushed through into soft waves.

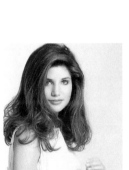

△ This alternative style was achieved by tonging. It could also be set on shapers.

△ Naturally wavy hair was lightly layered, then set on large rollers. When the hair was dry it was brushed lightly to give broken up-waves and curls.

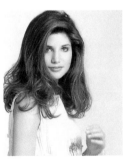

△ Thick hair was cut with graduated sides and a heavy fringe to give this 60s look. The hair can be blow-dried smooth or left to dry naturally.

△ Setting lotion was applied to clean hair, which was set on large rollers and heat-dried. When the hair was completely dry the rollers were removed and the hair gently back-combed at the roots to give even more height and fullness.

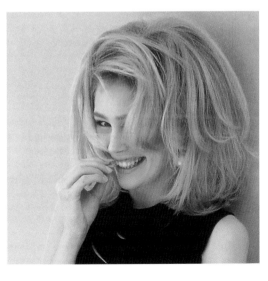

△ A thick graduated cut was given maximum lift by spraying the roots with gel spray and backcombing lightly, then brushing over the top layers.

# more sleek looks for long hair

One of the most important aspects of having long hair is keeping it in good condition, sleek and glossy, but once you have cracked that, long locks provide a wealth of opportunities when it comes to impeccable styling and making an impact.

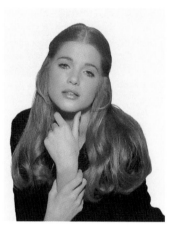

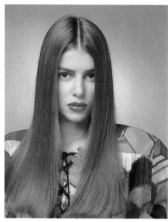

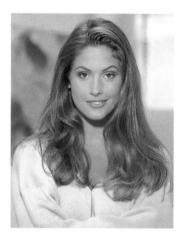

△ The hair was sprayed with styling lotion and set on heated rollers. When it was dry a bristle brush was used to smooth it into waves.

△ Straight hair was blunt-cut at the ends and simply styled from a centre parting.

△ To give one-length hair extra body the head was tipped forwards and the hair misted with sculpting lotion. The roots were scrunched a little with the hands before straightening the head.

# take one girl

The following styles illustrate how one-length hair can be transformed using different styling techniques.

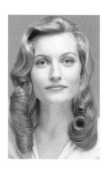

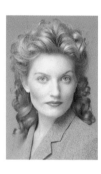

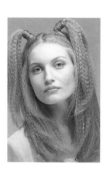

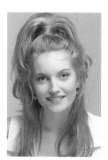

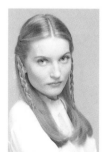

△ **1** Soft waves were created with rollers.

△ **2** The top hair was clipped up and the back hair tonged into tendrils.

△ **3** High bunches were carefully secured and the hair crimped.

△ **4** The top hair was secured on the crown. A band was wrapped with a small piece of hair and the length allowed to fall freely.

△ **5** The hair was clipped back and two simple braids were worked at each side.

# Style gallery, long hair for special occasions

These styles will inspire you when you want to transform your long hair for a glamorous party or special event.

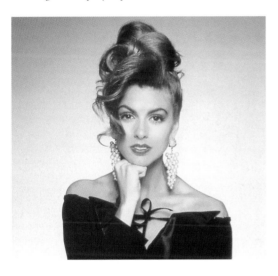

△ The hair was softly scooped into large curls and pinned in place. One tendril was left to fall free to soften the style.

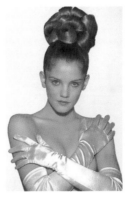

△ The hair was secured in a very high ponytail on the crown, then divided into sections and looped into curls. If your hair isn't long enough for this style, you could use a hairpiece.

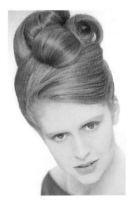

△ Vibrant blonde and copper lights add brilliance to the hair. The front hair was sectioned off and the back hair secured in a high ponytail. The hair was then divided and coiled into loops before pinning in place. The front hair was smoothed over and secured at the back.

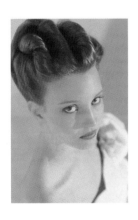

△ The foundation for this style came from a roller-set. The back hair was then formed into a French pleat and the top hair looped, curled and pinned into place.

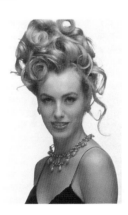

△ Very curly hair was simply twisted up at the back and secured with pins. Curls were allowed to fall down on one side to give a feminine look.

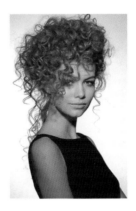

△ Long hair was scooped up, but the essence of this style is to allow lots of strands to fall in soft curls around the face.

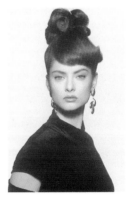

△ A high ponytail forms the basis of this style. The hair was then looped into curls and pinned, and the fringe (bangs) was combed to one side.

# Styling tools

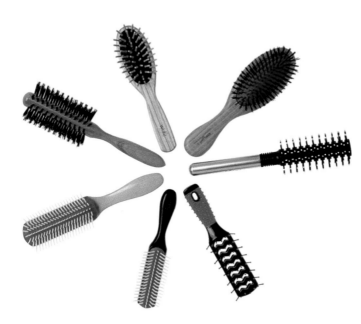

Brushes, combs and pins are the basic tools of styling. The following is a guide to help you choose what is most suitable from the wide range that is available.

## brushes

These are made of bristles (sometimes called quills or pins), which may be natural hog bristle, plastic, nylon or wire. The bristles are embedded in a wooden, plastic or moulded rubber base and set in tufts or rows. This allows loose or shed hair to collect in the grooves without interfering with the action of the bristles. The spacing of the tufts plays an important role – generally, the wider the spacing between the rows of bristles, the easier the brush will flow through the hair.

### the role of brushing

Brushes help to remove tangles and knots to smooth the hair. The action of brushing from the roots to the ends removes dead skin cells and dirt, and encourages the cuticles to lie flat, thus reflecting the light. Brushing also stimulates the blood supply to the hair follicles, promoting healthy growth.

△ **Choosing the right tools not only makes hairstyling fun, but also makes it much easier.**

### natural bristles

These bristles are produced from natural keratin (the same material as hair) and therefore create less friction and wear on the hair. They are good for grooming and polishing, and help to combat static on flyaway hair. However, they will not penetrate wet or thick hair and you must

use a softer bristle brush for fine or thinning hair. In addition, the sharp ends can scratch the scalp.

### plastic, nylon or wire bristles

These bristles are easily cleaned and heat resistant, so they are good for blow-drying. They are available in a variety of shapes and styles. Cushioned brushes give good flexibility as they glide through the hair, preventing tugging and helping to remove knots. They are also non-static.

A major disadvantage is that the ends can be harsh, so try to choose bristles with rounded or ball tips.

## types of brush

**Circular or radial brushes:** These come in a variety of sizes and are circular or semi-circular in shape. These brushes have either mixed bristles for finishing, a rubber pad with nylon bristles, or metal pins for styling. They are used to tame and control naturally curly, permed and wavy hair and are ideal for blow-drying. The diameter of the brush determines the resulting volume and movement, in much the same way as the size of rollers do.

**Flat or half-round brushes:** They are ideal for wet or dry hairstyling and blow-drying. Normally they are made of nylon bristles in a rubber base. Some bases slide into position on to the plastic moulded handle. Rubber bases can be removed for cleaning and replacement bristles are sometimes available.

**Pneumatic brushes:** These have a domed rubber base with bristles set in tufts. They can be plastic, natural bristle, or both.

**Vent brushes:** All these have hollow centres allowing the air-flow from the dryer to pass through the brush. Special bristle, or pin, patterns are designed to lift and disentangle

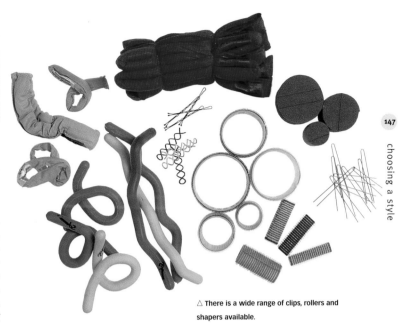

△ **There is a wide range of clips, rollers and shapers available.**

even wet hair. Vents and tunnel brush heads enable the air to circulate freely through both the brush and the hair so the hair dries faster.

## combs

It is advisable to choose good-quality combs with saw-cut teeth. This means that each individual tooth is cut into the comb, so there are no sharp edges that will damage your hair. Avoid cheap plastic combs that are made in a mold and so form lines down the centre of every tooth. They are sharp, and gradually scrape away the cuticle layers of the hair, causing damage and often breakage.

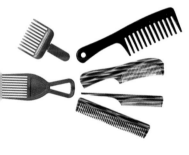

△ **A wide-toothed comb is ideal for disentangling and combing conditioner through the hair. Fine tail-combs are for styling. Afro combs are specially designed for curly hair.**

## pins and clips

These are indispensable for sectioning and securing hair during setting, and for putting hair up. Most pins are available with untipped, plain ends, or cushion-tipped ends. Non-reflective finishes are available, so the pins are less noticeable in the hair, and most are made of metal, plastic or stainless steel. Colours include brown, black, grey, blonde, white and silver.

**Double-pronged grips:** These are most frequently used for making pin or barrel curls. Grips give security to curls, French

pleats and all upswept styles. In North America they are known as "Bobby" pins, in Britain as "Kirbies". To avoid discomfort, position grips in the hair so that the flat edge rests towards the scalp.

**Heavy hairpins:** Made of strong metal, they are either waved or straight. These are ideal for securing rollers in place and when putting hair up.

**Fine hairpins:** Used for dressing hair, they are delicate and prone to bend out of shape, so they should be used to secure only small amounts of hair. These pins are easily concealed, especially if you use a matching colour. They are sometimes used to secure pin curls during setting, rather than heavier clips which can leave a mark.

**Sectioning clips:** These are clips with a single prong, and are longer in length than other clips. They are most often used for holding hair while working on another section, or for securing pin curls.

**Twisted pins:** Shaped like a screw, they are used to secure chignons and French pleats.

## rollers

These invaluable styling tools vary in diameter, length and the material from which they are made. Smooth rollers, that is those without spikes or brushes, will give the sleekest finish, but they are more difficult to

put in. More popular are brush rollers, especially the self-fixing variety that do not need pins or clips.

## shapers

These soft styling devices were inspired by the principle of rag-rolling hair. Soft "twist tie" rollers are made from pliable rubber, plastic or cotton fabric and provide one of the more natural ways to curl hair. In the centre of each roller is a tempered wire, which enables it to be bent into shape. The waves or curls that are produced are soft and bouncy and the technique is gentle enough for permed or tinted hair.

To use, section clean, dry hair and pull to a firm tension, "trapping" the end in a roller that you have previously doubled over. Roll down to the roots of the hair and fold over to secure. Leave in for 30–60 minutes without heat, or for 10–15 minutes if you apply heat. If you twist the hair before curling you will achieve a more voluminous style.

# Style easy

The combination of practice and the right styling products enables you to achieve a salon finish at home. The products listed below enable you to do it in style.

## gels

Sometimes called sculpting lotions and used for precise styling, gels come in varying degrees of viscosity, from a thick jelly to a liquid spray. Use them to lift roots, tame wisps, create tendrils, calm static, heat set and give structure to curls. Wet gel can be used for sculpting styles.

**GEL TIP**

A gel can be revitalized the following day by running wet fingers through the hair, against the direction of the finished look.

## hairspray

Traditionally, hairspray was used to hold a style in place; today, varying degrees of stiffness are available to suit all needs. Use hairspray to keep the hair in place, get curl definition when scrunching, and mist over rollers when setting.

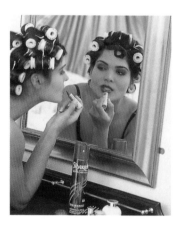

△ Hairsprays are available in a variety of formulations, including light and firm holds.

**HAIRSPRAY TIPS**

• A light application of spray on a hairbrush can be used to tame flyaway ends.

• Use hairspray at the roots and tong or blow-dry the area to get immediate lift.

## mousse

The most versatile styling product, mousse comes as a foam and can be used on wet or dry hair. Mousses contain conditioning agents and proteins to nurture and protect the hair. They are available in different strengths, designed to give soft to maximum holding power, and can be used to lift flat roots or smooth frizz. Use when blow-drying, scrunching and diffuser drying.

**MOUSSE TIPS**

• Make sure you apply mousse from the roots to the ends, not just in a blob on the crown.

• Choose the right type for your hair. Normal is good for a great many styles, but if you want more holding power, don't just use more mousse as it can make hair dull; instead, choose a firm or maximum-hold product.

## serums

Used to improve shine and softness by forming a microscopic film on the surface of the hair, serums, glossers, polishes and shine sprays are made from oils or silicones Formulations can vary from light and silky to heavier ones with a distinctly oily feel. They also contain substances designed to smooth the cuticle, encouraging the tiny scales to lie flat and thus reflect the light and make the hair appear shiny. Use these

**SERUM TIP**

Take care not to use too much serum or you will make your hair oily.

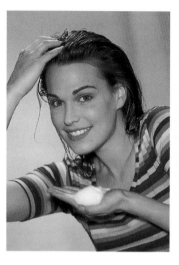

△ When applying mousse use no more than a "handful", and take care to ensure that you distribute it evenly.

products to improve the feel of the hair, to combat static, de-frizz, add shine and gloss, and temporarily repair split ends.

## styling or setting lotions

Containing flexible resins that form a film on the hair and aid setting, styling lotions protect the hair from heat damage. There are formulations for dry, coloured or sensitized hair; others give volume and additional shine. Use for roller-setting, scrunching, blow-drying and natural drying.

**STYLING LOTION TIP**

If using a styling lotion for heat-setting look out for formulations that offer thermal protection.

## waxes, pomades and creams

These products are made from natural waxes, such as carnauba (produced by a Brazilian palm tree), which are softened with other ingredients such as mineral oils and lanolin to make them pliable. Both soft and hard formulations are available. Some pomades contain vegetable wax and oil to give gloss and sheen. Other formulations produce foam and are water soluble, and leave no residue. Use for dressing the hair and for controlling frizz and static.

# Useful appliances

Heated styling appliances allow you to style your hair quickly, efficiently and easily. A wide range of heated appliances is available.

## air wavers

Air wavers combine the speed of a blow-dryer with the ease of a styling wand. They operate on the same principle as a blow-dryer, blowing warm air though the shaft. Many wavers are available with a variety of clip-on options, including brushes, prongs and tongs, some with retractable teeth. Use for creating soft waves and volume at the roots.

> **AIR WAVING TIP**
> Apply a styling spray or lotion before air waving, and style the hair while it is still damp.

## crimpers

These consist of two ridged metal plates that produce uniform patterned crimps in straight lines in the hair. The hair must be straightened first, either by blow-drying or using flat irons. The crimper is then used to give waves or ripples. Some crimpers have reversible or dual-effect styling plates to give different effects.

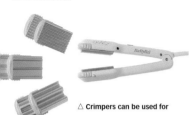

△ Crimpers can be used for special styling effects or to increase volume.

> **CRIMPING TIPS**
> • Do not use on damaged, bleached or over-stressed hair.
> • Brushing crimped hair gives a softer result.

> **BLOW-DRYING TIPS**
> • Always point the airflow down the hair shaft to smooth the cuticle and encourage shine.
> • Take care not to hold the dryer too near the scalp; it can cause burns.
> • When you have finished blow-drying allow the hair to cool thoroughly, then check that the hair is completely dry. Warm hair often gives the illusion of dryness while it is, in fact, still damp.
> • Never use a dryer without its filter in place – hair can easily be drawn into the machine.

## blow-dryers

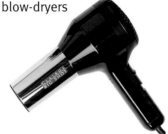

Choose a dryer that has a range of heat and speed settings so that the hair can be power-dried on high heat, finished on a lower heat, and then used with cool air to actually set the style. The average life expectancy of a blow-dryer is usually between 200 and 300 hours.

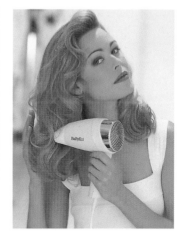

△ The blow-dryer is an essential piece of equipment, particularly when you need to dry your hair in a hurry.

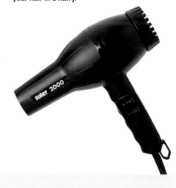

> **DIFFUSERS AND NOZZLES**
> Originally, diffusers were intended for drying curly hair slowly, in this way encouraging curl formation for scrunched styles. The diffuser serves to spread the airflow over the hair so the curls are not literally blown away. The prongs on the diffuser head also help to increase volume at the root and give lift. Diffusers with flat heads are designed for gentle drying without ruffling, and are more suitable for shorter styles. The newest type of diffuser has long, straight prongs which are designed to inject volume into straight hair while giving a smooth finish. Nozzles fit over the end of the barrel of the blow-dryer and are used to give precise direction when styling.

## heated rollers

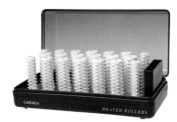

△ Heated rollers are available in sets, normally comprising a selection of 20 or so small, medium and large rollers.

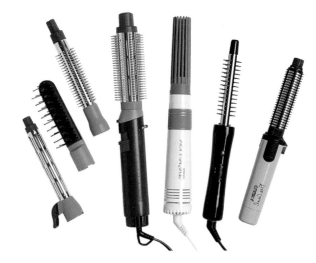

△ Easier to handle than tongs, hot brushes come in a wide range of sizes and are specially designed for creating curls of different sizes. Use for root lift, curl and movement.

Early heated rollers had spikes, which many women prefer because they have a good grip. New developments include ribbed rubber surfaces, which are designed to be kinder to the hair, curved barrel shapes that follow the form of the head, and clip fasteners.

### HEATED ROLLER TIP

Ten minutes is enough time in which to heat up a heated roller-set.

The speed at which the rollers heat up varies, depending on the type of roller. PTC (positive temperature co-efficient) element rollers heat up fastest because they have an element inside each roller, and the heat is transferred directly from the base to the roller. Wax-filled rollers take longer, around 15 minutes, but they retain their temperature over a longer period. All rollers cool down completely in 30 minutes. Use heated rollers for quick sets, to give curl and body. They are ideal for preparing long hair for dressing.

### REDUCING STATIC

Heat drying encourages static, causing hair to fly away. You can reduce static by lightly touching your hair, or misting your hairbrush with spray to calm the hair down.

## hot brushes

The most effective styling technique to use with a hot brush is to wind down the length of the hair, then hold it there for a few seconds until the heat has penetrated through the hair, then gently remove it. Cordless hot brushes, which use batteries to produce heat, are also available and are very convenient for taking on holiday or on business trips.

### HOT BRUSH TIP

Take neat, methodical sections when working with a hot brush or the hair may tangle. Use large clips to keep back the rest of your hair.

▽ When using a hot brush make certain you follow the manufacturer's instructions carefully.

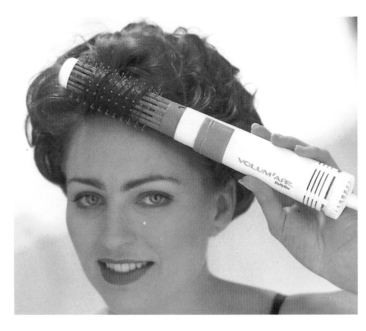

## straighteners

Ceramic straighteners are based on the same principle as crimpers but have flat plates to iron out frizz or curl. Use for "pressing" really curly hair. For the best results choose a ceramic rather than a ceramic-coated one. Some ceramic straighteners claim to seal in moisture and natural oils so they won't dry your hair. They smooth the cuticles and leave your hair soft and static-free.

**STRAIGHTENING TIPS**

• Use a styling spray before straightening.

• Straighteners are designed for occasional, not daily, use because they function at a very high temperature, which can cause damage to the hair.

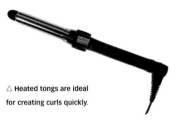

△ Heated tongs are ideal for creating curls quickly.

## tongs

Styling tongs consist of a barrel, or prong, and a depressor groove. The barrel is round; the depressor is curved to fit around the barrel when the tong is closed. The thickness of the barrel varies, and the size of the tong that is used depends on whether small, medium, or large curls are required.

**TONGING TIPS**

• Be careful when tonging white or bleached hair as it can discolour.

• Always use tongs on dry, not wet, hair.

• If curling right up to the roots, place a comb between the tongs and the scalp so the comb forms a barrier against the heat.

• Leave tonged curls to cool before styling.

## travel dryers

Specially made for taking on holiday, travel dryers are usually miniature versions of standard dryers, and some even have their own small diffusers. Check that the dryer you buy has dual voltage and a travel case.

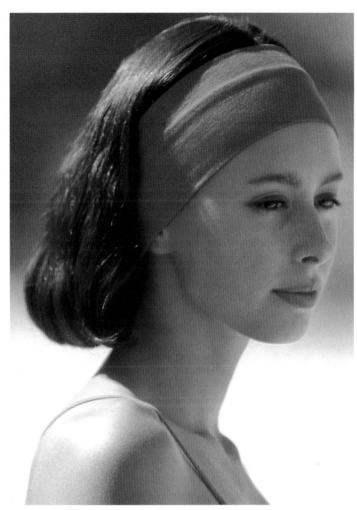

△ Keep holiday haircare to a minimum by making use of dual-purpose heated appliances. Don't forget to pack a universal plug when travelling abroad.

**SAFETY TIPS**

• Equipment should be unplugged when not in use.

• Never use electric equipment with wet hands, and don't use near water.

• Only use one appliance for each socket outlet – adaptors may cause overload.

• The cord should not be wrapped tightly around the equipment; coil it loosely before storing.

• Tongs can be cleaned by wiping with a damp cloth; if necessary use a little alcohol to remove dirt.

• All electrical equipment should be checked periodically to ensure that leads and connections are in good order.

• Untwist the cord on the dryer from time to time.

• Clean filters regularly – a blocked filter means the dryer has to work harder and will eventually overheat and cut out. If the element overheats it can distort the dryer casing.

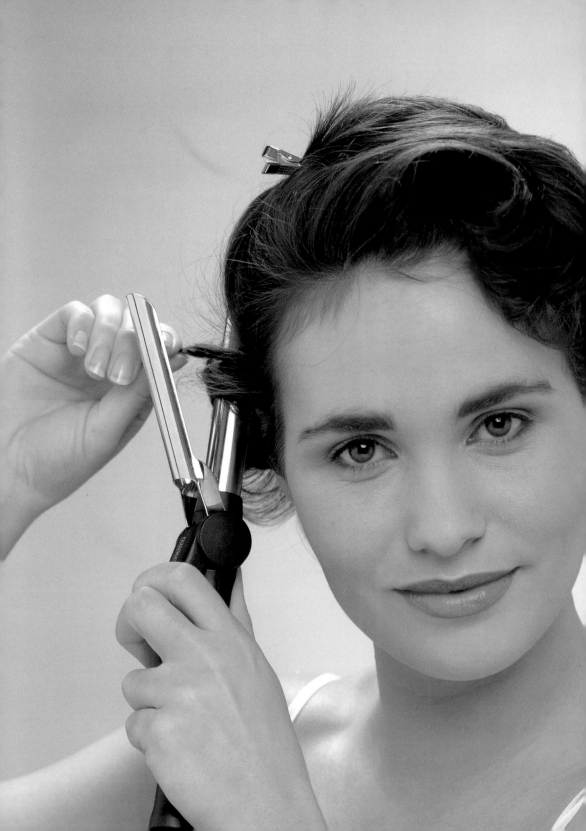

# Styling your Hair

This section tackles the basics of hair setting and drying techniques. Then you can use these skills to tackle the special projects, which show you how to create braids, chignons, French pleats (rolls), top knots, twists, coils and curls. By following the simple step-by-step pictures, you'll be amazed at how easy it is to transform your hair to suit almost every mood and occasion.

# Blow-drying

Follow these simple instructions to achieve the smoothest, sleekest blow-dry ever.

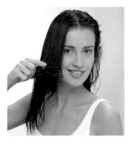

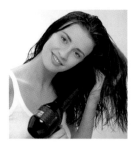

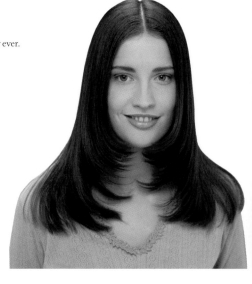

△ **1** Shampoo and condition your hair as usual. Then comb through with a wide-toothed comb to completely remove any tangles.

△ **2** Partially dry your hair, running your fingers through it as you work. This is just to remove the excess moisture.

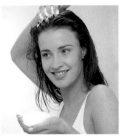

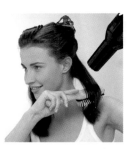

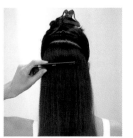

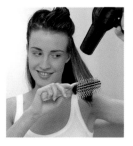

△ **3** Apply a handful of mousse to the palm of your hand. Then using your other hand, spread the mousse through the hair, distributing it evenly from the tips to the ends.

△ **4** Divide your hair into two main sections by clipping the top and sides out of the way. Then, working on the hair that is left free and taking one small section at a time, hold the dryer in one hand and a styling brush in the other. Place the brush underneath the first section of hair, positioning it at the roots. Keeping the tension on the hair taut (but without undue stress), move the brush down towards the ends, directing the airflow from the dryer so that it follows the downwards movement of the brush.

△ **5** Curve the brush under at the ends to achieve a slight bend. Focus on drying the roots first, repeatedly applying the brush to the roots once it has moved down the length of the hair. Continue this until the first section is dry. Repeat step 4 until the whole of the back section is completely dry.

△ **6** Release a section of hair from the top and dry it in the same manner. Continue in this way until you have dried all your hair. Finish by smoothing a few drops of serum through the hair to flatten any flyaway ends.

**STYLING CHECKLIST**

*You will need:*

- styling comb
- dryer
- mousse
- clip
- styling brush
- serum

**BLOW-DRYING TIPS**

- Use the highest heat or speed setting to remove excess moisture, then switch to medium to finish drying.
- Point the airflow downwards. This smoothes the cuticles and makes the hair shine.
- Ensure each section is competely dry before working on the next.

# Finger drying

This is a simple and quick method of drying and styling your hair. It relies on the heat released from your hands rather than the heat from a hairdryer. However, finger drying is only really viable for short to mid-length hair.

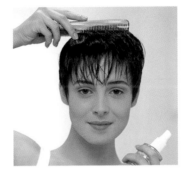

△ **1** Shampoo and condition your hair, then spray with gel and comb through.

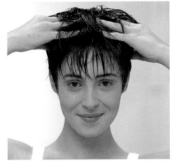

△ **2** Run your fingers rapidly upwards and forwards, from the roots to the ends.

**FINGER-DRYING TIP**
Finger-drying is the best way to dry damaged hair, or to encourage waves in naturally curly, short hair.

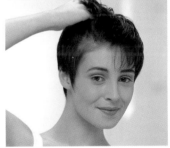

△ **3** Lift up the hair at the crown to give it volume and body at the roots.

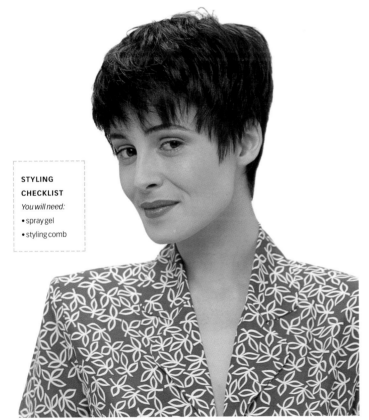

**STYLING CHECKLIST**
*You will need:*
• spray gel
• styling comb

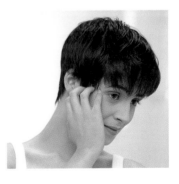

△ **4** Continue lifting as the hair dries. Use your fingertips to flatten the hair at the sides.

# Barrel curls

One of the simplest sets is achieved by curling the hair around the fingers and then pinning the curl in place. Barrel curls are a great way to create a natural, soft set.

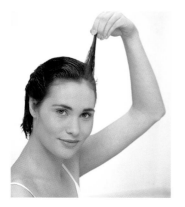

△ **1** Shampoo and condition; apply setting lotion and comb from the roots to the ends. Take a small section of hair (about 2.5cm/1in) and smooth it upwards.

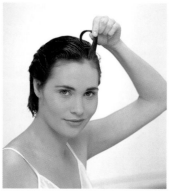

△ **2** Loop the hair into a large curl.

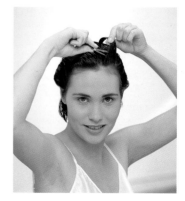

△ **3** Clip in place.

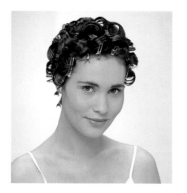

△ **4** Continue to curl the rest of the hair in the same way.

▷ **5** Allow the hair to dry naturally, or with a hood dryer, then carefully remove the clips. To achieve a natural tousled look rake your fingers through your hair. For a smoother finish use a hair brush.

**STYLING CHECKLIST**
*You will need:*
• setting lotion
• styling comb
• clips
• hood dryer (optional)

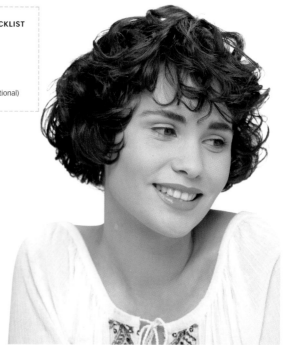

# Roll-up

A roller set forms the basis of many styles; it can be used to smooth hair, add waves or soft curls, or provide a foundation for an upswept style.

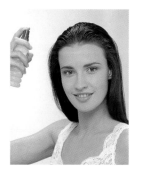

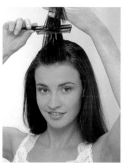

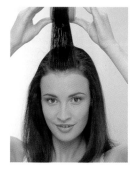

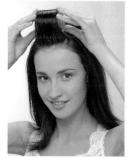

△ **1** Shampoo and condition your hair, then partially dry to remove excess moisture. Mist with a styling spray.

△ **2** For a basic set, take a 5cm/2in section of hair (or a section the same width as your roller) from the centre front and comb it straight up, smoothing out any tangles.

△ **3** Wrap the ends of the sectioned hair around the roller, taking care not to buckle the hair. Then wind the roller down firmly towards the scalp, keeping the tension even.

△ **4** Keep winding until the roller sits on the roots of the hair. Self-fixing rollers will stay in place on their own but if you are using brush rollers you will have to fasten them with pins.

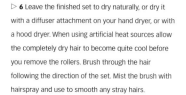

**STYLING CHECKLIST**

*You will need:*

- styling spray
- tail comb
- self-fixing rollers or brush rollers and pins
- hand or hood dryer (optional)
- hairspray

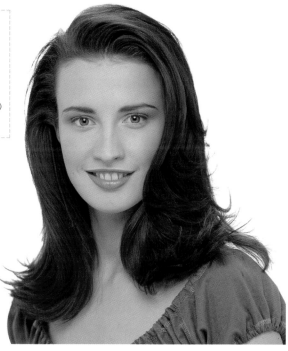

△ **5** Continue around the whole head, always taking the same width of hair. Re-mist the hair with styling spray if it begins to dry out.

▷ **6** Leave the finished set to dry naturally, or dry it with a diffuser attachment on your hand dryer, or with a hood dryer. When using artificial heat sources allow the completely dry hair to become quite cool before you remove the rollers. Brush through the hair following the direction of the set. Mist the brush with hairspray and use to smooth any stray hairs.

# Soft setting

Fabric rollers are the modern version of old-fashioned rags. Apart from being very easy to use they are kind to the hair and give a highly effective set.

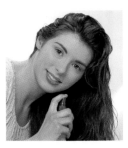

△ **1** Dampen the hair with styling spray, making sure you distribute it evenly from the roots to the ends.

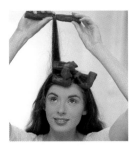

△ **2** Wind sections about 2.5cm/1in wide around fabric rollers. Wind the roller smoothly towards the scalp.

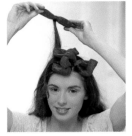

△ **3** Continue winding the roller gently and firmly, taking it right down to the roots.

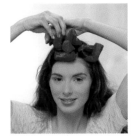

△ **4** To fasten, simply bend each end of the fabric roller towards the centre. This grips the hair and holds it in place.

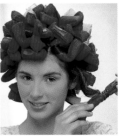

△ **5** Leave the completed set to dry. Then remove the rollers by unbending the ends and unwinding the hair.

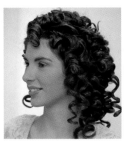

△ **6** When all the rollers have been removed the hair falls into firm corkscrew curls.

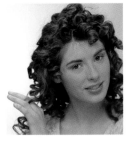

△ **7** Working on one curl at a time, rake and tease out each curl with your fingers for a full, voluminous finish.

**TIP**

For even more volume, twist each section of hair lengthwise before winding it into the fabric roller.

**STYLING CHECKLIST**

*You will need:*

- styling spray
- fabric rollers

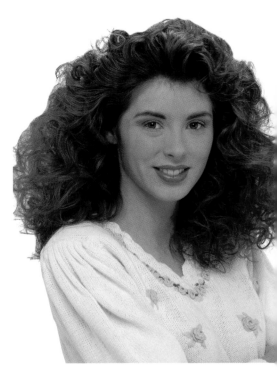

# Tong *and* twist

Tongs can be used to smooth the hair and add just the right amount of movement.

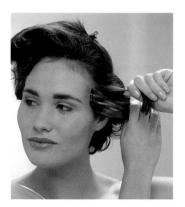

△ **1** Shampoo, condition and dry. Apply a mist of styling lotion. Avoid mousse as it sticks to the tongs and bakes into the hair. Divide off a small section.

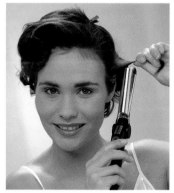

△ **2** Press the depressor to open the tongs.

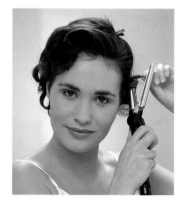

△ **3** Wind the whole section of hair around the barrel of the tongs.

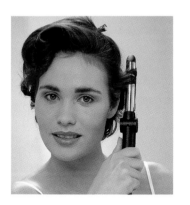

△ **4** Release the depressor to hold the hair in place and wait a few seconds for the curl to form. Remove the tongs and leave to cool as you work on the rest of the hair. Style by raking through with your fingers.

**TIP**
Never use tongs on bleached hair. The high heat can damage the hair, causing brittleness and breakage.

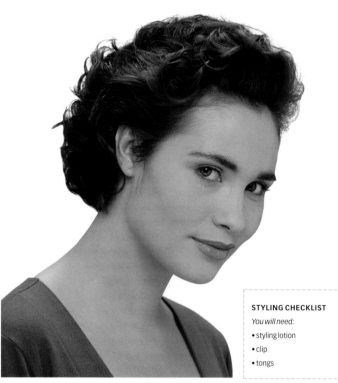

**STYLING CHECKLIST**
*You will need:*
- styling lotion
- clip
- tongs

# Style and go

Hot brushes with tong attachments enable you to create lots of styles. Here we show you two different techniques, which give two different looks.

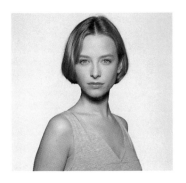

△ **1** Shampoo, condition and dry your hair.

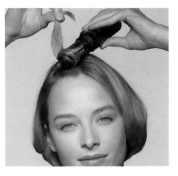

△ **2** Take a section of hair about 5cm/2in square, and apply some styling lotion. Using the brush attachment gently smooth the hair from the roots to the ends. Place the hot brush near the roots, twist the hair around the brush, and hold for a few seconds. Gently unravel the hair and hold without pulling.

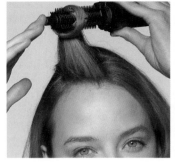

△ **3** Place the ends of the hair into the hot brush and wind halfway down the hair length.

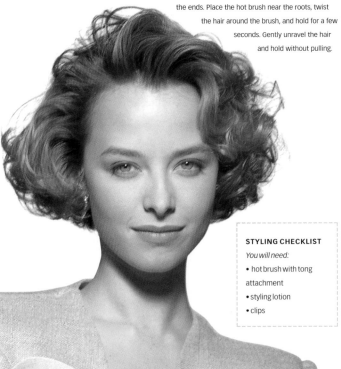

△ **4** Unwind and loop the hair into a barrel curl, securing with a clip. Repeat steps 2 to 4 until you have done the whole head. Remove the clips. Comb.

**STYLING CHECKLIST**
*You will need:*
- hot brush with tong attachment
- styling lotion
- clips

**TIP**
Play with the direction of the waves to see which way they fall best. Draw the fingers upwards from the back of the neck and through the hair for extra lift. Finish with a light mist of hairspray.

**STYLING TRICKS**

• Always use hot brushes on dry hair, never on wet hair.

• Don't use mousse or gel when heat styling. Instead, try special heat-activated styling lotions and sprays. These are designed to help curls hold their shape without making the hair sticky or frizzy.

• Bobbed styles can be smoothed down and the ends of the hair tipped under using tongs. Just section the hair and smooth the tongs down the length, curving the ends. It is important to keep the tongs moving with a gentle sliding action, twisting the wrist and turning the barrel of the tongs under.

• Unruly fringes (bangs) can be tamed by gently winding the fringe around the tong or brush and holding for a few seconds.

This style uses the tong attachment for a more sculptured, voluminous look.

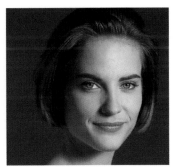

△ **1** Shampoo, condition and dry your hair.

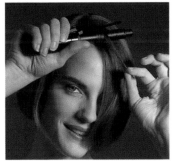

△ **2** Take a section of hair about 1cm/$^1$/$_2$in long and apply some styling lotion. Using the tong attachment on the styler, lift the depressor and keep it open. Slide the tongs on to the hair, just up from the roots. Holding the depressor open, wind the hair around the barrel, towards the face, ensuring the ends are smooth.

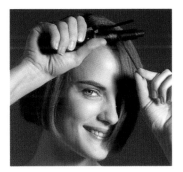

△ **3** Continue wrapping the hair down the length of the barrel, taking care not to buckle the ends of the hair. Hold for a few seconds to allow the curl to form.

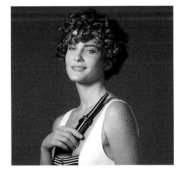

△ **4** Release the depressor and allow the spiral curl to spring out. Repeat steps 2 to 3 until you have curled the whole head, then rake through the hair with your fingers for a softly sculptured look.

**TIP**

After tonging, don't be tempted to brush your hair or you will lose the curl.

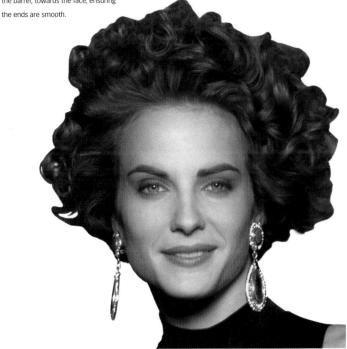

# Curl creation

A perm that is past its best can be revived using this diffuser-drying technique.

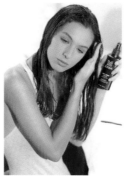

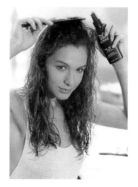

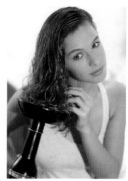

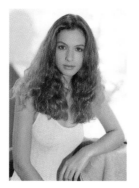

△ **1** The hair has the remains of a perm and is therefore flat at the roots with some curl from the mid-lengths to the ends.

△ **2** Wash, condition and towel-dry your hair, then apply curl revitalizer to the damp hair.

△ **3** Use a wide-toothed comb and work from the roots to the ends to ensure the curl revitalizer is distributed evenly.

△ **4** Attach the diffuser to the dryer and dry the hair, allowing the hair to sit on the prongs of the diffuser. This action enables the warm air to circulate around the strands of hair, encouraging the formation of curls. To maximize the amount of curl, use your hands to scrunch up handfuls of hair.

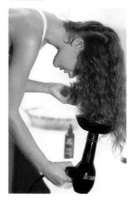

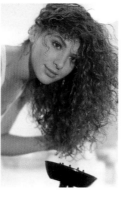

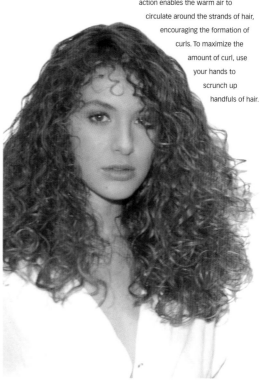

△ **5** Tip your head forwards, allowing the hair to sit in the diffuser cup. Do not pull the hair, simply squeeze curls gently into shape.

△ **6** Repeat steps 4 and 5 until all the hair is dry.

**TIP**

This technique works equally well on naturally wavy or curly hair, giving separation and definition to curls

**STYLING CHECKLIST**

*You will need:*

• curl revitalizer
• wide-toothed comb
• dryer with pronged diffuser attachment

# Smooth and straight

# Instant set

Volume can be added to long straight hair by using a dryer with a diffuser attachment that has long straight prongs.

Hair can be given lift, bounce and movement with a quick set using heated rollers.

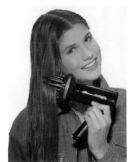

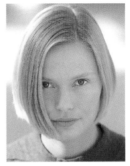

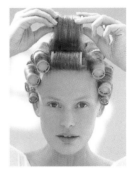

△ **1** Long thick hair often tangles easily and it is difficult to add volume and control.

△ **2** Shampoo and condition your hair, then part it down the centre. Attach a diffuser with long prongs to your dryer and, as the hair dries, comb the prongs down the hair in a stroking movement. This will direct the airflow downwards, smoothing and separating the hair.

△ **1** Shampoo and condition your hair. Apply mousse and blow-dry smooth. Heat the rollers according to the manufacturer's directions.

△ **2** Wind sections of hair (about 5cm/2in wide) on to rollers, taking care not to buckle the hair ends. Use medium and small rollers at the front and sides, larger rollers on the crown.

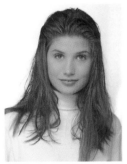

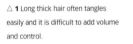

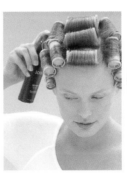

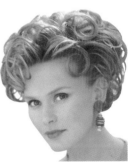

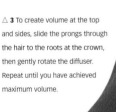

> **STYLING CHECKLIST**
> *You will need:*
> • comb
> • dryer with diffuser attachment with long straight prongs

△ **3** To create volume at the top and sides, slide the prongs through the hair to the roots at the crown, then gently rotate the diffuser. Repeat until you have achieved maximum volume.

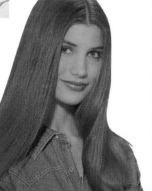

△ **3** Wind the rollers down towards the root, making sure that the ends are tucked under smoothly. Keep the tension even. Secure each roller with the clip supplied. Mist your set hair with a styling lotion.

△ **4** Allow the rollers to cool and then remove, taking care not to disturb the curls. To finish, loosen the curls by raking your fingers through them.

> **STYLING CHECKLIST**
> *You will need:*
> • mousse
> • styling lotion
> • heated rollers with clips

# Double-stranded
# braids

These clever braids have a fishbone pattern, which gives an unusual look.

# Dragged
# side-braids

Curly hair can be controlled, yet still allowed to flow free, by braiding at the sides and allowing the hair at the back to fall in a mass of curls.

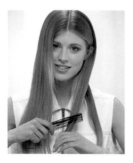 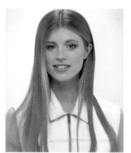

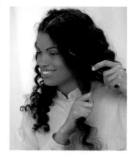 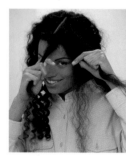

△ **1** Part your hair in the centre and comb it straight.

△ **2** Divide the hair on one side of your head into two strands, then take a fine section from the back of the back strand and take it over to join the front strand, as shown.

△ **1** Part your hair in the centre and divide off a large section at the side, combing it as flat as possible to the head.

△ **2** Divide the section into three equal strands and hold them apart.

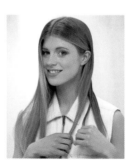

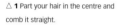

**STYLING CHECKLIST**

*You will need:*

- styling comb
- covered bands
- coloured feathers
- two short lengths of fine leather

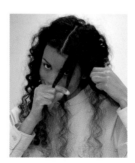 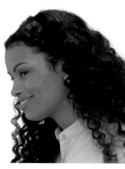

△ **3** Now take a fine section from the front of the front strand, and cross it over to the back strand. Take a fine section from the back strand again and bring it over to join the front strand. Continue in this way; you will soon see the fishbone effect appear. Secure the ends with covered bands and add feathers, tying in place with fine leather. Repeat on the other side.

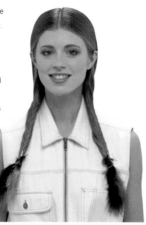

△ **3** Begin to make a dragged braid by pulling the strands of hair towards your face and then braiding in the normal way, that is, taking the right strand over the centre strand, the left strand over the centre, and the right over the centre again, keeping the braid in the position shown.

△ **4** Continue braiding to the bottom and secure the end with a covered band. Tuck the braid behind your ear and grip it in place, then make a second braid on the other side.

**TIP**

Encourage curls to form by spraying the hair with water and then scrunching with your hands.

**STYLING CHECKLIST**

*You will need:*

- styling comb
- 4 covered bands
- hair grips

# Ponytail styler

A simple ponytail can be transformed easily and quickly using this clever styler.

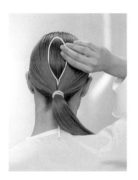

△ **1** Clasp the hair into a ponytail and secure it with a covered band. Insert the styler as shown.

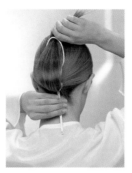

△ **2** Thread the ponytail into the styler and pull it through.

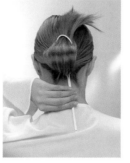

△ **3** Begin to pull the styler down…

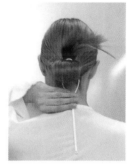

△ **4** …continue pulling…

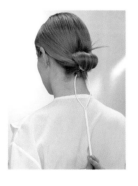

△ **5** …so the ponytail pulls through…

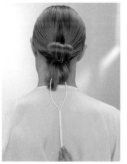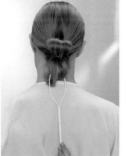

△ **6** …and emerges underneath.

**TIP**
To smooth any flyaway ends rub a few drops of serum between the palms of your hands and smooth over the hair.

**STYLING CHECKLIST**
*You will need:*
- covered band
- ponytail styler

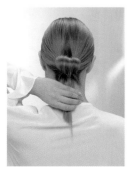

◁ **7** Smooth the hair with your hand and insert the styler again, repeating steps 2 to 6 once more to give a neat chignon loop.

**TIP**
The same technique can be used on wet hair as long as you apply gel first, combing it through evenly before styling.

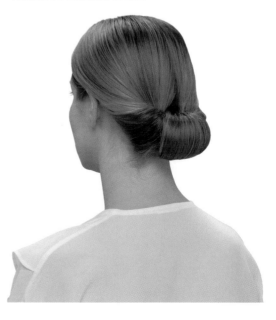

# Curly styler

The ponytail styler can also be used to tame a mass of curls, creating a ponytail with a simple double twist.

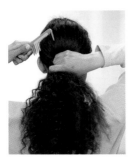

△ **1** Use a comb with widely spaced teeth to smooth the hair back and into a ponytail. Secure with a covered band.

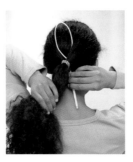

△ **2** Insert the styler as shown.

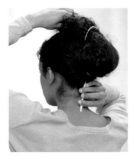

△ **3** Thread the ponytail into the styler and pull it through.

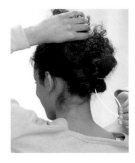

△ **4** Begin to pull the styler down…

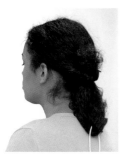

△ **5** …continue pulling…

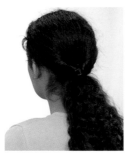

△ **6** …so that the ponytail pulls through.

**TIP**
When inserting the styler through a ponytail, carefully move it from side to side in order to create enough room to pull the looped end of the styler through more easily.

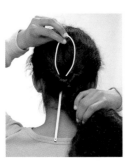

△ **7** Repeat steps 3 to 6.

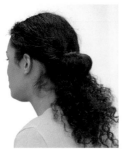

△ **8** Apply a little mousse to your hands and use it to re-form the curls, scrunching to achieve a good shape.

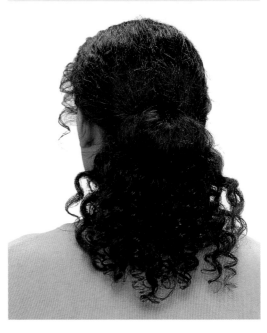

# Crown braids

By braiding the crown hair and allowing the remaining hair to frame the face you can achieve an interesting contrast of textures.

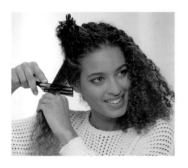

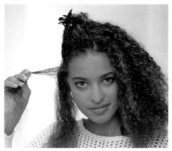

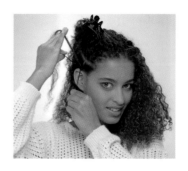

△ **1** Clip up the top hair on one side of your head, leaving the back hair free. Take a small section of hair at ear level and comb it straight.

△ **2** Start braiding quite tightly, doing one cross (right strand over centre, left over centre), and then gradually bringing more hair into the outside strands.

△ **3** Continue in this way, taking the braid towards the back of the head. Secure the braids with small covered bands.

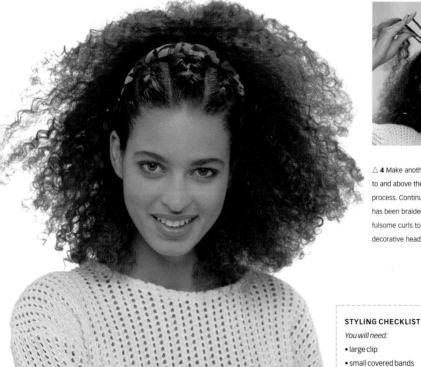

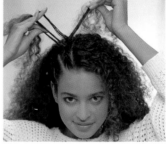

△ **4** Make another parting about 2.5cm/1in parallel to and above the previous braid, and repeat the process. Continue in this way until all the front hair has been braided. Scrunch the remaining hair into fulsome curls to increase the volume. Finally, add a decorative headband.

**STYLING CHECKLIST**

*You will need:*
- large clip
- small covered bands
- headband

**TIP**

The volume of the curls can be increased by tipping your head forwards, then applying styling spray and scrunching the hair lying underneath.

# Twist and coil

This style starts with a simple ponytail, is easy to do, and looks stunning.

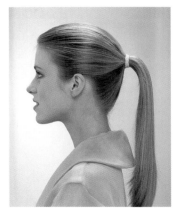

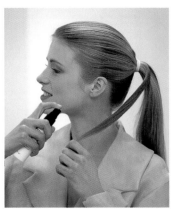

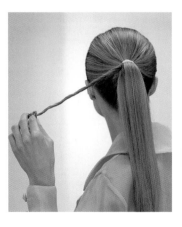

△ **1** Smooth the hair back and secure in a ponytail using a covered band.

△ **2** Divide off a small section of hair and mist with shine spray for added gloss.

△ **3** Holding the ends of a section, twist the hair until it rolls back on itself to form a coil.

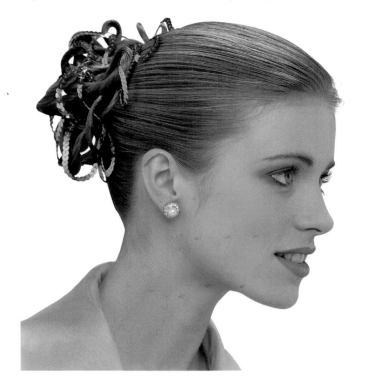

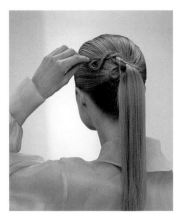

△ **4** Position the coil in a loop as shown and secure in place using hair pins. Continue until all the hair has been coiled. Decorate by intertwining with a strip of sequins.

---

**STYLING CHECKLIST**

*You will need:*
- covered band
- shine spray
- hair pins
- 1m/1 yd strip sequins

# Cameo braid

A classic bun is given extra panache with an encircling braid.

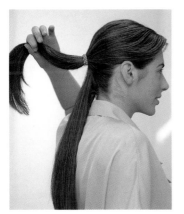

△ **1** Smooth the hair into a ponytail, leaving one section free.

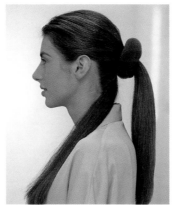

△ **2** Place a bun ring over the ponytail.

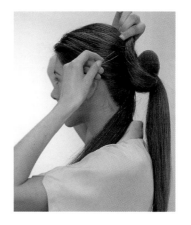

△ **3** Take approximately one third of the hair from the ponytail and wrap it around the bun ring, securing with pins. Repeat with the other two-thirds of hair.

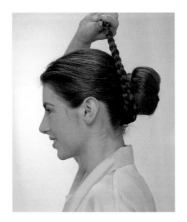

△ **4** Braid the section of hair that was left out of the ponytail, right strand over centre strand, left over centre and so on, and wrap the braid around the base of the bun, then secure with pins.

**STYLING CHECKLIST**

*You will need:*
- covered band
- bun ring
- hair pins

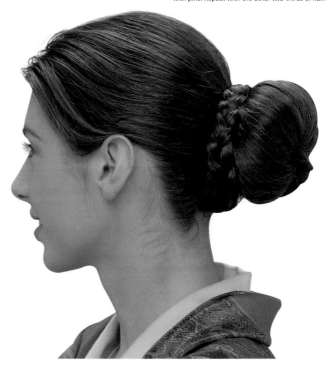

# Band braid

A plain ponytail can be transformed by simply covering the band with a tiny braid.

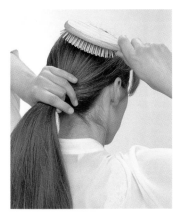

△ **1** Brush the hair back into a smooth, low ponytail, leaving a small section free for braiding. Secure in place with a covered band. Smooth the reserved section with a little styling wax.

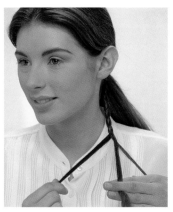

△ **2** Divide this section into three equal strands. Now, braid the hair in the normal way.

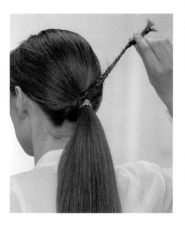

△ **3** Take the braid and wrap it tightly around the covered band.

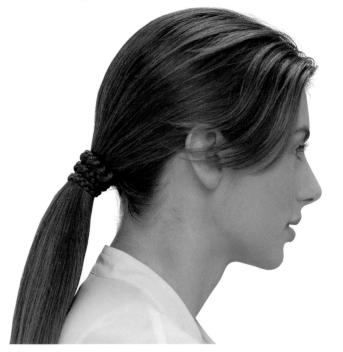

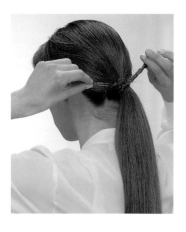

△ **4** Wind it as many times as it goes. Finally, secure with a grip.

---

**STYLING CHECKLIST**

*You will need:*

- brush
- covered band
- wax
- hair pin

# Clip up

Long, curly hair can sometimes be unruly. Here's an easy way to tame tresses but still keep the beauty of the length.

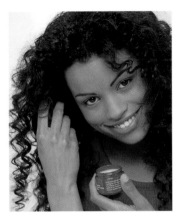

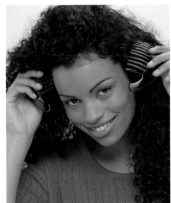

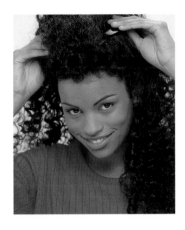

△ **1** Rub a little wax between the palms of your hands, then work into the curls with the fingertips. This helps give the curl separation and shine.

△ **2** Take two interlocking large curved combs and use them to push the crown hair up towards the centre.

△ **3** Push the teeth of the combs together to fasten on top of the head.

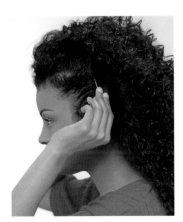

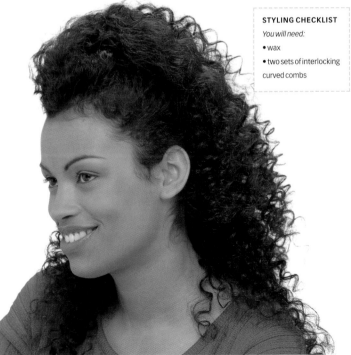

△ **4** Repeat with two more combs at ear level to secure the back hair.

**STYLING CHECKLIST**

*You will need:*

- wax
- two sets of interlocking curved combs

**TIP**

It's easier to disentangle curly hair if you use a comb with widely spaced teeth.

# Draped chignon

This elegant style is perfect for that special evening out.

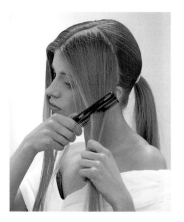

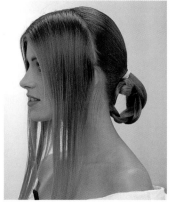

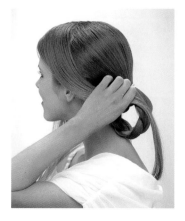

△ **1** Part the hair in the centre from the forehead to the middle of the crown. Comb the side hair and scoop the back hair into a low ponytail using a covered band.

△ **2** Loosely braid the ponytail – take the right strand over the centre strand, the left over the centre, the right over the centre, and so on, continuing to the end. Secure the end with a small band, then tuck the end under and around in a loop and secure with grips.

△ **3** Pick up the hair on the left side and comb it in a curve back to the ponytail loop.

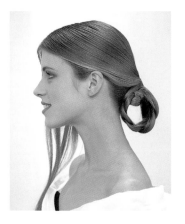

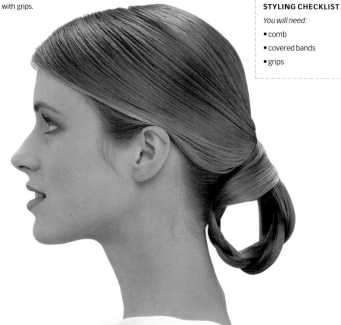

△ **4** Swirl this hair over and under the loop and secure with grips. Repeat steps 3 and 4 on the right side.

**STYLING CHECKLIST**
*You will need:*
- comb
- covered bands
- grips

**TIP**
Even long hair should be trimmed regularly, at least every two months, to keep it in good condition.

# City slicker

Transform your hair in minutes using gel to slick it into shape and add sheen.

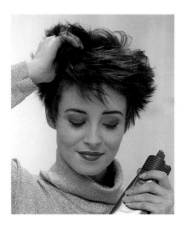

△ **1** Take a generous amount of gel and apply it to the hair from the roots to the ends.

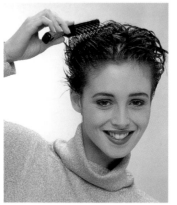

△ **2** Use a vent brush, a comb or your fingers to distribute the gel evenly through the hair.

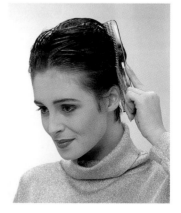

△ **3** Comb the hair into shape using a styling comb to encourage movement.

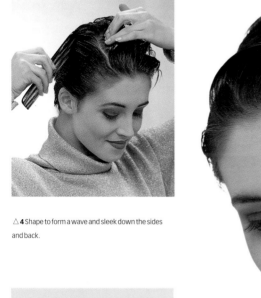

△ **4** Shape to form a wave and sleek down the sides and back.

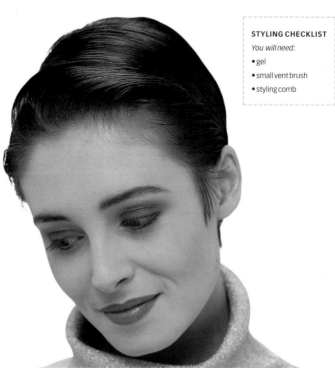

**STYLING CHECKLIST**
*You will need:*
- gel
- small vent brush
- styling comb

**TIP**
Make sure you distribute the gel evenly all over your hair before styling.

# Simple pleat

Curly hair that is neatly pleated gives a sophisticated style. The front is left full to soften the effect.

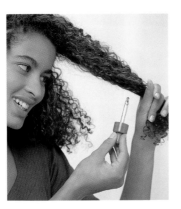

△ **1** Divide off a section of hair at the front and leave it free. Smooth with a little serum. Take the remaining hair into one hand, as if you were going to make it into a ponytail.

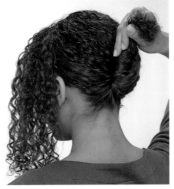

△ **2** Twist the hair tightly from left to right.

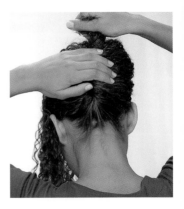

△ **3** When the twist is taut, turn the hair upwards as shown to form a pleat. Use your other hand to help smooth the pleat and at the same time neaten the top by tucking in the ends.

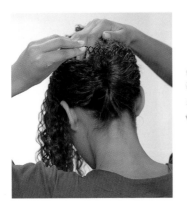

△ **4** Secure the pleat with hair pins. Take the reserved front section, bring it back and secure it at the top of the pleat, allowing the ends to fall free.

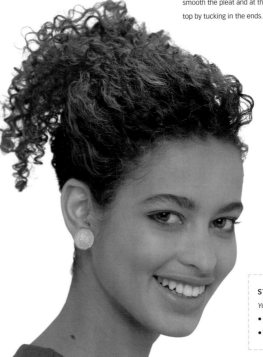

**STYLING CHECKLIST**

*You will need:*

• serum
• hair pins

# Looped curls

Two ponytails form the basis of this elegant style.

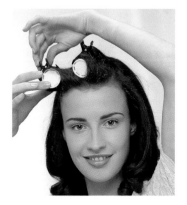

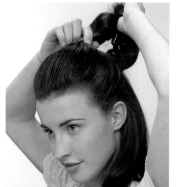

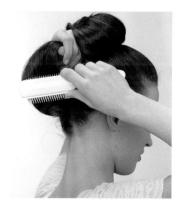

△ **1** Apply setting lotion to the ends of the hair only. This will give just the right amount of body and bounce to help form the curls. Set the hair on heated rollers. When the rollers are quite cool – about 10 minutes after completing the set – take them out and allow the hair to fall free.

△ **2** Divide off the crown hair and secure it with hair pins in a high ponytail. Apply a few drops of serum to add gloss, and brush the hair through.

△ **3** Place the remaining hair in a lower ponytail.

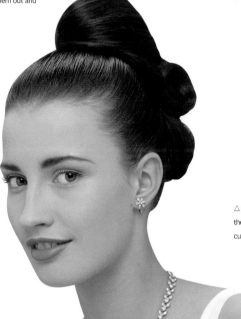

△ **4** Divide each ponytail in sections 2.5cm/1in wide, then comb and smooth each section into a looped curl and pin in place. Set with hairspray.

**STYLING CHECKLIST**
*You will need:*
- setting lotion
- heated rollers
- serum
- covered bands, hair pins

# French pleat

Mid-length to long hair can be transformed into a classic, elegant French pleat (roll) in a matter of minutes.

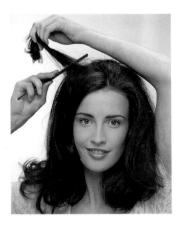

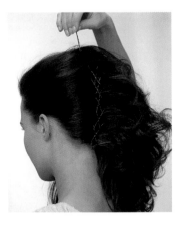

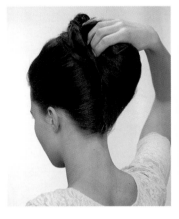

△ **1** Backcomb the hair all over.

△ **2** Smooth your hair across to the centre back and form the centre of the pleat by criss-crossing hair-grips in a row from the crown downwards, as shown.

△ **3** Gently smooth the hair around from the other side, leaving the front section free, and tuck the ends under.

**STYLING CHECKLIST**

*You will need:*

- comb
- hairgrips
- pins
- hairspray

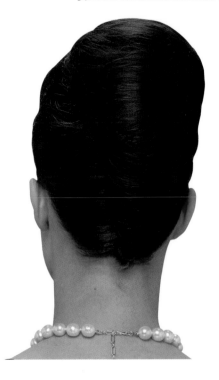

△ **4** Secure with pins, then lightly comb the front section up and around to merge with the top of the pleat. Mist with hairspray to hold.

# Short and spiky

Short hair can be quickly styled using gel and wax to create a cheeky, fun look.

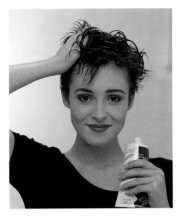

△ **1** Work a generous amount of gel through your hair from the roots to the ends.

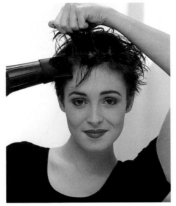

△ **2** Dry your hair using a directional nozzle on your dryer; as you dry, lift sections of the hair to create height at the roots.

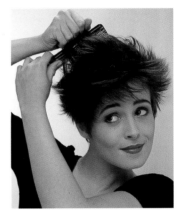

△ **3** When the hair is dry, backcomb the crown to give additional height.

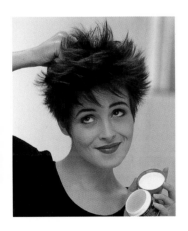

△ **4** To finish, rub a little wax between the palms of your hands, then apply it to the hair to give definition.

**TIP**
Gel can be reactivated by misting the hair with water and shaping it into style again.

**STYLING CHECKLIST**
*You will need:*
- gel
- blow-dryer
- comb
- wax

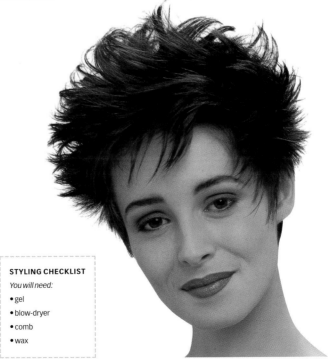

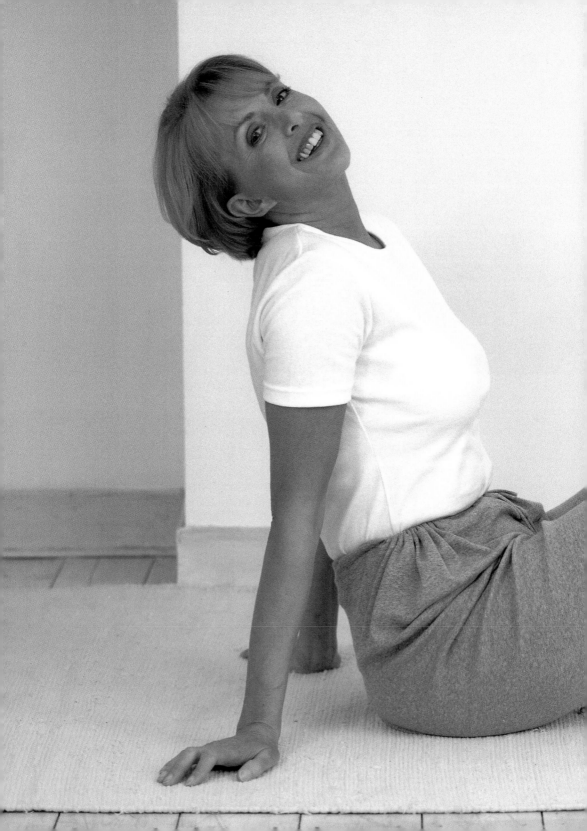

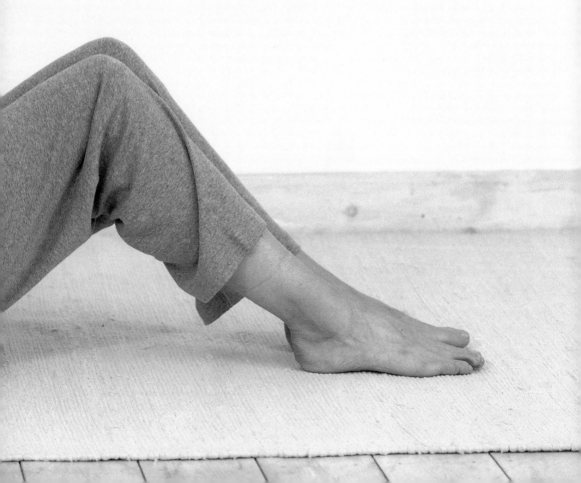

# EXERCISE AND HEALTHY EATING

# Health and fitness

Fitness is the key to a healthy mind and body. It is based on stamina, strength and suppleness – with better shape and self-esteem as the bonuses. Being fit improves your physical prowess and grace, and also makes you feel better overall. Most of us know that if we were fitter, we would have more confidence and greater zest for life. But although we are more health-conscious about our diet nowadays, regular exercise is still not a part of most people's daily lives. Surveys always draw the same conclusions as to the reasons for this: lack of time, energy, interest and confidence. Becoming fit is neither as difficult nor as time-consuming as it may appear to be: you can get fit – and get a better body into the bargain – more easily and enjoyably than you may think.

## how fit do you need to be?

There is no such thing as standard fitness – it depends on your personal make-up and why you want to be fit: being robust enough to run a marathon, for example, is different from honing stamina, strength and suppleness to gain improved physical shape and health. For exercise to be of any help, it should boost your metabolism and improve your cardiovascular (heart and circulation) and respiratory (breathing) systems.

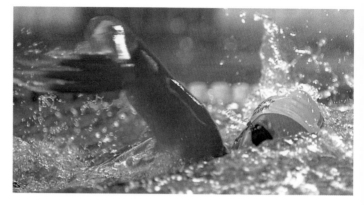

## making goals and recording results

Finding a goal that will inspire you is one of the secrets of success. To achieve that goal, you must have a motive that is important enough to give you an iron will, such as improving your figure for a special event (for example, your wedding and honeymoon), buying yourself a longed-for figure-hugging dress, or simply boosting your fitness levels generally. Set the deadline and stick to it. Depending on what you want to achieve, a three-week plan is ideal because it is not too long and if you persevere (take it week by week or day by

△ **Regular swimming sessions are a very effective way of keeping the whole body in good physical condition.**

day – whichever you find easiest), you will soon see results. However, be realistic: if your goals are too high you are more likely to fail; if they are too low, you will not have enough of a challenge.

Goals will inspire you, but speedy results are the key to keeping up regular exercise – it is perfectly natural that you will want to see rewards for all your hard work – although it is advisable to build up a pattern gradually. The minimum amount of exercise you need to do to improve your personal fitness is 20 minutes three times a week – the "3 x 20" maxim. This means three bouts of exercise vigorous enough to make you fairly breathless (but not gasping for breath). So if you do the general fitness exercises outlined in this book 3 times a week for 20 minutes you will get fitter. If you want to see fast results, though, you need to add extra activities – such as a couple of games of tennis, swimming, or brisk walking – to your exercise quota, so that you are actually exercising six days a week.

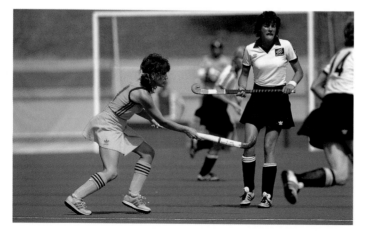

◁ **Hockey is a demanding sport that strengthens the legs, is beneficial to the heart and lungs, and significantly improves co-ordination.**

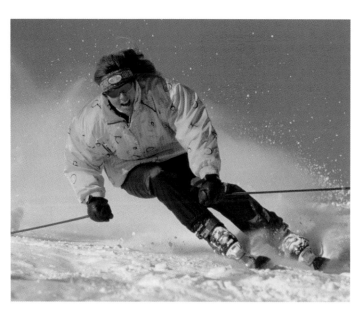

◁ In order to enjoy skiing you will need to be reasonably fit. Focus on improving the strength in your legs to take full advantage of this exhilarating winter sport.

heart rate into a certain range. These are the ideal exercise heart-rate ranges for the different ages:

| Age | Pulse Range |
|-----|-------------|
| 20+ | 130–160 |
| 30+ | 124–152 |
| 40+ | 117–144 |

To find out your active pulse rate per minute, rest two fingers lightly on your pulse immediately after exercising, count the beats for 10 seconds and multiply by 6.

## why bother with keeping fit?

Why are you reading this book? Are you fed up with lacking confidence? Are you tired of running out of puff, being out of shape or always feeling under the weather? Do you regularly suffer from colds, or experience bad pre-menstrual syndrome (PMS), stress or sleepless nights? These are just some of the signs of being unfit. So exercise is worth it, because when you are fitter, recurring problems such as these may ease or even completely disappear.

▽ A good many water sports demand strength, stamina and a fine sense of balance. Windsurfing is no exception to the rule.

**CAUTIONS**

Before taking up any form of rigorous exercise or training, you should consult your doctor – especially if any of the following conditions apply to you:

• diabetes or epilepsy

• over 35 years of age with a long history of inactivity

• cardiovascular or respiratory problems

• chronic joint or back problems.

• obesity

• pregnancy

• heavy drinking or smoking.

amount of exercise gradually. This will avoid any feelings of faintness that may be caused by the pooling of blood below the waist that occurs in the course of vigorous exercise.

## monitoring your pulse rate

Checking your pulse rate at regular intervals is crucial because it allows you to monitor whether you are exercising adequately. The maximum heart rate for an adult is approximately 220 beats per minute minus your age in years. The ideal heart rate during exercise is betweem 65 and 80 per cent of this figure. The aim of exercise is to get your

## warming up and cooling down

Warm-up activities are important because they ensure that your body is ready for exercise: they ease your muscles into action so that they react more readily to activity, and they also prepare you for a rise in heart rate and body temperature. Warm-ups should be done slowly and rhythmically for 5–10 minutes (depending on age and personal fitness).

In addition, it is very important to set time aside to cool down after exercising: keep walking or moving around slowly for at least 5 minutes. This cool-down period is vital because it allows you to decrease the

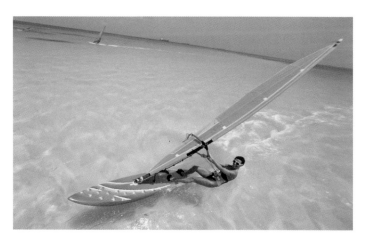

# Exercise and relaxation

We push ourselves at such a pace these days that feeling stressed can, at times, almost become the normal way to feel. A certain level of stress is necessary because it helps to keep us on the ball, but being under prolonged pressure, and ignoring physical signs such as shaky hands, hyperventilation and a fast heartbeat, is not at all healthy. So if any of these sensations sound familiar to you, resolve to make time every day to relax your body and free your mind of problems.

## how exercise helps you to relax

Exercise doesn't just tone your muscles, it also eases the muscular aches and pains that go hand-in-hand with stress; it also distracts your mind from the worries that make you tense. Regular exercise – and especially yoga – lifts your mood (remember how good you felt the last time you did some invigorating exercise?) and soothes your mind. As you become fitter, you will find that your ability to cope with the mundane problems that crop up improves.

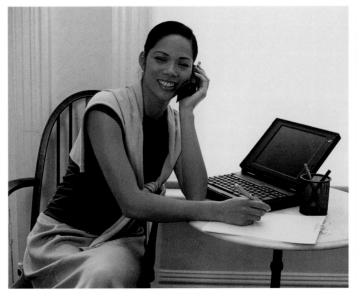

## yoga – a good route to relaxation

Yoga is an exercise technique and ancient doctrine based on achieving mental, physical and spiritual harmony. The belief is that when all these elements are in tune with each other, overall health is at a peak. As well as improving joint mobility, suppleness, shape and self-image, yoga can dispel the headaches and tiredness brought on by stress and nervous tension. The practice involves many active principles, but the most popular ones that are used in Western teaching are as follows:

**Asanas, or postures:** These are held for several minutes at a time and, together with the correct breathing, perfected to give certain physical, spiritual and emotional benefits before each new step is learned.

**Pranayama:** This is deep, slow breathing

△ Sitting at a desk hunched over a computer or talking on the phone, we often don't realize how tense our bodies become. It is important to take regular breaks away from your desk.

which is normally done while sitting – either in a lotus position or on a chair that allows your spine to stay straight. If you find it difficult to sit straight then lie down.

**Relaxation:** Up to 15 minutes is spent resting (usually lying flat on the floor) after yoga to help your mind and body unwind and recharge. Yoga principles and postures are best learned with a teacher, rather than out of a book.

## pilates – creating a relaxed, confident stance

In Pilates, controlled repetitive actions realign and re-educate the body. Mental focus and breathing techniques encourage flowing movements and increased awareness as well as improving body tone. Pilates combines stretches and strengthening exercises and is one of the safest forms of exercise.

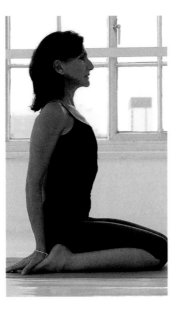

◁ There are many forms of yoga but they all emphasize the importance of good breathing and posture, of body awareness and of working within your own abilities.

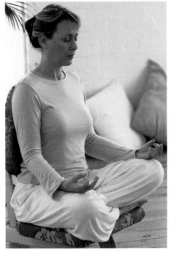

△ Meditation is a pleasant way to relax completely. The physical benefits include relaxation, improvement of sleeping patterns, lowering of high blood pressure and speedier recovery from fatigue.

◁ Lie comfortably on the floor for 15 minutes and focus on tensing and then totally relaxing every part of your body from top to toe.

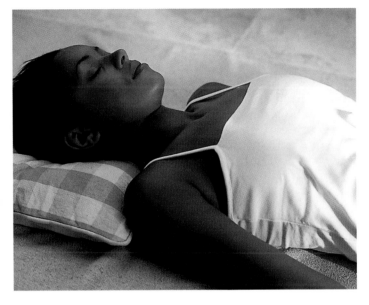

## neck and shoulders – tension focus

Anyone who has ever spent most of the day at their desk, or hunched over a computer keyboard for long periods without a break knows all about the discomfort that stiff neck, back and shoulder "knots" can cause. Our upper torso is usually the focal point for mental and physical stress, and the stiffness this causes can lead to headaches and back pain. One of the best ways to avoid and relieve this type of physical stress is to get up and walk around the room regularly, stretching and loosening your shoulders by circling them backwards and forwards as you go.

## improving respiratory awareness

Our emotional state is reflected by our breathing patterns. When we are under strain or nervous, we tend either to hyperventilate (over-breath) or to inhale short, shallow breaths – a habit that you can break only when your attention is drawn to it. Examine the way you are breathing now: is your breathing pattern regular and steady? If not, take a couple of slow, deep breaths and start again, and this time make a conscious effort to breathe steady, equal, calm breaths.

## instant relaxation

Stand by an open window and take deep breaths for a slow count of 10 or 12. Then hold your breath for about 10 seconds, and release with a long "aaah". (To begin with, do twice only or it might make you feel dizzy or faint.)

---

**RELAXATION CHECKLIST**

If you are aware of yourself becoming tense, set aside 10 minutes at the end of each day to relax (or make time in the middle of the day if you need it). The important thing is to run slowly through this progressive relaxation checklist step by step:

• **Be aware of your body:** Tense every little bit of your body, then make a conscious effort to relax every part. Bunch your toes, then free them; clench your thigh and buttock muscles, then let them relax; pull in your stomach muscles and let them go; hunch your shoulders, then relax them; clench and relax your hands several times.

• **Monitor your breathing pattern:** Take note of how you are breathing: is the pattern slow and regular? If not, inhale deeply and slowly, hold your breath for a couple of seconds, then release it again, letting your body relax completely as you exhale.

• **Correct your posture:** Sitting, standing and walking badly can also produce knots and tightness in the muscles in your back, neck and shoulders. It is vital that you study the way that you sit, stand and move and work on correcting any postures that cause tension in your body.

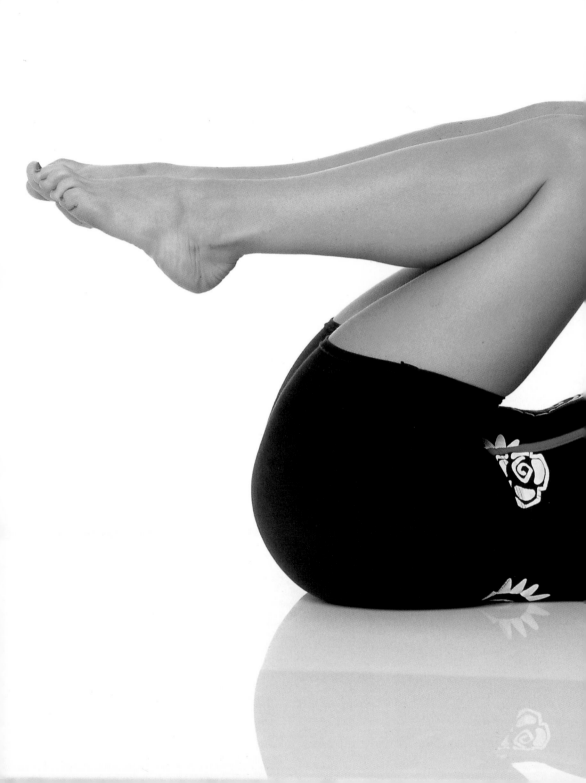

# Keeping Fit

Are you unfit and out of shape? You might blame your lifestyle because today everything is geared to make life as easy as possible, and you might find it hard to make time to take exercise. However, keeping fit does not need to be hard work and time-consuming. If you want a firmer, healthier body, simply follow the exercise sequences in this chapter.

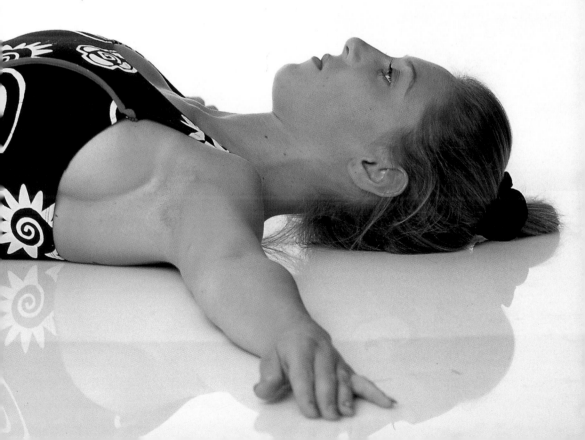

# Exercises for general fitness

This exercise routine helps to improve overall fitness and should take you roughly 30 minutes to complete. Aim to do the routine three times a week and try to fit in extra aerobic exercises – such as swimming, walking or cycling – on the other days (aerobic exercises include activities that can be done rhythmically and continuously and that boost the efficient uptake of oxygen).

**SOME POINTS TO REMEMBER BEFORE YOU EXERCISE**
- If you are not in the habit of exercising regularly, it is advisable to check with your doctor that this exercise routine is suitable for you.
- If you feel any pain or feel dizzy – or experience anything other than the normal sensation of muscle fatigue – stop exercising.
- Always work out at your own pace; don't feel you have to work faster than feels comfortable or do more than you feel capable of.
- It is advisable to avoid exercise if you are ill, or have a virus or a raised temperature.

## warm-up exercises

Before you start the general exercises, it is extremely important that you set aside the time to warm up your muscles. A warm-up routine can take as little as 2 or 3 minutes and the aim is to stretch and loosen your muscles. If they are feeling tight or stiff, it can be risky to start exercising vigorously immediately because this can result in strains and even injuries. You can follow the special warm-up exercises outlined on these pages, or carry out your own routine of stretches for a couple of minutes. If you do your own routine, remember to include exercises to warm up your whole body.

Think of warm-up exercises as a way of easing your body slowly and gently into increased activity. Focus on making the movements relaxed, slow and rhythmical, not sharp and jerky. Each of the exercises focuses on warming and stretching a particular area of the body. It is crucial that you take the time to repeat the sequences and make sure that you follow each movement exactly. Concentrate particularly on stretching and extending the neck, spine and legs, which are more susceptible to injury than other parts.

**Warm-up exercise A**

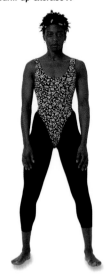 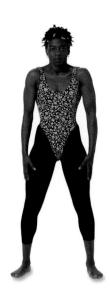 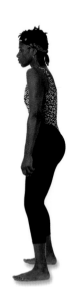 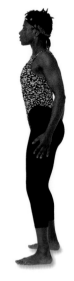

△ **1** Stand upright with your feet apart and in line with your shoulders, with your arms hanging loosely at your sides and your shoulders down.

△ **2** Bring your shoulders forwards.

△ **3** Then raise them as high as you can.

△ **4** Now move your shoulders back as far as possible. Finally, bring them back to the starting position.

## Warm-up exercise B

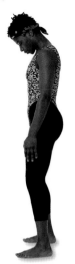

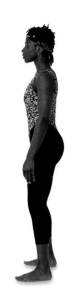

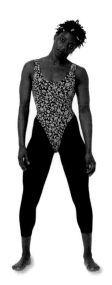

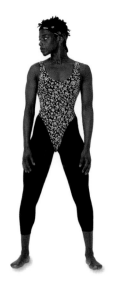

△ **1** Maintain an upright posture as in Exercise A. Tip your head forwards so that your chin is almost resting on your chest.

△ **2** Raise your head, stretching and lengthening your neck as you return to the upright position. Repeat 4 times.

△ **3** Tip your head to the left, keeping the shoulders down, then return to the centre, stretching to lengthen your neck. Repeat with your head to the right. Repeat 4 times on each side.

△ **4** Keep your head up and look over your left shoulder. Then face forwards and stretch to lengthen your neck. Repeat 4 times. Now do 4 times turning to the right. Repeat this sequence twice.

## Warm-up exercise C

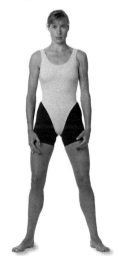

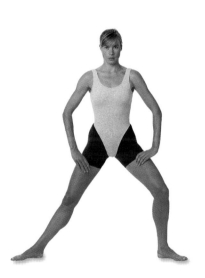

△ **1** Stand with your feet fairly wide apart; lean forwards slightly from your hips keeping your chest lifted and back straight.

△ **2** Rotate and bend your left leg out from the hip so your knee is over your left foot and pointing in the same direction. Keep your right leg straight. You will feel a stretch in the inner thigh; if not, move your feet wider. Repeat 5 times, hold for 5 seconds; swap legs and repeat.

### REPETITION GUIDE FOR GENERAL FITNESS EXERCISES

| Toning Exercises | Repeats/Time Allowance |
|---|---|
| Warm-ups | 5 minutes |
| Press-ups | 10 repeats |
| Lying Flies | 10 repeats |
| Squats | 10 repeats |
| Reverse Curls | 10 repeats |
| Sit-ups | 10 repeats |
| Cool-downs | 3–5 minutes |
| Aerobic Exercise | 20–30 minutes |

The recommended 10 repeats are for beginners – you should aim to repeat each exercise (from Warm-ups to Cool-downs) 15 times, or as often as is comfortable. Start by doing this set of exercises twice a week, then work up to three times a week and combine it with some other form of exercise – ideally aerobic – for the time suggested above.

# working on the chest, back and legs

Once you have warmed up properly, you are ready to begin these exercises which focus on your chest, back, legs and abdominal muscles. Read the instructions carefully and make sure you understand how to carry out each movement. If you follow this routine at least twice a week, and combine it with another form of exercise, you will soon have a fitter, firmer and healthier body.

## chest muscles: press-ups

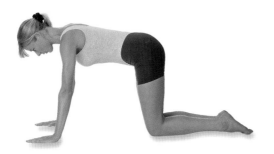

△ **1** Place yourself on all fours with your knees directly under your hips, your hands beneath your shoulders with your fingers pointing forwards, and your palms flat. Make sure your back is straight – that is, parallel with the ceiling – all the time. Achieve this by pulling your stomach in and tucking your pelvis under.

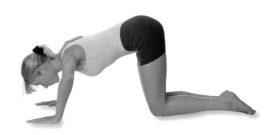

△ **2** Steadily lower yourself – nose first – towards the floor. Then raise yourself back to the starting position, breathing in as you go.

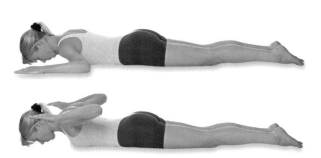

## upper back muscles: lying flies

◁ **1** Lie on your front on the floor with your hips down, and keep your body relaxed. Rest your forehead on the floor, your arms out on each side at right angles to your body, elbows bent.

◁ **2** Keeping your elbows bent, steadily lift both arms, making sure they are parallel to the floor. Lower your arms once again. Make sure you don't pull your elbows back; keep them in line with your shoulders and keep your hips and feet in contact with the floor all the time.

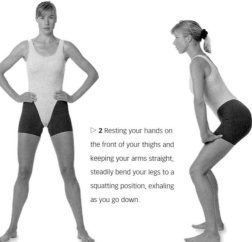

## leg muscles: squats

▷ **1** Stand up straight with your feet a little more than shoulder-width apart. If you stand on tiptoe, this exercise tones your calf muscles and your quadriceps, the muscles on the front of your thighs; if you angle your toes slightly outwards while on tiptoe, it benefits your inner thighs.

▷ **2** Resting your hands on the front of your thighs and keeping your arms straight, steadily bend your legs to a squatting position, exhaling as you go down.

▷ **3** Then, inhale as you rise steadily back to the starting position. When you do this exercise, it is important to keep your back straight and your knees flexible. Don't let your knees bend further forward than your toes.

# working on the abdominal muscles

When you carry out these exercises, you need to make sure that you keep your lower back pressed into the floor throughout and focus on working slowly, with total control. In the upper abdominals exercise, lift your head and shoulders as one unit, never separately. Roll up from the top of your head; you might find it helpful to imagine you are trying to hold a peach between your chin and your chest, as it is important to try to keep this gap constant throughout. Make sure your face muscles are completely relaxed all the time.

## lower abdominals: reverse curls

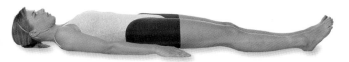

△ **1** Lie flat on your back on the floor, arms by your sides, palms flat on the floor beside you. Keep your shoulder blades down and relax your neck.

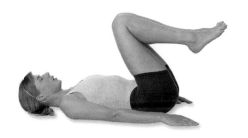

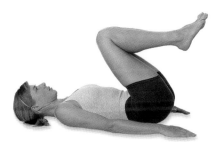

△ **2** While keeping your arms and hands flat on the floor, bring your knees in towards your chest one at a time, and once there, keep both knees together in the bent position.

△ **3** Breathe in and, keeping your spine firmly pressed into the floor, pull in your abdominal muscles while at the same time curling up your coccyx (tail-bone) to bring your knees closer to your chest. Keep your feet relaxed throughout. Lower your body to the starting position, exhaling as you go down.

## upper abdominals: sit-ups

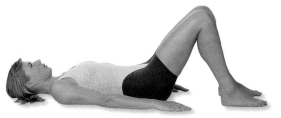

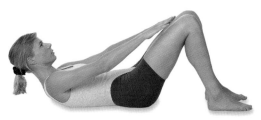

△ **1** Lying flat on the floor with your arms by your side, palms flat on the floor, bend your knees and keep your feet flat on the floor a little distance apart in line with your hips.

△ **2** Lift your head and shoulders – inhaling as you move up – and push your fingertips towards your knees keeping your arms straight. Lower your body back to the starting position, exhaling as you go down; repeat the movement.

# Choosing the right sport

Team sports and work-outs at the gym are fun; they also add to your exercise quota for the week, helping you reach your self-improvement goals that much faster. The benefits of taking part in specific sports and of working out are given here.

## make exercise easy to do

Your body cannot "store" fitness, so once you have started, you have to keep exercising regularly. Make your routine flexible: if you think it is going to be hard to maintain, don't choose an activity that requires good weather or a long detour from your office or home.

## sports and work-outs

**Badminton:** Aerobic; improves joint flexibility, stamina, leg and shoulder tone and strength; 30–40 minutes' continuous play burns up around 200–800 calories.

**Golf:** Anaerobic; improves arm, shoulder and leg tone, and strength (you walk 6.5–8km/4–5 miles when you do a round of golf and burn off around 100–200 calories).

**Jogging:** Aerobic; improves stamina and leg strength and tone; an hour's jogging burns up 200–350 calories. Before taking up jogging take the usual precautions: check with your doctor and, as with all aerobic exercise, increase the pace gradually.

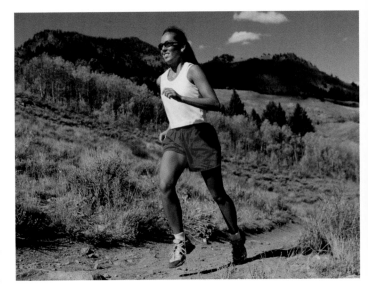

**Tennis:** Aerobic; boosts stamina and suppleness; strengthens and tones your shoulders, forearms, calves and thighs; if you play very energetically (with plenty of running around the court) at least twice a week for an hour, you will burn up around 300–400 calories per session.

△ When you go jogging always wear a good-quality pair of trainers and support bandages if your joints are weak.

**Brisk walking:** Aerobic; strengthens and tones your legs. (You should lose up to 100 calories per hour.)

**Cycling:** Aerobic; builds stamina; tones legs. (An hour's cycling could lose you 250–400 calories, depending on the terrain.)

**Skipping:** Aerobic; boosts stamina, strength and leg tone. Start with 3 skipping sets of 30 seconds with a 5-minute break after each;

---

**DIETING COMBINED WITH EXERCISE**

You will lose weight if you limit your food intake, but not as quickly or as evenly as you would if you combined a balanced weight-loss diet with regular exercise. This is because exercise increases your metabolism, and, if you want to lose weight more quickly, you need to exercise in conjunction with dieting.

---

**THE RIGHT FOOTWEAR**

What you wear on your feet is crucial to your performance and to the benefits you will get from exercise. Good sports shops will give advice on the right trainers to wear for different activities, but cross-trainers – designed to be worn for most sports – are probably your best investment because they are good all-rounders.

---

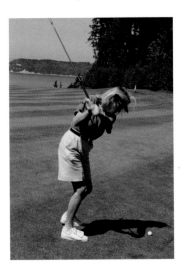

▷ Golf is a sport that particularly benefits shoulders, arms and legs. Playing a round of golf involves a good deal of walking.

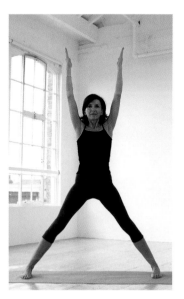

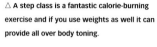

△ **A step class is a fantastic calorie-burning exercise and if you use weights as well it can provide all over body toning.**

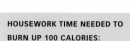

◁ **With minimal equipment and easy to fit into a daily routine, yoga is excellent for building up strength and tone thoughout the body.**

**HOUSEWORK TIME NEEDED TO BURN UP 100 CALORIES:**
Ironing: 50 minutes
Sweeping the floor: 40 minutes
Washing up: 60 minutes
Vacuuming: 30 minutes

then build up to skipping for 2 minutes with a 10-minute break and also increase the repetitions. (Expect to lose up to 500 calories per hour.)

**Rebounding:** Aerobic; bounding on a mini trampoline is a fun way to get fit at home. (In an hour expect to lose 300 calories.)

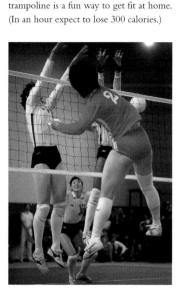

◁ **Taking part in a team sport once a week is a good idea:** not only will it make you fitter, slimmer and happier, but the competitive spirit will also strengthen your resolve.

**Swimming:** Aerobic; swimming is one of the fastest (and best) ways to boost overall fitness, muscle tone, joint flexibility and relaxation. Do 4 lengths of a 25m/25yd pool, rest for a minute and build endurance by reducing rest time and increasing your swim time; within a fortnight you will be noticeably fitter and firmer; an hour's breaststroke burns 500–800 calories.

**Football:** Aerobic; improves stamina; strengthens and tones your legs; an hour's play burns up around 250–1000 calories.

**Boxing:** Aerobic; tones and strengthens your chest, shoulders and arms; an hour's boxing burns up around 400–600 calories.

**Volleyball:** Aerobic; improves stamina; tones and strengthens the whole body, especially your legs and arms; mobilizes joints; an hour's play burns up 200–600 calories.

**Squash:** As above; an hour's play burns up 400–1000 calories.

**Aerobics:** Specific aerobics classes combine exercise with constant movement for up to an hour; fast fat-burners are an ideal activity to do regularly if you are after speedy results. In an hour-long class you would lose 250–500 calories, depending on intensity.

**Circuit, cross, resistance or weight training:** Aerobic; increase stamina, strength and suppleness; an hour of circuit training burns up 350–550 calories.

**Step classes:** Aerobic; improves stamina; tones and strengthens your lower torso (bottom, thighs and calves); an hour-long class burns up 500–800 calories.

**Yoga:** Improves posture; tones; strengthens and relaxes the body; loosens joints; an hour of yoga burns up about 200 calories.

**HELP FOR PMS**
Exercise is the last thing you feel like doing when you are pre-menstrual. However, it will make you feel more relaxed and relieve the symptoms. Swimming is particularly beneficial.

# Body shape

The shape of your body is unique, and it is important to remember that this is because the basic skeletal and muscular form that you have inherited is unchangeable. Features such as your height, foot size, shoulder width and the length and shape of your legs, nose, fingers and toes combine to produce a whole. Each person is an individual, with characteristics and features particular to their genetic make-up.

## body types

Although we come in a variety of shapes and sizes, the human body is cast from three basic moulds. Often, features from two or three of these body types are jumbled with our individual characteristics, but it is the more dominant features that slot us into one of the following groups: ectomorphs, mesomorphs and endomorphs.

Ectomorphs are usually small- and slender-framed with long limbs and narrow shoulders, hips and joints. They usually have little muscle or body fat. Mesomorphs have medium to large – but compact – frames with broader shoulders and pelvic girdle, and well-developed muscles. Endomorphs are naturally curvaceous, with more body fat than muscle, wider hips, shorter limbs and a lower centre of gravity than the other two body types.

## self-image

If you are a little overweight, it can be annoying to hear someone who you think is slim moaning about being overweight. Remember though that this stems from self-image. Very few of us actually see ourselves as we really are. We tend to misjudge our bodies with sweeping claims to fatness, even when we have only a spot of excess flab around our midriff to show for it. And although it sounds amazing, the way we behave in everyday life (and think others see us) often tallies with our self-image. It's a vicious circle: we think we don't measure up to the standard beauty ideal so our self-

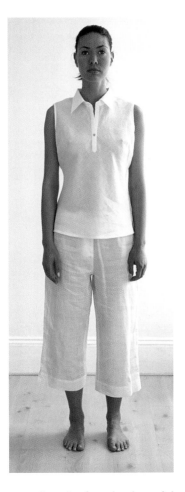

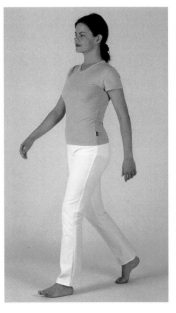

△ Alexander Technique focuses on improving posture and ease of movement during simple activities such as walking, bending and lifting. It explores how the mind and body work together to perform everyday tasks.

◁ We all have things about our bodies we would like to change. Standing up straight and feeling confident about how we look is vital for a positive self-image.

esteem dips again, often so low that we feel we will never have a better body. This in turn causes self-confidence to plummet further, we feel even worse, and so the vicious circle continues.

Taking control of your self-image brings enormous bonuses. And the faster you can do this, the greater the rewards, as speedy results boost your confidence more quickly. But before you undertake a scheme to get into better shape, you must work on your positive thinking: realize your potential by deciding on (and accepting) your body

model, then use this as your goal. Forget conventional beauty ideals – you don't have to have mile-long legs to have a good figure, and what you already have – your basic shape – is great. It just needs perfecting, and that is something that everyone can do.

## good posture

The difference that good posture makes to the look of our bodies is enormous, mainly because when we are standing properly our abdominal muscles are in their correct supporting role and the whole body is

▷ Improving self-image can be as simple as making positive affirmations while in a calm, meditative state. We all have qualities in which we can take pride and pleasure, and it is important to focus on these positive attributes.

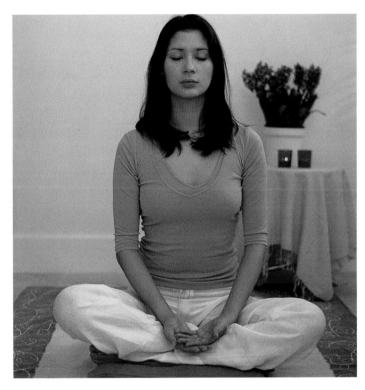

aligned so that it looks leaner and taller. Good posture is also beneficial for our mental and physical health; some alternative therapies (such as the Alexander Technique) are based on the principle of correct posture because it can be very helpful for easing back pain, stress and even headaches.

## STRAIGHTENING THE SPINE

This is a very simple exercise to carry out to improve your posture.

Kneel on the floor, take a deep breath in, and then on the out breath drop and relax your shoulders. Imagine your head is attached to a cord tied to the ceiling. Every time you breathe out imagine the cord pulling your head up, and your spine lengthening and straightening.

# neck care for improving posture

▽ A poor posture profile, such as a curved back, slumped shoulders and a head that juts forward, is commonplace. Stretching exercises can help reverse this trend before the poor posture becomes habitual.

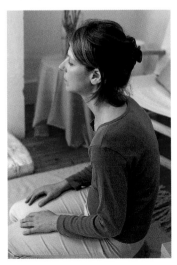

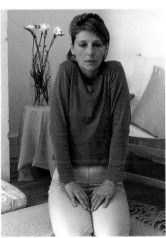

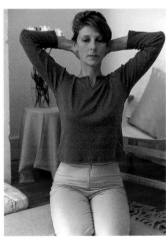

△ **1** Take a deep breath in and slowly begin to lift your shoulders up and back as far as they will comfortably go. On the out breath, slowly release, beginning the upward movement again on the next breath. As your shoulder blades come down, imagine them meeting in the middle of your back. Shoulder shrugs help to release tension in the large muscles of the upper back that pull on the neck.

△ **2** Centre your head and tuck in your chin. Put your hands behind your head, push your head against them and hold for 3–5 seconds. Repeat 10–20 times. Then place one hand on the side of your head. With your chin in, push your head against your hand and hold for 3–5 seconds. Repeat 10–20 times. Swap hands and repeat on the other side. These movements help to strengthen the neck muscles.

# Tackling problem areas

Very few people are able to say honestly that they are totally happy with their body. Everyone has at least one gripe – if it is not big feet, it is thin hair or knobbly knees. All these perceived "flaws" can be improved or disguised, but as anyone who has ever tried (and failed) to move the fat that sits on strategic points such as hips, thighs, stomachs and buttocks knows, it is much easier to hide the flaws than to tackle them. Trouble spots such as these are notoriously stubborn to shift, but it is possible to alter your outline with a combination of diet and exercise.

## common problems

Any of the following can be discouraging, but remember – each problem has a solution.

**Slack stomachs:** Our stomachs become flabby when the abdominal muscles slacken; this usually happens through lack of exercise. Your abdomen extends from just under the bustline to the groin, and it is packed with muscles that criss-cross to form a wall to hold the abdominal contents in place – a bit like a corset. Exercise is not the only way to keep your stomach flat though: weight is also an important factor and the long-term answer is both diet and exercise.

**Thunder thighs:** Like bottoms and busts, thighs are a great source of discontent, whether it is because they are too flabby, muscular or skinny. You inherit the basic shape of your thighs, but that does not

necessarily mean that you were born with the excess fat that may be covering them. Thigh size and tone can certainly be altered with the right diet, correct body care and regular exercise. Sports such as cycling, skiing, tennis, squash and riding (a great inner-muscle firmer) will tone your thighs, as will weight-training for specific areas of the body.

**Large bottoms:** There are three large muscles in our buttocks: gluteus maximus, medius and minimus. These create the shape, but not the size, of our rear ends. It is the tone of these muscles and the fatty tissue around them that gives us the bottoms we have. The good news is that buttock muscles respond well to exercise, which means that any effort you put into bottom-toning exercises will be rewarded quite quickly. Locomotive exercises – such as fast walking, running upstairs and jogging – are especially good bottom trimmers. Other exercises are given in the Exercises for Specific Problems.

**Slack upper arms:** Arms do not really change shape a great deal during our lives, unless we lose or gain a lot of weight. Muscle tone is the main problem, but, as in the case of thighs, exercise and specific weight-training will tone up and reshape flabby arms. It is very often the case that any changes in body shape that happen through exercise and diet are noticeable most quickly on your upper arms.

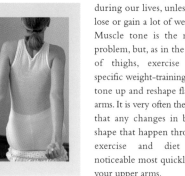

△ **The best way to assess your figure is to stand in front of a full-length mirror. Be honest with yourself, and look for areas that need improving.**

**Droopy breasts:** Breast shape and size only really change when our weight swings dramatically, during pregnancy, breast-feeding, menstruation, or if taking oral contraceptives. Gravity is the bust's worst enemy, especially if the breasts are not given proper support, because it literally drags the breasts down and slackens their tone. Although the breasts are supported by suspensory ligaments, they do not contain any muscle (the milk glands are buffered by protective fatty tissue) so you cannot noticeably reverse lost tone. However, if you exercise the pectoral muscles beneath your armpits you will give your breasts a firmer base and more uplift.

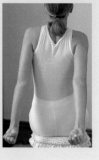

**FLABBY ARM FIXER**
To firm up flabby arms, add this exercise to your daily exercise routine, or spend five minutes doing it twice a day. Sit on a chair holding your hands in loose fists and, with your arms extended behind, make downwards punching movements backwards and forwards.

**TWO QUICK THIGH-TONERS**

If you do not have time to do a full exercise routine, grab 10 minutes in the morning and evening to warm up and do these two exercises.

**outer thighs**

Sit on the floor with your legs straight out in front and hold your arms out to the sides as shown. Roll sideways on to your bottom – go right over on to your outer thigh and then roll right over on to the other thigh. Do this 20 times.

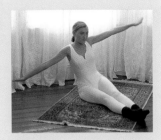

**inner thighs**

Stand upright and consciously tighten – and hold – your buttock muscles for a slow count of five. Repeat with your thigh muscles and then your calf muscles. You can do this while you are waiting for your bath to run, standing at the bus stop, and so on.

**Thick ankles:** Trim and slender ankles are seen to be a great asset. But if you are not blessed with these, or if your ankles tend to become stiff and puffy from fluid retention, you need to brush up on some ankle-improving exercises.

Assess the flexibility of your ankles by sitting on a chair or stool with your feet on the floor and, while keeping your heel down pull the rest of your foot up as far as it will go: if the distance between your foot and the floor measures 12–15cm/5–6in your joint flexibility is good; if it is between 10–12cm/4–5in it is fair; and if it is less than that, your joint flexibility is poor.

## improving your true form

Obviously there are certain things about your body shape that you will never be able to change. However, it is important to focus on your good points and remember that there is a great deal you can do to improve on your natural shape and form.

**Confront your body:** Go on, be brave. Strip to your underwear, stand in front of a mirror and have a good look at your body. Take your time and be tough but realistic. You may have disliked your thighs since you were 16 – and they will probably never be those of a supermodel – but if you look hard enough you might just find that they are not as bad as you have always thought, and that improving them is not going to be that hard after all.

**Write it all down:** Note down all the things that annoy you (and that you can do something about) as well as those that you like or do not mind. Then go through your list of dislikes, ticking the things that you really want to do something about. Also, make a mental note to start appreciating your good points: the more you focus on them the less you will notice the not-so-good zones.

**Make an action checklist:** Add a set of action points under the problem zones you have listed. If you want to firm up your arms for that sleeveless sundress you have been unable to wear for a decade of summers, make notes like this:

Flabby Upper Arms

Do Basic Exercises

Check diet

Exfoliate/moisturize.

Finally, add your goal(s) and your deadline to the top of the list and put it somewhere where you are going to see it frequently.

▽ **Making an action checklist will help you focus on your goals.**

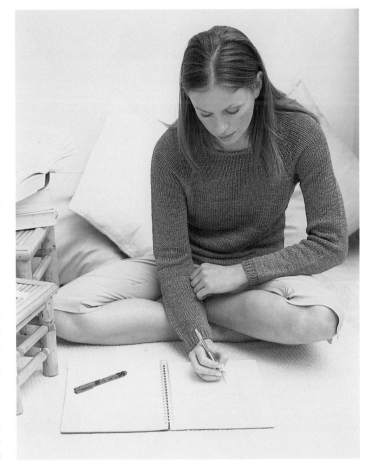

# Exercises for specific problem areas

Add these basic exercises to your general fitness routine to give special problem areas extra work, or do them on their own as an isolated routine. If you do them on their own, use the abdominal muscle exercises from the general fitness plan for your stomach – and remember to warm up first and cool down afterwards.

## thigh muscles

### exercise A

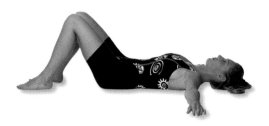

△ **1** Lie on your back on the floor with your arms resting straight out at right angles to your body and your feet apart in line with your hips.

△ **2** Hold a cushion between your knees and, keeping your back pressed into the floor, press your knees together 10 times quickly and 10 times slowly, keeping the cushion in place throughout.

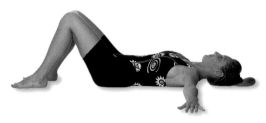

△ **3** Now repeat the sequence from step 2 again, but this time holding a tennis or golf ball between your knees.

### exercise B

▽ **1** Lie on your back on the floor with your legs straight and your lower back pressed to the floor. Put your arms along your sides, palms to the floor.

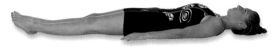

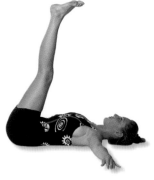

◁ **3** Keeping your legs together, steadily straighten them so that they are pointing up towards the ceiling. Keep your feet relaxed, do not point them.

▷ **2** Stretch your arms out to the side at right angles to your body. Bend your legs and bring your knees in towards your chest.

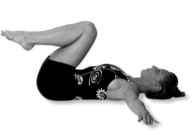

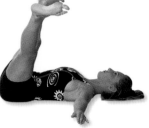

◁ **4** Slowly open your legs out sideways – as wide as you can – then close them again. Repeat the exercise 4 times. When you feel completely comfortable with this exercise, you can try doing it with small weights tied to your ankles.

### exercise C

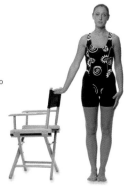
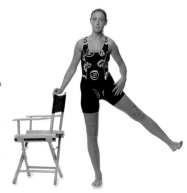

▷ **1** Stand alongside a chair or table (lightly holding the edge to maintain your balance), with your shoulders down and relaxed. Have your knees slightly bent and your feet facing forwards.

▷ **2** Lift your left hip slightly and slowly move your leg out and up (no higher than 45 degrees), keeping your foot and knee facing forwards. Make sure you do not let your body tilt – keep it as straight as possible. Carefully lower your leg. Repeat the whole exercise 10 times, then turn and repeat with the other leg.

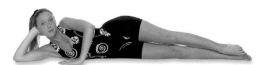
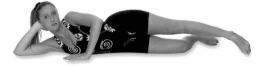

### exercise D

△ **1** Lie on your right side on the floor with your legs out straight. Support your head with your right hand.

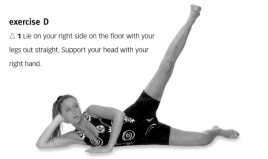

△ **2** Bend your lower leg behind you to maintain balance and tilt your hips slightly towards the floor; your head, hips, knees and feet should all be facing forwards. Balance yourself with your left hand on the floor in front of you.

◁ **3** Slowly lift your upper leg, then bring it down until it touches the lower one; raise it again and repeat this movement 6 times. Turn over and repeat steps 1–3 on the other side.

## ankles and calf muscles

### exercise A

▽ **1** Sit up straight on a chair, with your knees together and heels on the floor and slightly apart, in line with your hips. Bring your big toes up (as high off the floor as possible) and roll your feet in towards each other.

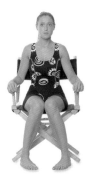
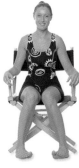

▷ **2** Now tilt and move both feet down and outwards from the ankle, keeping your big toes raised as much as possible as you roll your feet on to their outer edges. Repeat this 10 times.

### exercise B

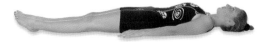

△ **1** Lie flat on your back on the floor with your legs straight.

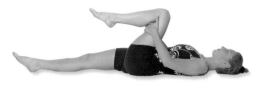

△ **2** Bring one leg up and hold it beneath the back of your thigh so that it is pulled towards your chest. Rotate your foot 10 times clockwise and 10 times anti-clockwise. Repeat with the other leg. Increase the number of repeats to 20 for each foot, working alternately in groups of 7.

# buttock muscles

### exercise A

▷ **1** Stand upright and lightly hold the back of a chair or the edge of a table with both hands to maintain your balance. Put your weight on your right leg and turn your left leg out from the hip.

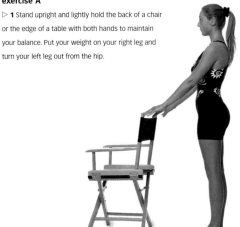

▷ **2** Keeping your foot flexed, take your left leg back as far as you can without bending it at the knee, forcing the movement or over-arching your back. Repeat with the other leg. Repeat 5 times for each leg and gradually build up to 20 repetitions.

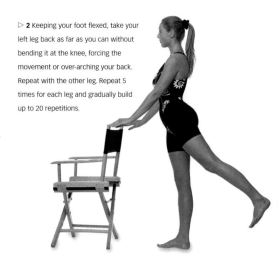

### exercise B

▽ **1** Lie on your back with your knees bent and your feet slightly apart, in line with your hips. Place your arms by your sides, palms flat on the floor.

▽ **2** Place your weight on your shoulders and upper back (not your neck), raise your bottom to a comfortable height and tighten your buttock muscles, keeping your feet flat on the floor and your arms by your sides. Hold for several seconds. Lower your bottom to the floor. Repeat 5 times, building up to 20 repetitions.

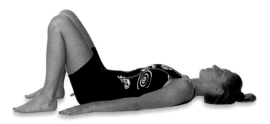
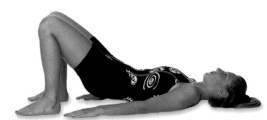

### exercise C

▽ **1** Kneel on all fours with your knees slightly apart, in line with your hips, but keeping them tucked right under your hips. Place your hands in front of you, shoulder-width apart and facing forwards. Bend your elbows so that you are leaning on your forearms.

▽ **2** Keeping your foot flexed, push your left leg out straight behind you, keeping your back and hips parallel. Bring your leg and foot down to the floor, keeping your foot flexed and your leg straight. Repeat 12 times. Return to the original position, then repeat the exercise with your other leg. Build up to 20 repetitions.

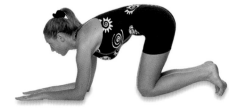
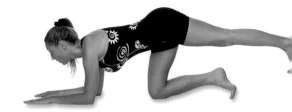

# upper arm muscles

▷ **1** Stand upright with your feet shoulder-width apart and your arms hanging loosely by your sides.

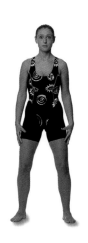

▷ **2** Lift your arms, flex your hands and make 5 small circles forwards and then backwards with both arms moving simultaneously. Aim to build up to 20 circles, and when you are used to the exercise, hold a can of beans in each hand and repeat. You can vary the exercise by bringing your arms around to the front and tracing the circles there as well. As you improve with practise, move your feet closer together.

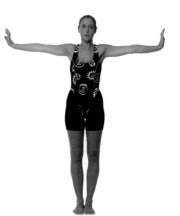

# bust (pectoral) muscles

**exercise A**

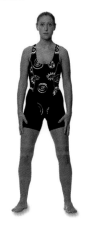

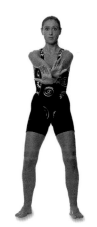

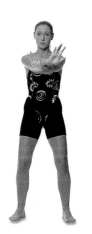

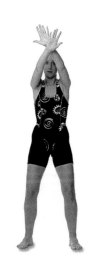

△ **1** Stand upright with your feet apart in line with your shoulders. Keep your shoulders up, back straight, bottom and stomach tucked in, legs slightly bent and arms loosely by your sides.

△ **2** Make a scissor movement across the front of your body (at waist-level) by crossing one hand over the other while holding your arms straight out in front.

△ **3** Raise your arms to chest level and repeat the action.

△ **4** Then repeat the action holding your arms at head level. Keep the scissor movements controlled as you swing; do 20 repetitions at each level.

**exercise B**

▽ **1** Kneel on all fours as if you were about to do press-ups, with your legs raised at the back and your feet crossed. Your arms should be straight.

▽ **2** Bend your arms as you lower your body to the floor. Do this 10 times to begin with, and build up to 30 repetitions. Remember to keep your back straight.

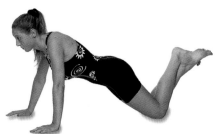

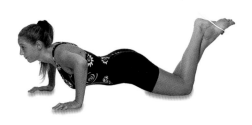

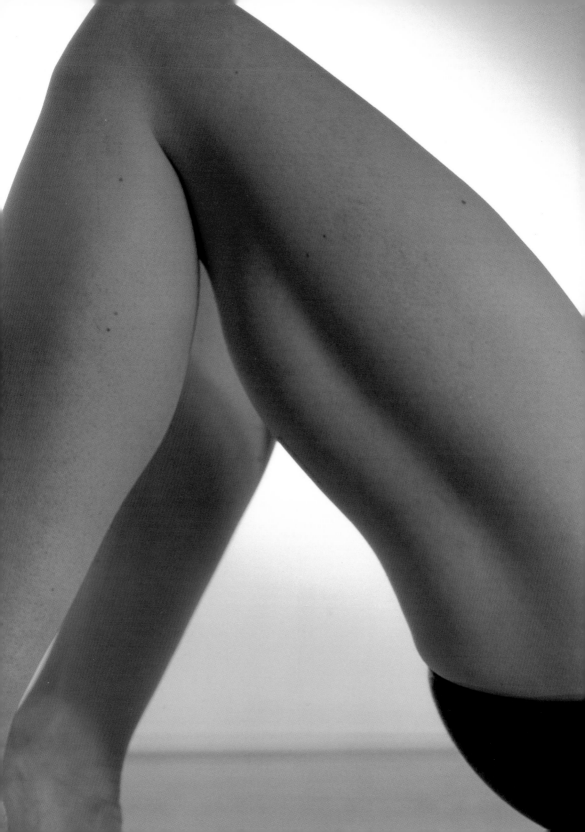

# Introducing Pilates

This section explores the benefits of Pilates and what you can expect to achieve. If you have tried other exercise programmes and wondered why your success was limited, find out why Pilates is different and why its practice will become an essential and enjoyable part of your life.

# The benefits of Pilates

This chapter explains the key elements of Pilates and takes you through a range of exercises. The programme aims to be user-friendly: it is designed for beginners but advanced variations of many exercises are included so that you can progress.

The "first position" in each exercise is the most basic. If you are new to Pilates, start with this one, or you will not master the control and focus needed to perform the exercise correctly. Your main concern is doing the movement correctly, not how many repetitions you can do. The "second position" should be attempted only when you understand the first position. For some people this may take two or more months. Others may take as little as three weeks. Just progress at your own rate. The "third position" is a more intense variation still.

## a holistic approach

It is important to look at exercise in a holistic way and to integrate it into your daily life with minimal disturbance. The programme does not set out to turn you into an Olympic athlete. It might, however,

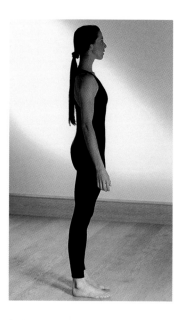

△ Pilates helps to re-define posture, creating a relaxed, confident stance. It is worth remembering that the correct posture can give an illusion of a 2kg/6lb weight loss.

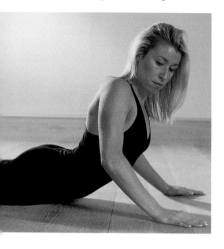

△ Pilates combines stretches and strengthening exercises, making it one of the safest and most effective forms of exercise.

give you that push you need to start exercising by explaining just why it is important, not just for aesthetic purposes but to help you avoid pain and injury, to make you feel good about your body and to increase your self-esteem.

We hope that the programme is clear, logical and simple to remember, so that it will be easy to make it a regular part of your daily routine – just like brushing your teeth – because exercise really should be a matter of course. It's just common sense.

## everyone can benefit

Pilates can benefit everyone, whatever your age or fitness level. Although you will get stronger all over, one of the main benefits of Pilates is to increase core strength. This is a phrase that is used a great deal in Pilates, and it refers to the important abdominal and

back muscles at your centre that support your whole body whether moving or at rest. As these muscles are strengthened, your posture will improve.

If you are new to Pilates, you will find these exercises different from others you may have tried. Pilates involves a series of movements that flow into one another without pauses, and concentrates on the body as a whole, stretching some muscles, strengthening others and, by helping you to function more effectively, reducing the risk of injury in everything you do.

In Pilates only a few repetitions are needed per exercise in comparison with other methods. If you are performing the movements correctly, up to 10 repetitions will be more than adequate. This means that you can give each repetition your full effort and concentration: you will maximize the potential of the exercise without growing tired or bored with continual repetitions.

## the importance of focus

Another distinguishing feature of Pilates is that to practise it you must be totally focused and concentrated. This concentration creates a mind–body connection. A Pilates sequence can help to still the insistent clamour of your daily life, acting like meditation to calm your mind and help you see things more clearly. This focus and attention to alignment and detail makes Pilates unique and very satisfying.

## correct, controlled movements

You should check throughout the exercises that your spine is in neutral (unless otherwise stated), that the abdominals are contracted, that you are not holding your breath at any time, that the muscles not involved in the movement are relaxed (it is common to hold tension in the jaw and shoulders) and that the movements are controlled. All these factors are the key elements that make Pilates so effective, and they are fully explained on the following pages.

▷ Pilates creates a strong, lean, balanced body. This reduces the risk of injury and helps to eliminate nagging aches and pains.

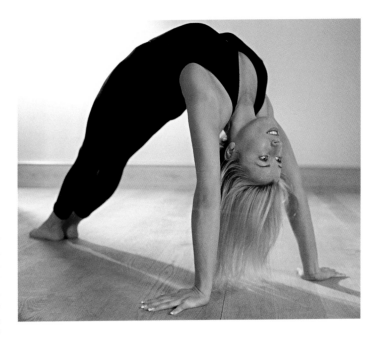

## stabilizing muscles

Muscle imbalances occur through repetitive strain or faulty mechanics, and result in an uneven pull of the muscles around a joint. This imbalance may cause injury to that joint. The pain that results inhibits the postural or stabilizing muscles around the joint and, as a result, these muscles weaken, making the injured joint more unstable and more susceptible to further injury and pain. And so the cycle repeats itself. Even when the area is no longer painful, these muscles do not automatically strengthen again. This is why injuries tend to recur. To recover fully, the muscles in that area need to be specifically strengthened and their co-ordination retrained.

Trunk or core stability requires strength, endurance and co-ordination of the stabilizing abdominal, pelvic floor and lower back muscles. Stability is vital to support and protect the lower back from injury, to help with general postural alignment and to allow the release of the hips for greater freedom of movement. So, better core stability can reduce the chance of injury. Improving it is often the way to get rid of back problems that you may have suffered from for years. Core stability exercises are a crucial part of Pilates, which focuses on improving the strength and control of stabilizing muscles.

## the endorphin effect

You may hear regular exercisers talking about the high they get from activity: this is the production of endorphins, chemicals in the brain that are stimulated by exercise and have similar effects to opiates. Tests have shown that people who suffer from illness and depression are significantly helped by taking exercise.

As well as describing each exercise in detail, this chapter gives advice on putting together a sequence to help you achieve the benefits you are seeking, and on incorporating Pilates into a fitness regime of exercise and healthy eating. Start investing in the present and future health of your body.

▽ Within weeks of beginning regular Pilates practice, you will see a clear improvement. Pilates creates long, lean muscles with no risk of developing a bulky, overdeveloped physique.

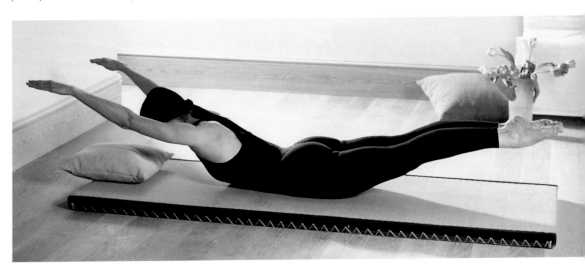

# The key elements of Pilates

Some concepts are referred to repeatedly in Pilates: these are the "key elements" that make it more than just a sequence of movements. Keep them in mind throughout your sessions, relating them to each exercise, and as you become more familiar with the technique they will start to make more sense to you. They will help you to get the most benefit from each movement, and also keep the exercises safe and comfortable. Some of these key elements will come more naturally to you than others, but do not feel discouraged. They will eventually become automatic and you will find yourself applying the same principles to other forms of activity, because they are based on attention to detail and alignment, safety and common sense.

## breathing

You breathe unconsciously, however, when you are completely relaxed and calm your breathing pattern is very different from when you are tense, anxious or negative.

At times of tension and stress, breathing is usually irregular and shallow, and does not completely meet your need for oxygen. If you learn to control your breathing while practising Pilates as well as during daily activity, it will help you to maintain your energy and stay relaxed.

Holding your breath causes tension in your muscles, which decreases when you exhale. For this reason, athletes learn to exhale when executing certain movements such as a tennis serve, a basketball dunk or a golf swing: they are programmed to exhale on the maximum effort. In sports that require a maximum effort during a longer period of time, such as power-lifting, elite athletes will hold their breath. This gives their muscles added stability but has several potentially negative effects on their blood pressure. Remember that these athletes are aiming at a particular goal: they want to win medals at all costs, sometimes even by endangering their health. You should never

hold your breath when exercising. In Pilates, it is sometimes difficult to gauge which of the movements is the one that takes maximum effort. Most of the movements maintain tension in the torso at all times, but your breathing should always be regular and relaxed.

When starting out on this or any other exercise programme, strive to master the general movement first, then focus on the breathing patterns. It is often the case that correct breathing patterns start to come naturally as the body tries to help itself, but you can practise breathing control exercises when you are not moving to help you learn the correct technique. During the exercises try not to let the ribs flare up (push upwards and outwards away from your spine), which sometimes goes hand in hand with arching the spine. Aim to keep the ribs the same distance from your hips, just sliding them out to the sides and then back again as you breathe. This is described as breathing laterally.

## breathing exercise

**Here is a simple breath-control strategy that you can practise at any time. Regulating your breathing will enhance your body awareness and control and make you feel calm and centred.**

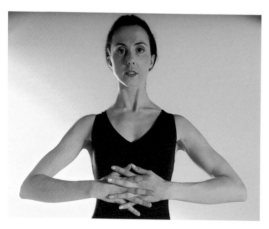

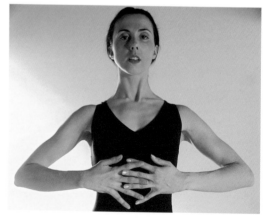

△ **1** Place your hands with your palms under your chest, on your ribs, and your fingers loosely interlocked. Inhale slowly and continuously through your nose, to a count of four. Do not strain, keep yourself relaxed.

△ **2** As you inhale concentrate on allowing your ribs to expand laterally: your fingers should gently part. Don't let your ribs jut forward. Exhale slowly, expelling all the breath from your lungs, then repeat.

## concentration

Your muscles respond better to a training stimulus if the brain is concentrated on the effort. Remember that it is the brain that sends out the signal to the muscle to contract. So, it is imperative that you concentrate on the work you expect the muscle to perform.

It is very easy to get distracted while exercising if you do not set the right mood, avoiding intrusive sounds or disturbances that will take your mind off what you are doing. It is also necessary to prepare yourself mentally to focus on your body and the work that it will be doing.

## control

All movements should be performed slowly and with absolute control. The faster you do anything, the less actual muscle mass you will use to do the exercise; instead, you will be using momentum. Most Pilates movements are not static; they should be continuous but at the same time controlled and precise.

## flow

Pilates movements cannot be likened to repetitions of a conventional exercise. They are continuous. Try to "link" one movement with the next, maintaining a steady flow of energy throughout the session. You will not be stopping and starting as in conventional exercise, but flowing like a steadily turning wheel.

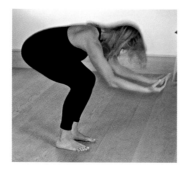

△ **Maintain a steady flow of energy, keeping movements graceful and fluid.**

## relaxation

Pilates is a gradual re-education of the body, and in order to benefit from it you must try not to create unnecessary tension. This would eventually create an imbalance in the body, which is the very thing you are trying to remedy. Watch especially for tension in the neck and jaw, but you may hold it anywhere – even in the feet. During a session, give yourself little mental checks from head to toe and you will start to see where you tend to hold tension. Awareness is half the battle.

## adherence

No exercise programme works unless you do it! Adopt this programme as part of your life and make it as much a part of your daily routine as brushing your teeth. Physical activity is as much a way of taking care of your body as personal hygiene.

▽ **The anterior and posterior views of the human muscular system show the main muscles of the front and back of the body. Although this is a simple diagram only, it will help you to gain a clear understanding of the location of the muscles used throughout your Pilates practice. Be aware, though, that Pilates uses many other supporting muscle groups during different phases of a movement.**

**THE MUSCULAR SYSTEM**

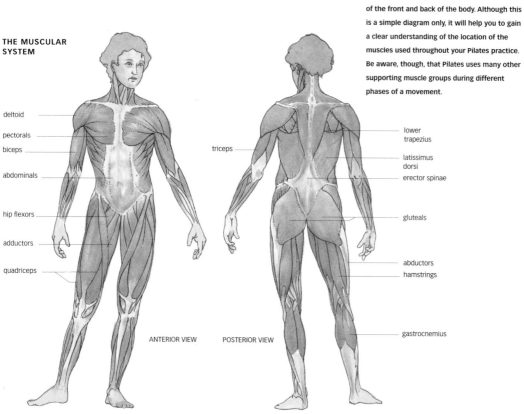

deltoid

pectorals

biceps

abdominals

hip flexors

adductors

quadriceps

triceps

lower trapezius

latissimus dorsi

erector spinae

gluteals

abductors

hamstrings

gastrocnemius

ANTERIOR VIEW          POSTERIOR VIEW

# Core strength

The principal aim of the exercises is to create core strength, which will be the powerhouse for the rest of your body. When you reach a level of understanding of core strength Pilates starts to feel like an altogether different form of exercise: you begin to get a feel for your body working as a whole in a very focused, concentrated way.

The abdominals and back form the centre of the body, from which all movements in Pilates are initiated. If you look at a ferris wheel in a funfair, there is movement around the wheel but the powerhouse is the centre because everything is controlled from there. This is how you should view your body. Your centre should be your first priority, because without sufficient strength in this area you are vulnerable to injury. So, what are these muscles and how do you locate them?

**THE KEY ABDOMINAL MUSCLES**

▷ The illustration displays the key abdominal muscles used in Pilates. These are the muscles used when we refer to "working from a strong centre" or developing "core strength".

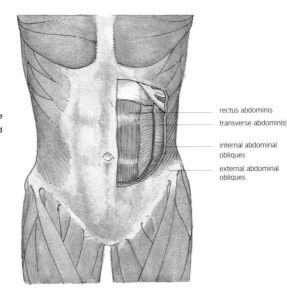

rectus abdominis
transverse abdominis
internal abdominal obliques
external abdominal obliques

## muscles that stabilize the torso

**Rectus abdominis**: This is a wide and long muscle that runs all the way down from the sternum (breast bone) to the pubic bone. The rectus abdominis helps to maintain correct posture and allows forward flexion.

**Obliques**: These are located at the waist, and there are actually two sets: the internal and external obliques. They allow you to rotate at the waist as well as flexing laterally (to illustrate this, imagine that you are picking up a suitcase by your side).

**Transverse abdominis**: This muscle is located behind the rectus abdominis, like a "girdle" wrapped around your stomach. It is used when you draw your navel towards your spine, and is the muscle that contracts when you cough.

## building core strength

By stabilizing the torso you are creating a "co-contraction" between the abdominal muscles and the back muscles. This means that all these muscles are working together to create a stable entity. In most people they are weak, and in the back they can be tense and tight. In this situation the spine may be pulled out of alignment, causing improper posture and risk of injury. When the back muscles and the abdominals are strong and flexible it becomes easier to maintain correct posture. Pilates strengthens and stretches these core muscles, helping to correct imbalances and reducing the chances of suffering back pain.

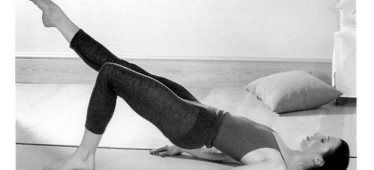

◁ Pilates exercises are designed to build up your core strength.

## locating the transverse abdominis

Sit or stand upright, inhale and pull your stomach towards your back, imagining that you are wearing very tight jeans and trying to pull your tummy away from the waistband. This is what you will be doing during all the Pilates exercises.

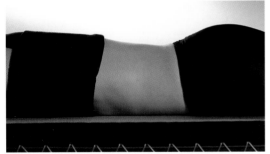

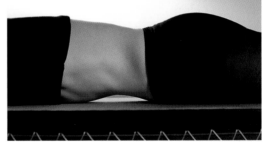

△ **1** Lie on your tummy with your head relaxed and supported on your folded hands or on a small cushion under your forehead. Keep your head in alignment with your back and the back of your neck long, without shortening the front. Try to keep your hip bones on the floor and relax your shoulders.

△ **2** Inhale, then as you exhale pull your navel towards your spine, trying to create an arch under your abdominals. You may not be able to lift very far up at first: this is not important as long as you understand the concept. Gently lift your shoulders back and draw your shoulder blades down your spine.

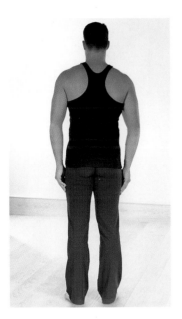

△ **If sliding your shoulder blades down your spine is a baffling request**, practise this subtle movement by standing up with your arms by your sides. Keeping your back straight, push your fingertips towards the floor. Do not force your arms down or lock them into position. Try to keep the shoulder blades close to the back of the ribcage. This is very useful for limiting tension around the shoulders, which tends to make you pull your shoulders up to your ears.

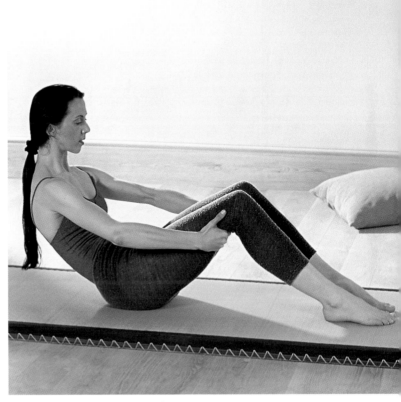

△ Every movement should be controlled via your abdominals. Keep bringing your attention and focus back to pulling your navel towards your spine.

# Neutral spine

A healthy spine has natural curves that should be preserved and respected but not exaggerated. The term "neutral spine" refers to the natural alignment of the spine. If you have any serious pain in your back, check with a physician before embarking on any exercise programme. The main curves are:

- **The cervical spine**: the area behind the head, along the back of the neck, is concave; it should curve gently inwards.
- **The thoracic vertebrae**: the largest area of the back curves very slightly outwards.
- **The lumbar spine**: the lower back should curve slightly inwards; it should not be flat or over-curved.
- **The sacral spine**: the sacral curve is at the bottom of your spine and curves gently outwards.

It is important to allow the spine to rest in its natural position to prevent stresses and imbalances. During Pilates movements you should ensure (unless otherwise directed) that your back is not flat or pushed into the

## Finding neutral spine

**The importance of neutral spine cannot be emphasized enough, as it allows your spine to elongate and relax. Before starting an exercise it can be helpful to roll gently between the two extreme positions and then try to fall comfortably between the two.**

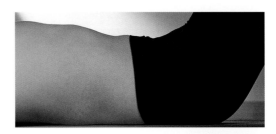

◁ **1** Tilt your pelvis, flattening your back into the floor.

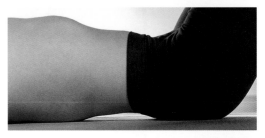

◁ **2** Tilt your pelvis in the opposite direction, creating an arch under your lower back. Make this movement slow and take care not to hold for too long or you may cause tension in your lower spine.

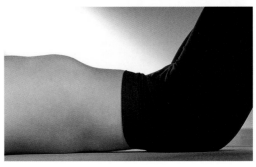

◁ **3** Find a position between these two extremes in which your back feels natural and comfortable: this is neutral spine. Unless otherwise stated, you should always work from this position during your Pilates routine.

**THE AREAS OF THE SPINE**

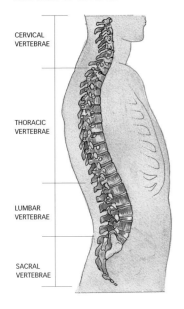

CERVICAL
VERTEBRAE

THORACIC
VERTEBRAE

LUMBAR
VERTEBRAE

SACRAL
VERTEBRAE

floor, although this can be tempting in order to achieve a flatter tummy. What you tend to do in this position is grip at the hip flexors (the muscles located at the top of the thighs) thus creating tension in a place that is commonly tight anyway. You must also try to avoid over-curving your spine, as this pushes the abdominals forwards and tightens the muscles around the spine. "Neutral spine" lies in between these two extremes and echoes the natural and safe position that your spine prefers.

◁ The diagram shows the four natural spinal curves. These curves help to cushion some of the shock from our daily activities – even walking creates some mild stress. One of the key elements of Pilates is the close attention given to the alignment of the spine during all movements.

# Planning a Pilates programme

To be effective any exercise needs to be organized into a programme that is easy to remember and that you will want to do regularly. At the end of this exercise section there is guidance on devising a successful Pilates programme that will help you achieve your goals. Keep your programme balanced and combine it with cardiovascular work and good nutrition to give you a total fitness plan.

With Pilates, it can be difficult to identify the muscles that are being challenged as most movements involve a combination of several muscle groups all working together. A Pilates exercise may be overtly working the arms or the legs and may also be demanding constant stabilization from the torso. So you will find that even though a movement is targeting a certain muscle group, you will often feel it in other parts of your body as well.

In general, Pilates movements can be divided into three main categories:

- **Strengthening exercises** that concentrate on making certain muscle groups stronger and more toned.
- **Flexibility exercises** that improve the range of motion around a joint.
- **Mobility exercises** that train the body to move more easily.

## exercise categories

The following list groups the exercises according to both the action that is being reinforced and the dominant muscles that are being used. Once you have worked through the exercises on the following pages, you can use it to plan a programme.

### exercises that strengthen the upper body

- Push-ups (deltoids, pectorals, biceps, abdominals and stabilizing back muscles)★
- Triceps push-ups (triceps, deltoids, abdominals and pectoral muscles)
- Leg pull prone (abdominals, stabilizing back muscles)★
- Triceps dips (triceps, abdominals)

### exercises that strengthen the lower body

- Cleaning the floor (quadriceps, supporting muscles of the feet and ankles, abdominals)
- Open V (adductors, abdominals, hip flexors and stabilizing back muscles)
- Outer thigh blaster (abductors, abdominals, adductors and hamstrings)
- One-leg kick (hamstrings, abdominals, lower gluteals and erector spinae)★
- Inner thigh lift (adductors and abdominals)

### exercises that strengthen the abdominals and back

- One-leg stretch (abdominals and stabilizing back muscles)★
- Side kick (hamstrings, hip flexors, abdominals, abductors and stabilizing back muscles)★
- Leg pull prone (abdominals and stabilizing back muscles)★
- Roll-up (abdominals and hip flexors)★
- Side bend (obliques, abdominals, stabilizing back muscles; stretches the latissimus dorsi)★
- Side squeeze (internal and external obliques, abdominals, shoulder stabilizers and abductors)
- Hundred (abdominals and stabilizing mid-back muscles)★
- Swimming (abdominals, gluteals and erector spinae)★

### exercises that promote flexibility

- Gluteals stretch (gluteals)
- Chest stretch (pectorals)
- Side stretch (latissimus dorsi)
- Hip flexor stretch (hip flexors)
- Spine twist (obliques, adductors and hamstrings; promotes thoracic mobility)★
- Abdominal stretch (abdominals)
- Spine stretch (erector spinae, hamstrings, adductors)★
- Deep chest and shoulder stretch (pectorals and latissimus dorsi)

- Lower back stretch (erector spinae and gluteals)
- Spine press (erector spinae)

### exercises that promote mobility

- Rolling back (spine)★
- Spine twist★ and Spine press (spine)
- Spine stretch (spine)★
- Rolling back (spine)★

## core exercises

These are marked with a star and you will get the best results if you choose a few "core" exercises – movements that are considered pure Pilates exercises – and concentrate on these for a period of time, say four to six weeks, giving your muscles a chance to adapt to the work. Start with these, and once you have mastered them (not necessarily advancing to a higher level, just feeling comfortable and confident about the movement) add on a few more.

▽ **Shoulder circles are a useful warm up exercise and a good way to relieve tension in the shoulders and upper back. Make the movement slow and controlled, keeping the spine in neutral.**

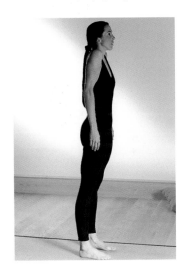

# Assessing common postural faults

The human body is a fantastic machine. It is designed to walk, run, jump, push and pull. It is autonomous and multifunctional and can adapt to many different situations - for instance, by strengthening or lengthening its muscles or adding a layer of fat to protect it from the cold. Unless you were born with a particular physical challenge, your body began life as a symmetrical and co-ordinated unit.

Unfortunately, in adult life many bodies are no longer aligned or symmetrical. The two sides function differently, with some muscles overworked and tight while others are weak and overstretched. So what does a perfectly balanced body look like? First, both sides of the body have equal strength and flexibility. The shoulders, hips and ankle joints are level and symmetrical and the shoulder blades are back and down.

## posture check

Stand in front of a full-length mirror and look at your reflection. Just relax and take up your usual stance without thinking about your posture. Assess your stance honestly – or ask a trusted friend for their assessment. Here are some common misalignments of the body. Do you recognize any of these?:

• The head may be tilted to one side, jut forward or tilt backwards.
• The legs may sway backwards.
• There may be a curved "C" shape in the spine.
• The back may be over arched.
• The shoulders are not level or parallel: one may be rotated forward or elevated or both shoulders may be rounded.
• The palms of the hands are turned backwards

• The hip joints are uneven, tilted backwards or forwards or to one side
• The knees and ankles may be rolling inwards or outwards and are asymmetrical
• The feet turn in or out
• The weight is not evenly distributed between the feet
• The arches in the feet are collapsed

There are many reasons why your body has become misaligned. When any part of the body becomes dysfunctional the whole unit is affected. Even though some muscles are not doing their job effectively, you still have to get on with your day-to-day life so other muscles compensate for weaknesses. Using your body in a faulty manner reinforces these imbalances. Eventually you may start to ache in those areas that need to compensate. Aches and pains are the body's

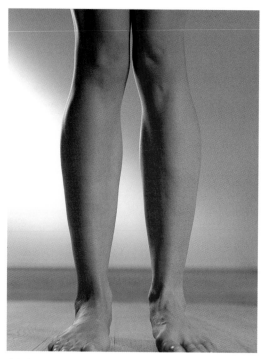

△ The knees or ankles may roll inwards or outwards, or may be asymmetrical

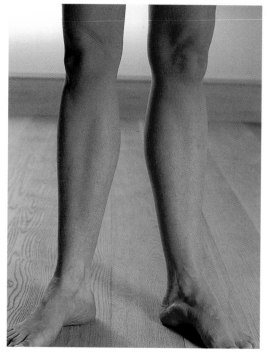

△ The feet may be turned inwards or outwards

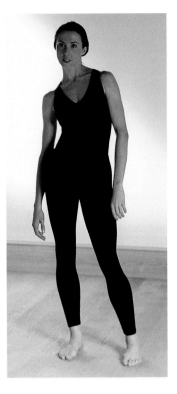

◁ **The hip joints may be uneven, with the weight unevenly distributed between the feet**.

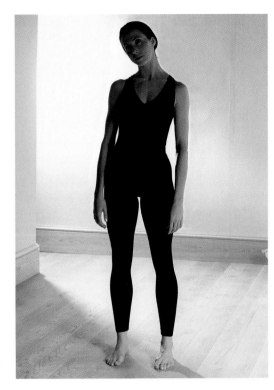

▷ **The head may be tilted to one side, creating muscular imbalances in the neck and back**.

way of alerting you to a problem. You may even get injured or at best suffer chronic pain, commonly in the neck, back, knees, hips or shoulders. It is advisable to get an accurate assessment of the imbalance from a trained professional whilst it is still in its early stages as it is best to try to remedy the problem before your body overcompensates.

Think about the way you feel when you sit for long periods of time. Is your neck sore on one side? Does your lower back ache? This is not the way you are supposed to feel. If your body is doing its job correctly, you should not be experiencing pain or discomfort at any one place in your back or neck from sitting or standing for long periods.

So why are our bodies not doing what they were originally intended for? Most people live in a stress-filled environment. Life has become faster, more is expected, and in order to cope many devices have been designed for increased convenience and reduced effort. Devices like remote controls, lifts and cars have meant that we are less physically active than previous generations.

This lack of activity has led to a rise in obesity levels and conditions such as heart disease. We can no longer rely on general activity to keep us healthy, so we have to look at increasing our exercise levels. Stress and tension in the body can be very damaging, causing imbalances that make muscles over-tight and this can lead to movement becoming restricted.

You can tell a lot about your body from your shoes. Look at a pair of your own shoes with leather (not rubber) soles. Are they more worn on the inside or the outside? Does the sole of one shoe look older than the other? Are the toes pushing against one side of only one of the shoes? Most people have slightly misaligned feet but, if this is a distinct pattern or causes discomfort, it may be worth checking with a qualified specialist. You may have an actual postural deviation that inhibits the maintenance of correct posture. If so, this should be dealt with by a medical practitioner.

▷ **The head may jut forward out of alignment with the spine**.

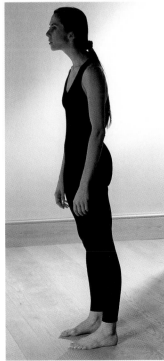

# Improving your posture with Pilates

The body must be re-educated to cope with the stresses of daily life. In cases where the postural fault is severe, or there is pain, you should see a specialist before attempting this or any other exercise programme. Pilates is not meant to be an alternative to the prescription of a medical professional, but it can be a useful tool to accompany the recommendations of a specialist.

Commonly when people train in a gym they tend to choose exercises randomly, concentrating on the areas of the body they like the least, or doing exercises that they find easy to do: this can reinforce existing misalignments. Unless the body is trained as a whole, as in Pilates, its weaknesses will only be reinforced. The regular practice of Pilates strengthens and stretches all the core postural muscles, making correct posture far less of a muscular effort and more of an unconscious act.

To understand the whole picture it is essential to realize the importance of the torso. Every step you take, every weight you

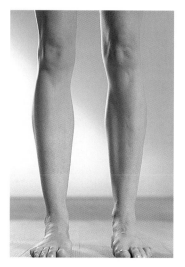

▷ When you are standing correctly, the knee and ankle joints are symmetrical and the knees face forwards.

lift and every movement you make must be stabilized by the muscles of the abdominals and the back to protect the spinal cord against injuries. It does not matter how strong your arms are, unless your torso can protect you by stabilizing internally, your strength will be limited. Think of your body as a chain of muscles: you are only as strong as your weakest link.

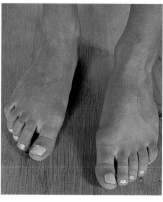

△ The weight of the body should be equally spread between all four "corners" of the feet. Weakened muscles or rapid weight gain may have led the arches in the feet to collapse.

If your posture is not good, your muscles will have been working in an incorrect manner for a long time. You cannot force them into place in a few sessions; there will be a period of adaptation. Always seek medical advice if you feel pain either during or after exercise. However, it is good to learn to differentiate between sore muscles and pain. Muscle soreness is par for the course

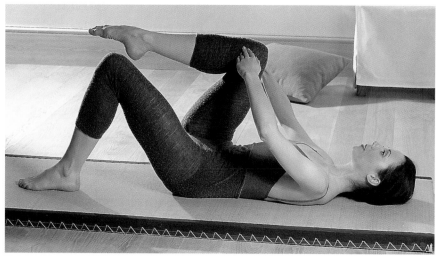

▷ Pilates works by strengthening the key postural muscles, making it physically more comfortable to maintain the correct alignment.

▷ Stand in front of the mirror and carefully check your posture. Pay special attention to your hips, arms, shoulders, spine and weight distribution

when you begin to exercise; you will feel it most about 48 hours later. Stretching out the muscles at the end of a session helps, as can a hot bath. You may also want to try some of the wide variety of gels and creams designed to ease muscular tension. Ask your pharmacist for a recommendation.

So take up your stance in front of the mirror again. Only this time adopt what you consider to be "good posture". You should note the following points. Can you see them in your reflection?:

• Shoulders are level
• Hip bones are equal and symmetrical
• The thumb side of the hand faces forward
• The knee joints are symmetrical and face forwards
• The ankle joints are symmetrical
• The weight of the body is equally distributed between all four "corners" of the feet
• You are lengthening through your spine

▽ Become aware of how people respond more positively to you as your posture changes.

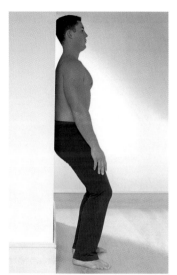

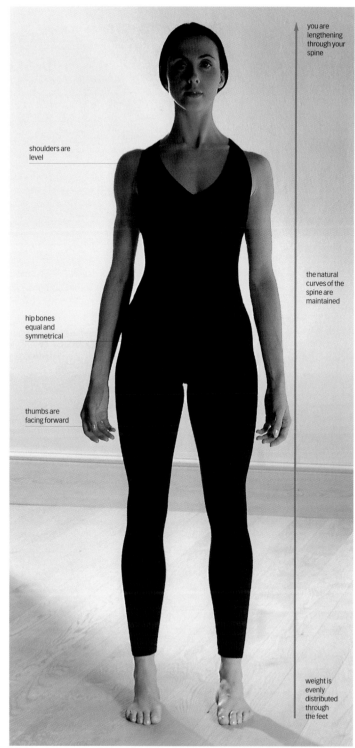

you are lengthening through your spine

shoulders are level

the natural curves of the spine are maintained

hip bones equal and symmetrical

thumbs are facing forward

weight is evenly distributed through the feet

# Pilates in everyday life

There would be little point in spending time exercising if you did not take a fresh look at your posture throughout the day, as you could still be reinforcing imbalances in the body that you are now dedicating time to amending. Pilates will help to strengthen and lengthen the muscles needed to maintain good posture but you also need to learn how to carry your body in the most efficient, safest way possible all the time.

Your posture, the way you hold yourself, says a lot about you. When you watch someone with very good posture enter a room, observe how your eye is drawn to them and the assumptions you can find yourself making about their lives. They seem to be in control, confident and capable.

Psychologically you are also affected by your own posture: notice how much more positive you feel when you sit or stand upright. Try this when on the telephone, it will immediately give you more confidence.

Posture is not just a question of how you walk or sit. To get maximum benefit from your exercise sessions, you need to get your whole body to work at maximum efficiency all the time so that it can cope with the daily demands placed on it. This means reducing imbalances throughout the body.

## sitting

If, like a large percentage of the population, you work in an office, you are likely to sit for long periods of time, usually in chairs that are not ergonomically correct.

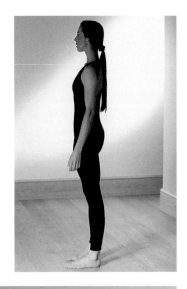

▷ Ask an honest friend to assess your posture as often we are unaware of our postural habits.

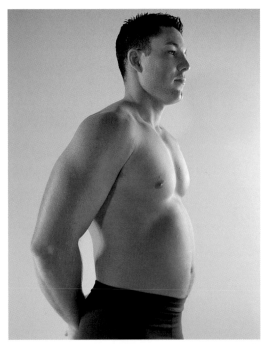

△ Posture has a dramatic effect on our appearance. In this picture, the tone of the abdominal muscles has been completely abandoned. This lack of tone makes the model look slightly overweight.

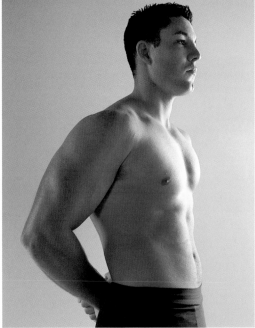

△ By correcting his posture and restoring tone in the abdominals, the model looks 5-6 lbs lighter. His whole appearance has changed, presenting a slimmer and more toned physique.

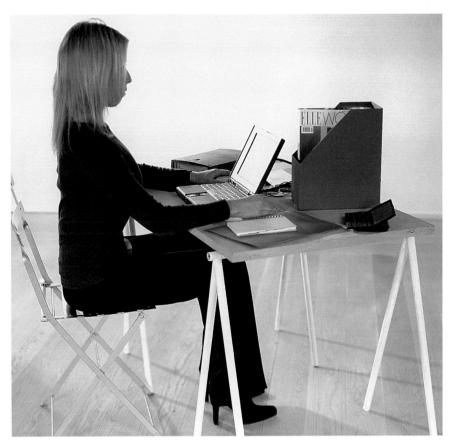

⊲ Avoid flexing for-
ward over your desk.
Lengthen up through
your spine with your
shoulders back and
down, and keep your
head in alignment. Do
not let the abdominals
sag. Your feet should be
flat on the floor, with
your knees directly
over them.

215

introducing Pilates

If you are working at a computer, writing or eating, you are likely to sit in a forward flexed position, with shoulders forward, head dropping, neck muscles tensed and spine arched. Over a period of time, this posture can become the one that you adopt every time you sit, reinforcing the muscular imbalances. It is really quite difficult to sit up straight. Your torso must be strong enough to maintain a static contraction in the back and abdominal muscles to hold your body in place. Correct alignment is the same whether you are sitting, standing or lying down: it should not change because you change positions. Whether you are standing or sitting, the shoulders should be back and down, the chest open, the abdominals contracted, the chin parallel to the floor, the feet flat on the floor.

Pilates will give you the strength to maintain correct alignment for prolonged periods of sitting. When sitting, the knees should be bent at right angles and the spine straight and lengthened but still in neutral. The legs should not be crossed. This posture can be especially difficult to maintain if you are concentrating on an activity in front of you, such as using a computer. VDU monitors that tilt and stools designed to make you sit correctly are worthwhile investments. A good way to remember your posture throughout the day is to simply write the word "posture" on your screen saver: notice the instant effect seeing the word has on you. You can also try to enrol the help of work colleagues: ask them to remind you throughout the day of your posture and to correct you if you slip into negative habits.

Whatever you are doing, stand and stretch at least once every hour. Raise your arms above your head and very gently arch and curve your back. You will feel an immediate relief in the lower back.

## standing

Very few people stand with their weight distributed evenly between both feet. Usually they favour one leg and then the other if they are standing for long periods of time. People with an exaggerated curve in the lower back quite often lock their knees and allow their stomachs to protrude. These habits usually result in back and knee pain. Here again, it is important to strengthen the torso in order to be able to maintain correct alignment. Refer back to the posture check and try to become aware of the way you stand throughout the day. Aim to lengthen up through your spine with your head in alignment and your spine in neutral. Make a list of your natural tendencies and aim to work on one thing at a time, until you gradually adjust your habits. If it helps, tell someone close to you that you are working on your posture and get them to remind you every time they see you slump or stand on one leg.

# Rolling back

As you work on these exercises that concentrate on the abdominals and back, feel the abdominals getting stronger and flatter as you progress. Your back will be free from the burden of aches and stiffness. Make sure you work on a mat that gives plenty of support, and once you have practised rolling down the spine with your hands on the floor, try

progressing on to rolling back: you may not roll back up on your first attempt, but keep practising. When pulling in abdominals, imagine you are squeezing a sponge held between your navel and your spine. Squeeze the sponge as hard as you can. Take care not to roll back on to your neck. Pay careful attention to the alignment of your body as you work.

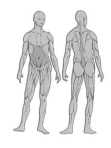

**Purpose:** To mobilize and massage the back and strengthen the abdominals

**Target muscles:** Erector spinae, abdominals

**Repetitions:** Repeat 6 times

### first position

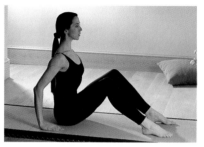 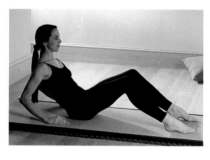

△ **1** Sit with your spine in neutral and your knees bent with both feet flat on the floor. Place your hands near your hips with your fingers facing your feet. Inhaling wide and full through the ribs, draw your navel towards your spine. Lower your chin towards your chest then, using your hands for support, start to roll down to the floor. Try to place each vertebra on the floor, one by one. To do this, tilt your pelvis and curve your spine into a C-shape.

△ **2** Once you have rolled down as far as you find comfortable, exhale and, using your core strength, return to the starting position. Pull up through the crown of your head to create a long spine, then repeat. Use your arms only as support and avoid transferring all your weight on to your triceps.

#### Checkpoints
- Keep your feet flat on the floor
- Lengthen up through the spine at the end of the movement
- Tilt the pelvis

### second position

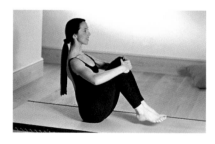 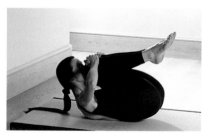

△ **1** Sit upright with your spine in neutral. Lengthen up through the spine and imagine your head floating up to the ceiling. Place your feet flat on the floor and your hands just below your knees. Don't overgrip; keep your elbows bent and your chest open. Take care not to tense or grip around your neck.

△ **2** Inhale as you tilt the pelvis and curve the spine into a C-shape to roll back, tucking in your chin and keeping your thighs close to your chest. As you exhale, use your abdominals to pull you back up to the starting position. Try not to use momentum, but make the movement flow at a consistent speed. Between each roll lengthen up through the spine.

#### Checkpoints
- Keep the chin tucked into the chest
- Do not grip the neck
- Use your abdominals to get you back to the starting position again

# The roll-up

In spite of the name of this exercise, you begin by rolling down. It is an excellent way to strengthen the abdominals but is very challenging, so ensure you are comfortable and confident with the first position before moving on. Although you are curving your spine do not collapse into the movement. Roll down only a little way at first to get the feel of the movement, then roll lower as you become stronger. At all times, do a mental check that you are not tensing other parts of your body, such as your neck or face. As you come back to an upright position imagine that you are sitting against a cold steel door.

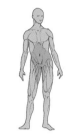

**Purpose:** To strengthen the abdominals
**Target muscles:** Abdominals, hip flexors
**Repetitions:** Repeat 10 times

**Checkpoints**
- Do not overgrip the legs, use them only as support
- Lengthen up through the spine in the starting position
- Feel the abdominals pull you up

## first position

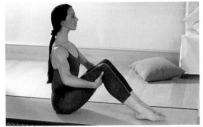

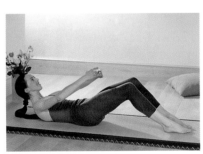

△ **1** Sit upright with your feet flat on the floor and your knees bent. Hold the back of your thighs, with your elbows bent and your arms open; don't overgrip. Your spine should be in neutral. Lengthen up through the spine but do not grip the neck. Slide the shoulder blades down the spine.

△ **2** Inhale and tilt your pelvis to create a C-shaped spine. Keeping your feet flat on the floor, roll down bone by bone, creating space between the vertebrae. Your hands are there to support you if you lose control but try to rely on abdominal strength to stabilize the movement. As you curl down, imagine your spine is a bicycle chain that you are placing down link by link. When you have lowered down as far as you can, exhale and contract the abdominals to roll back up to the starting position. Sit upright, keeping the spine in neutral.

## second position

**Checkpoints**
- Use the abdominals, not momentum, to pull you up
- Lower bone by bone
- Do not collapse into the movement
- Keep the feet on the floor

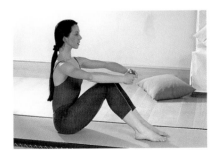

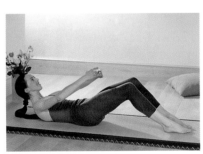

△ **1** This time, hold your arms directly in front of you, level with your shoulders. Your elbows should be bent, arms rounded. Let your shoulder blades glide down your spine and feel the crown of your head "float" up towards the ceiling. Inhale and tilt your pelvis to begin the downward roll as before.

△ **2** When you first progress to this position try a few small roll-downs to get the feel of the movement before going down further. Feel the support of the abdominals throughout the downward and upward roll. Keep your feet flat on the floor all the time.

# The hundred

This static contraction builds core strength and is one of the most commonly taught Pilates exercises. Challenge yourself to reach a hundred. The Hundred really tests your co-ordination. Try not to stagger your breathing as you count your taps: the breath should be flowing and even. Pay special attention to any tensing in the neck and face in this position. To help you do this exercise well, visualize a heavy weight balancing on your abdominals and pulling your navel down towards your spine.

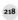

### first position

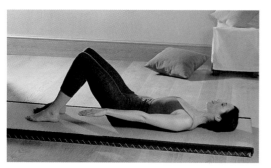

◁ Lie on your back with your knees bent, your feet flat and your head in alignment. The spine should be in neutral and the abdominals hollowed, drawing the navel to the spine. Your arms are by your sides, lifted off the mat. Slide your shoulder blades down your spine. Inhale as you count to five then exhale for five. Gently tap your fingertips on the floor and co-ordinate your breathing with your taps. Breathe steadily and laterally into your ribs.

**Purpose:** To strengthen core muscles, co-ordinate breathing patterns and build endurance.
**Target muscles:** Transverse abdominis, rectus abdominis, stabilizing mid-back muscles
**Repetitions:** 20 x 5 beats

Checkpoints
• Keep your arms lengthened
• Draw the shoulder blades down the spine
• Keep the abdominals hollowed

### second position

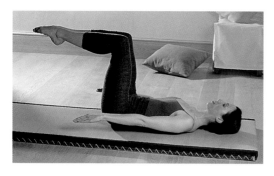

◁ When you feel confident about the first position, lift your feet off the floor. Your knees should be directly above your hips and your feet level with your knees. Do not allow your knees to fall away as this will cause your spine to curve. If this is too much of a challenge you can raise just one leg, but do not twist your hips. Repeat the breathing pattern as before. Keep the abdominals flat throughout and maintain the distance between your hips and ribs.

Checkpoints
• Glide your shoulder blades down your spine
• Keep your knees above your hips
• Toes are pointed
• Feet stay level with knees

### third position

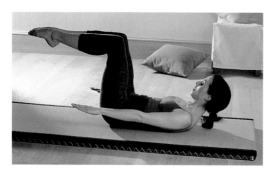

◁ Curl your upper body off the floor, dropping your chin towards your chest so that you are facing your thighs. Do not grip your neck and keep drawing your shoulder blades down your spine. Maintain the breathing pattern for a hundred beats as before. If you want a greater challenge, try straightening the legs. Lower your eyes in this position to check that your abdominals are flat and your ribs are not flaring up.

Checkpoints
• Release tension from the neck
• Do not clench your jaw
• Keep the abdominals flat

# The swimming

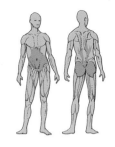

This exercise is a favourite with physiotherapists as it is a very effective way of developing strength in the core muscles. It is a very challenging exercise but is an easy one to cheat on, so read the instructions carefully to make sure that you are performing the exercise correctly. Ensure that you keep your abdominals lifted. Instead of just raising your arms and legs, visualize them lengthening away from your trunk. Do not try to lift them too high from the floor. Make your movements elegant and flowing and avoid throwing your arms and legs or collapsing back on to the floor on the way down. Take care not to lift your hips off the floor or to overbalance on to one side or the other.

**Purpose**: A strength exercise, challenging co-ordination and core strength
**Target muscles**: Abdominals, gluteals, erector spinae
**Repetitions**: Repeat 10 times

## first position

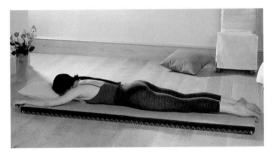

◁ Lie on your front, placing a small pillow under your forehead to keep your head in alignment with your spine, which is in the neutral position. Keep your neck long. Stretch your arms over your head and lengthen them away. Point your toes and lengthen your legs away. Breathe laterally, wide and full. Draw in your abdominals, imagining that there is a drawing pin on the mat that you are lifting away from.

**Checkpoints**
• Do not tip your head back
• Keep the abdominals lifted
• Breathe laterally

## second position

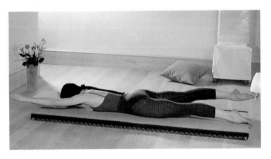

◁ Introduce a challenge to your core strength by lifting one leg. Exhale as you lift and inhale as you lower the leg. Keep both hips in contact with the floor, and do not try to lift the leg too high. Keep lengthening as you lift, maintaining the distance between the ribs and hips. Do not lose the lift in your abdominals. Take care not to twist the raised leg but keep your knee and foot in line with your hips. Repeat with the other leg.

**Checkpoints**
• Lengthen as you lift the leg
• Do not twist the hips

## third position

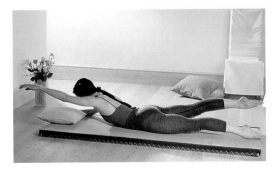

◁ As you exhale, lift your opposite arm and leg together. When you lift your arm raise your head and upper body with the movement, but keep facing the floor so that your head stays in line with your spine. Lengthen through your arms and legs and keep your hips in contact with the floor. Remember the drawing pin under your navel: if you lose the lift in your abdominals, continue to work in the second position for a while longer.

**Checkpoints**
• Keep your head in line with your spine
• Do not twist the torso
• Lengthen from a strong centre

# One-leg stretch

introducing Pilates

Do not be fooled into thinking that this is a relaxing leg stretch – it is actually a very challenging movement which builds core strength and is also good for improving co-ordination. Keep your hips still throughout as if they were being held in a vice. Take care not to curve your spine, and keep your shoulder blades pulled down your spine and close to the back of your ribs throughout. If you find the hand position difficult, you can lightly hold either side of your knee instead. Make sure that you are just making light contact and do not over-grip as this causes tension in the neck and jaw. Your upper body should be stabilized by your abdominal muscles.

**Purpose:** To strengthen abdominals and improve co-ordination
**Target muscles:** Abdominals, stabilizing back muscles
**Repetitions:** Repeat 10 times on each leg

### Checkpoints
• Hollow your tummy throughout
• Keep the hips still

## first position

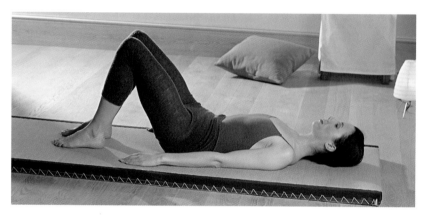

△ **1** Lie on your back with your knees bent and your feet flat on the floor. Your spine should be in neutral and your head in alignment: do not shorten your neck by tipping your head back or dropping your chin to your chest. Draw the navel to the spine.

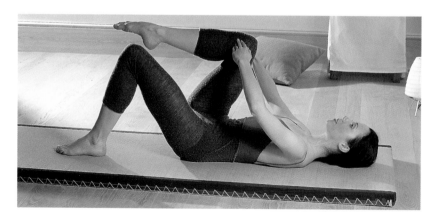

△ **2** Lift one foot off the floor, keeping the knee bent, and pull the leg gently towards you, supporting it at the knee. Try not to over-grip, causing tension in the neck, and keep your foot in line with your knee. Take care not to let the ribs flare up. Repeat with the other leg, inhaling as you lift and exhaling as you lower.

## second position

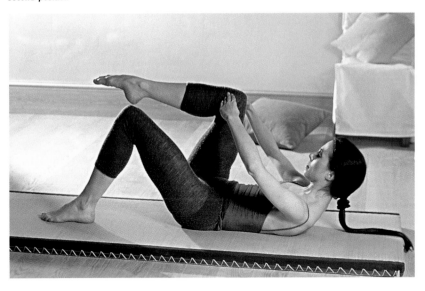

**Checkpoints**
• Do not tip the head forward
  or back
• Watch for tension in the neck

△ Once you understand the first position, curl the upper body off the floor and continue the same movement. Let the chin fall towards the chest, and try to limit tension in the neck. Keep the hips very still, controlling any movement from the hips via your abdominals. Breathe laterally. Keep the stomach hollowed throughout the movement, trying to make it as flat as possible.

## third position

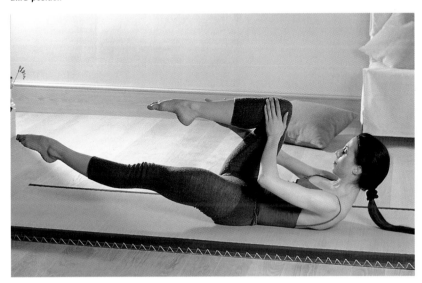

**Checkpoints**
• Pull the shoulder blades
  down your spine close to the
  back of your ribs
• Lengthen the legs away
• The lower your straight leg,
  the harder your abdominals
  have to work

△ This position really challenges your co-ordination. As you raise the right leg, place the right hand on the ankle and the left hand on the inside of the knee. Change hands as you change legs. As one leg comes in to the body the other leg lifts and lengthens away on an exhalation. Keep your toes pointed and stretch down through the straight leg. The movement is controlled by the abdominals: keep them hollowed, and maintain the distance between the ribs and hips. Do not twist the hips: imagine they are being held in a vice. Keep the pace slow and consistent.

# Leg pull prone

This is actually a yoga position as well as a modified Pilates one. You will gain a lot of torso strength and stability from this exercise, and if you do it properly it will feel as if every muscle in your body is being challenged. Remember to breathe freely throughout the exercise and do not hold your breath when holding the position. It is common to shrink down into your shoulders in this position so try to maintain the length in your neck throughout. Keep checking for tension around the neck, face and shoulders. Focus on your abdominals; they should be stabilizing your whole body. You could try to visualize a drawing pin inserted through your navel and attaching to your back.

**Purpose:** To strengthen the abdominals and spine and challenge the upper body
**Target muscles:** Abdominals, stabilizing back muscles
**Repetitions:** Repeat up to 10 times

### first position

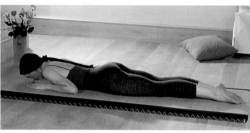

◁ Lie on your front with your head in line with your spine. Bend your arms and keep your upper arms close to your body. Lift the abdominals off the floor, imagining that you are creating an arch under your stomach. Breathe wide and full. Concentrate on this abdominal lift and aim to hold it for one minute before relaxing again.

**Checkpoints**
• Slide your shoulders down your spine
• Keep the upper arms close to your body

### second position

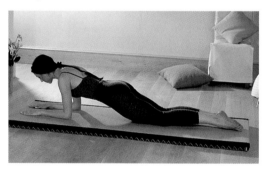

◁ Your elbows should be directly under your shoulders. Do not push your buttocks towards the ceiling or arch your spine. Keep your head in line with the spine and lengthen it away: don't sink into your shoulders or squeeze the shoulder blades together. Make sure that your hips stay square. The abdominals are lifted throughout. If this is too difficult, lower your hips and curl just your upper body off the floor. Try to hold this for one minute.

**Checkpoints**
• Maintain a straight line from your head to your knees
• Do not let the abdominals sag

### third position

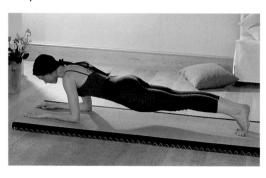

◁ Lift up on to your toes, straightening your legs. This is a real challenge, so be sure to have worked on the first and second positions for quite some time before progressing. Take care not to transfer all the weight into your shoulders or upper body, and keep your hips square. Pull your navel to your spine, maintaining the distance between your ribs and hips, and breathe laterally. Aim to hold for up to one minute.

**Checkpoints**
• Keep a straight line from your head to your heels
• Do not transfer all your weight into your upper body
• Draw your shoulder blades down your spine

# The side kick

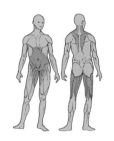

This is another good exercise for core strength, concentrating on the lower body. Have patience and work gradually through the progressions to achieve the best results. When performing the side kick take care not to use momentum to lift and lower your leg. It may help to visualize moving your leg through mud as this will slow you down.

Keep your foot or knee in line with your hip. Note the alignment of your hips and keep them stacked on top of one another as it is common for the hips to roll forwards and the posture to collapse. This is stabilized by the abdominals and the obliques (the muscles at the side of the waist). Try to keep a steady connection with their involvement.

## first position

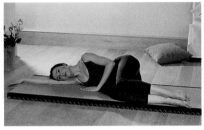

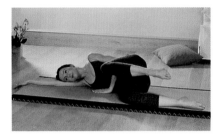

△ **1** Lie on your side, resting your head on your outstretched lower arm. Keep your head in line with your spine, which is in neutral, and your hips stacked vertically; they must not roll in or out. Your knees are bent, one on top of the other. Place your free hand in front for balance but do not lean into the supporting arm or transfer your weight forward.

△ **2** Lift the top knee directly above the other knee. Inhale and, with your toes pointed, move the knee back as you exhale until it travels behind your body. The challenge is to keep your hips stacked and your abdominals hollowed. Your shoulder blades should be pulled down your spine and your ribs should not be pushed up. You should feel this in your side. If you want to increase the challenge straighten the top leg, keeping the toe pointed.

**Purpose:** To challenge core strength and work the lower body
**Target muscles:** Hamstrings, hip flexors, abdominals, stabilizing shoulder muscles, abductors
**Repetitions:** Repeat 10 times each side

### Checkpoints
- Do not transfer all your weight on to the arm in front
- Keep your abdominals flat

## second position

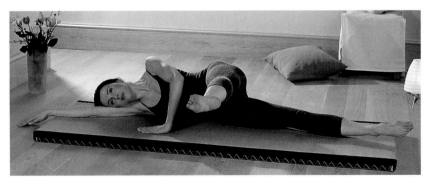

### Checkpoints
- Do not let the hips collapse
- Lengthen out through the legs

△ Straighten both legs. This is very challenging so be sure to advance only after working with the previous position. Bring the bottom leg forward slightly from your hip; it should not be in line with your spine. Keep the hips vertical and lengthen out through both legs. The control comes from your centre. Exhale as the leg travels backwards.

# The side squeeze

introducing Pilates

This exercise will shape the waist and abdominals, so it is especially good for the area that hangs over your waistband when you wear fitted clothes. As you lift, check for tension in your neck or other parts of your body, and watch that your ribs stay down. Do not let the abdominals sag but hold them taut throughout.

If you wish to add an extra challenge, raise the top knee, keeping it in line with your hips – no higher. Make this a slow, controlled movement. Take care not to overgrip with your hands. Perform the movement with flow, avoiding any jerk when lifting and lowering.

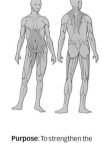

**Purpose:** To strengthen the waist and mid-section, stabilizing and improving balance
**Target muscles:** Obliques, shoulder stabilizers, abdominals and abductors
**Repetitions:** Repeat 10 times on each side

### Checkpoints

- Do not allow the abdominals to sag
- Keep your hips stacked
- Maintain the distance between your ribs and hips
- Really feel the muscles in your side working

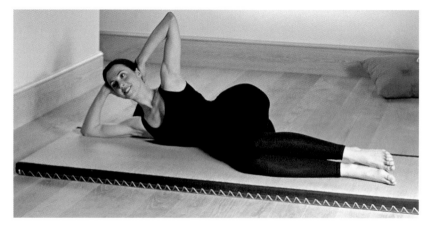

△ **1** Lie on your side with your knees bent and in line with your hips. Your hips are stacked and your abdominals hollowed. Place your hands on your head, directly opposite each other. Do not tip your head back or drop your chin to your chest. Breathe in.

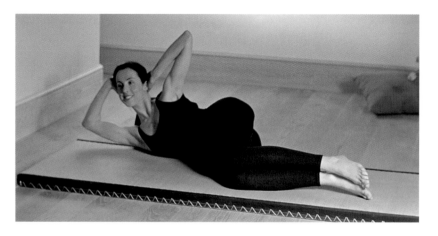

△ **2** Exhale as you lift your upper body off the floor and inhale as you lower. Make the lift slow and controlled. Don't jerk your neck or grip too hard with your hands. Maintain the length through your spine and take care not to let your hips collapse, but keep them stacked. Make sure your knees stay level with your hips. Draw your shoulder blades down your spine.

# The side bend

This movement may look simple but it creates a marked improvement around the waistline if you practise it regularly, as well as developing core stability and balance. Feel the movement being controlled by your torso. Take care in this position not to let the hips roll either inwards or outwards. Imagine that you have a red dot on your hips that should always face the ceiling as you lift. Maintain the length in your neck and avoid sinking into your shoulders. You may not be able to lift very far off the floor initially but do not worry as the real benefit comes from maintaining the correct alignment and performing the exercise accurately. You might find that this exercise is less challenging on one side than the other – it is common for one side to be a little stronger than the other.

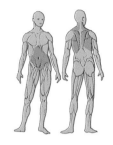

**Purpose:** To strengthen the abdominals and sides and improve balance
**Target muscles:** Obliques, abdominals, stabilizing shoulder muscles and latissimus dorsi
**Repetitions:** Repeat up to 10 times on each side

**Checkpoints**
- Initiate the movement via a strong centre
- Do not transfer all your weight on to your arms
- Keep the neck soft

### first position

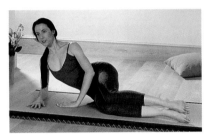

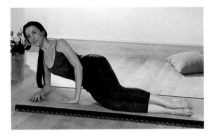

△ **1** Lie on your side with your legs bent, knees level with hips and feet in line with knees. Imagine there is a rod running vertically through your hips. Rest on your elbow, which should be directly under your shoulder, and bring the other arm in front for support. Resist the temptation to push all your weight on to the supporting hand or the resting elbow.

△ **2** Inhale, breathing into your sides, and as you exhale lift your hips off the floor. Use the muscles in the side closest to the floor to initiate the movement and control it via a strong centre. Hollow the abdominals, drawing navel to spine, slide your shoulder blades down your spine and ensure that your ribs are not pushing up.

### second position

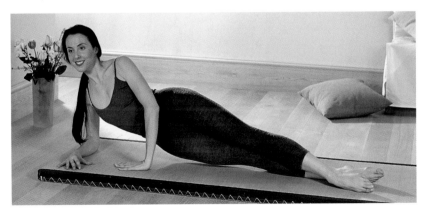

**Checkpoints**
- Make sure the hips do not collapse
- Keep the abdominals hollowed
- Lift straight up, not veering to either side
- Keep the movement flowing

△ Progress only after reaching a level of ease in the first position. If you feel ready, straighten your legs and lengthen them away. Cross one foot over the other, with the toes pointed, to support you as you lift your hips. Keep your head in line with your spine and lengthen up through the top of your head.

# Push-ups

These push-ups are great for shaping the upper body: the shoulders and biceps. If they are performed properly, your abdominals will get a workout too. Once you progress beyond the first position, if your previous exercise was a standing one you can preserve the flow of movement and loosen up the spine by using a transitional move to get to the floor. Follow the instructions for the mobilizing exercise called "Rolling Down the Spine" and, once your hands are hovering at floor level, bend at the knees, place your hands on the floor and move into the start position for push-ups.

In every position, pull the abdominals in tight, never allowing them to sag, and keep your spine in neutral. Check for tension in your neck. Build up gradually to the full push-up.

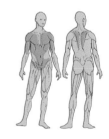

**Purpose:** To strengthen the upper body

**Target muscles:** Deltoids, pectorals, biceps, stabilizing back muscles and abdominals

**Repetitions:** Repeat up to 10 times

**Checkpoints**
- Keep your head in line
- Do not let the abdominals sag

## first position

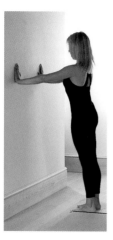

◁ **1** Stand facing a wall and place your hands on it. Your hands should be level with and just wider than your chest and flat against the wall, with the fingers pointing upwards. Your feet stay flat on the floor. Keep your spine in neutral and lengthen up your body, feeling your head "float" towards the ceiling.

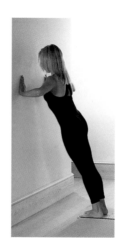

◁ **2** Bend at the elbows to bring your chest towards the wall. Keep your head in line with your body, slide your shoulder blades down your spine, and check that you are not pushing up your ribs. Push away from the wall to come back to your starting position. Keep the movement slow and controlled.

## second position

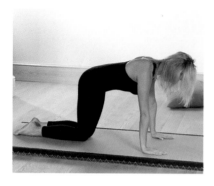

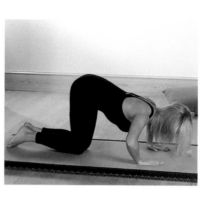

**Checkpoints**
- Do not lock the elbows
- Lower only as far as you can control
- Keep your chest at hand-level and your head in front of your hands

△ **1** Position yourself on all fours, knees directly under your hips and hands directly under your shoulders, with the fingertips facing forwards. Keep your spine in neutral and don't let your head sink into your neck.

△ **2** Keeping your head in line with your spine, exhale as you lower your chest to the floor between your hands by bending your elbows. Do not allow the abdominals to sag. As you push up, straighten the arms without locking the elbows.

## third position

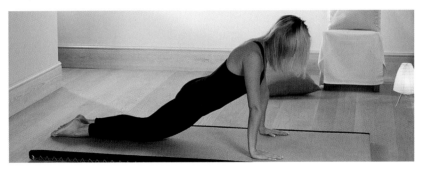

**Checkpoints**
- Keep a straight line from your head to your knees
- Do not let your buttocks stick up
- Do not arch or curve your back

**227**

introducing Pilates

△ **1** Drop your hips so that there is a straight line from your head to your knees. Your fingertips should be facing forwards and your hands directly under the shoulders. Keep the abdominals strong and your hips square.

▷ **2** Exhale as you lower and inhale as you lift. Keep your head in line with your spine and in front of your hands. Don't let your ribs flare up. Keep your weight evenly distributed between your knees and your hands.

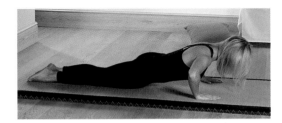

## fourth position

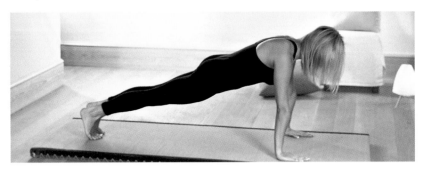

**Checkpoints**
- Keep your shoulder blades down the spine
- Make it a controlled, flowing movement
- Breathe laterally

△ **1** Form a straight line from your head to your feet, supporting yourself on your toes and hands. The fingertips should face forwards and your head should be in alignment with your spine.

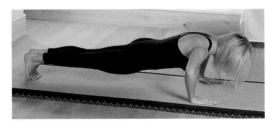

◁ **2** Lower your chest to the floor between your hands, then push up, keeping your elbows soft. Keep the movement controlled and continuous. Lower only as far as you can control.

# Tricep push-ups

A common complaint is the lack of muscle tone at the back of the upper arm; this is excellent for challenging this area. It works by adapting the classic push-up to work on the triceps. The movements may look the same but there are subtle – and very important – differences. The elbows stay close to the body this time. To help you keep your elbows by your sides, visualize doing the movement in a narrow space between two walls. Try to maintain a constant, slow speed throughout the exercise, although this can be very difficult to maintain on the last few repetitions.

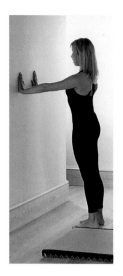

### first position

▷ **1** Stand facing a wall. Place your hands flat against the wall, fingers pointing upwards. Your hands should be level with and just wider than your chest. Your feet stay flat on the floor. Keep your spine in neutral and slide your shoulder blades down.

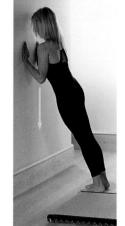

▷ **2** Bend at the elbows to bring your chest towards the wall as you exhale. Unlike in the classic push-up, your elbows should remain close to the body and pointing down at all times. Keep your head in line with your body and check that you are not pushing up your ribs. Push away from the wall to come back to your starting position.

**Purpose**: To strengthen the upper body and the abdominals
**Target muscles**: Triceps, pectorals, deltoids and abdominals
**Repetitions**: Repeat up to 10 times

**Checkpoints**
• Do not let your elbows "wing" out to the sides
• Watch for your shoulders moving up towards your ears
• Lengthen up through the top of your head

### second position

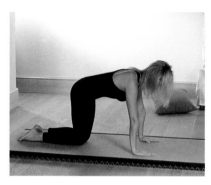

△ **1** Position yourself on all fours, with your hands directly under your shoulders, fingertips facing forwards. Keep your spine in neutral and maintain a straight line from your head to your hips. Don't let the abdomen sag.

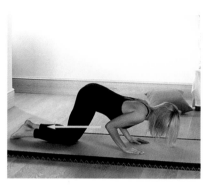

△ **2** Exhale as you lower your chest to the floor. This time, bend at the elbow and ensure that your elbows point towards your feet, with your upper arms staying close to your sides. As you push up, straighten the arms without locking the elbows.

**Checkpoints**
• Keep your chest level with your hands
• Keep your head in front of your hands
• Keep your feet flat on the floor

## third position

▷ **1** Drop your hips so that there is a straight line from your knees to your head. Glide your shoulder blades down your spine. Your fingertips should face forwards.

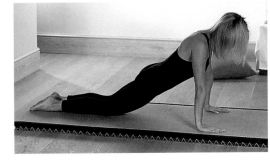

▷ **2** Exhale as you lower and inhale as you lift. Keep your head in line with your spine. Ensure that your head stays the same distance from your hands and that the elbows are pointing in the direction of your feet. Try to perform the exercise with flowing, continuous movements.

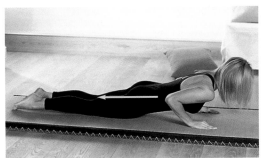

**Checkpoints**
• Do not let your buttocks stick up
• Feel the movement in the back of your upper arms
• Do not rely on momentum

**229**

introducing Pilates

## fourth position

**Checkpoints**
• You should really feel this in the triceps
• Keep your body in alignment
• Hollow the abdominals
• Maintain a straight line from your head to your feet

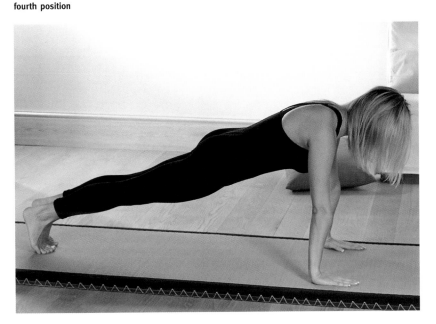

△ Make sure you have been practising the modified positions for some time before progressing to this position. This time your whole body should be in one straight line. Don't let your head sink into your shoulders. Lower the chest to the floor, keeping your elbows pointing towards your feet and using the same breathing pattern as for the previous positions.

# Tricep dips

This exercise is indispensable for firming up the muscles at the back of the arms. The tricep runs from the shoulder to the elbow and can be hard to work, but if neglected, this is the part of your arm that wobbles when you wave. Find a chair that offers support at the correct height and check that it will not slip away from you. Work through the full range of the movement by straightening the arms, but take care not to "lock out" the elbows. Lengthen up through the top of your head.

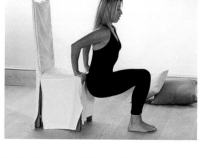

**Purpose**: To tone the triceps

**Target muscles**: Triceps, abdominals

**Repetitions**: Start gently but work up to 20 times

### Checkpoints
- Keep your back close to the chair
- Do not lock your elbows
- Keep your head in line

## first position

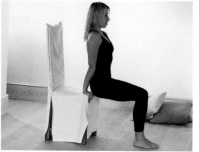

△**1** Place yourself in front of the chair with bent knees and feet flat on the floor. Support yourself on your hands with your fingers pointing down. Lengthen up through your spine, which is in neutral. This is your starting position. Make sure that your abdominals are hollowed throughout the exercise.

△ **2** Bend your elbows and lower your body as you inhale. Glide your shoulder blades gently down your spine and watch that your ribs do not push up. As you return to the starting position on an exhalation, take care not to "lock out" your arms, just straighten them. Keep your back close to the chair and make sure your elbows travel backwards rather than out to the sides. Execute the movement with control.

## second position

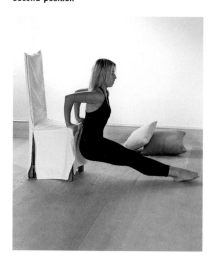

◁ Start in the same basic position as above, but this time put your legs straight out in front of you with your toes pointed. Keep your back close to the chair, your elbows pointing straight behind you and fingers pointing down. In this advanced position it is very tempting to let the elbows travel out to the sides, particularly if you are tired or not paying full attention. Ensure that your head does not sink into your shoulders. Your breathing should be wide and full allowing your ribs to expand fully, but keeping your abdominals hollowed out throughout the exercise. Aim to keep the movement flowing and continuous, and don't let the pace speed up or slow down. In this way you will work the triceps and abdominals harder and get the most benefit from the exercise.

### Checkpoints
- Do not use momentum
- Keep the abdominals hollowed
- Maintain an even flow

# Exercises for thighs

The following exercises pay attention to the inner thighs and hips. Although you will be predominantly toning the lower body, you should still focus on hollowing out the abdominals. Ankle weights can be added to both of these exercises. Alignment is very important for these exercises, so follow the directions carefully, letting the movements flow rather than "throwing" the leg.

## The outer thigh blaster

If practised regularly, this exercise will really firm up the outsides of the hips and thighs and strengthen the lower body. Do not let the abdominals sag, and slide your shoulder blades gently down your spine. Maintain a constant distance between your ribs and your hips and keep the hips square, moving only your leg. Watch for tension elsewhere in the body as you do the exercise.

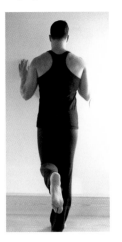

◁ **1** Stand facing the wall with your hands at chest level and flat against the wall. Bend one leg at the knee so that your foot is level with your knee and both knees are in line. Your spine should be in neutral and your foot flexed. Check that there is a straight line from your head to your feet, resisting the temptation to lean into the wall or bend at the hip.

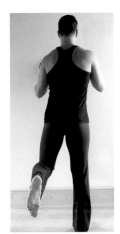

◁ **2** From this starting position, take your knee out to the side. It is important to keep your foot flexed and your knees aligned. Exhale as your leg travels away from your body, inhale as you bring it back. You should not swing the leg. Don't "sink" into the supporting leg, but keep lengthening up through the spine.

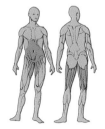

**Purpose:** To tone the hips and lower body
**Target muscles:** Abductors, abdominals, adductors and hamstrings
**Repetitions:** Repeat 10 times with each leg

**Checkpoints**

• Keep your lifted foot in line with your knee
• Keep the rest of your body still; move only the working leg

## The inner thigh lift

This is a popular exercise that is often done badly. However, when it is performed correctly it works wonders with that much complained about area, the inner thigh. To progress the exercise you could use ankle weights, but you should really get a feel for the inner thigh initiating the movement before moving on.

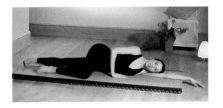

△**1** Lie on your side, supporting your head on your outstretched arm. Your hips should be stacked and your other hand can rest in front of you on the floor for support. Bend the top leg and rest your knee on the floor. Straighten the lower leg and lengthen it away on the floor with the foot flexed. Do not curve your back or allow your ribs to jut forwards. Glide your shoulder blades down your spine.

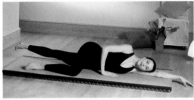

△ **2** Inhale, and as you exhale, lift the bottom leg as high as you can, keeping the abdominals hollowed all the time, then lower it. Make the movement flow, trying to avoid any jerky movements or, worst of all, swinging your leg. You should feel the muscle of the inner thigh doing the work. Take care not to twist the knee. Keep your foot in line with your leg; there is a tendency to lead with the toes in this position.

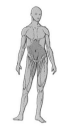

**Purpose:** To tone the inner thigh
**Target muscles:** Adductors and abdominals
**Repetitions:** Repeat 10 times with each leg

**Checkpoints**

• Do not roll hips
• Do not curve the spine

# The openV

This is not one of the most graceful-looking movements, but it works wonders for the thighs, especially the inner thighs, and also benefits the abdominals. It is very important to pay special attention to keeping your knees (and feet in the second and third positions) directly above your hips at all times. If your feet fall towards the floor, your lower back may curve upwards which could cause stress. Check that you are not holding any tension in the shoulders or neck. To create an extra challenge try placing a cushion between your knees. Of course, you won't be able to open your legs so far.

**Purpose:** To firm up the inner thighs
**Target muscles:** Adductors, hip flexors, abdominals and stabilizing back muscles
**Repetitions:** Repeat 10 times

**Checkpoints**
• Check that your feet do not drop down
• Keep your feet flexed
• Do not curve your spine

## first position

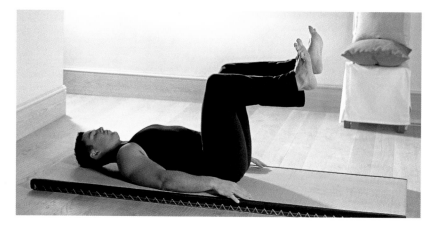

△ **1** Lie on your back, with your knees bent and directly above your hips, and your feet level with your knees. Your feet should be flexed. Your arms are on the floor, lengthening away, your shoulder blades slide down your spine, and your head is in alignment with your spine. Start with your knees apart.

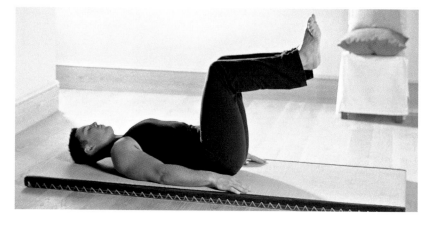

△ **2** Keeping your feet in line with your knees, bring your knees together and squeeze to feel your inner thighs working. Hold for a few seconds, then return to the starting position. Keep your abdominals hollowed throughout and your spine in neutral.

## second position

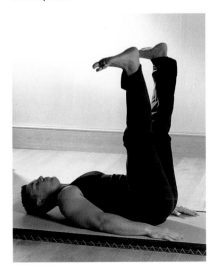 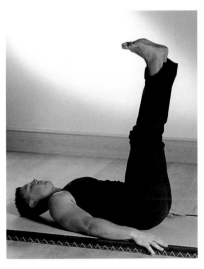

**Checkpoints**
- Do not allow the legs to drop away from your body
- Do not let the legs open too far
- Squeeze the knees together

△ **1** The basic movement is the same as before, but is done with straight legs. Lengthen up through your heels and keep your feet flexed. Start with your legs apart.

△ **2** Bring your legs together and squeeze to work your inner thighs. Keep the hips still via the abdominals, which are hollowed throughout. Keep your arms strong, and really feel your inner thighs working.

## third position

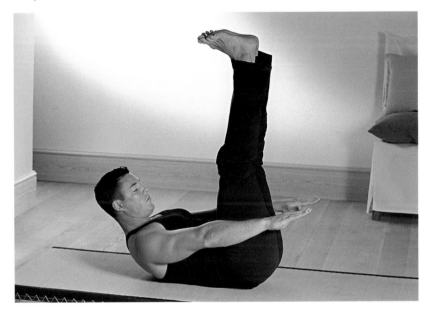

**Checkpoints**
- Watch for tension in the neck
- Lengthen the arms away
- Lengthen up through the heels
- Slide your shoulder blades down your spine

△ Curl your upper body off the floor, watching for tension in the neck and shoulders. Don't let your head sink into your shoulders, but glide your shoulder blades down your spine. Watch that your ribs do not flare up. Keep hollowing the abdominals; you can glance down and check that they are held flat. Squeeze the legs together as before.

# Cleaning the floor

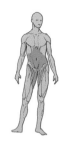

This movement will improve your balance and strengthen your lower body and all the small muscles in your feet and ankles – it is great for weak ankles. Initially, you may find the balance quite challenging. If so, it may help to look at a fixed point on the wall. It is common to find that your balance is better on one side than the other as most people favour one side. One of the objectives of this exercise is to balance any subtle differences in strength. Concentrate on maintaining the alignment between your foot and knees. If it helps, imagine that your supporting leg is held in a narrow gap between two walls.

**Purpose**: To strengthen the lower body, feet and ankles
**Target muscles**: Quadriceps, supporting muscles around feet and ankles, abdominals
**Repetitions**: Repeat up to 10 times with each leg

### Checkpoints
- Watch for your knees rolling inwards or outwards
- Keep your supporting foot flat on the floor
- Lengthen up through the spine
- Make the movement smooth and continuous

## first position

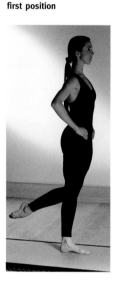

◁ **1** Stand up tall and imagine the crown of your head floating up to the ceiling. Feel your spine lengthening. It should stay in neutral throughout. Keep your abdominals as flat as possible. Place your hands on your hips and keep your head in line with your spine. Keeping your knees in line with one another, let one foot hover above the floor as you balance evenly on the other.

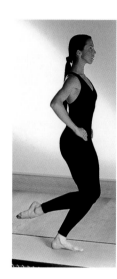

◁ **2** Bend the supporting leg and lower your body as far as you can control. Do not collapse into the movement. The supporting foot may feel a little wobbly at first. Check that the knee of the supporting leg stays in alignment with the foot. Inhale as you come back up to standing. Keep your upper body strong and watch that your ribs do not travel away from your hips.

## second position

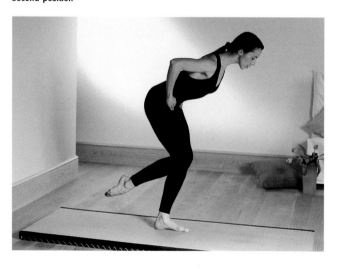

◁ Bend your knee and lower as far as you can into the position as before. This time, you are going to hold this position and then very carefully lower your chest towards the floor. Bend only a little initially. To get back to the starting position, straighten your torso first then come back up to standing. Keep your head in line.

### Checkpoints
- Do not try to lower too far
- Do not collapse into the movement
- Keep lifting the abdominals

# One-leg kick

This core exercise really challenges your co-ordination as you cannot see the movement – you just feel it. It is fantastic for toning up the lower body while challenging core strength. A good way to visualize the movement is to imagine that you are squeezing a pillow between your hamstrings and your calf. Try to resist just placing the leg: really feel the hamstrings working. This is a deceptively hard movement so do not worry if it takes practice. You may find it easier to get a feel for the movement first, then add the correct breathing pattern and work on lengthening down through the other leg.

**Purpose:** To tone the lower body and develop core stability and strength
**Target muscles:** Hamstrings, erector spinae (when upper body is lifted), abdominals, gluteals
**Repetitions:** Repeat 10 times with each leg

### first position

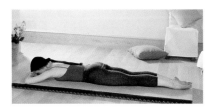

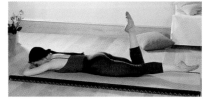

△ **1** Lie on your front, supporting your forehead on your folded hands to keep your head in alignment. Draw your navel to your spine, trying to form an arch under your abdominals.

△ **2** Relax the neck. Avoid clenching the jaw. Relax your shoulders and slide the shoulder blades down your spine. Bend one leg at the knee. This is your starting position.

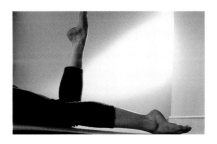

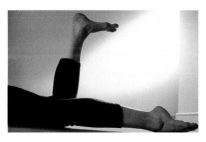

△ **3** Inhale, and as you exhale, point your toes and make a stabbing movement with your foot towards your buttocks. Keep your knees together and lengthen through the legs.

△ **4** Ease out of this position then repeat, this time with your foot flexed. Then extend your leg back to its original position. Meanwhile, the supporting leg on the floor should be lengthening away at all times.

#### Checkpoints
• Keep the movement swift and continuous
• Limit any movement by keeping the abdominals hollowed throughout
• Slide the shoulder blades down your spine

### second position

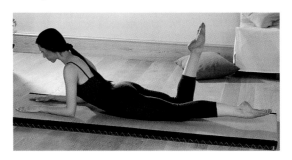

◁ Perform the same movements, but this time curl your upper body off the floor and rest on your elbows. Slide the shoulder blades down. Keep your neck long throughout and watch that your ribs do not travel away from your hips. Lengthen through the spine. If you feel a pinch in your spine in this position, stay with the first position for a while.

#### Checkpoints
• Keep your neck in line throughout the exercise
• Breathe wide and full
• Do not push all your weight on to your arms

# Spine stretch

If your back feels tight or if you just want a healthy and mobile spine then this is the stretch for you. You will feel longer, stretched and more flexible. This is a flowing movement, not a static stretch. To keep your spine lengthening up and to stop you collapsing into the stretch, imagine that you have a beach ball in front of you, and lift up and over the ball. As you come upright again, imagine that your back is rolling up a pole, vertebra by vertebra, and take care to keep this alignment from your head to your hips; do not lean forwards, or away from the imaginary pole.

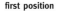

**Purpose:** To stretch the spine

**Target muscles:** Erector spinae, hamstrings, adductors and abdominals

**Repetitions:** Repeat 10 times

**Checkpoints**
- Do not collapse into the stretch
- Keep the movement flowing and continuous
- Let your head float up to the ceiling

## first position

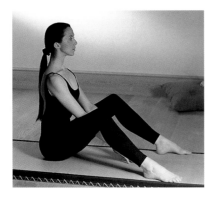

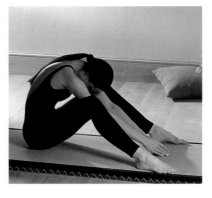

△ **1** Sit upright with your knees bent and your feet flat on the floor. Create as much length through your spine as possible. Keep the shoulders relaxed.

△ **2** Let your chin gently drop to your chest, then roll down bone by bone through your spine. As you do so, gently reach forwards with your hands. Keep your abdominals hollowed throughout. Roll back up to the starting position and lengthen up through your spine. Do not collapse into the stretch, but lift up through the abdominals and spine. Exhale as you lower into the stretch.

## second position

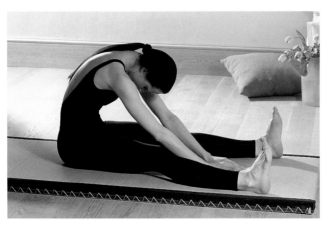

◁ The movement is the same as before, but this time straighten the legs and flex your feet, lengthening the heels away. Bend the knees slightly if you find this uncomfortable. The legs should be parted as far as is comfortable. As you roll up create as much length as possible between the vertebrae. Keep your buttocks on the floor.

**Checkpoints**
- Do not have the legs too far apart
- Visualize reaching up and over a beach ball
- Roll up vertebra by vertebra

# Spine twist

A deceptively challenging movement, this twist will stretch the waist and lower back while strengthening the abdominals. To gain the maximum benefit, it is important to keep your bottom on the floor throughout this movement. Let your head float up to the ceiling and pull your navel towards your spine. Try to keep the movement smooth and continuous. On your first attempts at this exercise you may be surprised at how hard it is to sit correctly aligned. We all develop certain postural habits and this exercise challenges them so it will feel intense at first. It gets easier with practice.

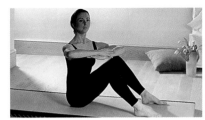

**Purpose**: To stretch the sides, strengthen the abdominals and promote thoracic mobility
**Target muscles**: Obliques, abdominals, adductors and hamstrings
**Repetitions**: Repeat 10 times on each side

## first position

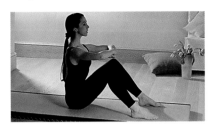

△ **1** Sit upright, lengthening up through the spine, with your knees bent and feet flat on the floor, legs slightly apart. Cross your arms loosely across your chest. Maintain a straight line from your head to your bottom.

△ **2** Breathing laterally, inhale and, as you exhale, turn the upper body to one side, keeping your buttocks firmly on the floor. Repeat on the other side. Remember that this is a flowing movement, not a static position.

**Checkpoints**
- Keep the movement flowing
- Hollow the abdominals
- Lengthen up through the spine

## second position

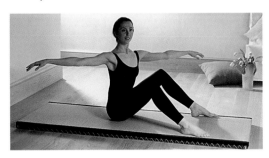

◁ The basic movement is the same but is performed with straight arms, lengthening out through the arms from the shoulders. Take care not to drop them. Now you are stretching in two directions: lengthening out through your arms and up through your spine. Slide your shoulder blades gently down your back and keep your feet flat on the floor.

**Checkpoints**
- Do not collapse into the movement
- Keep the whole of your buttocks on the floor
- Do not curve the spine

## third position

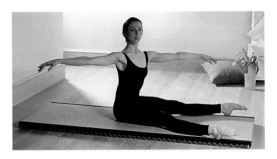

◁ The movement is the same but this time straighten the legs and point your toes. You are now stretching in three directions: up through your spine, out through your arms and through your legs. Be sure to keep your buttocks on the floor. You may be tempted to lean into one side as you turn.

**Checkpoints**
- Lengthen all the way to the toes
- Feel the abdominals working

# Lower back stretch

This is a good warm-up stretch. Taking deep breaths can help you to relax into the stretch and you may find your muscles becoming more pliable, allowing you to ease yourself further into the movement. The stretch is great for easing mild tension in the lower back, which is a common complaint. Some people find it beneficial to rock slightly from side to side while in this stretch as this can gently mobilize the lower back. To do this, keep your upper body on the floor and make the movement very subtle. Although a small number of repetitions are recommended, these are only a guideline until you are confident about your instincts. Hold the stretch for longer or repeat if you need to.

## first position

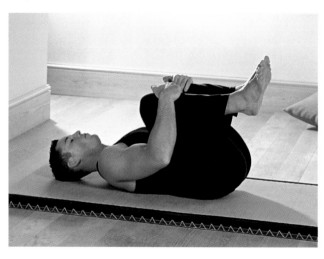

◁ Lie on your back and bring both knees up towards your chest. Support your legs with your hands, just below your knees. Relax your shoulders and feel the stretch in your lower back. Remember to keep your abdominals hollowed. Inhale to prepare and exhale as you lift your legs.

**Purpose:** To stretch the lower back

**Target muscles:** Erector spinae and gluteals

**Repetitions:** Stretch twice; hold for 30 seconds each

### Checkpoints

• Check for tension in the neck and shoulders

• Relax into the stretch

• Do not overgrip with your hands

## second position

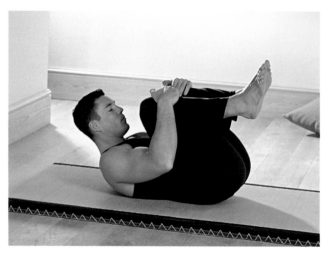

◁ Curl your head and shoulders off the floor, imagining curling up like a ball. Keep your neck soft: do not force your head forwards to your knees. Take care not to overgrip – keep your elbows open.

### Checkpoints

• Curl up and down slowly

• Make sure your mat is thick enough to protect your back

# Spine press

This movement mobilizes and stretches the lower spine. It is a good one to try whenever your lower back feels stiff, especially if you have been sitting for a long period, at your desk for example (and it can be done very discreetly). The curve of the spine should be very subtle. Take care not to over-curve your spine as you may "pinch" the muscles in the lower back. If it feels uncomfortable to curve your spine, or you have problems with your lower back, you may want to perform the second part of the movement only. When you tilt your pelvis, initiate the movement by imagining you are pressing your navel towards your spine. Avoid collapsing into the movement by lengthening your spine.

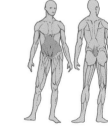

introducing Pilates

**Purpose:** To mobilize and stretch the lower back
**Target muscles:** Erector spinae and abdominals
**Repetitions:** Stretch twice; hold for 30 seconds each

### Checkpoints

• Do not over-curve your spine
• Keep the abdominals hollowed
• Keep your head in alignment

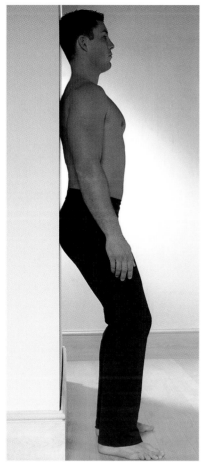

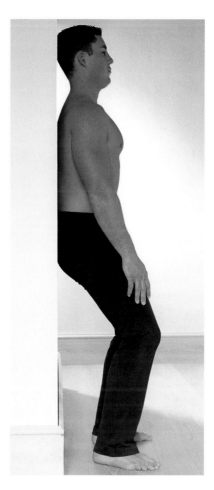

△ **1** Stand a short distance away from the wall, with your back against the wall, your knees bent and your arms by your sides. Lengthen up and glide your shoulder blades down your spine.

△ **2** Inhale, and as you exhale, push your spine flat against the wall by tilting your pelvis and contracting your abdominals. Keep your head in alignment. Try not to collapse into the movement: keep your abdominals hollowed.

# Simple stretches

The following stretches are great for lengthening fatigued, tense muscles. The two upper-body stretches are great for opening up the chest; this is ideal if you have been sitting at a desk for a long period of time. On the first Chest Stretch, the wrist is also being slightly stretched. If this is uncomfortable, turn your hand round so that your fingertips point to the ceiling. In the Deep Chest and Back Stretch, slightly bend your knees if your legs are stretched beyond the comfort zone. When performing the gluteals stretch, be sure to keep your bottom on the floor or you will not stretch enough.

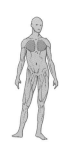

## chest stretch

**This feel-good stretch is great for relieving tightness in the chest and uses the wall for support. It can be done almost anywhere to relieve tightness in the chest.**

**Purpose**: To stretch the chest
**Target muscles**: Pectorals
**Repetitions**: Stretch twice; hold for 30 seconds each

**Checkpoints**
• Keep your spine in neutral
• Feel the stretch in your chest
• Relax your shoulders

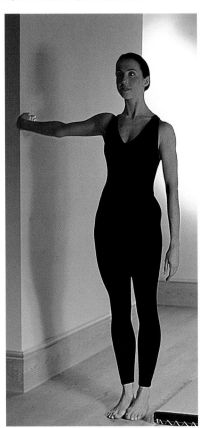

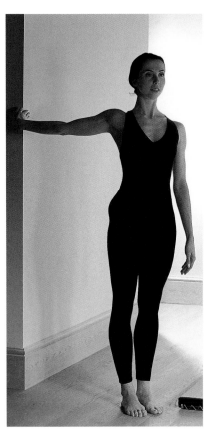

△ **1** Stand sideways to a wall. Extend one arm and place your hand flat on it. Keep your hand in line with your chest and your feet in line with your hips. Draw in your abdominals; your spine stays in neutral.

△ **2** Now turn your hips away from the wall, so that you feel a stretch in your chest. Relax your shoulders and enjoy the stretch. Change sides and repeat the movement.

## gluteals stretch

This stretch is reasonably easy to do and promotes a greater range of movement in the lower body. It is also a valuable stretch to do before many different sports that involve a lot of lower body work.

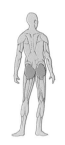

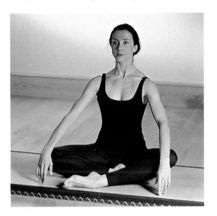

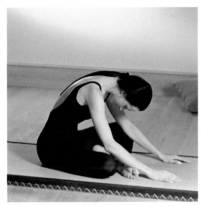

**Purpose:** To stretch the lower body
**Target muscles:** Gluteals
**Repetitions:** Stretch twice; hold for 30 seconds each

**Checkpoints**
- Keep your buttocks on the floor
- Replace the spine bone by bone
- Create length between the vertebrae

△ **1** Sit on the floor and position one leg in front of the other (the legs are not crossed). Relax your arms in front of you. Lengthen up through the spine, creating space between the vertebrae. Don't worry if your knees don't fall to the floor, just relax and let the knees fall into a natural position.

△ **2** Drop your chin towards your chest and curl down the spine while pushing the arms forwards and keeping your buttocks on the floor. Curl up again, switch the positions of the legs and repeat on the other side. Do not collapse into the movement; keep the abdominals pulled in throughout.

## deep chest and back stretch

This stretch is ideal for easing tightness in the chest and back. Try to relax your shoulders and neck into the stretch. If this stretch is too intense, you can bend your knees.

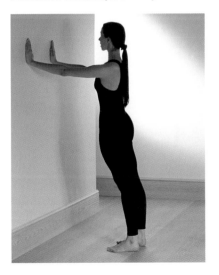

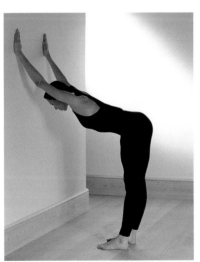

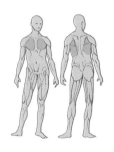

**Purpose:** To stretch the chest and shoulders
**Target muscles:** Pectorals and latissimus dorsi
**Repetitions:** Stretch twice; hold for 30 seconds each

**Checkpoints**
- Keep your head in line with your spine
- Keep your hips over your knees
- Bend the knees if necessary

△ **1** Stand facing the wall with your feet together and place your hands flat on the wall level with your shoulders, just wider than shoulder-width apart. Lengthen up through the spine.

△ **2** Inhale, then as you exhale, lower your chest by bending from the hips, to feel a stretch in your chest and back. Keep your head in line with your spine. Keep the spine lengthened and the abdominals hollowed.

▷

## abdominal stretch

This is a very popular stretch that is similar to the "cobra" in yoga. It is very good for stretching the abdominals after all the hard work they have done. Take care not to throw your head back in this stretch. Keep facing the floor and lengthen up through the top of your head to avoid sinking into the shoulders. If you feel any pinching in your lower back, ease gently out of the stretch.

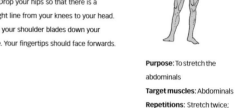

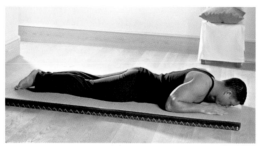

◁ **1** Drop your hips so that there is a straight line from your knees to your head. Glide your shoulder blades down your spine. Your fingertips should face forwards.

**Purpose:** To stretch the abdominals
**Target muscles:** Abdominals
**Repetitions:** Stretch twice; hold for 30 seconds each

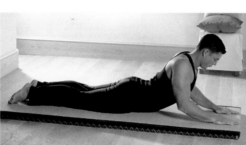

◁ **2** Inhale, and as you exhale, lift your upper body off the floor, resting the weight on your arms. Keep the abdominals hollowed and lifted, and take care not to over-curve the spine. Keep your hips on the floor. Do not sink into your neck, but lengthen up through your spine. Watch for tension in the neck. If you feel a pinch in your lower back, ease out of the stretch.

**Checkpoints**
• Do not over-curve your spine
• Keep your head in line with your spine
• Keep your hips on the floor

## hip flexor stretch

The hip flexors tend to be one of the tightest muscle groups, and when these muscles get overly tight they can cause discomfort and eventually imbalances. People involved in most sports benefit from this stretch, especially runners.

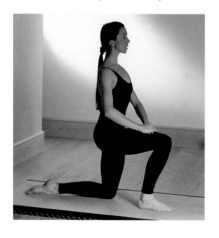

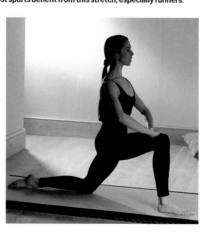

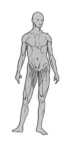

**Purpose:** To stretch the hip flexors
**Target muscles:** Hip flexors
**Repetitions:** Stretch twice; hold for 30 seconds each

**Checkpoints**
• Take care not to collapse into the stretch
• Lunge into the stretch
• Keep your head in alignment

△ **1** Kneel down on the floor and take one step forwards, using your hands for support. If you need extra cushioning, place a pillow under the supporting knee.

△ **2** Lunge carefully into the front leg, exhaling as you go forwards. Make sure your raised knee is directly over your foot. Lengthen up through the spine and keep the abdominals hollowed. You should feel this stretch at the top of the rear leg. Change legs and repeat.

# waist lifts

**This is a good movement to stretch and mobilize the spine. If it feels too intense or uncomfortable to have your arms overhead, then stretch with them by your side.**

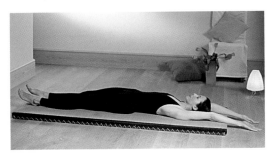

◁ **1** Lie on your back with your arms overhead or, if this is difficult, by your sides. Lengthen through your feet, spine and arms: visualize two cars pulling you in different directions. Draw the navel in to the spine.

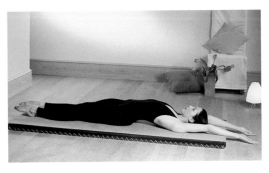

◁ **2** Carefully lift your waist. This is a very subtle movement; take care not to create a big curve in your spine. Keep the abdominals strong and the head in alignment. Watch for any gripping in your lower back. If you feel any pinching in your back, ease out of the stretch.

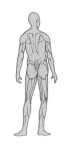

**Purpose:** To stretch and mobilize the spine
**Target muscles:** Erector spinae
**Repetitions:** Stretch twice; hold for 30 seconds each

**Checkpoints**

- Ease out of the stretch if any pinching occurs
- Keep the abdominals strong
- Lengthen out the spine

# side stretch

**This feels good at any time. No wonder cats and dogs are always stretching – it relieves the body of unwanted tension and liberates the spine and joints.**

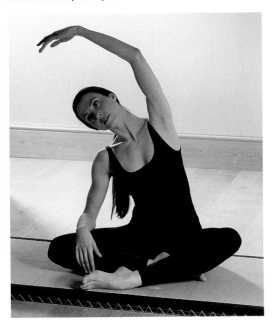

◁ Sit on the floor with one leg in front of the other (the legs are not crossed). Inhale as you prepare. Exhale as you raise one arm and lengthen up through the spine, then stretch into one side from a strong centre, taking care not to collapse into the stretch. Feel the stretch in your back. Pull the navel to the spine and keep your buttocks on the floor. If this leg positioning is uncomfortable, bend your legs and keep your feet flat on the floor.

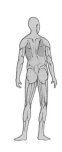

**Purpose:** To stretch the back
**Target muscles:** The latissimus dorsi
**Repetitions:** Stretch twice on each side; hold for 30 seconds each

**Checkpoints**

- Keep your buttocks on the floor
- Lengthen up through the spine
- Don't let the abdominals sag

# Sample programmes

To put together a programme that suits you, consult the chart on page 209, which shows the dominant muscles that are used. This will help you choose a selection of movements from each group to make a well-rounded programme. The majority of the exercises need to be repeated 10 times each (or, in the case of unilateral exercises, 10 times per side).

When putting together a programme, it is best to allow 5 minutes for each movement. A certain group of muscles may need more attention because of muscular imbalances or repetition of a certain activity. Also take into account the initial warm-up, final stretch and a relaxation period at the end. To get you started, two basic plans are suggested here.

Vary your programme from time to time so that you do not get bored. If you dislike an exercise or it does not feel right on a particular day, do a different movement that targets the same muscle groups. Always listen to your body. Most of the exercises have variations, so work your way progressively through the different levels of intensity.

## The short programme

If you don't have time for an hour-long session, you can plan a mini programme lasting 25 minutes. However, try to base most sessions on the hour-long plan and use the short plan only when necessary (25 minutes is better than skipping the session entirely). You will obviously have to shorten the length of time spent on each exercise, as well as doing fewer of them: aim to achieve five to seven repetitions of each movement.

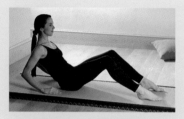

4
◁ **Rolling back**
3 minutes
(p.216)

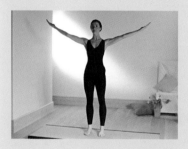

1
◁ **Warm-up**
8–10 minutes
ensures you are
warmed up
before you start
exercising (p.186).

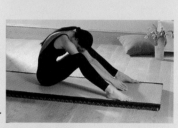

5
◁ **Spine stretch**
3 minutes
(p.236)

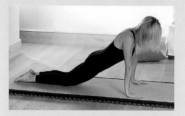

2
◁ **Push-ups**
3 minutes
(p.226)

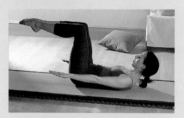

6
◁ **Hundred**
3 minutes
(p.218)

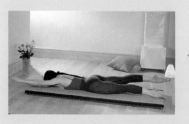

3
◁ **Swimming**
3 minutes
(p.219)

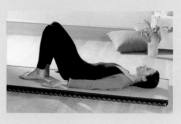

7
◁ **Relaxation**
Lie down and
relax for 2
minutes to finish
the session

# The one-hour programme

This sample format includes some of the "core" movements; this would be a good programme to start with while you are adapting to these exercises. As with most Pilates programmes, the emphasis is on strengthening the torso. After a few weeks, you can change some of these movements for others; try always to do some movements from each of the different categories so that you are working on all parts of the body and developing strength, flexibility and mobility.

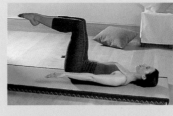

◁ **Hundred**
5 minutes
(p.218)

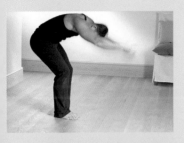

◁ **Warm-up**
8–10 minutes
ensures you are
warmed up
before you start
exercising (p.186).

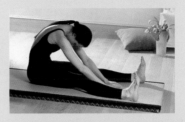

◁ **Spine stretch**
5 minutes
(p.236)

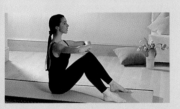

◁ **Spine twist**
5 minutes
(p.237)

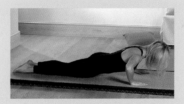

◁ **Push-ups**
5 minutes
(p.226)

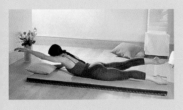

◁ **Swimming**
5 minutes
(p.219)

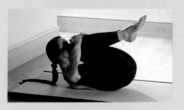

◁ **Rolling back**
5 minutes
(p.208)

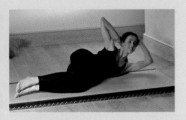

◁ **Side squeeze:
right side**
5 minutes
(p.224)

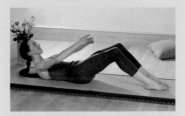

◁ **The roll-up**
5 minutes
(p.217)

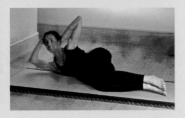

◁ **Side squeeze:
left side**
5 minutes
(p.224)

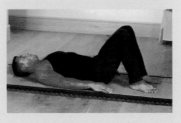

◁ **Relaxation**
Relax for
5 minutes to
finish the
session

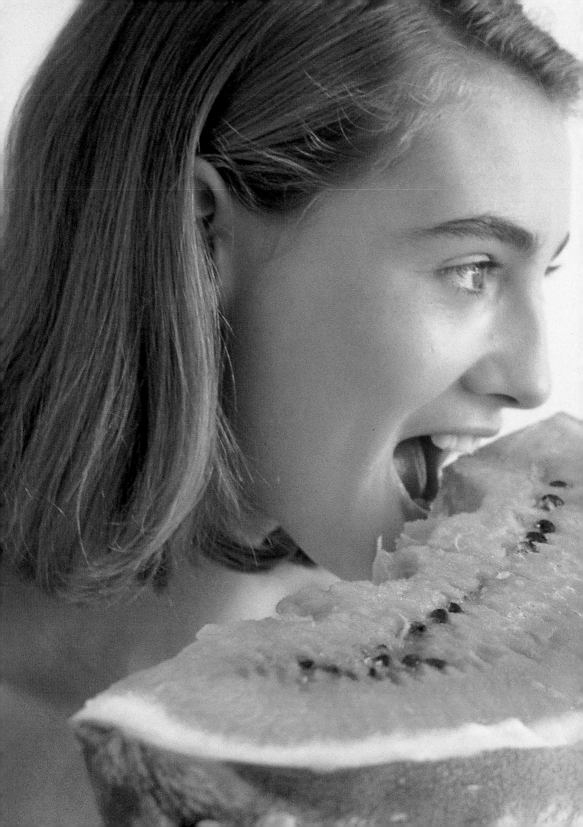

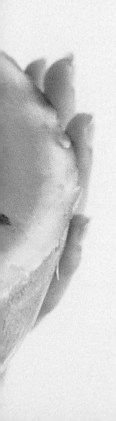

# Healthy Eating

Developing healthy eating habits plays a huge part in how your body performs and how you feel about it. Eating foods that promote good health makes sense, and is surprisingly simple. So take advantage of the latest nutritional research to improve your diet, your health and your beauty.

# A healthy balance

Balance is crucial to healthy eating, and understanding how to choose a healthy combination of foods is the first step towards improving your eating habits and lifestyle.

## vital vitamins

Vitamins are crucial for a number of processes carried out by the body. Usually only a few milligrams are required each day but they are essential for good health. Most vitamins cannot be made by the body so they must be obtained from food.

Vitamins have a wide variety of functions in the body. Some vitamins play a part in enzyme activity. Enzymes are protein molecules and they are responsible for every aspect of metabolism, the energy we produce. Producing plenty of enzymes improves the processes of digestion, detoxification and immunity, and also helps to slow down the aging process.

Vitamins A, C and E are antioxidants which protect body cells from damage. If the body is under stress, vitamin C (ascorbic acid) is used more quickly. Smoking is a form of stress for the body, and smokers should be particularly careful to make sure that they eat fruit and vegetables containing vitamin C.

## essential minerals

A wide variety of minerals is vital for good health, growth and body functioning. Some, such as calcium and iron, are needed in quite large amounts, and for some people there is a real risk of deficiency if they do not eat a healthy diet.

**Calcium:** A regular supply of calcium is vital because bone tissue is constantly being broken down and rebuilt. A calcium-rich diet is particularly important during adolescence, pregnancy, breastfeeding, the

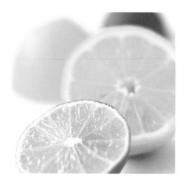

△ **Citrus fruits are a rich source of vitamin C. One orange a day provides an adult's daily requirement of vitamin C.**

menopause and old age. Smoking, lack of exercise, too much alcohol, high protein and high salt intakes all encourage calcium losses.

| VITAMINS | BEST SOURCES | ROLE IN HEALTH |
|---|---|---|
| A (retinol in animal foods, beta-carotene in plant foods) | Milk, butter, cheese, egg yolks, margarine, carrots, apricots, squash, red (bell) peppers, broccoli, green leafy vegetables, mango and sweet potatoes. | Essential for vision, bone growth, and skin and tissue repair. Beta-carotene acts as an antioxidant and protects the immune system. |
| B1 (thiamin) | Wholegrain cereals, brewer's yeast, potatoes, nuts, pulses (legumes) and milk. | Essential for energy production, the nervous system, muscles and heart. Promotes growth and boosts mental ability. |
| B2 (riboflavin) | Cheese, eggs, milk, yogurt, fortified breakfast cereals, yeast extract, almonds and pumpkin seeds. | Essential for energy production and for the functioning of vitamin B6 and niacin as well as tissue repair. |
| Niacin (part of B complex) | Pulses, potatoes, fortified breakfast cereals, wheatgerm, peanuts, milk, cheese, eggs, peas, mushrooms, green leafy vegetables, figs and prunes. | Essential for healthy digestive system, skin and circulation. It is also needed for the release of energy. |
| B6 (piridoxine) | Eggs, wholemeal (whole-wheat) bread, breakfast cereals, nuts, bananas, and cruciferous vegetables such as broccoli and cabbage. | Essential for assimilating protein and fat, to make red blood cells, and for a healthy immune system. |
| B12 (cyanocobalamin) | Milk, eggs, fortified breakfast cereals, cheese and yeast extract. | Essential for formation of red blood cells, maintaining a healthy nervous system and increasing energy levels. |
| Folate (folic acid) | Green leafy vegetables, fortified breakfast cereals, bread, nuts, pulses, bananas and yeast extract. | Essential for cell division. Extra is needed pre-conception and during pregnancy to protect foetus against neural tube defects. |
| C (ascorbic acid) | Citrus fruits, melons, strawberries, tomatoes, broccoli, potatoes, peppers and green vegetables. | Essential for the absorption of iron, and for healthy skin, teeth and bones. An antioxidant that strengthens bones. |
| D (calciferol) | Sunlight, margarine, vegetable oils, eggs, cereals and butter. | Essential for bone and teeth formation. Helps the body to absorb calcium and phosphorus. |
| E (tocopherol) | Seeds, nuts, vegetable oils, eggs, wholemeal bread, green leafy vegetables, oats and cereals. | Essential for healthy skin, circulation and maintaining cells – an antioxidant. |

▷ Not all fats are "bad" for you, but only small amounts are needed to stay healthy. Eat monounsaturated fats such as olive oil, and polyunsaturates such as sunflower oil, in preference to butter and other saturated fats.

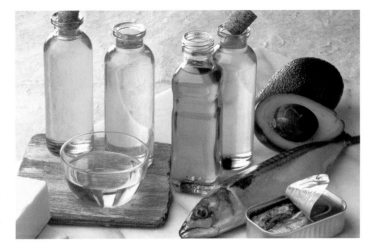

**Iron:** Only a fraction of the iron present in food is absorbed, although it is much more readily absorbed from red meat than from vegetable sources. Vitamin C also helps with absorption. Pregnant women, women who have heavy periods, and vegetarians should all be particularly careful about ensuring an adequate intake.

**Trace elements:** These include other essential minerals such as zinc, iodine, magnesium and potassium. Although important, they are needed in only minute quantities. They are found in a wide variety of foods and deficiency is very rare.

## fats – good and bad

Eggs, butter, milk and meat are a good source of energy, but we tend to eat too much fat which is why many of us are overweight: fat produces fat. Cut down on fat in your diet but do not cut it out completely: eat less fatty red meat and more fish and poultry; grill (broil), bake or stir-fry (using polyunsaturated and monounsaturated oils); eat eggs in moderation; and use semi-skimmed (low-fat) or skimmed milk instead of full-fat (whole) milk. Use margarine, or switch to a reduced fat olive-oil spread instead of butter; if you like butter, reserve it for special occasions.

Saturated fats come mainly from animal products (milk, butter, cheese and meat) and in excess are thought to contribute to raised cholesterol levels.

Polyunsaturated fats are found in vegetable oils such as sunflower, safflower, corn and soya-bean oils; they are also found in some fish oils and some nuts, and are said to help lower cholesterol levels.

Mono-unsaturated fats are found in olive and rapeseed oils; they are also said to lower cholesterol levels.

| MINERALS | BEST SOURCES | ROLE IN HEALTH |
|---|---|---|
| Calcium | Milk, cheese, yogurt, green leafy vegetables, sesame seeds, broccoli, dried figs, pulses, almonds, spinach and watercress. | Essential for building and maintaining bones and teeth, muscle function and the nervous system. |
| Iron | Red meat, egg yolks, fortified breakfast cereals, green leafy vegetables, dried apricots, prunes, pulses, wholegrains, tofu. | Essential for healthy blood and muscles. |
| Zinc | Peanuts, wholegrains sunflower and pumpkin seeds, pulses, milk, hard cheese and yogurt. | Essential for a healthy immune system, tissue formation, normal growth, wound healing and reproduction. |
| Sodium | Most of the salt we eat comes from processed foods such as crisps, cheese and canned foods. It is also found naturally in most foods. | Essential for nerve and muscle function and the regulation of body fluid. |
| Potassium | Bananas, milk, pulses, nuts, seeds, wholegrains, potatoes, fruits and vegetables. | Essential for water balance, normal blood pressure and nerve transmission. |
| Magnesium | Nuts, seeds, wholegrains, pulses, tofu, dried figs and apricots, and vegetables. | Essential for healthy muscles, bones and teeth, normal growth and nerves. |
| Phosphorous | Milk, cheese, yogurt, eggs, nuts, seeds, pulses and wholegrains. | Essential for healthy bones and teeth, energy production and the assimilation of nutrients. |
| Selenium | Avocados, lentils, milk, cheese, butter, brazil nuts and seaweed. | Essential for protecting against free radical damage and may protect against cancer. |
| Iodine | Seaweed and iodized salt. | Aids the production of hormones released by the thyroid gland. |
| Chloride | Table salt and foods that contain salt. | Regulates and maintains the balance of fluids in the body. |
| Manganese | Nuts, wholegrains, pulses, tofu and tea. | Essential component of various enzymes that are involved in energy production. |

## cereal grains

The seeds of cereal grasses, grains are packed with concentrated goodness and are an important source of complex carbohydrates, protein, vitamins and minerals. Grains are inexpensive and versatile.

Eat plenty of wholegrain foods such as brown rice, wholemeal bread, wholemeal flour and wholemeal pasta; they should form the bulk of a healthy diet.

## fruit and vegetables

Make a habit of eating lots of fresh fruit and vegetables: these are rich in carbohydrates, vitamins and minerals. Nutritionists recommend that every day you should aim to eat at least five portions of fruit (one portion could be a medium apple or orange, a wine glass of fruit juice, two plums or kiwi fruit or one large slice of melon or pineapple) and vegetables (aim to eat two large spoonfuls of vegetables – fresh, frozen, or tinned – with your main meal). Fruit and vegetables contain

phytochemicals, the plant compounds that stimulate the body's enzyme defences against carcinogens (the substances that cause cancer). The best sources are broccoli, cabbages, kohlrabi, radishes, cauliflower, brussels sprouts, watercress, turnips, kale, pak choi (bok choy), mustard greens, spring greens (collards), chard and swede (rutabaga).

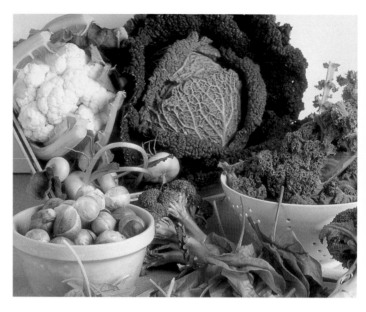

△ **One of the easiest ways to boost your intake of fibre, vitamins and minerals is to eat plenty of vegetables.**

## sugary foods

Many of us tend to eat too much sugar so try cutting added sugar out of your diet completely for 21 days (your body will still

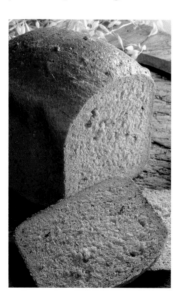

△ **Starchy carbohydrates should make up about 50 per cent of your daily diet.**

**FACTS ON FIBRE**

Fibre is important for a healthy diet. Your body cannot digest it, so, in rather basic terms, it goes in and comes out, taking other waste with it. Fibrous foods include bread, rice, cereals, vegetables, fruit and nuts. Aim for about 30g (just over 1oz) of fibre a day. These are some examples of good fibre sources:

| good sources | average portion | grams of fibre |
|---|---|---|
| wholemeal pasta | 75g/3oz (uncooked) | 9 |
| baked beans | 115g/4oz | 8 |
| frozen peas | 75g/3oz | 8 |
| bran flakes | 50g/2oz | 7 |
| blackberries | 90g/3 1/2 oz | 6 |
| raspberries | 90g/3 1/2 oz | 6 |
| muesli | 50g/2oz | 4–5 |
| baked jacket potato (with skin) | 150g/5oz | 3.5 |
| banana | average fruit | 3.5 |
| brown rice | 50g/2oz | 3 |
| cabbage | 90g/3 1/2 oz | 3 |
| red kidney beans | 40g/1 1/2 oz | 3 |
| wholemeal bread | 1 large slice | 3 |
| high-fibre white bread | 1 large slice | 2 |
| stewed prunes | 6 fruit | 2 |

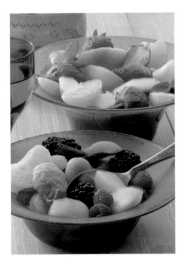

▽ Fresh fruit makes a healthy, low-calorie snack that is filling as well as delicious.

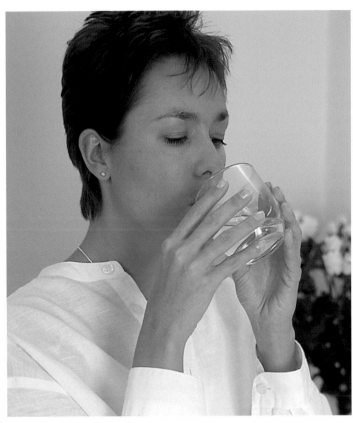

obtain it naturally from certain vegetables and fruit) and see how you feel. Even if you are not actively dieting you will probably find that you lose weight. Craving sugary foods when you are pre-menstrual is common, so try to eat little and often; snack on fruit with a high water content, such as watermelon and strawberries.

## salty issues

It is generally a good idea to eat less salt as too much may lead to high blood pressure. There are some good low-sodium salts available, so use these instead if you do need to season food with salt. Do not buy salted butter, avoid processed and smoked cheeses, add just a little salt (or none at all) to cooking water, and avoid processed foods.

## fluid intake

Drink plenty of water: your body loses 2–3 litres/3–5 pints of fluid every day, so drink no less than 1.5 litres/2$^{1}/_{2}$ pints of water daily. Once you get into the swing of it, consciously drinking water is an easy habit to maintain. Just keep some to hand and sip it slowly throughout the day.

## seeds, pulses and nuts

Pulses (legumes) are economical, easy to cook and good to eat. Low in fat and high in complex carbohydrates, vitamins and minerals, they are a valuable source of protein and good for diabetics, as they help to control sugar levels. Nuts are a good source of B complex vitamins and vitamin E, an antioxidant that has been associated with a lower risk of heart disease, stroke and certain cancers. They are a useful source of protein but are high in calories, so don't eat too many of them.

## sea vegetables

Sea vegetables such as arame, laver and kombu are an excellent source of betacarotene, and contain some of the B complex vitamins. They are rich in minerals – calcium, magnesium, potassium, phosphorous and iron are all present – and are credited with boosting the immune system, reducing stress and helping the metabolism to function efficiently. Eating sea vegetables regularly can improve the hair and skin, and the iodine they contain improves thyroid function.

△ As a rough guide you should aim to drink at least 8 glasses of water every day to keep your body properly hydrated.

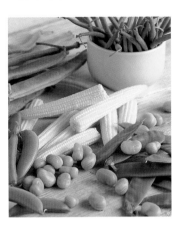

△ It is worth remembering that thanks to super-efficient harvesting methods many frozen vegetables are more nutritious than fresh ones.

# Eating for health and beauty

What we eat has a profound effect on our health and wellbeing. There is ample evidence of a link between poor diet and poor health, and this will affect the way you look. Shining hair, clear skin and strong nails are synonymous with good health.

Specific foods can have a positive impact on our skin, hair, bodies and overall wellbeing when eaten as part of a sensible, well-balanced diet.

## healthy hair and scalp

Aim for a balance of protein foods, including dairy produce, nuts and pulses (legumes). Your shopping list should include organic artichokes, sweet potatoes, carrots, spinach, broccoli, asparagus and beetroot (beet). Choose apricots, citrus fruits, kiwi fruit, berries and apples. Also eat plenty of oily fish and shellfish.

Dry hair and an itching, flaky scalp may be the result of zinc deficiency. Shellfish are good sources of zinc, as are red meat and pumpkin seeds. Essential fatty acids in vegetable oils, nuts and oily fish can also improve the condition of the scalp, while the minerals in sea vegetables, such as kombu and arame, help to make hair lustrous.

Vitamins A and B are important if hair is to be shiny and healthy. Eating liver once

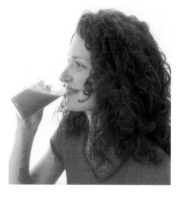

△ A glass of carrot juice contains a valuable supply of antioxidants.

a week is a great way of boosting your intake of vitamin A (retinol), provided that you are not pregnant. Fish liver oils are the richest source of retinol, but it can be obtained from eggs and full-cream (whole) milk. Also eat carrots, spinach, red (bell) peppers, sweet potatoes, peaches and dried apricots on a regular basis. These contain betacarotene, which the body converts to vitamin A.

## improving your skin

The skin is the largest organ in the body, and is especially vulnerable to the effects of modern living. The most important thing you can do to improve the quality of your skin is to drink water – ideally six to eight large glasses every day.

Regular exercise and plenty of fresh air combined with a healthy diet will work wonders on your skin.

If you have a specific skin condition, such as eczema or acne, it is important to consult your doctor, but if you merely think your skin is looking a bit lifeless and could do with a lift, you may find the following advice helpful.

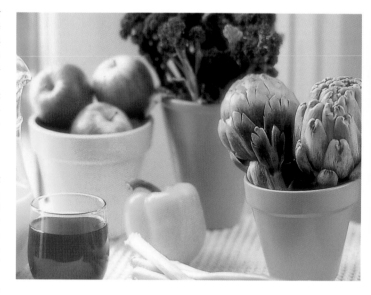

△ Eating plenty of fresh fruit and vegetables is vital for maintaining a healthy immune system.

Eat fresh vegetables such as carrots, spinach, broccoli and sweet potatoes which deliver the antioxidant betacarotene. Citrus fruit, kiwi fruit, berries, avocados, vegetable oils, wholegrains, nuts, seeds and types of seafood provide the antioxidant vitamins C and E, selenium and zinc, which all help to transport nutrients to the skin and maintain collagen and elastin levels. Zinc-rich foods such as liver, pâté and eggs can improve conditions such as psoriasis and eczema. Apples are rich in pectin, which helps to cleanse the liver, and so aids skin detoxification.

Artichokes are good liver cleansers, too, along with asparagus and raw beetroot. Fish, meat and eggs provide B vitamins, which promote supple, glowing skin. Similar benefits can be gained from eating oily fish such as mackerel, salmon, tuna, sardines and herrings. The fatty acids these fish contain (also found in nuts, seeds and vegetable oils) soften and hydrate the skin.

▷ Healthy, shining hair not only feels and looks great, it also reflects good physical wellbeing and conscientious maintenance.

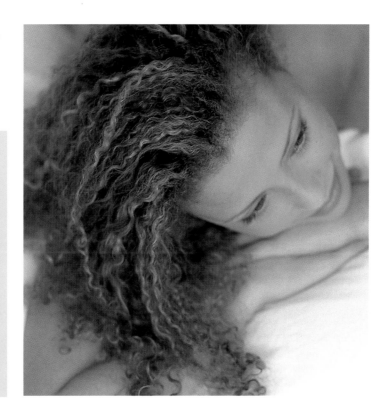

## maximizing nutritional value

To obtain the most nutritional value from your food, especially fruit and vegetables, it should be as fresh as possible, and preparation or cooking should ensure that as many nutrients as possible are retained.

• If you grow your own fruit and vegetables, or buy from a farm where the produce is picked or pulled as needed, freshness is guaranteed. If not, make sure your supplier has a rapid turnover.

• Transport produce home quickly. Remove any plastic wrapping. Store produce in a cool larder or in the refrigerator crisper.

• Avoid buying fresh produce from a supermarket or store that has installed fluorescent lighting over displays, as this can cause a chemical reaction, depleting nutrients in fruit and vegetables.

• Buy organic produce where possible, and avoid peeling if you can, since nutrients are concentrated just below the skin. Instead wash thoroughly. Prepared vegetables are convenient, but don't peel or slice produce until you are ready to use it, as the nutritional value diminishes rapidly after preparation.

• Try to eat the majority of your vegetables and fruit raw. Otherwise, use a steamer in preference to boiling because during this process soluble vitamins, such as thiamine, vitamin C and B vitamins leach into the water. If you must boil vegetables, use just a little water, and save the water to use in a soup or sauce.

• Buy nuts and seeds in small quantities.

Store them in airtight containers in a cool, dark place. Herbs, spices, pulses, flours and grains should be kept in the same way. Store oils in a cool, dark place to prevent oxidation.

▽ Strawberries are rich in B complex vitamins and vitamin C. They contain potassium, and have good skin-cleansing properties.

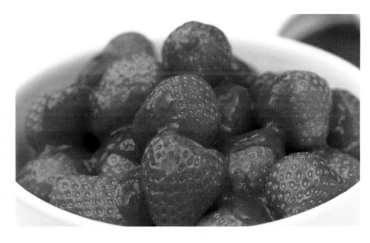

# Eating for energy

How often do you feel tired and lethargic? Does your energy dip dramatically in the afternoons, making you feel dozy (even if you have not washed down a three-course lunch with a bottle of wine) and in need of 40 winks? If your life is regularly disrupted by fatigue and you want to take action, one of the wisest things to do is to look at your eating habits and, if necessary, change what you eat and how you eat it.

## off to a good start

If you start the day with a substantial breakfast your body will get all the energy it needs early on. It is also true that those who fail to eat something sustaining for breakfast are more likely to snack mid-morning and this is unlikely to be a good nutritional choice. A bowl of muesli or porridge with fruit is a good slow-release option that will energize you to start your day.

## changing your eating habits

You are most likely to succeed in changing your diet if you eat regularly, in moderation, and slowly – and savour every mouthful. Although the bonuses of eating in a balanced way do not come instantly, if you take stock now and concentrate on eating

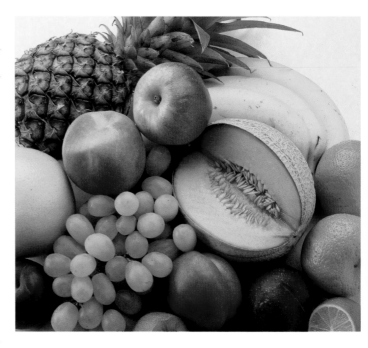

the fresh foods suggested below, as well as avoiding high-fat, sugar-rich foods such as cakes, pastries and salty snacks, you will probably notice a marked difference in your energy levels within a couple of weeks.

If your energy levels take a dive because your blood sugar is low, don't reach for chocolate or a rich biscuit. The quick energy boost these give will be followed by a slump, and you may end up far more tired than you were at the start. Eat a wholemeal salad sandwich instead; the carbohydrate in the bread will give you a more efficient energy fix that will be more prolonged and even.

## vitality foods for extra energy

A diet that makes you feel more energetic is based on natural, wholesome foods that are nutritious, rather than fatty and fast foods. If you want to boost your energy levels, stock up on fresh and dried fruits that are high in natural sugars, such as pears, kiwi

△ **Fruit is the ultimate convenience food. Packed with natural sugars it is ideal for giving you a boost when energy levels are low.**

fruit and apricots, vegetables such as peas, spinach, cabbage, onions, oily fish, poultry, and red meats such as game and lean beef. Eat nuts, brown rice, seeds, pulses (legumes), wheatgerm, wholegrains, and foods that contain minerals such as magnesium, phosphorous, and zinc, and water-soluble vitamins B and C. Use cold-pressed oils such as grapeseed, olive, sesame, sunflower, hazelnut and walnut to dress salads; do not skip dairy foods but use milk and natural yogurt (preferably low-fat); replace sliced white loaves with bread made from wholemeal flour.

## superfoods

Some foods are such a super-rich source of concentrated nutrients that they have earned themselves the title "superfoods".

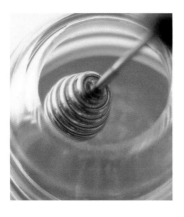

△ Honey is a good source of natural sugar and is gently energizing.

▷ Fresh fruit and vegetable juices have a powerful effect on the body, stimulating the whole system, flushing out the digestive system and encouraging the elimination of toxins.

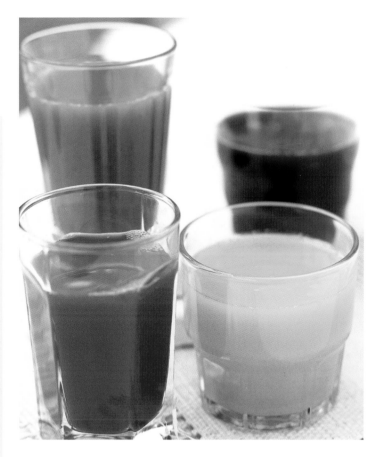

## VITAMIN-PACKED JUICES

Drinking freshly made juices is a quick and easy way to increase your nutrient intake and boost your energy levels without placing the digestion under any strain. Here are some good juices to try:

• Apple, orange and carrot: packed with vitamin C and energizing fruit sugars to give you a lift.

• Papaya, melon and grapes: papaya is soothing to the stomach, and this juice can help the liver and kidneys.

• Carrot, beetroot (beet) and celery: a good juice to kickstart the system in the morning. Try using 90g/3¹/₂oz beetroot to three carrots and two celery sticks.

• Cabbage, fennel and apple: a cleansing juice with antibacterial properties. Use half a small red cabbage, half a fennel bulb, 2 apples and 15ml/1 tbsp lime juice.

• Grapefruit, orange and lemon: this refreshing juice is great for boosting the immune system. Use 1 pink grapefruit, 1 blood orange and 30ml/2 tbsp lemon juice.

## ENERGY-BOOSTING SMOOTHIES

Homemade fruit juices and milk- or yogurt-based drinks are energy-boosting alternatives to commercially prepared drinks, and are easy to make. They are quick, low in fat, high-vitality and a great way of boosting your fruit intake. Choose sweet fruits such as mango, banana and apricots – these have a naturally high sugar content – then switch on the juicer or blender and drink them chilled. Here are two energizing smoothies to try:

• This smoothie is full of energizing natural sugars. Use 1 mango, 2 slices of pineapple, 1 banana, 150ml/¹/₄pint/²/₃cup semi-skimmed or skimmed (low-fat) milk or a small carton of natural (plain) low-fat yogurt and 2.5ml/¹/₂tsp honey (optional).

• For a more zesty energy-boosting smoothie use a handful of raspberries and strawberries, 2 apricots and 120ml/4fl oz/ ¹/₂cup milk or natural low-fat yoghurt.

Some, such as tofu, are old favourites, while others, such as quinoa, have only recently acquired widespread acclaim. Recent scientific research has discovered that plants contain thousands of different chemical compounds, and each of these compounds – known collectively as phytochemicals – has its own function. It is believed that some of them play a crucial role in preventing diseases such as cancer, heart disease, arthritis and hypertension.

To get the best from phytochemicals you need to eat at least five different types of fruit and vegetables daily, plus wholegrains, pulses, nuts and seeds. A number of phytochemicals also have antioxidant properties.

Antioxidants are vital for limiting damage to body cells by unstable molecules known as free radicals. The main antioxidant nutrients are vitamins A, C and E, and the minerals zinc and selenium. Good sources of antioxidants are: sweet potatoes, carrots, watercress, broccoli, peas, citrus fruit, watermelon, strawberries, and nuts and seeds.

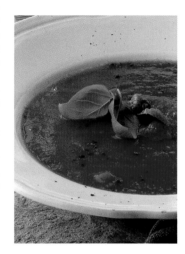

▷ Fresh tomato soup is packed with valuable antioxidant vitamins, while a sprinkle of basil aids digestion and calms the nervous system.

# Eating for weight loss

People tackle weight loss in ways that suit their lifestyles. But the safest and best way to shift excess pounds is to combine regular exercise with a balanced calorie-controlled diet. What you eat when you are trying to take off weight should not be that different from a normal eating plan – except for the amount you consume. If you have only a small amount to lose and you cut your calorie intake by 1,000 from the recommended 2,300 calories per day, you will lose weight; if you are aiming to lose a significant amount, stick to 1,200 calories a day and you will get there. Your basic weight-loss ethos is less sugar and saturated fats, more fibre and starch; the calories you eat should come from foods that supply you with the right number of nutrients to keep your body functioning properly.

## mind over matter

Quick weight loss is inspiring, but it is important to think ahead too; you need to retain your palate and eating habits and reassess your physical activity so that you can lose weight and stay slim. You cannot expect to achieve miracles in a few days, but

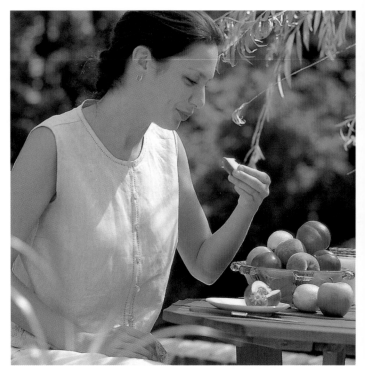

△ **Fruit is the ideal snack when you are dieting. It is very low in fat and calories and provides vitamins and minerals as well as energizing natural sugar energy.**

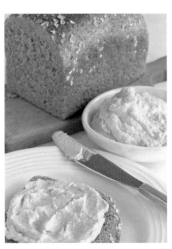

△ **For an excellent high-fibre snack, hummus is delicious spread on wholegrain bread or toast.**

you will see a difference within three or four weeks if you eat properly and exercise regularly. Losing weight successfully is like getting fitter: you need a horizon – or goal – ahead of you to help spur you on.

## healthy weight loss

To lose weight you have to eat fewer calories than your body burns up every day, but the amount varies from person to person. The exact amount depends on your personal composition – how much fat your body has, your metabolism and how much you weigh to begin with. As a rule of thumb though, the heavier you are when you start slimming, the more weight you are likely to lose within 21 days or a month. When you lose weight it comes off all areas of your body, but it can take longer to shift from certain areas, such as your arms and legs.

This is where exercise is particularly helpful, because working on specific trouble spots will usually encourage the weight to come off more quickly.

## weight gain and giving up smoking

You may put on a small amount of weight at first but if you are a smoker, stopping is the biggest leap you can make towards living a healthier lifestyle. If you think that kicking the smoking habit will make you pick at food all day, keep lots of raw vegetables and raisins on hand to munch on.

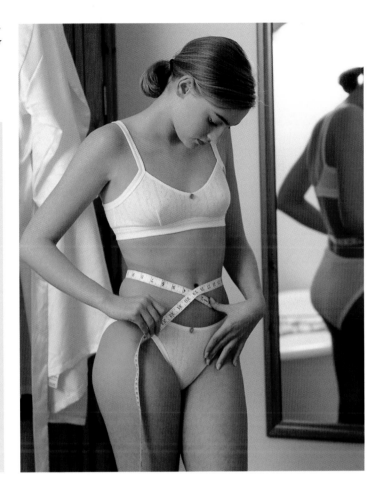

▷ Keeping a record of your measurements is one way of calculating weight loss. It may take longer to shift weight from certain areas, and this will also help you work out which areas you need to focus on when you exercise.

**TIPS FOR WEIGHT LOSS**

• If you can, it is better to eat more at the start of the day to give you energy and time to burn off the calories.

• Do not be tempted to skip meals. Skipping meals makes you crave and overeat at the next meal, and it slows down your metabolism, which ultimately hinders weight loss.

• Eat little and often to stop hunger pangs.

• Drink lots of water.

• If you want to snack, keep a supply of fruit, raw vegetables and raisins nearby.

• Don't be tempted to take slimming pills, diuretics or laxatives to speed up weight loss; they upset the body's natural equilibrium – something that can take considerable time to rebalance.

• Exercise regularly; extra activity uses up calories, and this is essential to weight loss.

• Don't give up if you lapse: it is quite normal to veer off track every so often, and as long as you get back on course as soon as you can, all your hard work will not be ruined.

## eating out – and staying on course

The best way to solve the problem of dining out without lapsing – without drawing attention to yourself and still being able to enjoy yourself – is as follows:

• Order a salad starter.

• Skip bread or breadsticks, or eat a piece of bread without butter – if it's good bread it can be just as delicious.

• Drink one glass of wine, and lots of water.

• Choose a simple main course, something like grilled fish or chicken; avoid rich sauces and lots of butter.

• Choose a simple, low-fat dessert: a sorbet would be ideal.

• Finish with herbal tea (peppermint is refreshing and settles your stomach after eating); or, choose espresso or black coffee, not cappuccino.

## gauging weight loss

You may choose to weigh yourself once a week first thing in the morning. Drawing up a goal chart to record any weight losses (and gains) may help to keep you inspired. Don't be tempted to weigh yourself too often because you are more likely to get discouraged; once a week is enough. Or, if you prefer, ignore the scales and just focus on how you feel by keeping a check on how your clothes feel. When tight clothes become more comfortable this is a sure sign that you are losing weight. Alternatively, you may prefer to keep a record of your measurements (bust, waist and hips) and see how they alter over the 21-day period. Do whatever works best for you, and when you have lost a little weight reward yourself with a treat such as new make-up, a manicure or a massage.

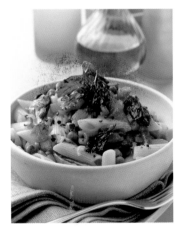

△ **Nutritious, starchy foods such as pasta are not fattening if eaten with low fat sauces, and starchy foods stop you feeling hungry for longer.**

# Detoxing for health

A detox is thought to cleanse and rejuvenate your body, improve the circulation and metabolism, and strengthen the immune system. It can also improve the condition of your skin, hair and nails, and slow down the aging process. As well as the physical benefits, a detox can improve your ability to cope with stress, clear your mind and lift your mood.

Fast foods, sugary or salty snacks, alcohol, coffee and tea all contain toxins, which can build up in the body and cause us to feel lethargic and unhealthy. Even if you have a healthy lifestyle, you are still exposed to poisonous substances in the atmosphere. The air that we breathe contains chemicals, gases and dust particles, and it can pollute our land, water and food.

The body is a highly efficient machine, and it is constantly working to remove toxins from the circulation. However, an unhealthy diet, stress and late nights all put the body under pressure, and can affect how well its elimination systems work. Regular exercise supported by a healthy diet and a weekly detox massage regime will help improve your circulation, eliminate waste from the muscles and keep the detoxifying organs in good working order.

It is also vital that you drink plenty of water. We lose fluid through the natural processes of urination, defecation and sweat. This fluid needs to be replaced. To maintain good health and an efficient detox system we should drink at least 6–8 large glasses of water each day.

## the art of detoxing

There are different approaches to detoxing. The most extreme method is fasting – which involves abstaining from all foods and drinking only water, herbal tea and juices over a short period.

Fasting has a tendency to slow the digestive system, so it can be counter-productive and is not recommended for most people. Your body is more likely to benefit from a gentle programme that does not place it under pressure. A detox is most effective if it is done over a day or two. During this time eat little and often, having only fibre-rich, healthy foods such as raw or lightly cooked fruits, vegetables and grains. Do several sessions of gentle exercise and rest as much as possible. Drink plenty of water to help flush toxins away. You can also drink fresh juices and herbal teas.

Massage can help to speed up the detox process, and brings a pleasurable, relaxing element to the day.

## one-day mono-diet

A good introduction to detoxing, a one-day mono-diet is based on eating just one type of raw fruit or vegetable for a whole day. A one-day mono gives your digestive system a rest, allowing it to concentrate on eliminating stored toxins. You are unlikely to experience any dramatic side-effects but a mono-diet will have a noticeable positive effect on your health and wellbeing.

Raw fruit and vegetables have a powerful cleansing effect on the body and also supply plenty of vitamins, minerals and fibre. If possible, choose a day when you are not working, to make sure that you have time to rest, relax and sleep.

### preparation

Choose just one of these fruits or vegetables:
- grapes
- apples
- pears
- pineapple
- papaya
- carrots
- cucumber
- celery

It is best to choose organic produce and you will need:
- 1–1.5kg/2–3lb of your chosen fruit or vegetable
- 2 litres/3$^1$/$_2$ pints/8 cups still mineral water or filtered water
- herbal teas or fresh herbs to infuse

### the days before detox

Prepare for your detox by cutting down on meat and dairy products, salt, wheat, tea, coffee and sugary foods. Avoid alcohol and cigarettes. The evening before, eat a light evening meal. A vegetable and bean soup or a stir-fry would be perfect. Have an aromatherapy bath and go to bed early.

### detox day

**Morning:** Start your day with the juice of half a lemon in a cup of hot water. This

△ A cup of hot water and lemon juice will stimulate the liver and the gallbladder to kickstart the detoxing process.

**HOW TO CUT DOWN TOXIN CONSUMPTION**
- Buy organic foods whenever possible.
- Avoid drinking unfiltered tap water.
- Reduce intake of processed and packaged foods.
- Cut back on the amount of sweet, fatty and salty foods you eat.
- Always wash and peel non-organic fruit and vegetables.
- Cut down consumption of dairy products and meat. However, make sure that you eat other foods to obtain the calcium your body needs.
- Drink less tea, coffee and fizzy drinks.
- Read labels carefully to avoid artificial additives and genetically modified ingredients.

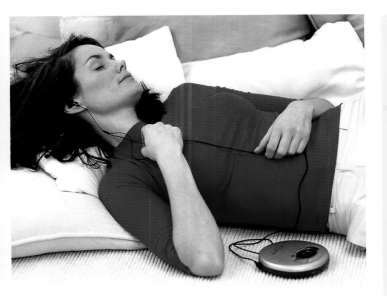

△ **You will benefit more from the detox if you take the day off so that you have time to rest, relax and sleep.**

kickstarts the liver. Do some simple stretching exercises. Give yourself a dry skin brush to stimulate the circulation before you shower or bathe. For breakfast, prepare your chosen fruit or vegetable. Sip water at regular intervals throughout the day.

**Late morning**: Have a massage or try out some relaxation techniques. Eat some of your fruit or vegetable and drink plenty of water.

**Lunch**: Prepare and eat your fruit or vegetable. Drink plenty of water.

**Afternoon**: Try doing some gentle exercises, such as yoga, Pilates or body conditioning, or brisk walking, cycling or swimming. Follow this exercise with some of your fruit or vegetable and herbal tea.

**Evening**: Finish off your quota of fruit or vegetable. Meditate or practise a relaxation technique, such as visualization. Pamper yourself with a manicure or pedicure. Listen to some calming music. Have an Epsom salts bath to encourage the elimination of toxins through your skin. Pour 450g/1lb of salts into a warm bath. Go to bed early.

**the day after**

It is important to ease your body out of a detox gradually. Start the following day with a cup of hot water and lemon juice and some simple exercises. For the first few days keep to cleansing foods and simple recipes. Try not to over-exert yourself.

## lymphatic drainage massage

Lymphatic drainage massage is one of the most gentle forms of massage. It works on the lymph system, and since lymph vessels are close to the surface there is no need for heavy pressure. The lymphatic system of the body is a secondary circulation system which supports the work of the blood circulation. The lymphatic system has no heart to help pump the fluid around the vessels, and therefore it must rely on the activity of the muscles to aid movement.

Lymphatic massage involves using sweeping, squeezing movements along the skin. The action is always directed towards the nearest lymph node. The main nodes used when treating the foot are located in the hollow behind the knee. Lymphatic drainage massage is hugely beneficial in helping to eliminate waste and strengthen the body's immune system. It is a useful exercise to perform on your detox day.

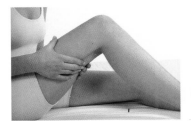

△ **1** To improve lymphatic drainage to the feet and legs, try a daily skin "brush" using your fingertips. Begin by working on the thigh. This clears the lymphatic channels ready to receive the lymph flood from the lower legs. Briskly brush all over the thigh from knee to top, three or four times.

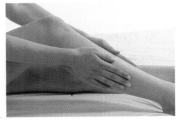

△ **2** Work on the lower leg in a similar way. Brush either side of the leg from ankle to knee, then treat the back of the leg. Follow this by brushing along the top of the foot, continuing up the front of the leg to the knee. Brush over each area twice more, making three times in total.

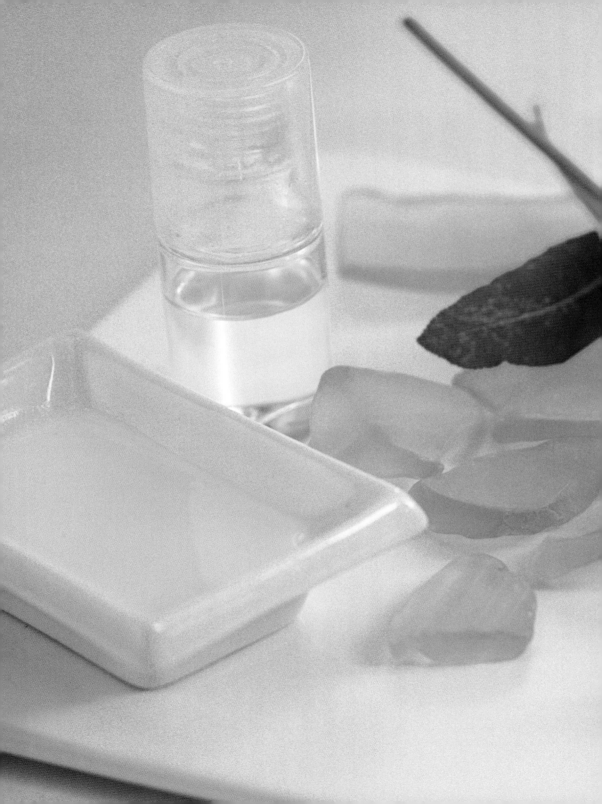

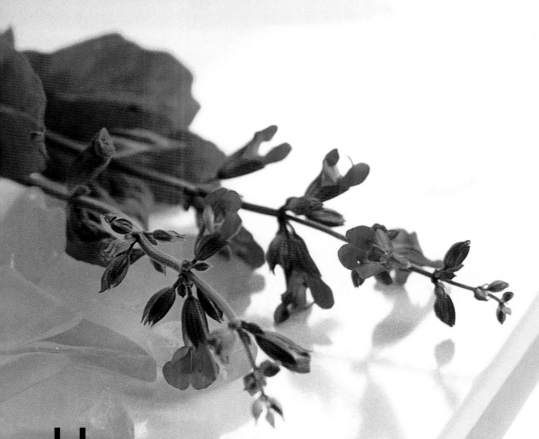

# HEALING
# AROMATHERAPY

# What is aromatherapy?

Many books have been written on the subject of aromatherapy. This section aims to be a little different in that it will illustrate how any woman can benefit from using essential oils throughout the stages of her life – beginning with the onset of puberty, through pregnancy and her reproductive years, on to the menopause and beyond. The section gives profiles of some of the most commonly used oils and describes how they can be used to treat physical and emotional conditions and to alleviate stress. It gives an overview of essential oils and offers advice for the best methods of use in the home. It also describes how oils can be incorporated into a woman's daily skin and beauty regime. First though, it is important to understand what is meant by aromatherapy, as well as something of how it works.

A popular conception of aromatherapy is as a "massage using essential oils". Although there is a connection between massage and aromatherapy, it is not strictly correct to define one in terms of the other.

Aromatherapy has been defined as "the controlled and knowledgeable use of essential oils for therapeutic purposes". These oils are powerful substances and they should always be handled with care, with professional advice taken where necessary. The essential oils used in aromatherapy are not the same as those used by the perfume and food industries, which standardize or adulterate them for commercial interest. Essential oils for aromatherapy should be natural, with nothing added or taken away.

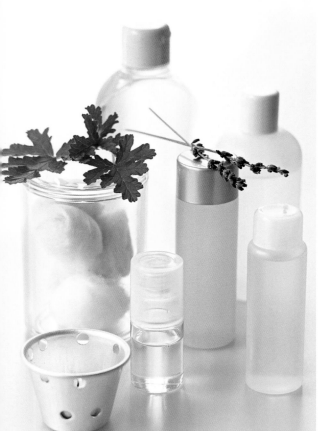

◁ **Many different plant extracts are used in beauty products. An extract is chosen not only for its fragrance, but also for its healing properties.**

▷ **Essential oils can be applied on a compress. Cut up pieces of cotton material and soak them in an oil and water preparation.**

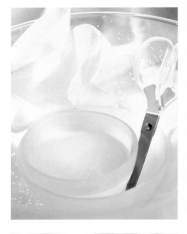

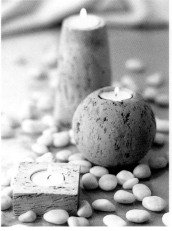

▷ **Vaporizing special aromatherapy candles is an easy way to set the mood for any occasion.**

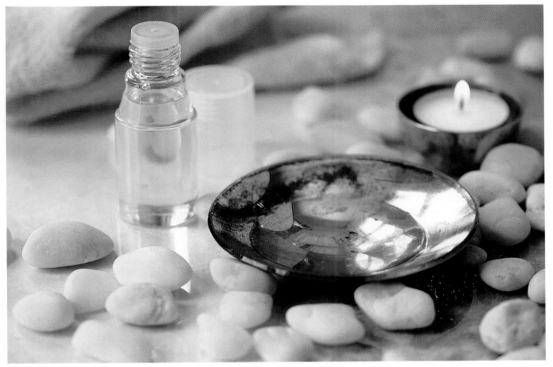

△ Adding a few drops of essential oil to a saucer of water and heating it over a candle flame causes the oil to vaporize and release its aroma into the room.

## HOW TO USE THIS SECTION

When essential oils are used for pleasure alone, the choice of oil is usually based on an individual's preferred aroma, and the properties and effects of the oil are not a priority. However, when used to maintain or improve health, the properties and effects are an important part of the choice.

Each essential oil has many properties, and these can affect both body and mind in more than one way. For example, rosemary essential oil has analgesic properties which will benefit headaches, painful digestion and muscular pain. However, rosemary is also a neurotonic, and can relieve general fatigue and stimulate the memory.

At the end of each chapter of this section is a list of essential oils recommended to help problems associated with that stage in life. Next to each one, from the oil's many assets, are shown the properties relevant to the par-

ticular problem. As an example, where geranium is suggested for athlete's foot, its antifungal quality is listed because this is the property required. In another case, where geranium is suggested for diarrhoea, its anti-inflammatory, antispasmodic and astringent properties are given because these are the relevant properties.

An enhanced result can often be obtained by selecting and using more than one essential oil (two, three or even four different essential oils can be used to make up the required number of drops). The synergy of the blended oils will result in an increase of energy within the mix, when compared to the energy available from one single essential oil.

Having selected the oils you want to use, the chapter on Aromatherapy Techniques will show you how to prepare them for use. The

application techniques suitable for use at home are shown here – application to the skin in a carrier oil, which takes the oils into the bloodstream and all around the body, or by inhalation alone. When we breathe in, some essential oil molecules travel to the lungs to be absorbed into the blood. Other molecules go directly to the brain. This is the quickest route and the most effective way to heal weak or fragile emotions and states of mind, such as stress and depression. The nose not only warms and cleans the inhaled air, but it also enables us to identify substances by their smell. Tiny hairs in the human nose, called cilia, send information via receptor cells to the brain to identify the inhaled molecules. The brain then releases neurochemicals, and these have either a sedative or a tonic effect, depending on the aroma.

# The essential oils

Essential oils are powerful agents and all of them – even those nominated as safe – must be used in the correct amounts and for the conditions to which they are best suited. One or two pure essential oils, and most synthetic and adulterated ones, may cause irritation and skin sensitivity. The botanical varieties chosen for this book have been carefully selected from those which do not present this problem. However, these varieties are not always commonly available in the shops and appropriate cautions are included here for the sake of safety.

Except in emergencies, as in cases of burns, stings or wounds, essential oils should not be applied undiluted to the skin, but should be mixed first in a base carrier oil. Citrus oils are photosensitive and should not be used before sunbathing. If you are unsure about the suitability of an oil, always seek the advice of a qualified aromatherapist.

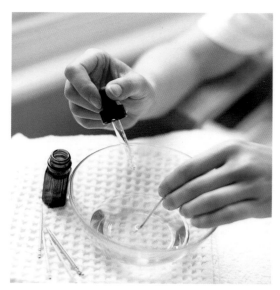

◁ Prepare a compress for treatment at home by blending your favourite essential oils and adding them to water.

▽ Setting the scene at home will contribute to the benefits of aromatherapy. Choose a quiet part of the house and light candles to help you relax.

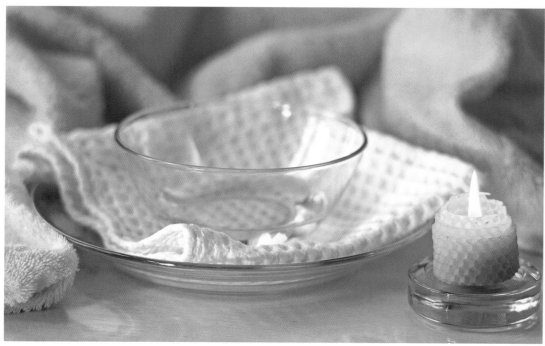

## Boswellia carteri – frankincense
family *Burseraceae*

### properties
analgesic, anti-infectious, antioxidant, anticatarrhal, antidepressant, anti-inflammatory, cicatrizant, energizing, expectorant, immunostimulant

These small trees, also known as olibanum, grow in north-east Africa and south-east Arabia. Cuts are made in the tree bark from which a white serum exudes, solidifying into "tear drops". When distilled, these produce a pale amber-green essential oil. Frankincense, an ancient aromatic product once considered as precious as gold, has been burnt in temples and used in religious ceremonies since Biblical times.

Frankincense is a gentle oil which is particularly useful for emotional problems, where it allays anger and irritability and soothes grief.

### safety
• No known contraindications in normal aromatherapy use.

### features in
Beauty and Well-being, The Reproductive Years, The Sunset Years.

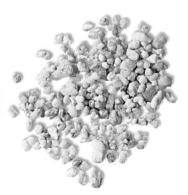

△ **Boswellia carteri –**
**frankincense**

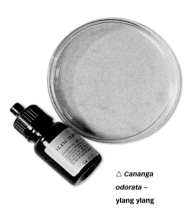

△ *Cananga*
*odorata –*
**ylang ylang**

## Cananga odorata – ylang ylang
family *Annonaceae*

### properties
antidiabetic, antiseptic, antispasmodic, aphrodisiac, calming and sedative, hypotensive, general tonic, reproductive tonic

Ylang ylang trees, with their long, fluttering yellow-green flowers, are native to tropical Asia: ylang ylang is a Malay word meaning "flower of flowers". The blooms are picked early in the morning and steam-distilled to yield an oil with an exotic and heady aroma.

Widely reputed for its aphrodisiac qualities, ylang ylang is said to counter impotence and frigidity. It can help emotional problems such as irritability and fear; and is effective against introversion and shyness. Ylang ylang also helps to regulate cardiac and respiratory rhythm.

### safety
• No known contraindications in normal aromatherapy use.
• Use in moderation. Excess can lead to nausea and headaches.

### features in
The Teenage Years, Beauty and Well-being, The Sunset Years.

## Cedrus atlantica – cedarwood
family *Pinaceae*

### properties
antibacterial, antiseptic, cicatrizant, lipolytic, lymph tonic, mucolytic, stimulant

There are 20 or more species of the trees which yield an oil of cedar. This particular tree, the Atlas cedarwood, grows in the Atlas mountains of north Africa. The first oil extracted was used by the Egyptians for embalming. Most of the oil was taken from wood chippings left from making boxes and furniture (King Solomon used cedarwood extensively when building the temple at Jerusalem). Cedarwood oil is now obtained by steam distillation. It has a pleasant, sweet, woody aroma and can be used in a variety of ways.

Cedarwood is effective for oily skin and scalp disorders, and its antiseptic properties and cleansing aroma are beneficial to bronchial problems.

### safety
• Unsuitable for pregnant women and small children.
• Should not be taken internally.

### features in
The Teenage Years, Beauty and Well-being.

▽ *Cedrus atlantica –*
**cedarwood**

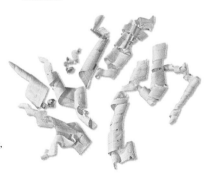

## Chamaemelum nobile –
## chamomile (Roman)
family *Asteraceae*

### properties

antianaemic, anti-inflammatory, antineuralgic, antiparasitic, antispasmodic, calming and sedative, carminative, cicatrizant, digestive, emmenagogic, menstrual, vulnerary, stimulant, sudorific

Roman chamomile is native to the British Isles and is a small perennial with feathery leaves and daisy-like flowers. The essential oil is a pale blue-green colour because of the chamazulene content (see *Matricaria recutica* – German chamomile).

The oil is gentle, soothing and calming. It is suitable for children and babies for irritability, inability to sleep, hyperactivity and tantrums. Roman chamomile is also useful for a range of adult complaints, including rheumatic inflammation, indigestion and headaches.

### safety

• No known contraindications in normal aromatherapy use.

### features in

Beauty and Well-being, The Reproductive Years, The Sunset Years.

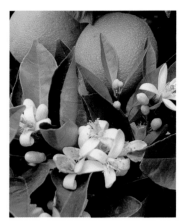

△ *Citrus aurantium* var. *amara* – neroli

## Citrus aurantium var. amara –
## neroli
family *Rutaceae*

### properties

antidepressant, aphrodisiac, sedative, uplifting

Neroli oil is the distilled oil from the blossoms of the bitter orange tree. It has a soft, floral fragrance, and is the most costly of the orange oils.

Neroli is beneficial for the skin and helps improve its elasticity. It is good for scars, thread veins and the stretch marks of pregnancy and has a sedative and calming effect on the emotions.

### safety

• No known contraindications in normal aromatherapy use.

### features in

Beauty and Well-being, The Reproductive Years.

## Citrus aurantium var. amara –
## orange (bitter)
family *Rutaceae*

### properties

anti-inflammatory, anticoagulant, calming, digestive, sedative, tonic

Oranges have a long tradition in both therapeutic and culinary use. A variety of essential oils are obtained from the fruit, flowers and leaves of both bitter (Seville) and sweet orange trees: neroli oil from the flowers, petitgrain from the leaves, and orange oil from the peel. Bitter orange is expressed from the peel of Seville oranges (most orange marmalades are also made from the peel of Seville oranges).

Bitter orange can be helpful for poor circulation, digestive problems and constipation. It has antidepressant qualities, and will promote positive thinking and cheerful feelings.

### safety

• Photosensitizer. Do not expose the skin to sunlight or a sunbed for at least two hours after use.
• No known contraindications in normal aromatherapy use.

### features in

The Reproductive Years, The Sunset Years.

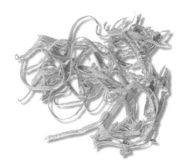

△ *Citrus aurantium* var. *amara* –
**bitter orange**

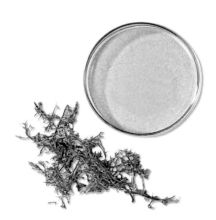

△ *Chamaemelum nobile* –
**Roman chamomile**

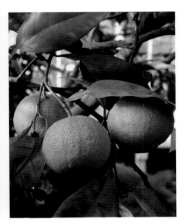

△ *Citrus aurantium* var. *amara* – petitgrain

## *Citrus aurantium* var. *amara* – petitgrain
family *Rutaceae*

### properties
antibacterial, anti-infectious, anti-inflammatory, antispasmodic, calming and energizing

Taken from the leaves of the bitter orange tree, petitgrain's aroma is a cross between the delicate fragrance of neroli oil and the fresh aroma of bitter orange peel. A good petitgrain oil, distilled with some of the blossoms also, is often referred to as the "poor man's neroli" because of its enhanced aroma. Unlike the oil from the fruit, which is expressed, petitgrain oil is obtained by distillation.

Petitgrain is balancing to the nervous system and is recommended for infected skin problems. Emotionally, it can help with anger and panic.

### safety
• No known contraindications in normal aromatherapy use.

### features in
The Teenage Years.

## *Citrus bergamia* – bergamot
family *Rutaceae*

### properties
antibacterial, anti-infectious, antiseptic, antispasmodic, antiviral, calming and sedative, cicatrizant, tonic, stomachic

The main area of bergamot production is southern Italy, although it is also grown on the Ivory Coast. The greenish essential oil is expressed from the peel of this bitter, inedible citrus fruit, which in Cyprus is often crystallized and eaten with a cup of tea. Traditionally, bergamot is a principal ingredient in eau-de-cologne because of its refreshing aroma, and is famous for its use as the flavouring in Earl Grey tea.

Bergamot is useful both in the treatment of digestive problems, such as colic, spasm and sluggish digestion, and for calming emotional states, such as agitation and severe mood swings. It is effective on cold sores but use with extreme caution if in strong sunlight.

### safety
• Photosensitizer. Do not expose the skin to sunlight or a sunbed until at least two hours after using.
• Bergapten-free bergamot is an adulterated oil and should not be substituted for the whole essential oil. If not going into the sun, bergamot can be used in the same way as any other oil without risk.

### features in
Beauty and Well-being, The Sunset Years.

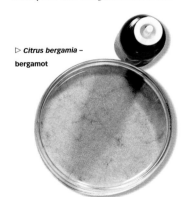

▷ *Citrus bergamia* – bergamot

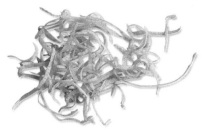

△ *Citrus limon* – lemon

## *Citrus limon* – lemon
family *Rutaceae*

### properties
antianaemic, antibacterial, anticoagulant, antifungal, anti-infectious, anti-inflammatory, antisclerotic, antiseptic, antispasmodic, antiviral, calming, carminative, digestive, diuretic, expectorant, immunostimulant, litholytic, phlebotonic, stomachic

Lemon juice and peel are widely used in cooking, and the essential oil is expressed from the peel of fruit not sprayed with harmful chemicals. Natural waxes in the oil may appear if it is kept at too low a temperature, but this does not detract from its quality or effectiveness.

Oil of lemon is an underestimated and extremely useful oil. It has an anti-infectious and expectorant effect on the respiratory airways and can help to eliminate the toxins which cause arthritic pain. It is also good for greasy skin. The clean, lively scent can lift the spirits, dispel sluggishness and indecision and relieve depression. Oil of lemon can also help to dispel fear and apathy.

### safety
• Photosensitizer. Do not expose the skin to sunlight or a sunbed for two hours after using.

### features in
The Teenage Years, Beauty and Well-being, The Reproductive Years, The Sunset Years.

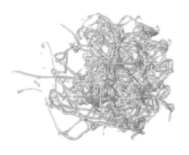

△ *Citrus paradis* –
grapefruit

## *Citrus paradis* – grapefruit
family *Rutaceae*

### properties
antiseptic, aperitif, digestive, diuretic

Originating in tropical Asia and the West Indies, the grapefruit tree is now cultivated mainly in North and South America. The yellow oil, produced mainly in California, is obtained by expression of the peel and has a sweet, citrus aroma.

It is effective in caring for oily skin and acne, and regular use twice daily is helpful for cellulite, water retention and obesity. Its antiseptic property is particularly useful in a vapourizer to disinfect the air of a sickroom. It is useful to add a little (4 drops per litre) to spring water when travelling to help prevent digestive problems.

### safety
• No known contraindications in normal aromatherapy use.

### features in
The Teenage Years, Beauty and Well-being, The Sunset Years.

## *Citrus reticulata* – mandarin
family *Rutaceae*

### properties
antifungal, antispasmodic, calming, digestive

The mandarin orange tree originates in China, and its fruit was named after the Chinese Mandarins. The fruit of the mandarin tree is very similar to the tangerine and oils from both fruits may be sold as mandarin. The essential oil is expressed from the peel.

Mandarin oil has digestive properties, and is excellent for treating both adults and children with indigestion, stomach pains and constipation. It can be very useful for over-excitement, stress and insomnia. It is often popular with children because of its gentle action and familiar orangey aroma.

### safety
• No known contraindications in normal aromatherapy use.

### features in
The Reproductive Years, The Sunset Years.

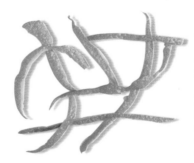

△ *Citrus reticulata* –
mandarin

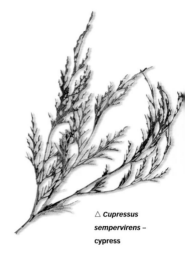

△ *Cupressus*
*sempervirens* –
cypress

## *Cupressus sempervirens* – cypress
family *Cupressaceae*

### properties
antibacterial, anti-infectious, antispasmodic, antisudorific, antitussive, astringent, calming, deodorant, diuretic, hormone-like, neurotonic, phlebotonic, styptic

Cypress oil is distilled from the leaves, cones and twigs of the cypress tree. *Sempervirens* is Latin for evergreen, and the resinous wood of this ancient tree has long been used as an aromatic.

The astringent action of cypress oil helps to regulate the production of sebum, reduce perspiration (even of the feet) and to staunch bleeding. It is reputed to help calm the mind where grief is present, and to induce sleep.

### safety
• No known contraindications in normal aromatherapy use.

### features in
Beauty and Well-being, The Reproductive Years, The Sunset Years.

## Eucalyptus smithii – eucalyptus
family *Myrtaceae*

### properties
analgesic, anticatarrhal, anti-infectious, antiviral, balancing, decongestant, digestive stimulant, expectorant, prophylactic

Known as gully gum, this tree is native to Australia. The oil distilled from its leaves is equally beneficial to, and much gentler than, the more common *Eucalyptus globulus*, or blue gum, which needs care in use. Because of its gentle action, gully gum eucalyptus is ideal for children; its aroma is also not as piercing as blue gum eucalyptus, which is usually rectified to increase its cineole content.

Eucalyptus is good for muscular pain and is effective against coughs and colds, both as a preventive and as a remedy. *E. smithii* oil has great synergistic power.

### safety
• No known contraindications in normal aromatherapy use.
• Keep to the recommended dilution when using as an inhalant for children.

### features in:
Beauty and Well-being, The Reproductive Years, The Sunset Years.

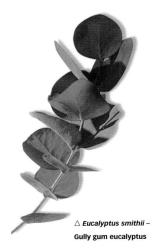

△ **Eucalyptus smithii –**
**Gully gum eucalyptus**

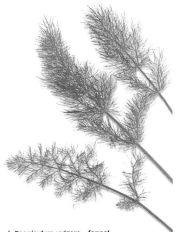

△ *Foeniculum vulgare* – fennel

## Foeniculum vulgare – fennel
family *Apiaceae* (or *Umbelliferae*)

### properties
analgesic, antibacterial, antifungal, anti-inflammatory, antiseptic, antispasmodic, cardiotonic, carminative, decongestant, digestive, diuretic, emmenagogic, lactogenic, laxative, litholytic, oestrogen-like, respiratory tonic

Fennel is widely grown in the Mediterranean area and the essential oil is distilled from its seeds. The delicate flower heads of all this family resemble umbrellas, as indicated by the original family name, *Umbelliferae*.

Fennel is recommended for lack of breast milk and because it is oestrogen-like, it can be valuable for PMS, the menopause and ovary problems. It will also work efficiently as a diuretic.

### safety
• Safe in normal aromatherapy amounts.
• Should not be used during pregnancy before the seventh month.

### features in
Beauty and Well-being, The Reproductive Years.

## Juniperus communis – juniper
family *Cupressaceae*

### properties
analgesic, antidiabetic, antiseptic, depurative, digestive tonic, diuretic, litholytic, sleep-inducing

The juniper tree is a small evergreen from the same family as cypress. The essential oil, distilled from the dried ripe berries (and sometimes the twigs and leaves), has a sweet fragrant aroma. Take care when buying juniper oil, as the berries are used to flavour gin and the residue is often distilled to produce a poor quality essential oil. Even genuine juniper oil can be frequently adulterated.

Juniper oil has a strong diuretic action which is useful for treating cystitis, water retention and cellulite. It has a cleansing, detoxifying action on the skin, and is useful for oily skin problems, such as acne. It is especially good for feelings of guilt and jealousy, and for giving strength when feeling emotionally drained.

### safety
• No known contraindications in normal aromatherapy use.
• May be neurotoxic if used without due care and attention.

### features in
The Teenage Years, Beauty and Well-being, The Reproductive Years, The Sunset Years.

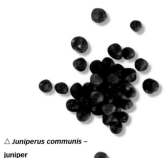

△ *Juniperus communis –*
**juniper**

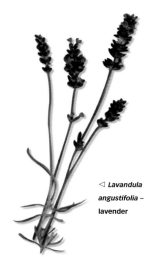

◁ **Lavandula angustifolia** – **lavender**

## Lavandula angustifolia – lavender
family *Lamiaceae*

### properties
analgesic, antibacterial, antifungal, anti-inflammatory, antiseptic, antispasmodic, calming and sedative, cardiotonic, carminative, cicatrizant, emmenagogic, hypotensive, tonic

Lavender is the most widely used aromatherapy oil. It is obtained from the plant's flowering tops, and grows wild throughout the Mediterranean region, although it is now cultivated worldwide. In spite of this, it is not easy to find a quality oil. Lavandin, a cheaper oil from a hybrid plant, is often substituted for true lavender.

Lavender is a skin rejuvenator, and helps to normalize both dry and greasy skins. It works in combination with other oils to alleviate arthritis and rheumatism, psoriasis and eczema. It aids sleep, relieves tension headaches, and is good for calming nerves, lifting depression, relieving anger, and soothing fear and grief.

### safety
• No known contraindications in normal aromatherapy use.

### features in
The Teenage Years, Beauty and Well-being, The Reproductive Years, The Sunset Years.

## Matricaria recutica – chamomile, German
family *Asteraceae*

### properties
antiallergic, antifungal, anti-inflammatory, antispasmodic, cicatrizant, decongestant, digestive tonic, hormone-like

German chamomile, an annual herb, grows naturally in Europe and its small white flowers are widely used in teas and infusions to aid relaxation and induce sleep. When the flowers are distilled a deep blue oil is produced. The blue colour is produced by the presence of chamazulene, a chemical not present in the plant but formed during the distillation process.

Chamazulene, in synergy with the other components of the oil, is a strong anti-inflammatory agent, which is especially useful for skin problems (particularly irritated skin) and rheumatism, when a compress is most effective. The oil is recommended for premenstrual syndrome, and for calming anger and agitated emotional states.

### safety
• No known contraindications in normal aromatherapy use.

### features in
Beauty and Well-being, The Reproductive Years, The Sunset Years.

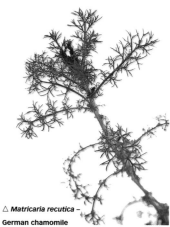

△ **Matricaria recutica** – **German chamomile**

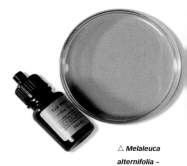

△ **Melaleuca alternifolia** – **tea tree**

## Melaleuca alternifolia – tea tree
family *Myrtaceae*

### properties
analgesic, antibacterial, antifungal, anti-infectious, anti-inflammatory, antiparasitic, antiviral, immunostimulant, neurotonic, phlebotonic

The tea tree plant is native to Australia. Traditionally, a type of herbal tea is prepared from its leaves, and the oil has long been recognized by the Australian Aborigines for its powerful medicinal properties.

Essential oil of tea tree has strong antiseptic properties with a matching aroma, and has excellent antimicrobial and antifungal action. It is a powerful stimulant to the immune system. The unadulterated essential oil has been found to be non-toxic and non-irritating to the skin, and is one of the few essential oils that can be applied directly and undiluted on the skin and all mucous surfaces. The antifungal activity of tea tree oil is much used against *Candida albicans*. It is also effective against some viruses, such as enteritis.

### safety
• No known contraindications in normal aromatherapy use.

### features in
The Teenage Years, Beauty and Well-being.

## Melaleuca viridiflora – niaouli
### family *Myrtaceae*

### properties

analgesic, antibacterial, anticatarrhal, anti-infectious, anti-inflammatory, antiparasitic, antipruritic, antirheumatic, antiseptic, antiviral, digestive, expectorant, febrifuge, hormone-like, hypotensive, immunostimulant, litholytic, phlebotonic, skin tonic

Niaouli trees originate from the region of Gomene in the South Pacific island of New Caledonia, hence "gomenol" became an alternative name. The trees are large with a bushy foliage and yellow flowers. The steam-distilled leaves and young stems yield an essential oil, which has a eucalyptus-type aroma. The majority of the oil is produced in Australia and Tasmania and very little is exported, making the genuine oil hard to find.

Niaouli is useful for a range of problems experienced by women. It is also a powerful antiseptic and anti-inflammatory agent, and is effective for respiratory problems, such as bronchitis and colds. Its properties suggest it will help against grief and anger.

### safety

• No known contraindications, but pregnant women and children should use with care.

### features in

Beauty and Well-being, The Reproductive Years, The Sunset Years.

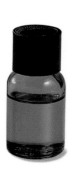

◁ *Melaleuca viridiflora –* niaouli

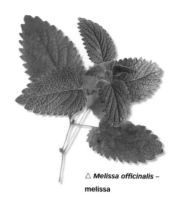

△ *Melissa officinalis –* melissa

## Melissa officinalis – melissa
### family *Lamiaceae*

### properties

anti-inflammatory, antispasmodic, antiviral, calming and sedative, choleretic, digestive, hypotensive, sedative, capillary dilator

Melissa, also known as lemon balm, is a small herb with tiny, white flowers originating from southern Europe. A daily drink of tea prepared from the fresh leaves is supposed to encourage longevity. The distilled yield from the leaves is tiny, making it a very expensive oil. Much of the melissa oil sold commercially is blended with cheaper essential oils and achieves a similar aroma.

Melissa's sedative action relieves headaches and insomnia and is particularly beneficial for a problematic menstrual cycle. It is also a tonic for the heart, calming the turbulent emotions of grief and anger and helping to relieve fear.

### safety

• Photosensitizer. Do not expose the skin to sunlight or a sunbed for two hours after using.
• It is difficult to obtain pure melissa oil, and many fakes contain skin irritants.
• No known contraindications in normal aromatherapy use.

### features in

Beauty and Well-being, The Reproductive Years, The Sunset Years.

## Mentha piperita – peppermint
### family *Lamiaceae*

### properties

analgesic, antibacterial, antifungal, anti-inflammatory, antimigraine, antilactogenic, antipyretic, antispasmodic, antiviral, carminative, decongestant, digestive, expectorant, liver stimulant, hormone-like, hypotensive, insect repellent, mucolytic, neurotonic, reproductive stimulant, soothing, uterotonic

The peppermint plant has dark green leaves from which its essential oil is distilled. The oil has a strong, refreshing aroma and is used extensively in the food and pharmaceutical industries, particularly for toothpaste, chewing gum and drinks.

Peppermint is renowned not only for its beneficial effect with digestive problems, such as indigestion, nausea, travel sickness, and diarrhoea, but also for respiratory problems. It can help to clear congestion or catarrh and is useful for bronchitis, bronchial asthma, sinusitis and colds. It helps to clear the mind, and will aid concentration and overcome mental fatigue and depression. It is also useful against anger, guilt and apathy. This is a good essential oil to keep to hand in the first aid cabinet.

### safety

• Use sparingly and keep to recommended dilution.
• May counteract homeopathic remedies.

### features in

Beauty and Well-being, The Reproductive Years, The Sunset Years.

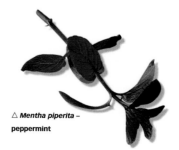

△ *Mentha piperita –* peppermint

## *Ocimum basilicum* var. *album* – basil
family *Lamiaceae*

### properties

analgesic, antibacterial, antifungal, anti-inflammatory, antiseptic, antispasmodic, antiviral, cardiotonic, carminative, digestive tonic, nervous system regulator, neurotonic, reproductive decongestant

Basil oil has a distinctive aroma and is distilled from the whole plant. Several varieties of basil, with different chemical composition, grow in warm Mediterranean climes (especially France and Italy), with leaves that vary in both size and colour, from green to a deep purplish red. The preferred variety for aromatherapy is *album*, as it is not likely to have a neurotoxic effect.

Basil is known mainly for its effect on the nervous system. It is a good tonic and stimulant and is helpful in coping with unwanted emotions, such as fear and jealousy. Its analgesic property makes it useful in cases of arthritis. It is also good for muscle cramp. Basil is an effective insect repellent, particularly against house flies and mosquitoes.

### safety

• No known contraindications in normal aromatherapy use.
• May be neurotoxic if used without due care and attention.

### features in

Beauty and Well-being, The Reproductive Years, The Sunset Years.

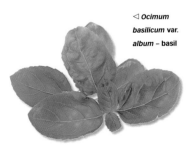

◁ *Ocimum basilicum* var. *album* – basil

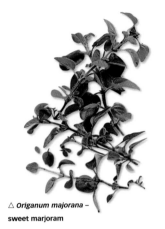

△ *Origanum majorana* – sweet marjoram

## *Origanum majorana* – sweet marjoram
family *Lamiaceae*

### properties

analgesic, antibacterial, anti-infectious, antispasmodic, calming, digestive stimulant, diuretic, expectorant, hormone-like, hypotensive, neurotonic, respiratory tonic, stomachic, vasodilator

Sweet marjoram is a popular culinary herb and has a reputation for promoting long life. The plant grows in the Mediterranean regions and has tiny, white or pink flowers: the oil is distilled from the plant's leaves and flowers. Sweet marjoram should not be confused with the sharp-smelling Spanish marjoram (*Thymus mastichina*), which is a species of thyme.

Sweet marjoram has been shown to be antiviral and is useful for cold sores. It can ease tension and irritability, lift headaches (especially those connected with menstruation) and promote sleep. It is useful for grief and anger, and its ability to calm and uplift makes it useful to combat moodiness.

### safety

• No known contraindications in normal aromatherapy use.

### features in

Beauty and Well-being, The Reproductive Years, The Sunset Years.

## *Pelargonium graveolens* – geranium
family *Geraniaceae*

### properties

analgesic, antibacterial, antidiabetic, antifungal, anti-infectious, anti-inflammatory, antiseptic, antispasmodic, astringent, cicatrizant, decongestant, digestive stimulant, haemostatic, styptic, insect repellent, phlebotonic, relaxant

The geranium plant is cultivated in Egypt, Morocco, the Reunion Islands and China. The oil is distilled from the aromatic leaves, the aroma of which depends on the variety of the plant and where it is grown. Some geranium oils have a definite rose-like smell and are often referred to as rose geranium. More correctly, rose geranium is when a tiny percentage of rose otto is added to the geranium oil.

Geranium will reduce inflammation and is good for acne, herpes, diarrhoea and varicose veins. It is also a relaxant, and will help grief and anger. It is useful for general moodiness and to balance the mood swings associated with PMS.

### safety

• No known contraindications in normal aromatherapy use.

### features in

The Teenage Years, Beauty and Well-being, The Reproductive Years, The Sunset Years.

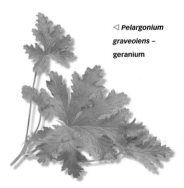

◁ *Pelargonium graveolens* – geranium

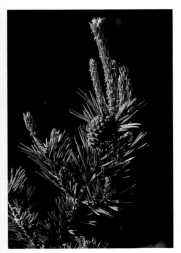

△ *Pinus sylvestris* – pine

## *Pinus sylvestris* – pine
family *Pinaceae*

### properties

analgesic, antibacterial, antifungal, anti-infectious, anti-inflammatory, antisudorific, balsamic, decongestant, expectorant, hormone-like, hypotensive, litholytic, neurotonic, rubefacient

Pine-needle essential oil has a warm, resin-like aroma and is distilled from the Scots-pine tree, which grows widely throughout Europe and Russia.

Pine is an excellent disinfectant and air-freshener: when dispersed in the air, its antiseptic qualities help to prevent the spread of infections. It is recommended for respiratory tract infections and hay fever, while its anti-inflammatory action makes it useful for cystitis and rheumatism. Pine is an excellent pick-me-up for general debility and lack of energy, and is said to dispel melancholy and pessimism.

### safety
• No known contraindications in normal aromatherapy use.

### features in
Beauty and Well-being, The Reproductive Years, The Sunset Years.

## *Pogostemon patchouli* – patchouli
family *Lamiaceae*

### properties

antifungal, anti-infectious, anti-inflammatory, aphrodisiac, cicatrizant, decongestant, immunostimulant, insect repellent, phlebotonic

The plant grows mainly in East Asia and its essential oil has a soft, balsamic aroma. The leaves are cut every few months as the newest ones yield the most oil. Patchouli oil improves with age and has a musty, exotic aroma that is very penetrating.

Patchouli is particularly valuable for broken, chapped and cracked skin, as well as inflamed skin, eczema and acne. It promotes the growth of new skin cells, which makes it helpful in reducing scar tissue. It is beneficial against haemorrhoids and varicose veins. It has a sedative effect on the emotions; its anti-inflammatory property helps calm anger and its antifungal property is useful for jealousy. It is said to help soothe an overactive mind.

### safety
• No known contraindications in normal aromatherapy use.

### features in
Beauty and Well-being, The Reproductive Years.

▷ *Pogostemon patchouli* – patchouli

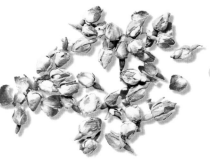

△ *Rosa damascena* – rose otto

## *Rosa damascena* – rose otto
family *Rosaceae*

### properties

antibacterial, anti-infectious, anti-inflammatory, astringent, cicatrizant, neurotonic, sexual tonic, styptic

The much-prized rose otto, also known as attar of roses, is distilled from the deep pink rose petals of this flowering shrub. The genuine, pure oil is extremely expensive as the petals contain very little oil. Roses for distillation are cultivated chiefly in Bulgaria, Turkey and Morocco. Rose absolute is extracted from the petals by a different process, and is a cheaper oil.

Rose otto has been favoured by women through the ages for its gentle action and fragrant aroma. It is said that rose otto balances the hormones and that it is helpful for irregular periods. Rose soothes the skin, lifts depression, and calms inflamed emotions, promoting feelings of happiness and well-being.

### safety
• No known contraindications in normal aromatherapy use.

### features in
Beauty and Well-being, The Reproductive Years, The Sunset Years.

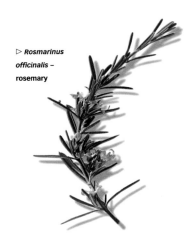

▷ *Rosmarinus officinalis –* rosemary

## *Rosmarinus officinalis –* rosemary
family *Lamiaceae*

### properties
analgesic, antibacterial, antifungal, anti-infectious, anti-inflammatory, antispasmodic, antitussive, antiviral, cardiotonic, carminative, choleretic, cicatrizant, venous decongestant, detoxicant, digestive, diuretic, emmenagogic, hyperglycaemic, blood pressure regulator, litholytic, cholesterol-reducing, mucolytic, neuromuscular effect, neurotonic, sexual tonic, stimulant

Native to the Mediterranean region, rosemary has a long history of culinary and medicinal use. This oil, with an impressive list of helpful properties, is obtained from the pale-blue flowers of the aromatic plant.

Rosemary is helpful for respiratory problems, arthritis, congestive headaches and constipation. It is also a tonic for the liver. This oil stimulates both body and mind. It lifts depression, clears the mind, and is an excellent memory aid.

### safety
• No known contraindications in normal aromatherapy use.

### features in
The Teenage Years, Beauty and Well-being, The Reproductive Years, The Sunset Years.

## *Salvia sclarea –* clary sage
family *Lamiaceae*

### properties
antifungal, anti-infectious, antispasmodic, antisudorific, decongestant, detoxicant, oestrogen-like, neurotonic, phlebotonic, regenerative

The strong smelling essential oil of clary sage is distilled from the dried clary sage plant and is used in eau-de-cologne, lavender water, muscatel wines and vermouth. It should not be confused with sage oil and is not a substitute for it.

Clary sage is excellent for all menstrual complications; its oestrogen-like qualities make it good for hormonal problems. It encourages menstruation and is useful for the hot flushes of the menopause. Clary sage is helpful for depression and fear, and during general convalescence.

### safety
• No known contraindications in normal aromatherapy use.
• Prolonged inhalation may cause drowsiness.
• Avoid alcohol consumption for a few hours before or after use.

### features in
The Teenage Years, Beauty and Well-being, The Reproductive Years, The Sunset Years.

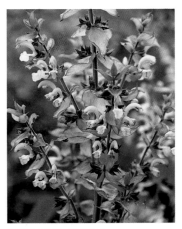

△ *Salvia sclarea –* clary sage

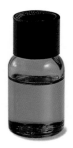

▷ *Santalum album –* sandalwood

## *Santalum album –* sandalwood
family *Santalaceae*

### properties
anti-infectious, astringent, cardiotonic, decongestant, diuretic, moisturizing, nerve relaxant, sedative, tonic

The sandalwood tree is native to India, and its cultivation is controlled by the government of that country – for each tree felled, another is planted. The offcuts and wood chips from the sandalwood furniture industry in India, together with the tree roots, are distilled to obtain the essential oil. The sweet, woody aroma of the oil has a soft and therapeutic effect.

Sandalwood, although a gentle oil, is important in the treatment of genito-urinary infections, especially cystisis. It is used for its effect on the digestive system, relieving heartburn and nausea, including morning sickness. It has been found to benefit both acne and dry skin (including dry eczema), as well as being useful for haemorrhoids and varicose veins. Its tonic properties are thought to be helpful in cases of impotence. Sandalwood can also be useful against fear.

### safety
• No known contraindications in normal aromatherapy use.

### features in
The Teenage Years, Beauty and Well-being, The Reproductive Years, The Sunset Years.

## Thymus vulgaris – thyme, sweet
family *Lamiaceae*

### properties
antifungal, anti-infectious, anti-inflammatory, antiseptic, antispasmodic, antiviral, diuretic, immunostimulant, neurotonic, sexual tonic, uterotonic

Thyme is native to the Mediterranean region and is a well-known culinary herb. The essential oil is distilled from its leaves and tiny purplish flowers. There are many different varieties of thyme oil, some of which need careful handling. The alcohol chemotypes of thyme (linalool and geraniol) are the safest for general use.

Sweet thyme is useful for respiratory problems, infections, and digestive complaints. It is especially helpful for insomnia of nervous origin. Sweet thyme is a safe, uterotonic oil to use towards the end of pregnancy and during labour, and it is known to facilitate delivery.

### safety
• No known contraindications in normal aromatherapy use.

### features in
Beauty and Well-being, The Sunset Years.

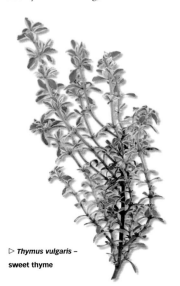

▷ *Thymus vulgaris –*
**sweet thyme**

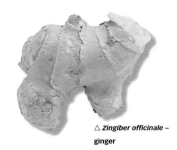

△ *Zingiber officinale –*
**ginger**

## Zingiber officinale – ginger
family *Zingiberaceae*

### properties
analgesic, anticatarrhal, carminative, digestive stimulant, expectorant, general tonic, sexual tonic, stomachic

This perennial herb is native to the tropical parts of Asia. The root, which is used in cooking, is renowned for its heat and for its digestive properties. Its yellow oil is distilled from the roots and, although it has a spicy aroma, the heat does not come through into the essential oil during distillation.

Ginger essential oil has properties which alleviate most digestive problems, including flatulence, constipation, nausea and loss of appetite. Its ability to dull pain is beneficial to muscular pain and sciatica, while its tonic properties are useful for emotions like fear and apathy, and will also help to draw out a reticent, withdrawn personality.

### safety
• No known contraindications in normal aromatherapy use.

### features in
The Reproductive Years, The Sunset Years.

## Special essential oils

*Myristica fragrans* – nutmeg
*Pimpinella anisum* – aniseed
*Salvia officinalis* – sage
*Syzygium aromaticum* – clove bud

There are some highly beneficial, but very powerful oils which are recommended in this book for special use only. These are used in pregnancy to facilitate delivery. However, their use is not advised without training in aromatherapy or aromatic medicine.

### safety
• These oils must only be used in the manner and amounts advised.
• Always seek advice from a qualified aromatherapist before home use.

### featured in
The Reproductive Years.

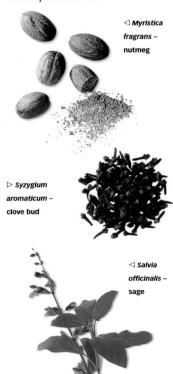

◁ *Myristica fragrans –* **nutmeg**

▷ *Syzygium aromaticum –* **clove bud**

◁ *Salvia officinalis –* **sage**

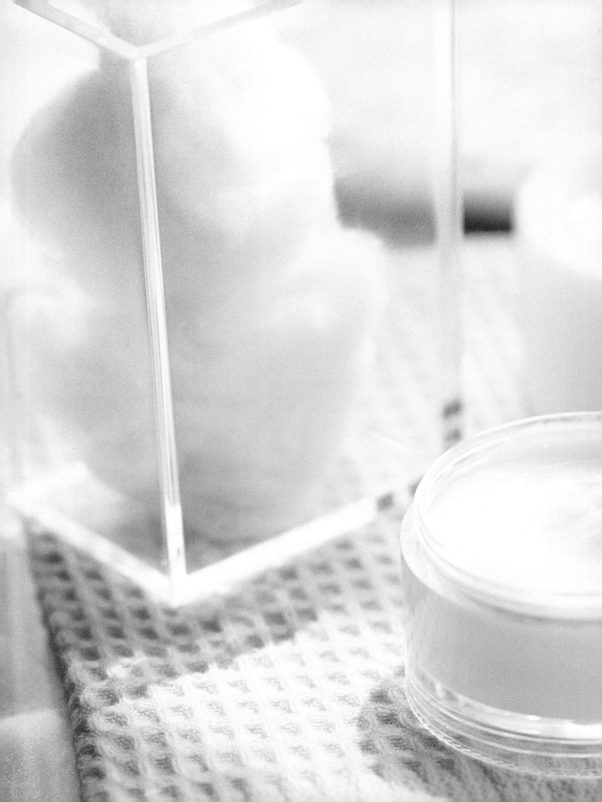

# Aromatherapy
# Techniques

Gentle, simple application techniques mean
that aromatherapy can be used safely at home
by women of all ages. Essential oils can be used
in baths, drinks, inhalations, gargles, vaporizers,
compresses and massage for complete beauty and
well-being treatments.

# Using inhalations and baths

aromatherapy techniques

Essential oils are rarely used in their original, concentrated form but are always taken into the body via a carrier substance. This can be anything which takes the oils into the body: air, water, vegetable oils, lotions and creams are all carriers.

## inhalation

When we breathe in the fragrance of an essential oil, some of its molecules travel to the lungs, pass through the lining and into the bloodstream, where they travel around the body. Other molecules take an upward route to the brain, which receives a healing message – to relax or energize, for example – and transmits the appropriate signal along the nerve channels of the body.

Inhalation is the quickest way for oils to enter the body, and is the most effective way to deal with fragile emotions, and negative states of mind such as stress and depression. It is very useful for respiratory conditions, especially those that may present an emergency situation, such as bronchitis or asthma. Although essential oils may be inhaled directly from the bottle, other methods are preferred.

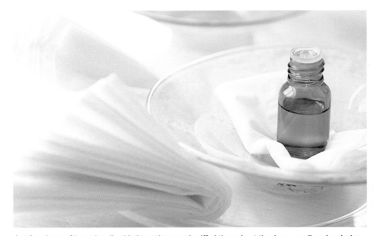

△ A few drops of lavender oil, added to a tissue and sniffed throughout the day, can relieve headaches.

### the hands

This method is useful for emergencies. Put one drop of essential oil into your palm and rub your hands briefly together. Now cup your hands over your nose, avoiding the eye area, and take a deep breath.

### a tissue

Place a few drops of essential oil on to a tissue and take three deep breaths. The tissue can then be placed on your pillow or inside your shirt, so that you will continue to benefit from the oil's aroma.

### steam inhalation

Fill a basin with hot water and add no more than 2-3 drops (use 1-2 drops for children and the elderly) of essential oil. Keeping your eyes closed to protect them from the powerful vapours, lower your head over the bowl and breathe in deeply.

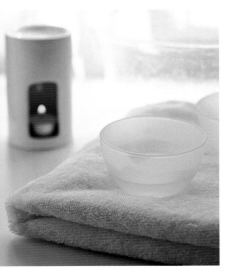

◁ Using an oil burner is a popular way of vaporizing essential oils. Keep enough water in the top to stop it drying out.

▷ A steam inhalation using eucalyptus oil can help to relieve head colds and sinus congestion.

### a vaporizer

This is one of the most popular methods of all for oil inhalation. Electric vaporizers are available, and are the safest types to use. Night-light vaporizers (or oil burners) are inexpensive and readily available in different sizes and designs. The basic model involves a night-light candle standing under a tiny

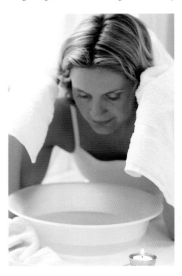

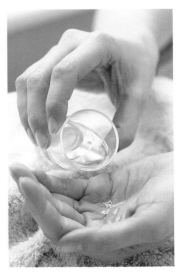

△ **Dry skin will benefit from an essential oil mix:
it is best massaged on to your body after a bath.**

cup filled with water, to which a few drops of oil are added. Keep the vaporizer out of the reach of children and pets. Top up the water and add more oils as necessary.

Use a vaporizer to keep infections at bay, to relax after a stressful day, or to set the mood for a party or a romantic evening. The number of oil drops is not critical and really depends on the size of the room.

### safety
• The quantities of essential oils given above for inhalations are suitable for children and the elderly unless otherwise stated.

## bathing
Essential oils do not dissolve well in water, and it is important that the molecules are evenly distributed. Bathing can enhance the effects of essential oils: the oils are not only absorbed through the skin but their aroma is also inhaled. There are several ways to enjoy bathing with essential oils.

### bath
Run the water in the bath to a comfortable temperature. Next, add 6–8 drops of oil, then swish the water thoroughly to disperse

▷ **Pamper yourself and unwind with a relaxing
aromatherapy bath at the end of a tiring day.**

the oil. Sit in the bath, and for maximum benefit, stay in the water for at least ten minutes to allow the oil to penetrate your skin and to enjoy the benefits of its aroma.

If you prefer, the oils can be mixed with 15 ml/1 tbsp dairy cream or honey before being added to the bath. This will help to disperse the oils. Alternatively, you can mix the oils into powdered milk, adding water to make a paste, before adding the mixture to the bath water. Bath oil prepared from vegetable oil and mixed with essential oils is fine for dry skin, but will feel greasy on normal skins.

### foot and hand bath
For sprains, localized swelling, bruising, or similar general discomforts, ten minutes in a foot or hand bath containing 6–8 drops of your chosen oils will bring welcome relief. Remember to keep a kettle of warm water nearby to add to the water in the bowl before it cools too much for comfort.

### sitz-bath
For vaginal thrush, a sitz-bath with essential oils is an effective treatment. Fill a large bowl one-third full with warm water and add 3–4 drops of your chosen oil. Sit in the bath for ten minutes.

### showers
It is not as easy to benefit from essential oils in the shower. However, you can add some oils to your shower gel or put some on to a sponge. Rub this over your body in the shower, or before you get into it. Make the most of the aroma, breathing deeply and rubbing with your sponge or hands while slowly rinsing. If you wash off the oils too quickly, you won't feel the benefit. Finish with a body lotion mixed with an oil.

### safety
• For children and the elderly the essential oil quantities should be halved.

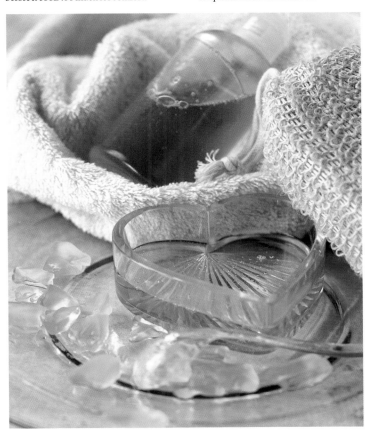

# Using compresses, gargles and drinks

Further effective ways of carrying essential oils into the body, using water as the carrier, are with compresses, gargles, mouthwashes and drinks. For the latter, it is important that the essential oils used, and the number of drops, are exactly as recommended.

## compresses

A compress brings effective relief in cases such as insect bites, arthritic joints, period or stomach pain, headache, sprains and varicose veins. Use a cold compress if there is inflammation and/or heat, and a warm compress if there is pain or a dull ache.

To make the compress, you need a piece of clean material and a container of water. Soft cotton or linen are the best materials to

▽ **A compress is a simple way to use essential oils, and the result can be very soothing.**

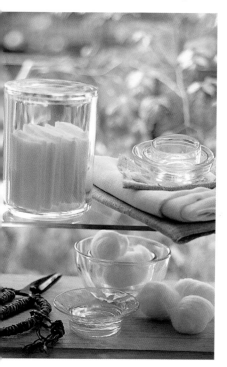

use. The container should be big enough to hold just enough water to soak into the compress: for example, an egg cup will be big enough for a finger compress, and a small bowl is suitable for an abdomen compress. Add your chosen essential oils to the water: 2 drops of oil is enough for a finger compress, and up to 8 drops of oil is enough for larger body compresses.

Stir the water in the container to disperse the essential oils, then gently lower the compress material on top to allow it to absorb the oils. When the material is wet, squeeze it lightly, position it on the area to be treated, and cover with cling film (plastic wrap) to hold it firmly in place.

For a cold compress, place a sealed, plastic bag of frozen peas or crushed ice cubes over the treatment area and hold in place. For a warm compress, wrap a strip of material such as a scarf, thermal garment or a small towel around the cling film. To keep a compress in place on an arm or leg, an old sock or pair of tights is ideal. Leave the compress in place for at least an hour, or overnight for a septic wound.

## gargles and mouthwashes

For sore throats, voice loss and colds which may go on to the chest, gargling with one or more essential oils can be very helpful. Put 2–3 drops of antibacterial essential oils into a glass and half-fill with water. A drop of a soothing oil can also be added. Stir well, take a mouthful, gargle and spit out. Stir again and repeat. It is important to stir the mixture before each mouthful so as to redisperse the oils. Gargling should be done twice a day for best results.

The procedure for mouthwashes is the same as for gargling, except that the liquid is swished around inside the mouth (rather than at the back of the throat) for 30 seconds before spitting out.

▷ **Adding a few drops of an antibacterial oil to a glass of water makes an effective gargle mix.**

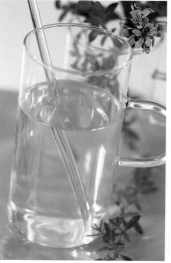

△ **When using a mouthwash, make sure the oils are well stirred in the water before each sip.**

### safety
• For children and the elderly the essential oil quantities should be halved.

## drinks

To use essential oils in drinks, the oils must be organic and mixed in a suitable carrier.

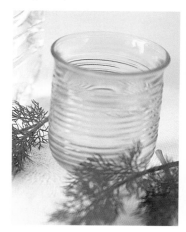

▷ Organic plants are grown without the use of chemicals. When taking oils internally, it is important to use only those of therapeutic and certified organic quality.

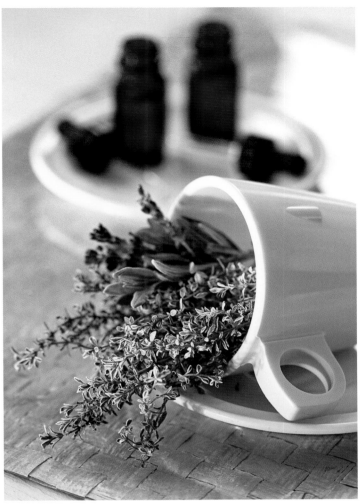

You are advised first to consult a qualified aromatologist or an aromatherapist working alongside a medical doctor. If you wish to use essential oils in water or tea at home without taking professional advice, it is imperative that the essential oils, and the dosage and time scales recommended in this book are strictly adhered to.

## water

Drinking plenty of water is good for us. If you are not fond of water as a drink, put 2 drops of an essential oil such as lemon or orange into 1 litre (1¾ pints) of water in a bottle and shake well. For a healthy digestive system, use 1 drop each of peppermint and fennel oil and mix as before. Shake the bottle before drinking. In conjunction with healthy eating habits, 1 drop each of grapefruit and/or cypress, used as before, can help weight loss as part of a slimming and exercise programme.

## teas

Only aromatologists are able to prescribe essential oils for internal, medicinal use. Tea is not a medicine, however, but a pleasant drink. If the tea tastes too strong when the oils are added, dilute it with more water.

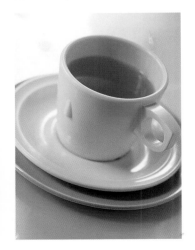

Tannin-free china tea or rooibos (red bush) tea make the best bases. Put 2-3 drops of essential oil on to the tea leaves or tea bag, add 1 litre (1¾ pints) of hot water, stir well, then remove the tea leaves or bag. The tea will taste better without milk. Never pour essential oil directly into tea: it will be too strong, and the oils will not disperse. Any tea not drunk immediately can be stored in the fridge and reheated as necessary.

For digestive disorders, a cup of tea drunk two or three times a day is a very gentle and effective remedy. Common

◁ Teas made with essential oils can be a pleasant way of enjoying the healing properties of plants.

urinary tract problems, such as cystitis, respond well, as do insomnia and pain from arthritic joints.

## safety

• Use only organic essential oils of therapeutic quality for adding to drinks.
• Absolutes or resins should never be ingested.
• These methods should not be used on children, but are suitable for the elderly.
• Never put essential oils directly into a cup of tea or glass of water. Otherwise, the drink will taste far too strong and will be very unpleasant. The oils should be used only by the methods stated.

# Aromatherapy massage techniques

Touch is the most basic human impulse, and massage is a therapeutic extension of touch dating back to ancient times. Hippocrates said that "rubbing loosens a joint that is too rigid", and when we hurt ourselves, our first reaction is to rub the pain away.

To experience a massage under qualified and caring hands is a relaxing experience in itself and it can only be enhanced by the addition of essential oils. If you cannot have treatment by a professional aromatherapist, there are some simple massage techniques

you can practise at home on yourself or on a partner, using essential oils for beneficial results. In the following pages are three simple self-massage techniques together with useful tips for blending essential oils at home.

## Neck and shoulder treatment

**Day-to-day stresses and anxieties often manifest themselves as tension in the neck and shoulder muscles, and treating this area can bring immediate benefits. One of the best times to work on your neck and shoulders is just before going to bed, especially if stress or insomnia are a problem. This will help to relax you and will put your body into a healing mode. Prepare your choice of essential oils with a carrier lotion or oil (*see* Preparing Oils for Application). Wear loose clothing or a towel and remove all jewellery for comfort. Apply a little of the oil mix to both shoulders and begin the massage.**

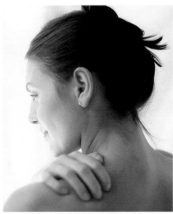

◁ **2** Keeping your hand in this position (palm on collarbone and fingers on shoulder muscle), feel with your fingers for any hard tension spots along the muscle and apply firm circular pressure to these with the pads of your three middle fingers. Be careful not to exceed an acceptable pain threshold.

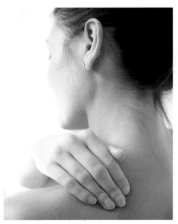

◁ **3** Take your fingers up your neck, repeating the circular movements with your three fingers where there are painful nodules. Repeat steps 2 and 3 if the area is still painful, and finish with several firm circles, as in step 1. Repeat the massage on the opposite shoulder, using your other hand.

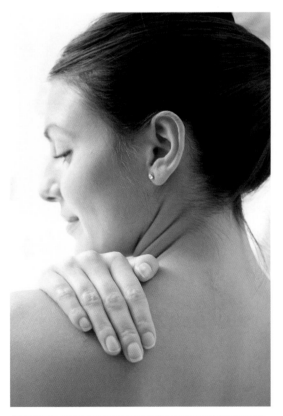

△**1** Resting the whole of your relaxed hand gently over the point of your opposite shoulder, move your hand firmly along the top of the shoulder until you reach the neck, then return to the shoulder point. Repeat this circle several times.

## Headache treatment

**It is instinctive to rub your temples or forehead when you have a headache. Giving yourself a head massage with one or more appropriate essential oils in a carrier lotion or oil can make the massage more effective.**

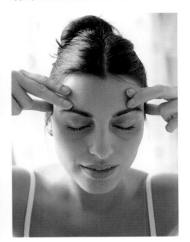

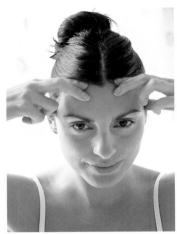

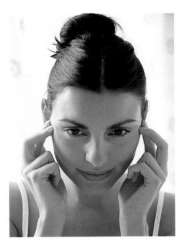

△ **1** Dab a little of the essential oil mix on your fingertips and place your fingers and thumbs at the temples. Place the length of your fingers on to your forehead and move them firmly from the centre towards the temples, returning back to the centre. Repeat several times.

△ **2** Keeping your thumbs in the same position, make circular movements from the centre of the top of your forehead to the upper temple, using only the cushions of your three middle fingers.

△ **3** Repeat these circles 1 cm (½ in) lower down the forehead, again moving from the centre to the temples. Repeat the circles, doing the last one at eyebrow level. With thumbs positioned as before, "glue" your fingers in the temple hollows and make firm circles which move the skin of the temples over the bone beneath. Repeat step 1.

## Scalp treatment

**A scalp massage is not only very relaxing, but is also very helpful for anyone who is worried about thinning hair, as it stimulates the hair roots. The roots can become starved of nourishment when the scalp muscle becomes too tight – such as through stress, for example – causing the hair to become thin and weak.**

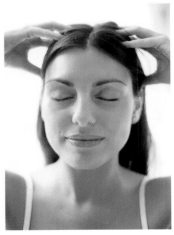

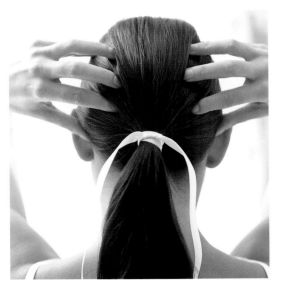

◁ **2** Place the hands on another part of the scalp and repeat. Carry on until the whole scalp has been covered. Repeat steps 1 and 2 several times.

△ **1** Place the thumbs at the top of the ears and "glue" the fingers to the scalp, moving it firmly and slowly over the bone beneath.

# Preparing oils for application

Essential oils can be added to a range of carrier bases: vegetable oils, unscented lotion or cream. The choice of base depends on how the mixture is to be used, and is also a matter of personal preference.

## types of carrier oil

There are many suitable vegetable oils, each with its own benefit. Unrefined, cold-pressed oils are the best for aromatherapy. The basic oils are widely available, while special and macerated oils are available from suppliers. As a guide, use 15–20 drops of essential oil in 50 ml of the base oil for mixtures to be applied to the skin. Reduce the ratio to 1:10 for preparations to be used on the face.

### basic oils

#### Sunflower *Helianthus annuus*

This oil is taken from the seeds of the giant yellow sunflower. It can relieve eczema and dermatitis, lower blood cholesterol, soothe rheumatism, and ease leg ulcers, sprains and bruises. It may also have diuretic properties.

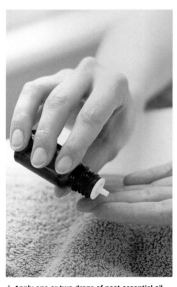

△ **Apply one or two drops of neat essential oil direct to the skin to soothe cuts, bites and stings.**

### Sweet almond *Prunus amygdalis* var. *dulcis*

Almond oil is taken from the kernel of the almond nut, but it is difficult to obtain cold-pressed almond oil. This oil alleviates inflamed and irritated skin, helps to relieve constipation, lowers blood cholesterol, and is good for eczema, psoriasis and dry skin.

### special oils

These can all be used alone or as 25 per cent of a basic carrier oil.

### Evening primrose *Oenethera biennis*

Yellow evening primrose flowers open at dusk, one circle of flowers at a time. The flowers open so quickly that the buds can be watched as they open. The flowers' seeds are cold-pressed when the stem has finished flowering. Evening primrose oil will relieve arthritis, lower blood cholesterol, help PMS, and soothe wounds. It is excellent for eczema, psoriasis and dry skin, and is said to have a beneficial effect on wrinkles.

### Hazelnut *Corylus avellana*

Cold-pressed hazelnuts yield an amber coloured oil. Hazelnut oil has astringent properties and can be used to relieve acne, stimulate circulation and protect against the harmful effects of the sun.

### Jojoba *Simmondsia chinensis*

Jojoba is not an oil but a liquid wax, which gives it excellent keeping qualities. Jojoba is an analgesic with anti-inflammatory properties, and it will soothe arthritis and rheumatism, acne, eczema, psoriasis, dry skin and sunburn. Jojoba is good for the scalp, and is a useful addition to shampoo.

### Rose hip *Rosa canina*

These small berries produce a syrup, a rich source of Vitamin C, and a golden-red oil. Rose hip oil is anti-aging and will help to regenerate tissue. It softens mature skin, and is good to use for burns, scars and eczema.

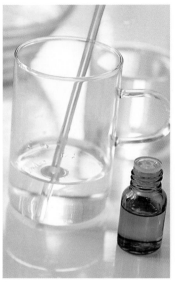

△ **Essential oils can be added to cold spring water to make your own customized skin toner. Choose the right oils for your skin type.**

### macerated oils

The process of macerating (soaking) plants in olive or sunflower oil enhances base oils with the plants' therapeutic properties. These macerated carrier oils can be added to a base vegetable oil, lotion or cream to enrich it. Macerated melissa and lime oils can also be used to enrich base oils.

### Calendula *Calendula officinalis*

Often referred to as marigold (although it is not related to French marigold, *Tagetes minuta*), Calendula has anti-inflammatory and astringent properties, and can relieve broken and varicose veins. Apply directly in undiluted form to ease sprains and bruises.

### St John's wort *Hypericum perforatum*

With its analgesic and anti-inflammatory properties, St John's wort will help to relieve haemorrhoids, sprains, bruises and arthritis, and can heal burns, sunburn and wounds.

## carrier lotion and cream

Unperfumed lotion, which is made from emulsified oil and water, can be used instead of vegetable oil as a carrier base. Lotion is particularly good for all self-application techniques as it is non-greasy. Use a cream if a base richer than a lotion is needed.

To prepare a blend for use on the body, mix 15–20 drops of essential oil with 50 ml (2 fl oz) of lotion or cream. For a blend to be used on the face, mix 5 drops of essential oil per 50 ml (2 fl oz) lotion or cream. Always ensure the jar or bottle you are using for your blend is completely clean and dry.

### safety note

Use only half the specified quantity of essential oils in any base carrier – vegetable oil, lotion or cream – if the mixture is to be used on children and the elderly. Pregnant women should always consult a qualified practitioner before using essential oils.

## Preparing a blend for the body using vegetable oil

**Vegetable oils are excellent carriers for massage. The essential oils readily dissolve in them, and they allow the hands to move continuously on the skin without dragging or slipping. Mineral oil, such as baby oil, is from a mineral, not a vegetable source. It aims to protects the skin by keeping moisture out and will not allow essential oils to penetrate: it is not suitable as a base oil.**

### ingredients
- essential oils
- vegetable carrier oil

### equipment
- screw-top bottle
- label and marker pen

### BLENDING TIPS

Care should be taken not to use too much of the mixed oil as it can stain sheets and clothes. To stop too much oil coming out at a time, place your fingers over the top of the bottle, tipping it against them. Apply the fingers to the area to be treated, repeating only if you need more oil.

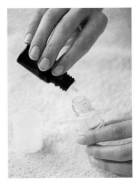

△ **1** Pour 15–20 drops of your chosen essential oil or oils into a 50 ml (2 fl oz) screw-top bottle.

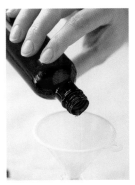

△ **2** Fill the bottle to within 2 cm (¾ in) of the top with your chosen vegetable carrier oil. Use a funnel, if preferred, to avoid any unnecessary spillage.

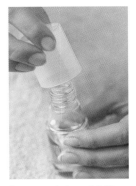

△ **3** Screw on the top and label the bottle with the quantity of each oil used, what the mixture is to be used for, your name and the date.

## Preparing a blend for the body using lotion

**A bland, non-greasy lotion is preferable to oil as it is less messy and is absorbed quickly by the skin. A lotion base is better for self-application techniques, as a vegetable oil bottle will become greasy and can easily slip through your fingers.**

### ingredients
- bland white lotion
- vegetable oil (optional)
- essential oils

### equipment
- screw-top jar or bottle
- label and marker pen

### BLENDING TIPS

Prepare a blend with a cream base in the same way. For a preparation to use on the face, mix 50 ml (2 fl oz) of the base lotion or cream with only 5 drops of your chosen essential oil.

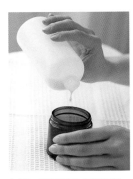

△ **1** For a lotion to use on the body, fill a 50 ml (2 fl oz) jar or bottle three-quarters full with an unperfumed white lotion, or a lotion mixed with a little vegetable oil, if preferred.

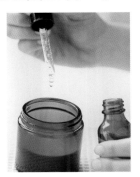

△ **2** Add 15–20 drops of the chosen essential oil or oil blend. Screw on the top and shake thoroughly. Add the rest of the lotion but do not fill right to the top, to allow room for reshaking.

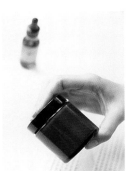

△ **3** Screw the top on firmly and shake again. Label with the contents, use, your name and the date. For a facial lotion, mix 50 ml (2 fl oz) of the base lotion with 5 drops of essential oil.

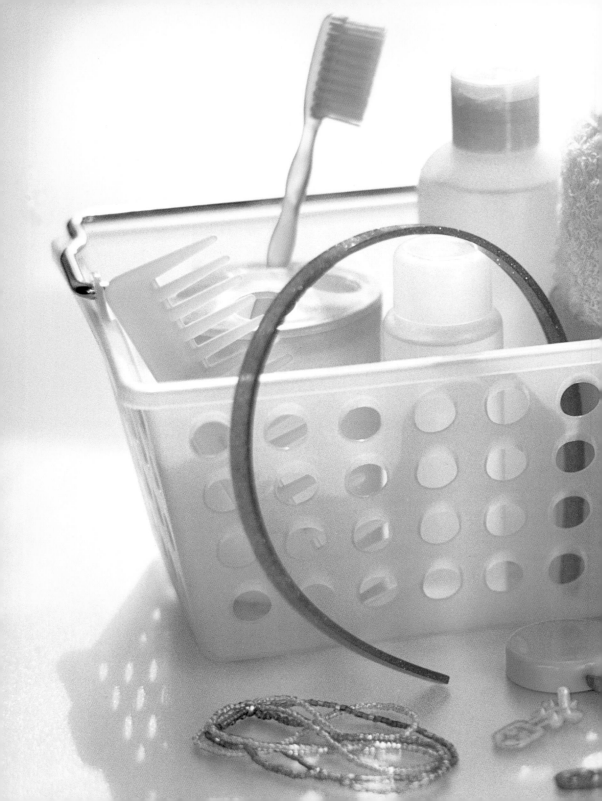

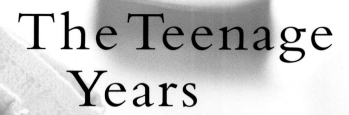

# The Teenage Years

Adolescence is a time of change, both physically and emotionally. Aromatherapy can help smooth the transition from childhood to becoming a young woman with gentle cleansing applications and soothing inhalations.

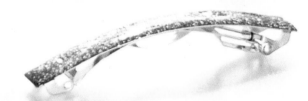

# Aromatherapy in adolescence

The actual rate at which children grow up varies greatly and there can be several years difference in the age at which individual children reach puberty. With the advent of puberty, both health and emotional patterns begin to change. The pituitary gland, responsible for the body's physical growth, begins to release hormones which stimulate the ovaries or testicles to produce eggs or sperm. As soon as these hormonal changes begin to take place, the girl starts to become a young woman and the boy a young man.

For a girl, one of the more obvious signs of becoming a young woman is marked by her developing breasts and by the onset of her periods. This can be a difficult time as she either adjusts to the physical changes that are taking place, or worries because they are happening too fast or not fast

▷ Being a teenager is not always easy. Hormone imbalances can lead to extreme mood swings and problems with both the hair and the skin.

**ESSENTIAL OILS AND THE SKIN**

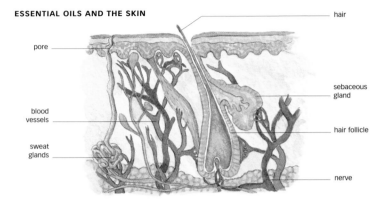

pore

blood vessels

sweat glands

hair

sebaceous gland

hair follicle

nerve

enough. Essential oils can be extremely useful to alleviate some of the physical discomforts and emotional aspects often associated with puberty and menstruation (*see* The Reproductive Years).

△ **A basic understanding of how the skin operates will help you to take care of it.**

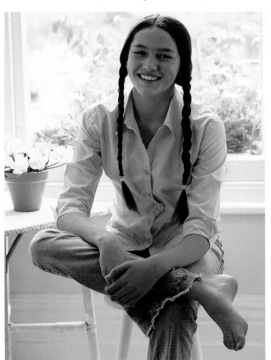

The teenage years are typically turbulent times. A girl's body is rapidly growing and changing in new and startling ways, and her hormones are likely to be affecting both her body and her mood. Hormonal changes trigger an imbalance of sebum in the skin (usually increasing the amount produced), which can lead to greasy skin and hair. This can be awkward at a time when a young woman is becoming aware of her appearance, and of the effect she has on the opposite sex, and feelings of inadequacy are common. The associated emotions of anxiety, resentment, fear and jealousy can all increase stress levels and trigger further reactions in the hair, skin and/or nails.

Essential oils can be very useful both in alleviating unsettled emotional states and treating the skin and hair problems themselves. Aromatherapy, used correctly, forms just one part of a holistic approach to health, and this approach should take into account the girl's nutrition and lifestyle habits, as well as any stressful or worrying external circumstances or events in her life, before the essential oils can be chosen. Now that she is no longer a child, a teenager needs to feel in control of her life, and looking after her health is a good way to begin.

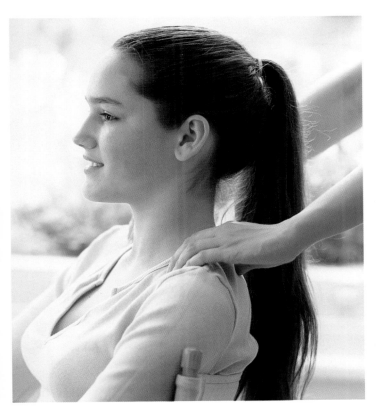

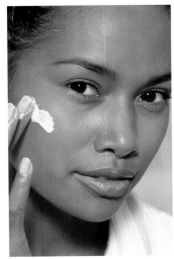

△ Receiving a shoulder masage is a pleasant and effective way of relieving stress and tension in the neck and shoulders. Ask a friend to gently rub and knead any knotty or tight areas.

△ Experiment with adding oils to your own skin creams and see which combinations work best.

## stress and anxiety

Apart from the changes taking place within her own body, life in the outside world can also be problematic for today's teenager. External circumstances, which are beyond her control, can be difficult to manage. If a parent changes job, for example, the family may have to move house and area. This means a new school, with a new teacher, and no immediate friends – all at a time when the academic workload is increasing and exams are becoming a reality. School may also be stressful because of bullying. This affects many teenagers, who exist in a perpetual state of fear and feel they are unable to talk to anyone about it.

There may also be problems within the family: heavy arguments between parents, between the teenager and her parents, or between siblings. For example, teenagers may feel rivalry or jealousy towards a brother or sister who seems to be given more of a parent's love and attention, and receives special treats and favours.

In many societies, the divorce rate is increasing and many modern-day children are "shared" between parents. It is debatable whether it is more stressful to the child to live with parents who don't get on and who argue, or to be caught between two homes.

Growing up involves finding out who you are and having your own ideas and opinions. Problems can arise when parents and their teenage daughter don't see eye-to-eye, and angry fights at home become a routine part of life. Teenagers face strong peer pressure to conform to current trends. This usually involves wearing the "right" clothes, and going to the "right" places for entertainment and holidays. All of these things cost money and can cause tension within the family.

Whatever the reason for stress or anxiety there are numerous relaxing essential oils which can help (*see* Coping with Stress and Emotions). These are best used in the bath or, for more immediate results, by inhalation (*see* Aromatherapy Techniques).

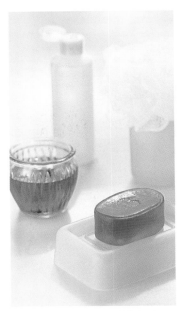

△ Now is a good time to start a daily beauty regime and have fun taking care of yourself.

# Everyday skincare

Embarrassing and unsightly skin conditions can be improved by following a healthy diet and a regular skin-cleansing routine using suitable products. The important thing is to follow both of these recommendations if you want to see positive, lasting results.

## lifestyle changes

A good starting point is to make a record of your dietary intake each day for a week. By studying this, you will be able to make any necessary adjustments. Try substituting fresh fruit for crisps and chocolate, or fresh juices and/or mineral water for carbonated, sugary drinks. At the same time, monitor improvements to your skin.

If you support yourself by taking aromatherapy baths to relieve stress and follow the skin-cleansing regime below, you should see visible results within a week. If you do not, it may be because the diet and/or care treatments have not been strictly followed.

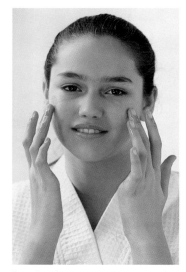

△ **Regularly cleansing and moisturizing your face will keep your complexion at its best**.

Remember, too, that acne is often worse just before menstruation, and that teenage acne usually subsides by the early twenties.

## problem skin

The hormonal changes of puberty lead to increased production of sebum by the sebaceous glands in the skin. From the normal, peach-like skin of childhood, a young woman may find her skin (particularly on her face) changing in texture. The pores become enlarged and more open and the skin becomes oily – particularly on the forehead and in a "T-panel" leading down the nose and on to the chin. These open pores are a breeding ground for bacteria, leading to spots, pimples and blackheads, which is why a regular and effective skin-cleansing routine becomes so important.

A spotty skin can become a problem if it develops into acne (*Acne vulgaris*). This is a medical condition and requires special care.

## Daily skincare routine

**To see an immediate improvement to the skin, a five minute skincare routine should be established and carried out twice a day. Essential oils added to unperfumed creams or lotions can be useful for treating difficult skin conditions and to help with the added emotional difficulties of low self-confidence. With perseverance (and improved lifestyle habits), this routine has proved to be extremely effective. Once the skin begins to improve, stress is reduced and a positive, rather than a negative, cycle is created.**

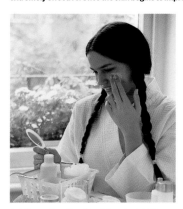

△ **1** Cleanse the skin with a light, water-soluble cleansing milk. Make your own by blending 1 drop each of rosemary, lavender and geranium oils into 30 ml (2 tbsp) base lotion. Rinse off with cold water.

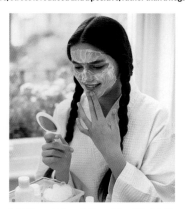

△ **2** Make a gentle, purifying mask by adding 2 drops each of cedarwood, juniper and lemon essential oils to 30 ml (2 tbsp) base cream. Apply to face and leave for ten minutes. Rinse off thoroughly with cold water.

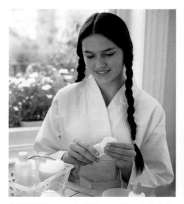

△ **3** Add 3 drops each of lemon and geranium oils to 50 ml (2 fl oz) distilled water. Wipe over the face and neck as a tonic. Follow with a moisturizing lotion mixed with 2 drops of hazelnut oil.

▷ The feet are prone to patches of dry, rough skin. Moisturizing your feet on a regular basis will help to keep them smooth and soft.

▽ Drinking plenty of mineral water can vastly improve your overall health and vitality.

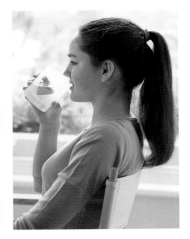

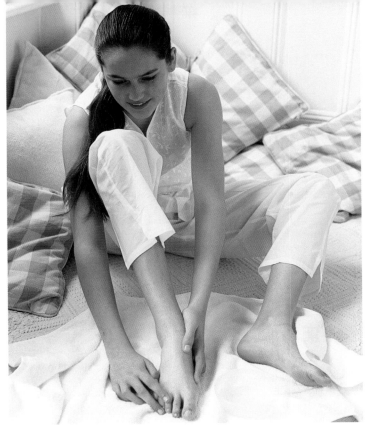

### teenage acne

Acne is caused when excessive amounts of sebum form a blockage at the skin's surface on the face, shoulders and back. Cysts, blackheads and red pustules develop, which can lead to pockmark scars. It is difficult to improve the skin once these scars appear.

The rise in the incidence and severity of teenage acne seems to be connected with some aspects of today's modern culture.

Insufficient fresh fruit and vegetables in the diet, chemical additives in food, and air pollution all cause a toxin overload which puts extra strain on the body. Taking good care of your skin and body will really help.

### tips for healthy skin

- Stick to a suitable daily skincare routine.
- Exercise for half an hour three times a week.
- Eat lots of fresh fruit and vegetables.
- Drink 6–8 glasses of mineral water a day.

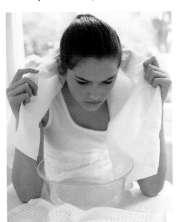

△ Regular steam inhalations with juniper can help clear blocked pores or blackheads.

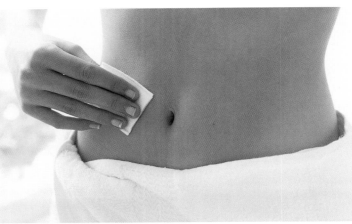

△ Stomach ache or period pains can be treated by applying a compress using basil, lavender and sweet marjoram. A piece of soft cotton or linen soaked in a water-oil mix makes a good compress.

# Caring for hair and nails

Both the hair and nails are made of keratin, a modified skin tissue, and both are present to protect us from harm. The hair and nails benefit from good nutrition, and care with essential oils can improve their appearance.

## teenage hair

Hair problems for teenagers will often mean greasy hair. Greasy hair needs frequent washing with a suitable shampoo to prevent the excess oil from causing spots around the hairline. However, the rubbing action on the scalp stimulates the sebaceous glands to produce more sebum and can make the problem worse. If you have greasy hair, shampoo it no more than once a day. Add an astringent essential oil to an unperfumed shampoo for your own aromatherapy treatment at home. Take care to apply the shampoo to the hair and not the scalp.

▷ **If your hair lacks lustre, try adding the appropriate oils to an unperfumed conditioner base. After shampooing, gently comb the mix through to the ends of your hair.**

Hair loss can also be a problem for some young women. This can be brought on by the stress of exams and personal worries, and also by harsh treatment of hair that is already weak, such as dragging it back too tightly from the forehead with hairbands. Mixing essential oils with your shampoo can help to strengthen weak hair. Handle hair with care, and ease it forward slightly before adding hairbands and accessories.

## conditioning

The condition of our hair is crucial to how we look, and good hair treatment brings its own rewards. Hair should be trimmed regularly – with no more than 1 cm (½ in) removed – to keep the ends strong. This is especially important with long hair: the more often long hair is trimmed, the faster it will grow and the better it will look.

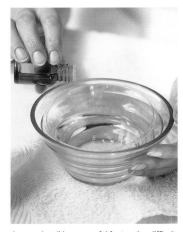

△ **Lavender oil is very useful for treating difficult nail conditions. Add a 2–3 drops to 5 ml (1 tsp) carrier oil and use as required.**

If your hair is in poor condition, use a separate conditioner: products which aim to combine a shampoo with a conditioner are rarely effective as they cannot do both jobs well. Add the essential oils your hair needs to an unperfumed, basic conditioner. Apply the mixture to your hair and scalp after shampooing and towel-drying. Cover with a plastic bag to keep in the heat, and leave for 30 minutes before rinsing well.

### tips for healthy hair

• Add 8–10 drops of essential oils to 50 ml (2 fl oz) of unfragranced shampoo (not baby shampoo – it is not especially mild).
• Give yourself a daily scalp massage with soothing essential oils to arrest and prevent early hair loss.

### nailcare

Nail-biting is often connected to stress and has a strong emotional component. It can be a difficult habit to break. Because teenage girls are often concerned with appearance, the desire for beautiful, manicured nails may help to overcome the problem.

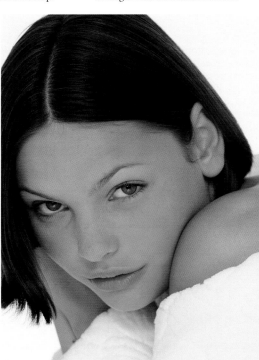

▷ Strong and beautiful nails begin at the cuticle. Use an oil mix and gently massage it on to the cuticle and surrounding area daily. After three months, you will see improvement in your nails.

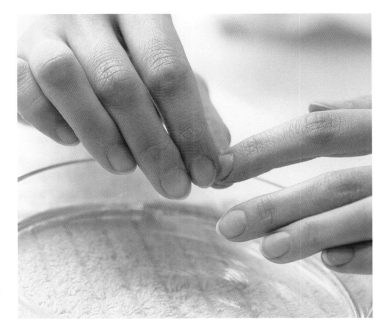

To encourage strong, healthy nails, you have to care for the cuticle as well as the nail, as this is where nail growth begins. Health disorders can cause ridging and thinning of the nails. Psoriasis and fungus under the nail tips can be treated with lavender or geranium oils. As with skin and hair, the nails give an indication of inner health.

**tips for healthy nails**
• Discourage nail-biting by coating the nails daily with neat lavender oil. The unpleasant taste of the oil will stop the chewing.
• Apply neat lavender oil daily to the nail cuticle to improve the condition of weak nails. Results will show in three months.

# Useful essential oils

| ESSENTIAL OIL | TREATMENT |
| --- | --- |
| **hair** | |
| Caraway *Carum carvi* | stimulant, encourages hair growth, aids scalp problems. |
| Cedarwood *Cedrus atlantica* | antiseptic and stimulant to scalp, reduces greasy dandruff, helps to renew hair growth |
| Clary sage *Salvia sclarea* | regenerative, improves poor hair growth |
| Juniper *Juniperus communis* | antiseborrhoeic (greasy dandruff), antiseptic (greasy scalp) |
| Lemon *Citrus limon* | antibacterial, astringent (reduces greasy dandruff) |
| Rosemary *Rosmarinus officinalis* | stimulating to circulation, helps renew hair growth |
| Ylang ylang *Cananga odorata* | tonic to scalp, aids hair growth |
| **nails** | |
| Geranium *Pelargonium graveolens* | antifungal (athlete's foot, skin and nail fungi) |
| Lavender *Lavandula angustifolia* | antifungal (athlete's foot, skin and nail fungi), healing (strengthens weak nails) |
| Tea tree *Melaleuca alternifolia* | anti-infectious, antifungal (skin and nail infections) |

| ESSENTIAL OIL | TREATMENT |
| --- | --- |
| **skin** | |
| Geranium *Pelargonium graveolens* | cicatrizant (healing), useful for open acne |
| Juniper *Juniperus communis* | antiseborrhoeic, antiseptic |
| Lavender *Lavandula angustifolia* | antiseptic, cicatrizant (healing) |
| Lemon *Citrus limon* | antibacterial, astringent |
| Petitgrain *Citrus aurantium* var. *amara* (fol) | anti-inflammatory, antiseptic, useful for infected acne |
| Cedarwood *Cedrus atlantica* | antiseptic, cicatrizant, stimulant (skin and scalp problems) |
| **stress** | |
| Clary sage *Salvia sclarea* | calming |
| Geranium *Pelargonium graveolens* | relaxant (agitation, anxiety) |
| Lavender *Lavandula angustifolia* | calming and sedative |
| Lemon *Citrus limon* | calming and sedative |
| Petitgrain *Citrus aurantium* var. *amara* (fol) | balancing and calming |
| **emotions** | |
| Bergamot *Citrus bergamia* | sedative, neurotonic, cicatrizant, antispasmodic (anxiety, agitation, grief, fear, mood swings) |

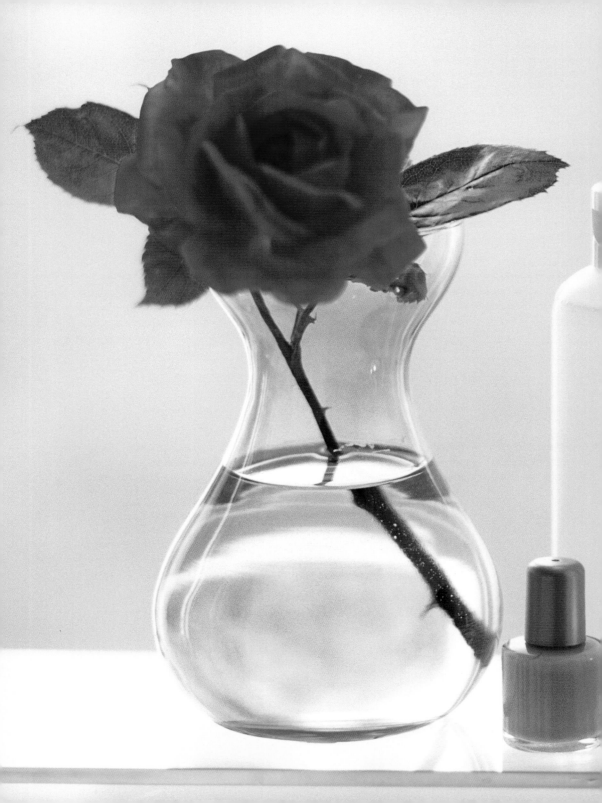

# Beauty and Well-being

Aromatherapy works on every level to cleanse the body and balance the mind. Use aromatic essential oils in your daily cleansing and moisturising routines for smoother skin, stronger nails and better-conditioned hair. The healing properties of plants can also play an effective role in stimulating the immune system to strengthen the body against disease.

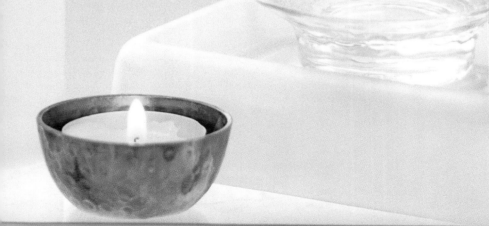

# Looking after yourself

Looking and feeling good is important for most women. Commercial products can do much to treat beauty emergencies, but the only effective, long-term solution is optimum health in body and mind.

## beautiful skin

A good complexion is a huge beauty asset: it helps a woman to look good and this, in turn, will boost morale. The skin is the largest organ of the body. It is always on display to the outside world and is worth taking care of. The skin has a slightly acid mantle, which keeps out harmful bacteria, and it is not a good idea to use excessively alkaline cleansers, such as soap, to wash the skin, as these destroy the necessary acid balance. The condition of the skin is a good indicator of general health within the body.

## lifestyle

The condition of our skin is affected by our lifestyle and general well-being, including our diet, how much exercise we take, our work, our family and our mental attitude.

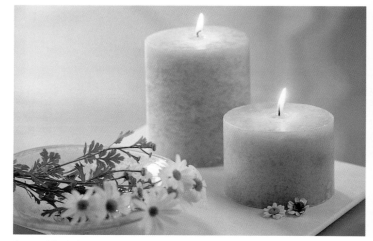

△ By carefully placing objects of natural beauty in your home, you can help your mind to relax and unwind. Soft candlelight is traditionally associated with feelings of peace and harmony.

To some extent, we are what we eat. Our circulatory system carries the nutrients from our food around the body: without a healthy diet, the body's cells receive insufficient nutrition. Regular exercise is also important. A sedentary lifestyle, when combined with a lack of exercise, means that food nutrients are not transported around the body efficiently, and toxins in the lymphatic system are not completely eliminated. This can lead to cellulite and other problems in the body and with the skin. A diet which includes plenty of water, fresh fruit and vegetables will help to keep our bodies free from toxins and promote a blooming, clear complexion.

Our day-to-day environment can also affect our bodies. Most homes and offices are centrally heated, and this has a drying effect on skin and hair. Keeping a bowl of water beside each radiator will help to increase humidity. Women who spend a great deal of time outdoors should take care

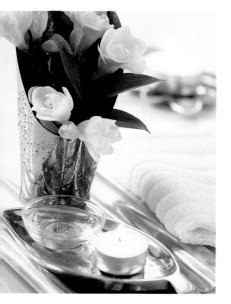

◁ Strategically placed oil and water mixes can increase humidity levels and also release aromas.

to protect their skin from excessive exposure to the sun, rain and wind: these are all damaging to the skin, and will promote wrinkles and early aging. Protect your skin from exposure to harmful ultraviolet rays, on the sunbed or outdoors, to reduce the risk of skin cancer.

Whether you are a working mother, a full-time mother, or a full-time career woman, feeling happy with what you do is important. This, in turn, is reflected in the condition of the skin, hair and nails. When we are unhappy, we tend to feel negative about ourselves and are more likely to focus on our tiny imperfections. This can leave us feeling even worse and creates a vicious cycle which can lead to depression. With a positive mental attitude, on the other hand, we feel happier and more buoyant, our stress levels decrease, and we look and feel in a healthier state.

## the aging process

Like all other organs, the skin deteriorates with age. Typically this is characterized by the slowing down of cell regeneration, and

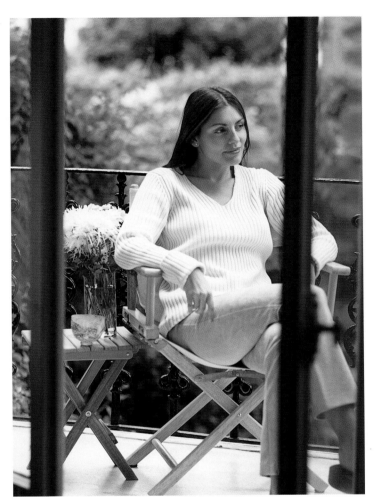

the fact that dead skin cells gradually take longer to be discarded. As we grow older, our skin becomes less moist and loses its elasticity. Facial expressions are more likely to develop into wrinkle lines. As oestrogen production decreases during the menopause years (*see* The Sunset Years), there is a thinning and dehydration of the epidermis (the outer layer of the skin).

Many factors play a part in skin aging: heredity, menopause, occupation, exposure to the sun and wind, poor diet, alcohol-consumption, smoking, prolonged stress, insufficient sleep, even crash diets (which can cause wrinkles) and excessive washing (which can dehydrate the skin). The aging process is also partly due to the formation of free radicals in the body, developed from a reaction between sunlight and oxygen. These molecules are unstable and, in their search to stabilize, reactions occur in the body which can cause cellular destruction, resulting in skin aging and internal disease.

Aging is beyond our control, but we can help to minimize its effects by giving our bodies the best attention possible. Lifestyle factors need to be addressed and then supported by a daily care regime with suitable lotions and creams, which can help to improve the elasticity and appearance of the skin, hair and nails. Protection can be taken against the negative effects of the weather and central heating.

It has been shown that essential oils can be used successfully to combat the effects of aging. Research studies have shown that many essential oils have cell regenerative properties, and essential oil products help to promote a much healthier, younger-looking skin. The essential oil molecules penetrate the skin and are able to work at the germinative layer, where the new cells are formed. These improved cells eventually reach the surface of the skin where the appearance is vastly improved.

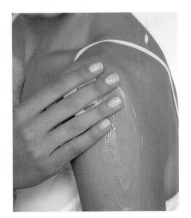

△ Apply a lotion containing analgesic essential oils to relieve aches and pains in the shoulders.

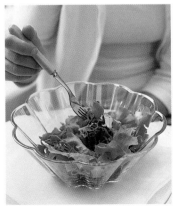

△ Eating plenty of fresh raw vegetables, fruits and salads will keep your energy levels high.

# Daily skincare

The sooner a woman begins a good skincare routine, the more she will reap the benefits as she gets older. A good moisturizer is arguably the most important item in a woman's wardrobe – you can replace your clothes, but not your skin. It is well worth investing in an efficient, quality moisturizer that you like to use.

There is a vast array of commercial products available, designed for every skin permutation imaginable: teenage, normal, dry, oily, mature, sensitive, and allergy-prone skins. Although well-formulated cosmetics without essential oils may benefit the skin, a natural, quality range with added essential oils will increase the benefits.

## choosing products

With aromatherapy, you should only have to choose between two basic product types because all essential oils are normalizing,

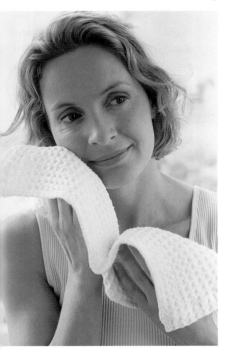

giving exceptional care to the skin. If the skin is normal to oily, then look for a cleansing milk and moisturizing *lotion*. Choose cleansing and moisturizing *creams* when the skin is more dry and in need of nourishment. Look for products which have good quality bases and which don't contain alcohol, lanolin or other animal products. Night creams containing lanolin make your skin greasy, as the molecules are actually too big to penetrate the skin, and the cream will "sit" on top of your face all night, rubbing off on the pillow. Prepare your products with well chosen essential oils in a concentration of 0.5 per cent.

### tips for healthy skin

If you wear make-up, it is important to cleanse your skin thoroughly before bed. In the morning, toner on cotton wool (cotton ball) is usually sufficient. Give yourself a treatment mask once a week. After a mask, you should moisturize twice, as masks draw out moisture as well as toxins. If you don't wear any make-up, a mask once a fortnight is usually sufficient.

If you don't wear make-up, use a mild toner only at night-time after cleansing. Moisturize first thing in the morning, after cleansing and toning.

### creating your own products

To make your own skincare products, use unperfumed bases, adding the appropriate essential oils, 1 drop for each 10 ml (2 tsp) of carrier. Cold spring water is an excellent basic toner.

### oily skin or acne

*daytime* base lotion with 10 per cent spring water added slowly while stirring.
*night-time* base lotion with 10 per cent hazelnut oil added slowly while stirring.

◁ **Always pat your face dry with a soft towel after rinsing. The skin on the face needs careful handling, whatever our age.**

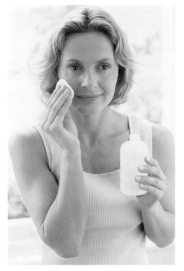

△ **Spring water can be used as a basic toner for all types of skin. Add your chosen essential oils.**

### dry or mature skin

*daytime* base lotion with 25 per cent rose hip or jojoba oils added slowly while stirring.
*night-time* base cream with 50 per cent rose hip or jojoba, or the macerated oils of lime blossom or melissa added while stirring.

### at the menopause

Try using hormone-like essential oils such as clary sage and niaouli which both have oestrogen-like properties.

## skin disorders

A skin problem can arise from many causes, some of which may be more obvious than others. It may stem from an internal physical problem, such as poor digestion or painful periods, or from a mental problem, such as deep-rooted anxiety or grief. The effects of on-going mental and emotional stress can also cause skin problems, which in turn may aggravate the condition as we become worried, anxious and embarrassed about how others see us.

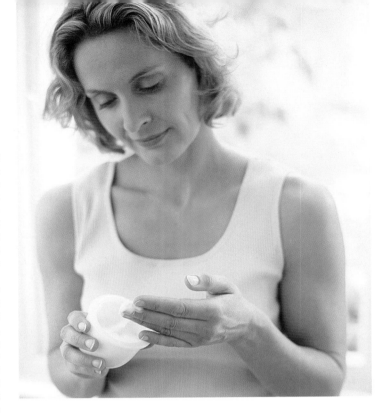

▷ Roman chamomile is excellent for soothing dry, irritable and inflamed skin. Try adding a few drops to your moisturizer and apply daily.

## aromatherapy treatment

Aromatherapy can play an important part in the treatment of skin disorders. The oils are not only able to treat the physical symptoms but, through their aromas, can also affect the mental state of the sufferer. For example, many people suffering chronic, painful skin conditions, such as eczema and psoriasis, may have high stress levels because of the impact of the disease on their physical appearance.

Essential oils are able to break this cycle effectively, lightening the mind as well as tackling the physical symptoms. Where the skin is already being moisturized, whether on the face, hands and/or body, it is easy enough to combine appropriate essential oils with the existing treatment for a two-in-one effect. For example, arthritis oils added to a hand and body lotion base reduce pain and inflammation at the same time as making the skin less dry and scaly.

For severe eczema it is very beneficial to change your diet to one that is dairy-free, eliminating cow's milk and related products from what you eat. This is usually enough to cure the condition, although it can take a few months for the results to be evident. Meanwhile, correct use of the appropriate oils will bring relief from the symptoms.

*Acne rosacea*, a form of acne which usually attacks women over 30, has similar symptoms to *Acne vulgaris* (*see* The Teenage Years). It seems to affect women who like highly seasoned foods and drink large amounts of tea and coffee. Dietary changes will be highly beneficial in all cases, while the use of aromatherapy treatments will improve the condition of the skin.

## Blending essential oils with a moisturizer

**For customized skincare, select the appropriate essential oils and add them to a good quality, bland base cream. Add a little rose hip carrier oil if your skin is particularly dry.**

### ingredients
- 40 ml (8 tsp) unperfumed base cream
- rose hip oil (optional)
- blend of appropriate essential oils

### equipment
- small jar
- swizzle stick or teaspoon
- spatula (optional)

### BLENDING TIP
Always apply creams to the face with clean hands, and best of all using a spatula, to avoid transmitting germs from your fingernails to the cream, and possibly to your skin.

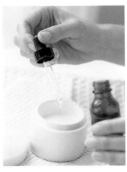

△ **1** For dry skin, add 5 ml (1 tsp) rose hip oil to a jar containing 40 ml (8 tsp) base moisturizing cream.

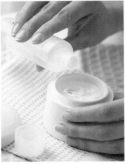

△ **2** After blending your own selection of appropriate essential oils, add 5 drops to the moisturizing cream.

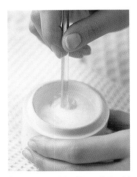

△ **3** Stir thoroughly with a swizzle stick or the handle of a clean teaspoon to blend the mixture.

# Daily hand, foot and nail care

Our hands are exposed daily to the elements and to household detergents, and our feet carry us wherever we want to go. Both deserve as much attention as the face, and will benefit greatly from aromatherapy.

## hand care

It is said that there are two ways to tell a woman's age: by her neck and by her hands. Our hands, like our necks and faces, are always exposed to the air and are always on visible display. However, it is easy to neglect them when leading a busy life.

### treatment

Essential oils can be added to a base lotion and used after each time you wash your hands. Patchouli is one of the best oils for cracked, dry skin, and clary sage helps delay cellular aging. If your hands are neglected and in need of a boost, try giving them an exfoliating "mask" treatment before going to bed. After using an exfoliating face mask on your hands, apply your hand lotion. Cover your hands with cling film (plastic wrap) and pull on a pair of cotton gloves, or cotton socks, over the cling film. Keep the mask in place for an hour before rinsing off.

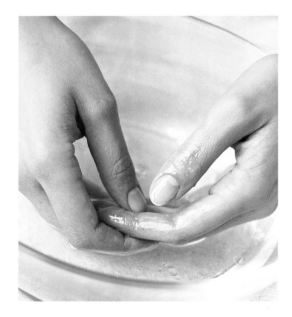

◁ Having well-cared for hands is a beauty asset. To give your hands a treat, prepare a mix using oils of geranium and rose otto and work well into the skin.

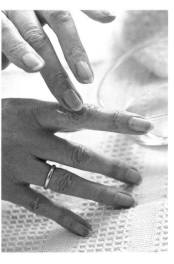

◁ For cracked knuckles, try patchouli oil mixed in a carrier cream or lotion base and applied to the affected area on clean, dry hands.

## foot care

Think of the amount of work our feet have to do – we walk on them daily, often in inappropriate footwear, and yet we give them surprisingly little care and attention.

### treatment

Spend some time each week giving your feet a thoroughly relaxing massage which benefits your feet and the rest of your body at the same time. Keep them as scrupulously clean as your face, regularly removing dead skin at the heels and drying properly between the toes.

Watch for any broken skin between the toes as this may be an early sign of athlete's foot – a fungal condition which can be difficult to treat once it takes hold. Plastic shoes are a common cause of athlete's foot as they create moisture and cause the feet

to sweat, creating the ideal conditions for fungus to develop. Essential oils can be used to treat all fungus-type infections as well as viral ones, including warts and verrucas. You will also need to address the underlying causes. These may be related to stress and poor nutrition, and will be helped with relaxing essential oils.

## nail care

Strong, well-manicured nails on the hands and feet play an important role in a woman's appearance. Brittle, damaged or weak nails can detract from this. Essential oils can be used to improve nail condition.

### treatment

Essential oil of lavender is particularly good for strengthening nails. Each evening, put your finger on to the nozzle of a bottle of lavender oil, tip the bottle, and rub the oil into the cuticles. After two or three months you should see some improvement as the treated nail grows through.

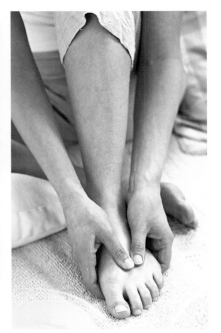

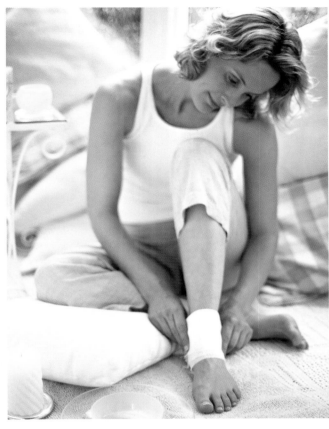

△ Giving yourself a foot massage not only feels good but also energizes the many reflex points on your feet, which in turn correspond to different parts of the body.

▷ For tired or swollen ankles, a cool compress soaked in Roman chamomile and lavender oil is both soothing and refreshing and can also alleviate any inflammation.

## Nail treatment

Pampering your nails with this weekly treatment will keep them healthy and strong. If your nails are particularly weak and damaged, you may prefer to apply this quick treatment every evening. Because nail growth is a slow process, the results are not immediate – it will be a couple of months before you see any improvement, but it will be worth the wait.

### ingredients
- warm water
- lavender essential oil

### equipment
- bowl
- cuticle stick
- cotton bud (Q-tip)

**NAIL-STRENGTHENING TIP**

Sucking a jelly cube each day is said to strengthen the nails. If you often have white flecks across your nails, increasing the calcium in your diet could also help.

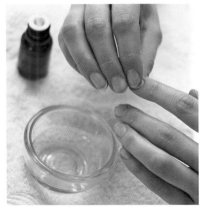

△ **1** Soak your fingertips in warm water before gently cleaning the surplus cuticle from the nails.

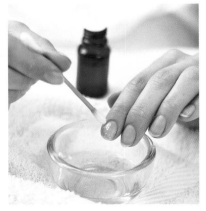

△ **2** Use a cotton bud (Q-tip) to apply neat lavender oil to each cuticle to strengthen them.

# Daily bodycare

Our bodies are protected for much of the time with clothes, and because of this, the skin of our torso is usually in a better condition – softer and smoother – than that of our arms and legs, which are more frequently exposed to sunlight.

## conditioning treatments

The arms and legs benefit hugely from the daily use of creams and lotions containing essential oils; improvements are particularly apparent when moisturizing bath or shower oils or gels have not been used as a matter of course. If your skin is dry or flaky, put your essential oils into a carrier oil to add a gleam to your skin. (*See* Preparing Oils for Application to select the most beneficial oil for your skin type.)

For a bath treatment for dry skin, grate 15 g (½ oz) unscented, non-alkaline soap into 120 ml (½ cup) boiling water, and stir to dissolve the soap. When cool, add 8 drops of your favourite essential oil or oil mix. Hold your mixture under the running tap to dissolve in the bathwater and make some bubbles. If you prefer lots of bubbles, add essential oils to a non-drying bubble bath.

If you have normal to oily skin, which is not known to be sensitive, give yourself a body rinse before leaving the bath or

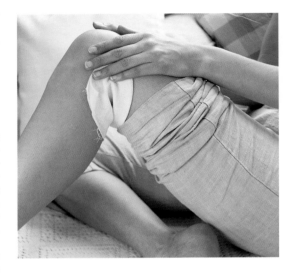

shower. Dissolve your essential oil or oils into 15 ml (1 tbsp) vodka, and mix with 1 litre (1¾ pints) spring water. Add 120 ml (½ cup) white wine or cider vinegar to the spring water mixture for an extra zingy feel.

If you have a problem with body odour, use the vodka rinse above, but without the vinegar. Add 3 drops of nutmeg essential oil and 3 drops of cypress essential oil; both of these have deodorizing properties.

For hard, rough skin on elbows and heels, use a facial exfoliating mask, followed by a moisturizing body lotion or oil to which 2–3 drops of essential oil have been added.

Cellulite is caused by ineffective blood circulation, which leads to poor lymphatic drainage and fluid retention. Aromatherapy can help with a daily regime. Pummel the area vigorously before applying essential oils in a carrier lotion or oil.

◁ Varicose veins can be painful and unsightly. A cool compress, made with cypress, clary sage or niaouli oil and applied to the affected area, can help.

## Varicose vein treatment

**Apply the essential oil blend or lotion mix to the whole leg before following the directions below. Upward strokes are important to help the blood move towards the heart. Use phlebotonic oils such as clary sage, cypress and niaouli.**

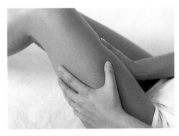

△ **1** Massage the upper half of the leg first with upward movements. This clears the valves to allow the blood to pass more easily from the lower leg.

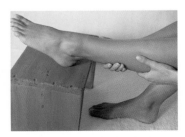

△ **2** Massage in an upward direction only, using the palms of both hands. Make long, firm strokes alternately with each hand up the calf muscle.

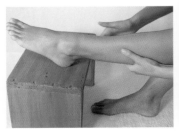

△ **3** Take the fingers of both hands alternately up the calf muscle. Complete the sequence by repeating step 2.

## Anti-cellulite treatment

**Cellulite is recognized by its resemblance to orange or grapefruit peel. A daily aromatherapy treatment, along with an improved diet and a thorough exercise plan, will boost the circulation and improve lymphatic drainage, helping to disperse the cellulite.**

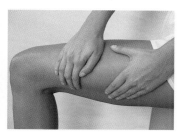

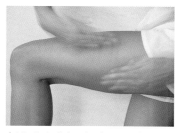

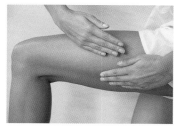

△ **1** After firmly rubbing in your prepared oil mix or lotion, take both hands alternately up the outside of the leg. Use a loofah or bristle brush if preferred.

△ **2** Use the heel of your hands to pummel the cellulite vigorously. This stimulates the circulation and allows quicker penetration of the essential oils.

△ **3** Continue to work over the cellulite area using the heels of both hands alternately. Maintaining the firmness of the strokes, repeat step 1.

# Useful essential oils

| ESSENTIAL OIL | TREATMENT |
|---|---|
| **skin types** | |
| **DRY SKIN** | |
| Chamomile (Roman) *Chamaemelum nobile* | anti-inflammatory (irritable skin) |
| Geranium *Pelargonium graveolens* | anti-infectious, cicatrizant |
| Lavender *Lavandula angustifolia* | antiseptic, anti-inflammatory, cicatrizant (healing) |
| Patchouli *Pogostemon patchouli* | anti-inflammatory, cicatrizant |
| Rose otto *Rosa damascena* | anti-inflammatory (blotchy skin), cicatrizant |
| **OILY SKIN** | |
| Cedarwood *Cedrus atlantica* | antiseptic, antibacterial, cicatrizant. |
| Lemon *Citrus limon* | astringent, antibacterial, anti-inflammatory |
| Ylang ylang *Cananga odorata* | tonic, balancing, calming, hypotensive |
| **MATURE SKIN** | |
| Clary sage *Salvia sclarea* | regenerative (cellular aging) |
| Frankincense *Boswellia carteri* | antioxidant (combats aging process), cicatrizant |
| **anti-aging** | |
| Clary sage *Salvia sclarea* | oestrogen-like, regenerative (counteracts cellular aging) |
| Frankincense *Boswellia carteri* | antioxidant (combats aging process) |
| Lemon *Citrus limon* | antisclerotic (combats aging process) |

| ESSENTIAL OIL | TREATMENT |
|---|---|
| **skin conditions** | |
| **PSORIASIS (INCLUDING NAILS)** | |
| Bergamot *Citrus bergamia* | cicatrizant |
| Lavender *Lavandula angustifolia* | cicatrizant |
| **ECZEMA** | |
| Bergamot *Citrus bergamia* | anti-infectious (weeping eczema), cicatrizant |
| Geranium *Pelargonium graveolens* | analgesic, anti-infectious, anti-inflammatory, cicatrizant |
| **ACNE *ROSACEAE*** | |
| Chamomile (German) *Matricaria recutica* | anti-inflammatory, cicatrizant |
| Chamomile (Roman) *Chamaemelum nobile* | anti-inflammatory, cicatrizant |
| Frankincense *Boswellia carteri* | analgesic, cicatrizant |
| **ATHLETE'S FOOT AND NAIL FUNGI** | |
| Clary sage *Salvia sclarea* | antifungal (skin conditions) |
| Geranium *Pelargonium graveolens* | antifungal, anti-infectious |
| Lavender *Lavandula angustifolia* | antifungal, antiseptic |
| **CELLULITE** | |
| Cypress *Cupressus sempervirens* | diuretic |
| Fennel *Foeniculum vulgare* | diuretic, circulatory stimulant |
| Juniper *Juniperus communis* | diuretic, lypolytic |
| **VARICOSE VEINS** | |

See The Reproductive Years for relevant essential oils.

# Coping with stress and emotions

There is increasing evidence to suggest that stress features significantly in the lives of many women, whether they are single, married or co-habiting, and whether or not they have children. Many women are finding it increasingly difficult to manage work and home commitments, leisure time and relationships, and these stresses are often multiplied when a woman has children.

Perhaps stress can be defined as having too much to do, in too short a time, and without the necessary resources. When such a situation goes on and on over a period of time, it can have an adverse effect on health. However, when we are unhappy, or under too much pressure for an extended period of time, our body's cells generate a negative, health-reducing effect and stress-related conditions may begin to show: insomnia, tension headaches, chronic back problems, digestive disorders, skin problems and other diseases in the body.

## the use of aromatherapy

Essential oils have been proved to have an influence on the central nervous system, which varies depending on the essential oils

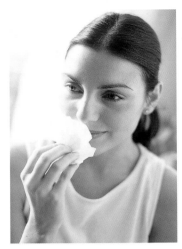

△ Sniffing a tissue prepared with essential oils is a handy method for improving concentration.

selected. Good use of aromatherapy can improve general health and well-being, helping us to cope with the physical and emotional aspects of stress.

If you are finding it difficult to concentrate on your work, prepare a tissue with a blend

of rosemary and peppermint essential oils, and sniff at intervals throughout the day. Both of these oils are decongestants and mental stimulants, and they should help to clear congested or conflicting thoughts and mixed emotions. Add lemon oil to the blend if you work on a computer. In one Japanese study, it was revealed that 54 per cent fewer typing errors were made by staff who had been exposed to a lemon aroma, compared to those who had not.

**TIPS FOR COPING WITH STRESS**
- Take regular exercise: join a gym, take up yoga, or go for long walks.
- Put aside some quiet time each day for yourself, for reading, reflection, meditation, visiting friends, or simply doing nothing at all.
- Eat a healthy diet, avoiding snacking on processed foods.
- Devise a schedule at home which means that everyone takes part in running the household.
- If you have a partner, make sure you spend at least one evening a week on your own together.
- Unwind in an aromatherapy bath with a favourite essential oil every evening: this promotes a refreshing sleep, which will help to prepare you for the next day.

## emotional insecurity

The emotions we express or feel can be separated into two groups: primary and secondary. Some primary emotions are positive, such as feelings of love, tolerance, and happiness, and these are not a problem. Difficulties arise with the negative primary emotions, such as fear, anger, guilt and

◁ **Inhalation is the fastest way for an essential oil to reach the brain. Vaporize ylang ylang for its balancing and calming properties.**

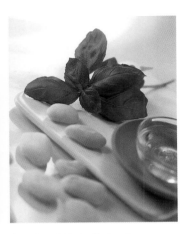

△ Basil is useful for its effects on the nervous system. It can help to dispel fear and jealousy.

jealousy. Secondary emotions are usually concerned with our personality. These may be shown as moodiness, confusion, timidity and inferiority, for example.

Essential oils are very useful for treating emotional problems. The oils are selected on the basis of their properties which relate to the emotion being expressed. For example, essential oils which have relaxing and anti-inflammatory properties are known to be soothing for anger, while oils with stimulating and digestive properties are better able to overcome fear.

## anger

The state of anger can range from mild irritability and impatience at one end of the scale to explosive outbursts and fury at the other. The ability to cope with anger varies from person to person, depending on the personality. When under stress, anger is more easily aroused and our ability to deal with our own feelings may be severely tested. It is important to have the ability to handle our anger in a positive, constructive way. The oils which help are, principally, calming, antispasmodic, anti-inflammatory and healing.

## fear

Stress and fear are sometimes related, and can be acute or chronic. If you oversleep and are running late for an important meeting, for example, your body goes into a temporary state of fear and your adrenal

glands produce extra adrenalin to help you deal with the situation. However, if the state of fear is long-lasting, it can become a chronic condition that can lead to illness. Living in a state of fear creates tension and anxiety which have a detrimental effect on our outlook and upon our bodies. The helpful essential oils are those which are analgesic, calming and soothing, and those which are stimulating to the mind, as well as to the respiratory and digestive systems.

## jealousy

Most jealous feelings are negative. Jealousy is often linked with anger and/or resentment, and may arise out of an inability to share our friends, family and possessions, or else out of a craving for things that we do not have, which other people seem to have. Although jealousy is often the most difficult emotion to admit to, it is one of the most deadly, where we can hurt not only others but also ourselves. Positive thinking and the use of essential oils which will detoxify or destroy fungi and kill viruses can help to overcome this self-destructive emotion.

Secondary emotions can also be helped by essential oils and are sometimes linked with a primary emotion like fear. Lack of confidence or a sense of under-achievement may involve fear, and mood swings may involve anger and/or irritability.

## lack of confidence

Many women suffer from a lack of self-confidence. Positive thinking is necessary here, along with neurotonic essential oils which will boost your morale by strengthening the nervous system. These stimulate the mind and will help you to achieve things you never thought were possible. Sweet thyme may help to promote bravery and instil drive and assertiveness due to its many tonic properties. The most effective methods of use are by tissue or vaporizer inhalation, and in the bath.

## moodiness

As well as being able to relax or stimulate the nervous system, essential oils can also induce slight mood changes. This makes

▷ Water with lemon and peppermint can help to dispel apathy and lift feelings of depression.

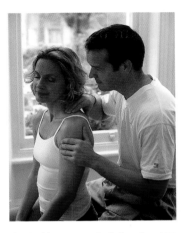

△ A shoulder massage using juniper oil can help when you are feeling emotionally drained.

the use of essential oils suitable for women who are inclined to be temperamental, and for the unpredictable mood swings and irritability suffered during PMS.

## loss of sensual awareness

Feelings of indifference, apathy and general loss of libido can be directly related to stress and/or overwork. Taking an essential oil bath or vaporizing some oils an hour before bedtime will help you to unwind, physically and emotionally. You and your partner may like to give each other aromatherapy back or shoulder massages to help each other relax and to prepare for love-making. Use essential oils which are renowned for their aphrodisiac and uplifting effects.

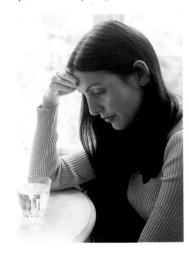

# Common health problems

There are several relatively common health problems which can occur at any age and with varying degrees of severity. Stress generally makes all these conditions worse.

## irritable bowel syndrome (IBS)

This disorder of the lower bowel usually occurs between 20-40 years of age. The usual symptoms are colicky pains, diarrhoea and/or constipation, and distension of the abdomen, giving rise to noisy rumblings and wind. Emotional factors can play an important part in this disorder, and those who are anxious and over-conscientious are the most likely sufferers. Symptoms can be worse just before a period, especially if PMS is present.

It is useful to experiment with diet. Exclude cow's milk and its products and monitor the result. Foods which contain wheat can also cause problems, as can the caffeine in tea and coffee. Try essential oils which balance the digestive system, used in a variety of ways: by ingestion (*see* Aromatherapy Techniques), by application of oils in a carrier base, rubbed on to the abdomen twice daily in a clockwise direction, and by compresses placed over the abdomen.

▷ An application of fennel, peppermint and/or rosemary can be helpful with IBS. Use in a carrier oil or compress applied to the abdomen area.

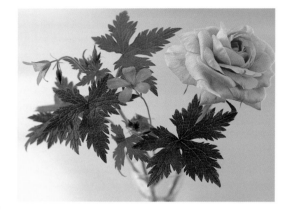

◁ The heady yet gentle aroma of rose is a favourite with almost every woman. Rose helps to lift the spirits and promote feelings of well-being.

## cystitis

This is a common problem that can occur after sex and during pregnancy. Cystitis is an infection and inflammation of the bladder and urethra. It is characterized by a frequent, painful urge to go to the toilet. Treatment is with antibacterial and antiseptic essential oils which have an affinity to the kidneys. Cystitis has been treated successfully using a tea with the relevant essential oils added (*see* Aromatherapy Techniques) and by application of the same oils in a carrier base to the abdomen and lower back.

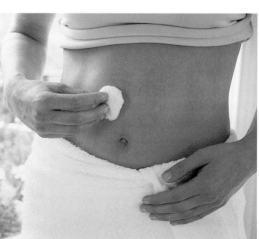

## sinusitis

Inflammation of the sinus area around the nose and/or eyes can occur at any time in life after puberty and is often difficult to cure, even with an operation. It causes chronic congestion, catarrh and sometimes headaches. Fortunately, sinusitis can be helped easily and successfully by adding the appropriate essential oils to your regular moisturizer. Allergic reactions or colds can exacerbate the condition, in which case neat essential oils should be inhaled on a tissue or used in the bath. Pressing on the sinus-pressure points on the feet (*see* Swiss Reflex Therapy) every night while symptoms persist is also helpful.

## vaginitis

Inflammation of the vagina, with accompanying irritation, can be caused by leaving a tampon in too long or through use of the contraceptive pill. The most frequent cause is when a yeast-like substance, called *Candida albicans*, a normal inhabitant of the mouth and bowel (and, in women, of the vagina) becomes infected. When symptoms first appear, immediate treatment with essential oils will help. Provided a tampon was not the cause of the inflammation in the first place, try a tampon with 2 drops of tea tree oil inserted into the vagina and left in overnight. Alternatively, taking regular sitz-baths for ten minutes at a time, using a synergistic mix of appropriate essential oils, can also help.

## thrush

Infected *Candida albicans* can show as white ulcerous spots inside the mouth (thrush), which can be dealt with using a mouthwash including anti-infectious essential oils. The vagina can also be affected with thrush, giving rise to itching and discomfort. Thrush usually affects women with a low immune system, where it can be due to stress, the overuse of antibiotics or diabetes. Additional symptoms which can present themselves at this time include cystitis, depression and headaches.

With thrush it is helpful if the intake of sugar and refined carbohydrates in the diet is reduced immediately. If the condition worsens, an effective form of aromatherapy treatment involves eating live yogurt containing suitable essential oils: 20 drops of oil to 100 ml (6–7 tbsp) of yogurt and, if possible, inserting some of this mixture into the vagina with a tampon applicator.

## endometriosis

This condition is when tissue similar to that of the lining of the uterus is found elsewhere – mostly in the ovaries. The tissue swells and bleeds, causing severe pain before a period and excessive blood loss during it. Conventional treatment may recommend removal of the ovaries (and therefore the

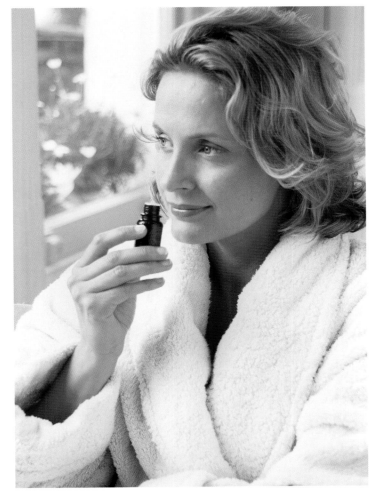

△ **Peppermint is useful for relieving nasal congestion and treating general sinus problems.**

hormone production) so that the uterus is no longer stimulated to produce the extra tissue. The contraceptive pill is often prescribed but this is not always successful.

Some women prefer to avoid surgery if possible, in which case it is worth trying hormone-like and decongestant essential oils first, as they have been known to help. If surgery is inevitable, then oestrogen-like essential oils will help the body to readjust itself to the loss of the ovaries.

◁ **A compress of clary sage and cypress can be used for problems associated with the ovaries.**

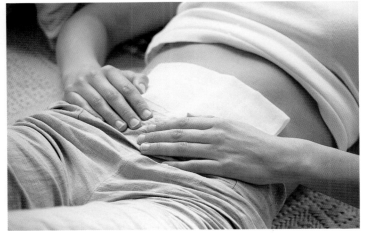

# Useful essential oils

| ESSENTIAL OIL | TREATMENT |
|---|---|
| **stress** | |
| Chamomile (Roman) *Chamaemelum nobile* | calming |
| Lemon *Citrus limon* | calming, hypotensive |
| Melissa *Melissa officinalis* | calming, sedative |
| Ylang ylang *Cananga odorata* | balancing, calming, hypotensive |
| **depression** | |
| Basil *Ocimum basilicum* var. *album* | neurotonic |
| Frankincense *Boswellia carteri* | energizing, immunostimulant |
| Juniper *Juniperus communis* | neurotonic |
| Neroli *Citrus aurantium* var. *amara* | tranquilizing (nervous depression, fatigue) |
| Niaouli *Melaleuca viridiflora* | tonic |
| Peppermint *Mentha x piperita* | neurotonic |
| Pine *Pinus sylvestris* | neurotonic |
| Rosemary *Rosmarinus officinalis* | neurotonic, sexual tonic |
| **stress with depression** | |
| Bergamot *Citrus bergamia* | balancing, calming, sedative, tonic to central nervous system |
| Clary sage *Salvia sclarea* | balancing, relaxing, neurotonic |
| Cypress *Cupressus sempervirens* | balancing, calming, neurotonic |
| Geranium *Pelargonium graveolens* | balancing, relaxing, stimulant (nervous fatigue) |
| Lavender *Lavandula angustifolia* | balancing, calming, sedative, tonic |
| Marjoram *Origanum majorana* | balancing, calming, neurotonic |
| Rose otto *Rosa damascena* | balancing, relaxing, neurotonic, sexual tonic |
| **poor concentration** | |
| Basil *Ocimum basilicum* var. *album* | neurotonic |
| Bergamot *Citrus bergamia* | balancing, tonic |
| Thyme (sweet) *Thymus vulgaris* | cardiotonic, neurotonic, immunostimulant |
| **irritable bowel syndrome** | |
| Fennel *Foeniculum vulgare* | analgesic, antispasmodic, digestive (constipation, diarrhoea, flatulence) |
| Peppermint *Mentha x piperita* | analgesic, anti-inflammatory, digestive (diarrhoea, flatulence) |
| Rosemary *Rosmarinus officinalis* | analgesic, antispasmodic, digestive (constipation, flatulence) |

| ESSENTIAL OIL | TREATMENT |
|---|---|
| **thrush (*Candida albicans*) and vaginitis** | |
| Lavender *Lavandula angustifolia* | analgesic, antifungal, anti-inflammatory |
| Pine *Pinus sylvestris* | analgesic, antifungal, anti-infectious, anti-inflammatory, neurotonic |
| Tea tree *Melaleuca alternifolia* | analgesic, antifungal, anti-infectious, anti-inflammatory, immunostimulant, neurotonic |
| Thyme (sweet) *Thymus vulgaris* | antifungal, anti-infectious, anti-inflammatory, immunostimulant, neurotonic |
| **cystitis** | |
| Eucalyptus *Eucalyptus smithii* | anti-infectious, antiseptic |
| Juniper *Juniperus communis* | anti-inflammatory, antiseptic |
| Lavender *Lavandula angustifolia* | anti-inflammatory, antiseptic |
| Thyme (sweet) *Thymus vulgaris* | anti-infectious, anti-inflammatory, antiseptic |
| **sinusitis** | |
| Eucalyptus *Eucalyptus smithii* | anti-inflammatory, antiseptic |
| Lavender *Lavandula angustifolia* | anti-inflammatory, anti-infectious, antiseptic |
| Peppermint *Mentha x piperita* | anti-inflammatory, anti-infectious |
| **endometriosis** | |
| Clary sage *Salvia sclarea* | decongestant, oestrogen-like, phlebotonic |
| Cypress *Cupressus sempervirens* | astringent, hormone-like (ovary problems), phlebotonic |
| Geranium *Pelargonium graveolens* | analgesic, astringent, cicatrizant, decongestant, phlebotonic, styptic |
| Rose otto *Rosa damascena* | astringent, cicatrizant, neurotonic, styptic |

Sweet scents are the swift vehicles

of still sweeter thoughts.

*Walter Savage Landor, 1775–1864.*

**ESSENTIAL OIL**       **TREATMENT**

## anger, fear and jealousy

The following essential oils given can benefit all of these emotions. The properties required for each condition are listed first, the oils which follow show the properties each possesses relevant to that particular emotion.

### ANGER

| | |
|---|---|
| Look for oils which are | analgesic, anticatarrhal, anti-inflammatory, antispasmodic, calming, carminative (relieving flatulence), cicatrizant, sedative |
| Basil *Ocimum basilicum* var. *album* | analgesic, anti-inflammatory, carminative, calming to the nervous system |
| Bergamot *Citrus bergamia* | antispasmodic, calming, cicatrizant |
| Geranium *Pelargonium graveolens* | analgesic, anti-inflammatory, antispasmodic, cicatrizant, relaxant |
| Juniper *Juniperus communis* | analgesic, anticatarrhal, anti-inflammatory |
| Lavender *Lavandula angustifolia* | analgesic, anti-inflammatory, antispasmodic, calming and sedative, cicatrizant |
| Lemon *Citrus limon* | anti-inflammatory, antispasmodic, calming, carminative |

### FEAR

| | |
|---|---|
| Look for oils which are | antispasmodic, cardiotonic, calming and soothing, digestive, hypotensive, mental stimulant, nausea relief, nerve tonic, respiratory tonic, sedative |
| Basil *Ocimum basilicum* var. *album* | antispasmodic, cardiotonic, neurotonic |
| Bergamot *Citrus bergamia* | antispasmodic (indigestion), calming, sedative (agitation), nerve tonic |
| Geranium *Pelargonium graveolens* | antispasmodic, relaxant |
| Juniper *Juniperus communis* | digestive tonic, nerve tonic |
| Lavender *Lavandula angustifolia* | antispasmodic, calming, cardiotonic, hypotensive, sedative |
| Lemon *Citrus limon* | antispasmodic (diarrhoea normalizing), calming, hypotensive, nausea relief |

The flowers anew, returning seasons bring

But beauty faded has no second spring.

*From The First Pastoral, Ambrose Philips, 1675–1749.*

**ESSENTIAL OIL**       **TREATMENT**

### JEALOUSY

| | |
|---|---|
| Look for oils which are | antibacterial, antifungal, antiviral, cicatrizant, detoxifying, litholytic |
| Basil *Ocimum basilicum* var. *album* | antibacterial, antiviral, decongestant (uterine) |
| Bergamot *Citrus bergamia* | antibacterial, antiviral, cicatrizant |
| Geranium *Pelargonium graveolens* | antibacterial, antifungal, cicatrizant, decongestant (lymph) |
| Juniper *Juniperus communis* | detoxifying, litholytic |
| Lavender *Lavandula angustifolia* | antibacterial, antifungal, cicatrizant |
| Lemon *Citrus limon* | antibacterial, antifungal, antiviral, litholytic |

## irritability

| | |
|---|---|
| Chamomile (Roman) *Chamaemelum nobile* | calming |
| Cypress *Cupressus sempervirens* | calming |
| Rose otto *Rosa damascena* | calming |

## lack of confidence

| | |
|---|---|
| Basil *Ocimum basilicum* var. *album* | neurotonic |
| Bergamot *Citrus bergamia* | balancing, tonic to central nervous system |
| Lavender *Lavandula angustifolia* | balancing, tonic |
| Marjoram *Origanum majorana* | balancing, neurotonic |
| Rosemary *Rosmarinus officinalis* | neurotonic |
| Thyme (sweet) *Thymus vulgaris* | cardiotonic, neurotonic, immunostimulant |

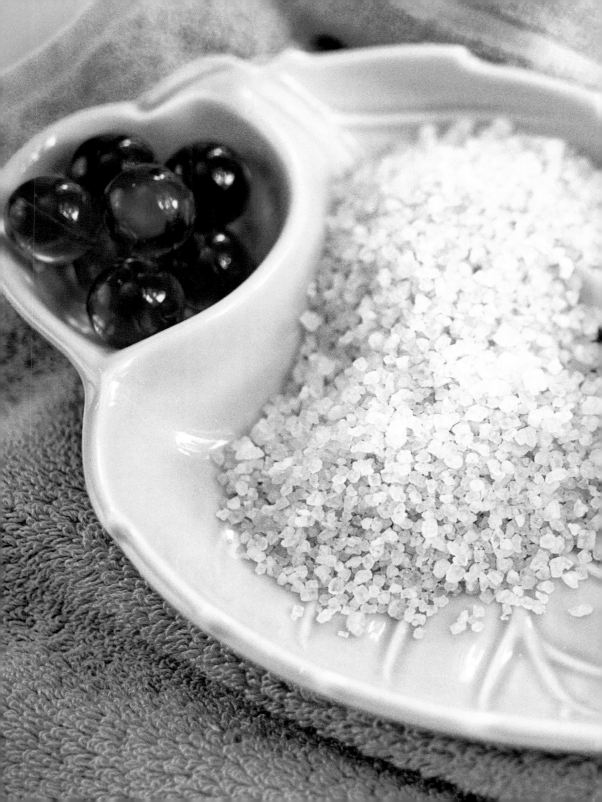

# The Reproductive Years

The gentle, calming effects of essential oils lend themselves perfectly to alleviating the physical discomforts of menstruation and pregnancy. Aromatic baths, soothing compresses and relaxing massage treatments can all help a woman stay naturally healthy throughout her reproductive years.

# Coping with menstruation

When a girl reaches puberty, her previously dormant ovaries begin to release eggs for potential fertilization in the uterus. The ovaries take it in turns, approximately once a month, to release one, or sometimes two, eggs. The length of this cycle varies between individuals, from three to five weeks on average. The menstrual cycle is controlled by several hormones released by the endocrine system: these include oestrogen and progesterone, the latter being responsible for the thickening of the uterus lining, ready to welcome and feed a fertilized egg. At the same time, the breasts begin to swell a little, as they prepare to produce milk-forming tissue, and congestion occurs, particularly in the area between the nipples and the armpits.

If the egg is not fertilized within a few days, it dies and, together with the lining of the uterus, is rejected by the uterus two weeks after its arrival. The result is a flow of blood lasting, on average, between three and five days. Once finished, it can take up to three weeks before the next egg is released, depending on the individual.

This hormonal activity can cause period pain (dysmenorrhoea), irregularity, a heavy blood flow (menorrhagia), hardly

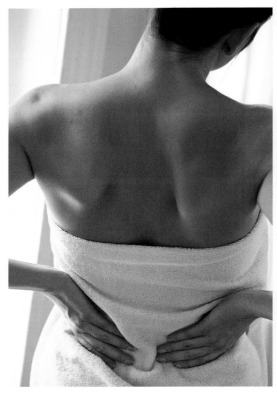

▷ **For some women, their periods are marked by a dull backache. Sweet marjoram, rosemary and pine can be applied on a warm compress to the painful area.**

△ **Peppermint is useful for treating nausea and headaches. It can be taken internally in water.**

any flow (oligomenorrhoea) or perhaps no flow at all (amenorrhoea). Other symptoms may appear, and can vary from water retention, constipation, backache, tiredness, nausea, headaches and migraine, to tender breasts and premenstrual syndrome (PMS). This emotional complication of PMS can adversely affect the rest of the family as well as the sufferer. PMS should not be confused with period pains or any of the other symptoms experienced during menstruation, as the moment blood flow begins, PMS symptoms disappear.

## painful periods

These are caused by congestion of blood in the uterus. Symptoms can range from a slight discomfort to a heavy, dragging pain in the abdomen. For some women, period pains may also affect the lower back.

### treatment

Apply analgesic and decongestant essential oils in a vegetable oil or lotion carrier-base, in a clockwise direction, over the entire abdomen, daily at bedtime, eight to ten days before your period is due. When you have pain or tender breasts it is beneficial to apply a warm compress, using the same essential oils as above (*see* Aromatherapy Techniques). Exercise can be helpful as it stimulates the blood circulation and relieves congestion. After childbirth, period pains usually diminish or disappear.

## irregular, infrequent or lack of periods

This can be very frustrating from the point of view of planning your life, especially if you are trying to conceive a child. The problem is due to hormonal imbalance. Worry can make things worse, so stress-relieving essential oils, when used regularly, can be beneficial.

### treatment

Roman chamomile, melissa and rose otto essential oils can be blended together in a carrier-base oil or lotion and rubbed into the abdomen, in a clockwise direction. The appropriate, hormone-like, essential oils should also be used.

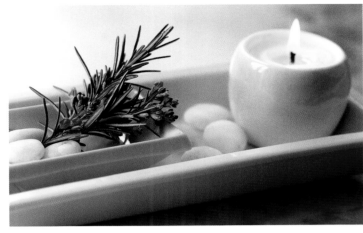

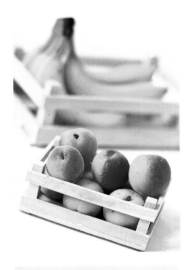

## scanty and heavy periods

These may be due to an imbalance of prostaglandin in the body, a hormone which affects the uterus. With heavy periods, the lining of the uterus is over-thick.

### treatment

Use hormone-like essential oils.

## other symptoms

Constipation, tiredness and backache can all arise as a result of period problems. Other

△ **Rosemary is a good choice to help with period problems, relieving constipation and fatigue.**

symptoms which can arise around the time of menstruation are associated with PMS.

### treatment

Many oils are effective against backache, and it is probably best to experiment until you find the ones you like best. Rosemary and mandarin, used together, are known to be effective for constipation.

◁ **Include plenty of fresh fruit in your daily diet. Healthy eating can alleviate period problems.**

**LIFESTYLE TIPS FOR MENSTRUAL PROBLEMS**

• Foods to avoid: excess sugar, salt, chocolate

• Foods to eat: liver, fish, fresh fruit (especially bananas), nuts, pulses, raw or cooked fresh vegetables (especially greens), salads (with evening primrose oil), diuretic vegetables, such as fennel, cucumber and cabbage (try cooking cabbage in a minimum amount of water and drink the water that is left after cooking).

• Drinks to avoid: excess caffeine found in tea, coffee and cola.

▷ **Experiment with making your own lotions. Choose the oils most suited to your symptoms and have a bottle made up and ready to use.**

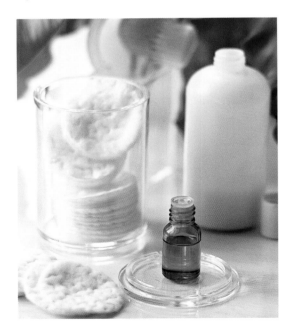

# Pre-menstrual syndrome (PMS)

Some researchers estimate that PMS affects up to half of adult women living in modern society. No one knows exactly the cause of PMS, but it is believed that the lowered hormone level in the body after the egg has been released is mainly responsible for the collection of mental and physical symptoms which can become apparent eight to ten days before menstruation. Contributory factors include poor nutrition and stress: women often juggle many responsibilities at the same time, with insufficient time to eat properly and relax.

## excessive water retention

Fluid retention is thought to be a crucial factor in PMS, as it affects all the cells in the body. PMS may be accompanied by weight gain and shows itself in the swelling of the abdomen, ankles and breasts, which can become very tender and swollen.

### treatment

Diuretic and decongestant essential oils can be used to help reduce swelling.

## persistent headaches and sleep disturbances

Both a lack of sleep and regular headaches are draining on the body, and will increase stress levels and the inability to cope.

### treatment

Calming, neurotonic and decongestant essential oils can be used to relieve the headaches and/or insomnia by balancing the whole body.

## emotional instability

Many women suffer from depression and irritability every month. In some cases, this can be severe and can lead to arguments and difficulties at home and at work.

### treatment

Antidepressive and calming essential oils, taken as inhalations and baths, can help.

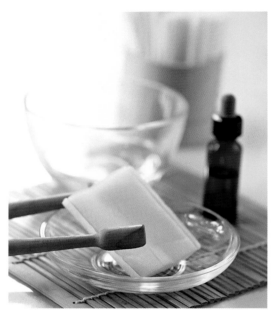

◁ To make a compress, add a few drops of your chosen oil blend to a bowl of water and mix well. Place a piece of cloth on the water's surface and let the oil soak into it. Use as needed.

▽ For sleepless nights, headaches, and irritability prepare a mix of Roman chamomile, melissa and lavender. It may be handy to keep some by your bedside.

**LIFESTYLE TIPS FOR PMS**

For the most effective results, a holistic approach to PMS is essential.

- Amend your diet to boost your general health and vitality
- Exercise to stimulate your blood circulation and to relieve congestion: try walking, cycling and swimming.
- Avoid stressful situations wherever possible, and ask for help if home or work responsibilities become too much
- Take your favourite relevant essential oils to work for instant therapy

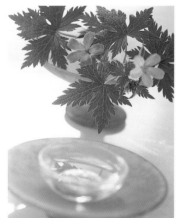

**hormonal treatment**

Some essential oils have a tendency to normalize hormonal secretions, including those involved in the reproductive system. Cypress is helpful for all ovarian problems. Clary sage and niaouli are oestrogen-like, which makes them useful for the stages in a woman's life when oestrogen production is unstable. To balance your hormones, these oils should be used in applications, baths and inhalations ten to 12 days before the expected start of a period.

# Useful essential oils

| ESSENTIAL OIL | TREATMENT |
|---|---|
| **hormone-like essential oils** | |
| Chamomile (German) *Matricaria recutica* | decongestant, hormone-like |
| Clary sage *Salvia sclarea* | decongestant, oestrogen-like |
| Cypress *Cupressus sempervirens* | hormone-like (ovarian) |
| Niaouli *Melaleuca viridiflora* | oestrogen-like (regularizes menses) |
| Peppermint *Mentha x piperita* | hormone-like (ovarian stimulant), neurotonic |
| **painful periods and backache** | |
| Basil *Ocimum basilicum* var. *album* | analgesic, antispasmodic, decongestant |
| Eucalyptus *Eucalyptus smithii* (not *Eucalyptus globulus*) | analgesic, decongestant |
| Geranium *Pelargonium graveolens* | analgesic, antispasmodic, decongestant |
| Lavender *Lavandula angustifolia* | analgesic, antispasmodic, calming, sedative, tonic |
| Marjoram (sweet) *Origanum majorana* | analgesic, antispasmodic, calming, neurotonic |
| Peppermint *Mentha x piperita* | analgesic, decongestant, hormone-like (ovarian stimulant) |
| Pine *Pinus sylvestris* | analgesic, decongestant |
| Rosemary *Rosmarinus officinalis* | analgesic, antispasmodic, decongestant |
| **irregular, scanty and/or lack of periods** | |
| Mix a blend using the hormone-like essential oils (above). Other possibilities include: | |
| Chamomile (Roman) *Chamaemelum nobile* | calming, menstrual regulator, nervous menstrual problems |
| Melissa *Melissa officinalis* | calming, sedative, regularizes secretions |
| Rose otto *Rosa damascena* | general reproductive system regulator |
| **heavy periods** | |
| Cypress *Cupressus sempervirens* | astringent, phlebotonic, hormone-like (ovary problems) |
| Melissa *Melissa officinalis* | calming, sedative, regularizes secretions |
| **fluid retention** | |
| Cypress *Cupressus sempervirens* | diuretic (oedema, rheumatic swelling) |
| Fennel *Foeniculum vulgare* | diuretic (cellulite, oedema) |
| Juniper *Juniperus communis* | diuretic (cellulite, oedema) |
| Sage *Salvia officinalis* | decongestant, lypolytic (cellulite) |

| ESSENTIAL OIL | TREATMENT |
|---|---|
| **low spirits (depression) and fatigue** | |
| Basil *Ocimum basilicum* var. *album* | nervous system regulator (anxiety), neurotonic (convalescence, depression) |
| Chamomile (Roman) *Chamaemelum nobile* | calming (nervous depression, nervous shock) |
| Clary sage *Salvia sclarea* | neurotonic (nervous fatigue) |
| Geranium *Pelargonium graveolens* | relaxant (anxiety, debility, nervous fatigue) |
| Juniper *Juniperus communis* | neurotonic (debility, fatigue) |
| Marjoram (sweet) *Origanum majorana* | neurotonic (debility, mental instability, anguish, nervous depression) |
| Pine *Pinus sylvestris* | neurotonic (debility, fatigue) |
| Rosemary *Rosmarinus officinalis* | neurotonic (general debility and fatigue) |
| **tender, congested breasts** | |
| Eucalyptus *Eucalyptus smithii* (not *Eucalyptus globulus*) | analgesic, decongestant |
| Geranium *Pelargonium graveolens* | analgesic, decongestant |
| **headaches** | |
| Chamomile (Roman) *Chamaemelum nobile* | antispasmodic, calming, sedative |
| Lavender *Lavandula angustifolia* | analgesic, calming, sedative |
| Marjoram (sweet) *Origanum majorana* | analgesic, antispasmodic, calming |
| Melissa *Melissa officinalis* | calming, sedative |
| Peppermint *Mentha x piperita* | analgesic, antispasmodic |
| Rosemary *Rosmarinus officinalis* | analgesic, antispasmodic, decongestant |
| **insomnia** | |
| Basil *Ocimum basilicum* var. *album* | nervous system regulator (nervous insomnia) |
| Chamomile (Roman) *Chamaemelum nobile* | calming, sedative |
| Lavender *Lavandula angustifolia* | calming, sedative |
| Lemon *Citrus limon* | calming |
| Melissa *Melissa officinalis* | calming, sedative |
| **irritability** | |
| Chamomile (Roman) *Chamaemelum nobile* | calming, sedative |

# Preparing for pregnancy

Once the menstrual cycle begins, becoming pregnant is a possibility until periods end at the menopause. Once an egg is fertilized, the body's hormones begin to change and can give rise to many symptoms, some of which can be helped with essential oils.

## after conception

A normal pregnancy lasts approximately nine months. It is divided into three periods of approximately three months, known as trimesters. Once you realize that you are pregnant, you may experience a variety of emotions, ranging from joy and delight to fear and apprehension. Towards the end of the first trimester your breasts may feel tender and your appetite may increase. At this stage you may develop a heightened sense of smell, and this may start to affect your food preferences.

The second trimester is probably the most enjoyable, as you gradually become accustomed to the physical and emotional aspects of having a baby. During this time, you can benefit from using essential oils to help with some of the stresses and strains you may be experiencing as you adjust to

the changes that are taking place in your body. Remember that any essential oils you use for yourself will also reach your baby, and they should be used with care and common sense if you are both to reap the benefits.

By the third trimester you will look well and truly pregnant and your body will start to feel heavy and cumbersome. During this time you need more rest, preferably with your feet up, and you will be starting to make preparations for labour.

Throughout the pregnancy be sure to eat well. You also need to look after your teeth: your baby will take from you what-ever nutrition he or she needs and it is you who will be deprived of essential nutrients such as calcium and iron. Listen to your body: a food craving can often indicate your baby's and your own body's needs. For example, a craving for cheese could mean your body needs more calcium and protein.

## cautions during pregnancy

You may not know you are pregnant until two months have already passed. If you are trying to conceive, you should use only the

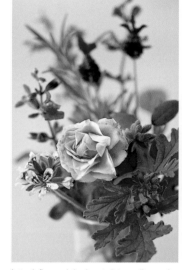

△ **Fresh flowers bring beauty into our lives and stimulate feelings of happiness and well-being.**

more popular essential oils, in general use, at this time. By the fifth month of pregnancy, the baby should be firmly attached to the uterus, and any essential oils can be used. All essential oils should be used only in the recommended dosage.

Some essential oils have components in them which may induce a period or which can affect the nervous system if overused. Some of these oils may help to stimulate the uterus into action, and they should be used only when labour commences, to relieve labour pains. Used correctly, essential oils can alleviate many of the minor discomforts of pregnancy. Many women also find them invaluable during labour to ease pain and to facilitate delivery. However, some controversy exists surrounding the use of some essential oils during pregnancy.

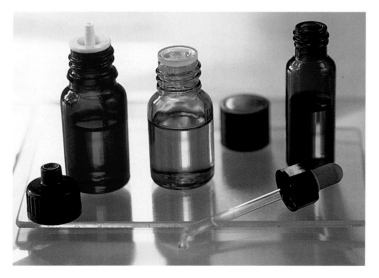

◁ **Two essential oils can be mixed together in an easy-to-use dropper bottle for effective self-treatment at home.**

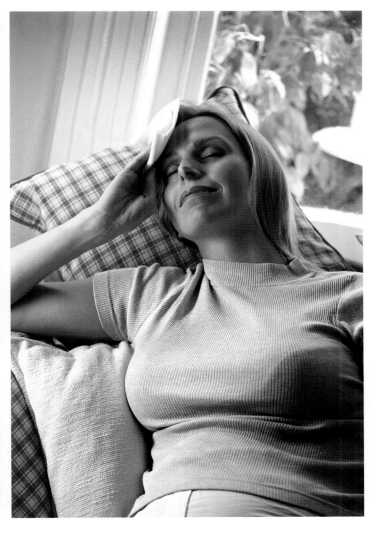

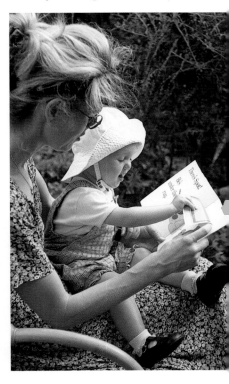

◁ A cool lavender compress can ease a tension headache. Lie or sit quietly in a place where you won't be disturbed and apply the compress to your temples or forehead until relief is felt.

▽ Whether this is your first pregnancy or whether you are already a mother, preparing for a new baby is an exciting time for all the family.

A few essential oils have the ability to stimulate uterine contractions, and could possibly cause miscarriage if taken in excessive amounts or taken internally during the first three to four months of pregnancy. Other oils can have an effect on the nervous system and the liver, and could be toxic when taken in too high a dose.

When oils are used correctly, the risks are very slight because of the low dosage involved (generally, five to ten drops at any one time). Women who have a history of miscarriage may be most at risk but, in any case, it is always better to err on the side of safety. Use only those essential oils which do not appear in any literature as being hazardous during pregnancy. There are many oils which will do you no harm at all but, if you are in any doubt about using an essential oil while pregnant, you should consult a qualified aromatherapist.

Whether pregnant or trying to start a family, the important thing to remember is that anything taken into the body, whether it is food, drink, nicotine, alcohol, or any other substance, will have an effect upon the system. Sensible eating with plenty of sleep and regular exercise is the best way to look after yourself and prepare your body and mind for motherhood.

### OILS TO AVOID DURING THE FIRST HALF OF PREGNANCY

Although all essential oils are safe when used with care and knowledge, it is advised that you avoid the following oils, which can promote menstruation:

- aniseed *Pimpinella anisum*
- fennel *Foeniculum vulgare*
- nutmeg *Myristica fragrans*
- sage *Salvia officinalis*
- yarrow *Achillea millefolium*

In addition, avoid any essential oil that is new to you at this time.

# Using aromatherapy in pregnancy

Essential oils can bring relief from the many minor troubles which can occur during pregnancy. Discomforts commonly experienced by women include morning sickness, backache, oedema (swollen legs and ankles), constipation, varicose veins, digestive problems (including heartburn), leg cramps and exhaustion. Coping with these discomforts can be especially difficult while the woman is working or if there is a small child or children to look after in the home. Essential oils are also useful during labour, to ease pain and to facilitate delivery.

## morning sickness

Nausea, which typically occurs in the morning, is often one of the first signs that a woman is pregnant. Inhalations with a vaporizer can be helpful at bedtime and first thing in the morning. The oils can be left to vaporize overnight in the bedroom. If the sickness persists through the day, prepare a tissue with the relevant oils, and keep it with you at all times.

## constipation

This is also another early sign of pregnancy. Prepare essential oils in a suitable carrier base and apply them to the abdomen in a

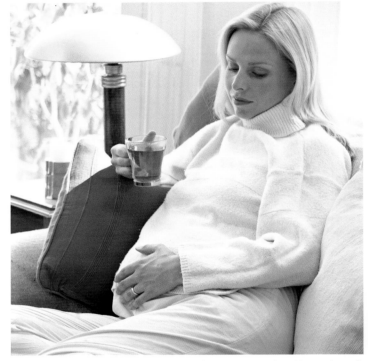

△ As your pregnancy proceeds, you will feel your baby's first movements. Setting aside some time each day to relax and be with your unborn child can help the mother-child bonding process.

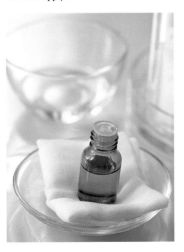

◁ Add a few drops of bitter orange to a bowl of water and make a compress to ease constipation.

clockwise direction. Alternatively, use the oils in the bath and/or on a compress. Eating a healthy diet and drinking plenty of water will help to reduce the risk of constipation.

## stretch marks

By the beginning of the second trimester, your clothes will be feeling tighter as your abdomen swells. Halfway through this trimester you will be able to feel the baby's first movements (an exciting moment). Start using essential oils at this time to prevent stretch marks on the skin of the abdomen. Through the correct and diligent

application of appropriate essential oils it is possible to maintain a supple and undamaged skin, and you will greatly appreciate your efforts after the baby is born.

Prepare a carrier base (include calendula oil) containing oils with regenerative and skin-toning properties. The mixture should be applied to the abdomen twice daily, morning and night. The area to be covered increases as the pregnancy proceeds, and will include the sides of the body, the groin and on and above the breasts.

## backache

As your baby grows, so the likelihood of backache increases. Sitting and standing with correct posture can go a long way to minimize backache, but it will usually occur at some stage and can be helped with essential oils when it does. Prepare a carrier base, then add the appropriate oils and ask a friend or your partner to give you a back massage, ideally at bedtime. Try using the same essential oils (but without the carrier oil) in the bath. Include basil and marjoram in the massage-mix; these can also be used if you suffer from leg cramps later on.

## heartburn

The growing baby may also put pressure on your stomach, causing indigestion and heartburn. For heartburn, add 2 drops each of mandarin and peppermint oils to 10 ml (2 tsp) carrier base and apply to the painful area. These oils can also be inhaled neat from a tissue or cupped hands, breathing deeply.

## varicose veins, swollen legs and ankles

It is as well for all women to watch out for early signs of these conditions through-out pregnancy. Resting with the feet and legs raised is beneficial for all leg conditions. Although the essential oils are different for each condition, the method of use is the same. Prepare a carrier base and add the oils.

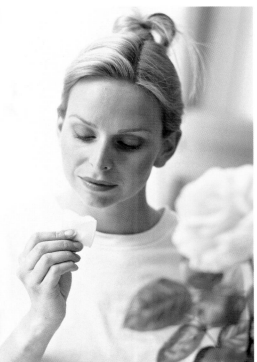

◁ **Your growing baby can cause painful heartburn. Put two drops each of mandarin and peppermint on a tissue and sniff throughout the day.**

▽ **Backache is a common complaint of pregnancy. Ask your partner for a back massage, using basil and marjoram, before going to bed.**

Apply the mixture to the whole leg, then bring your hands firmly from the foot up to the knee, before returning to the foot to start again. Massage only in an upward direction, to encourage blood flow to the heart. For varicose veins on the upper leg, massage upwards, going only from knee to groin – not back again – several times.

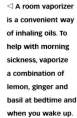

◁ **A room vaporizer is a convenient way of inhaling oils. To help with morning sickness, vaporize a combination of lemon, ginger and basil at bedtime and when you wake up.**

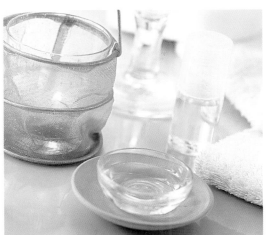

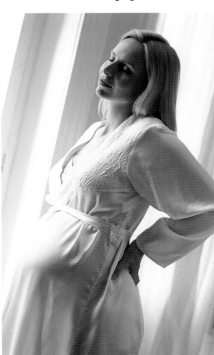

# Ante-natal bodycare

During the last trimester of pregnancy, it is a good idea to prepare for labour and to discuss with your midwife or doctor how you would like the birth to proceed. It is helpful to attend prenatal classes, especially if it is the birth of your first child. The classes teach useful exercises to help you relax when the time for labour comes.

## preparing for labour

Much of the pain of childbirth, particularly with a first child, is due to the muscles at the neck of the uterus and the perineum being tense and/or inflexible, which means they can tear when stretched. This can be eased by the application of muscle-relaxing essential oils in a vegetable carrier oil. If application is begun daily from several weeks before the expected birth date, the area can be made supple and soft. This will prepare it for the enormous amount of expansion needed for the baby to be born.

Massage a little of the mix twice daily around the perineum area, and try inserting your fingers into the neck of the womb to stretch it, thus helping to prevent tearing.

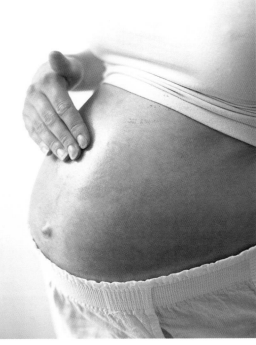

◁ To prevent stretch marks, geranium and frankincense, in a calendula oil carrier, should be massaged on to the abdomen area twice daily.

▽ Massage the lower leg in an upwards direction to relieve aches and oedema.

As you get heavier, remember to keep increasing the area to which you are applying your essential oil blend to prevent stretch marks, taking your mix round the sides of your body, on to the upper part of your thighs and above your breasts. It is also important at this time to rest your legs at regular intervals (from every five minutes to half an hour, if you suspect you are likely to develop varicose veins).

As the time for the birth approaches, you may experience conflicting emotions and mood swings. Using uplifting essential oils can give you inner strength to cope with all that is in store for you during this very exciting time in your life.

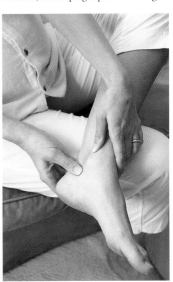

◁ Make regular checks for oedema on your feet and ankles as your pregnancy progresses. If symptoms occur, a massage plan can help.

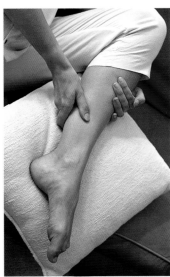

# Relief treatments for labour

There are some oils which are particularly useful in labour. In the past, these were limited to lavender and clary sage for their calming and relaxing effects. However, there are a few oils with womb-stimulant and analgesic properties, and these can help with contractions: aniseed, clove bud, nutmeg and sage. These oils are *absolutely not* advocated for the first four months of pregnancy and should not be used until the last week, when labour is about to begin. Used correctly, these oils can help to make the birth easier and quicker, especially for a first-time mother. They are used to relieve pain and induce sleep, and will have a soothing, dulling, lulling effect. Clove bud is particularly analgesic and nutmeg is an effective sedative.

## treatment

Try a mix of two drops each of any two of the oils with four drops of lavender on a tissue, and inhale between contractions. Some women like to put the tissue into the switched-off gas and air machine, which seems to have the psychological effect of making the oils more efficient.

Alternatively, blend three drops each of aniseed, nutmeg and peppermint with eight drops of lavender into 50 ml (2 fl oz) carrier oil, and ask your partner to massage your feet and lower legs every half hour. Apply the same mix to your own hands and shoulders, if preferred.

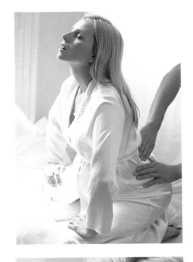

▷ **Lower back pain can be eased by massage. Ask your partner to rub the painful areas.**

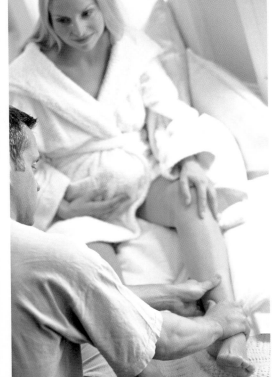

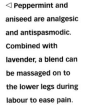

◁ **Peppermint and aniseed are analgesic and antispasmodic. Combined with lavender, a blend can be massaged on to the lower legs during labour to ease pain.**

▷ **Inhalation is the fastest method for an oil's aroma to reach the brain. Aniseed and lavender are calming and can help with contractions.**

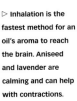

▷ **Nutmeg is a very useful oil for the last stages of labour as it relieves pain and can facilitate delivery. Consult a qualified aromatherapist if you wish to use it.**

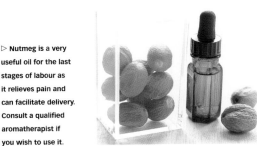

# Post-natal bodycare

Essential oils can be used to help with the common emotional stresses and physical problems arising as a result of the birth.

Use 6 drops of the appropriate essential oils blended in 20 ml (4 tsp) of calendula oil for application. Alternatively, use them on their own for inhalation or in the bath.

## birth wounds

During the birth, the perineum may be bruised and/or torn, and can be very painful afterwards. Using the three perineum oils, gently apply them several times a day. If the area is too painful to touch, use a compress (see Aromatherapy Techniques).

## breast feeding problems

Always apply the appropriate essential oils immediately after each feed, so that they are completely absorbed by your body before the baby's next feed is due.

**Insufficient milk:** Fennel oil encourages milk production. Fennel will also help to keep the baby's excreta normal and can help to relieve any wind.
**Too much milk:** 2 drops of peppermint oil with 4 drops of geranium oil can be used in a massage all over the breasts.
**Cracked nipples or mastitis:** Use 2 drops of each essential oil listed opposite.

## emotional difficulties

After the birth, it will take a while before your hormones return to normal. This can be a stressful time as you have a new baby to care for just when you are feeling in need of care yourself. Fatigue, anxiety, despondency and emotional imbalances are common. Essential oils can help before post-natal depression sets in. Blend oils for use by inhalation, in the bath or by application.

## treating your baby

Essential oils can help you and your baby cope with the everyday, minor ailments which many babies are subject to, such as

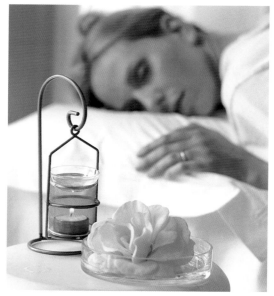

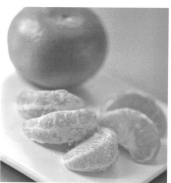

△ The gentle action of mandarin makes it a good choice for treating colic and digestive disorders.

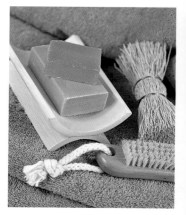

◁ After a long and exhausting labour, and with a new baby to look after, make sure you get enough sleep. Burn lavender through the night to relax and refresh you.

▽ Once your baby is born, pamper yourself and invest in some good quality skincare products.

indigestion, colic, constipation and/or diarrhoea, minor infections and nappy rash. For nappy rash, use 15 ml (3 tsp) base lotion with 5 ml (1 tsp) calendula oil, mixed with one drop of peppermint and up to three drops of any other selected oils.

Babies can benefit from massage with essential oils. The massage will relax them and can help to strengthen the bond between mother and child. For application to babies, use one drop of essential oil per 5 ml (1 tsp) carrier lotion or oil. For sleep problems, try two to three drops of oil in a vaporizer in the baby's room, or try them on a tissue which is pinned to the baby's clothes or placed inside the pillowcase.

# Useful essential oils

| ESSENTIAL OIL | TREATMENT |
|---|---|
| **hormone-like essential oils** | |
| Chamomile (German) *Matricaria recutica* | hormone-like |
| Clary sage *Salvia sclarea* | oestrogen-like |
| Niaouli *Melaleuca viridiflora* | oestrogen-like (regularizes periods) |
| **backache** | |
| Basil *Ocimum basilicum* var. *album* | analgesic, antispasmodic |
| Lavender *Lavandula angustifolia* | analgesic, anti-inflammatory, antispasmodic |
| Marjoram (sweet) *Origanum majorana* | analgesic, antispasmodic |
| **constipation** | |
| Ginger *Zingiber officinale* | analgesic, digestive stimulant |
| Mandarin *Citrus reticulata* | antispasmodic, calming, digestive stimulant |
| Orange (bitter) *Citrus aurantium* var. *amara* | calming, digestive stimulant |
| Rosemary *Rosmarinus officinalis* | analgesic, digestive stimulant |
| **nausea** | |
| Basil *Ocimum basilicum* var. *album* | digestive tonic, nervous system regulator |
| Ginger *Zingiber officinale* | digestive |
| Lemon *Citrus limon* | anticoagulant, antispasmodic, calming, digestive |
| **stretch marks** | |
| Frankincense *Boswellia carteri* | cell regenerative, cicatrizant (scars) |
| Geranium *Pelargonium graveolens* | cell regenerative, cicatrizant (stretch marks) |
| Lavender *Lavandula angustifolia* | cicatrizant (scars) |
| **fluid retention** | |
| Fennel *Foeniculum vulgare* | diuretic (cellulite, oedema) |
| Juniper *Juniperus communis* | diuretic (cellulite, oedema) |
| Lemon *Citrus limon* | diuretic (obesity, oedema) |
| **varicose veins** | |
| Clary sage *Salvia sclarea* | phlebotonic (circulatory problems, haemorrhoids, varicose veins) |
| Cypress *Cupressus sempervirens* | phlebotonic (haemorrhoids, poor venous circulation, varicose veins) |
| Niaouli *Melaleuca viridiflora* | phlebotonic (haemorrhoids, varicose veins) |

| ESSENTIAL OIL | TREATMENT |
|---|---|
| **labour** | |
| Aniseed *Pimpinella anisum* | analgesic, antispasmodic, calming (gentle narcotic), emmenagogic, oestrogen-like, uterotonic |
| Lavender *Lavandula angustifolia* | analgesic, antispasmodic, calming (anxiety), sedative |
| Nutmeg *Myristica fragrans* | analgesic, sedative (narcotic), neurotonic, uterotonic |
| Peppermint *Mentha x piperita* | analgesic, antispasmodic, hormone-like (ovarian stimulant), neurotonic, uterotonic (facilitates delivery) |
| **perineum** | |
| Geranium *Pelargonium graveolens* | analgesic, cicatrizant (wounds) |
| Lavender *Lavandula angustifolia* | analgesic, antiseptic (bruises) |
| Rosemary *Rosmarinus officinalis* | analgesic, anti-inflammatory |
| **breast milk** | |
| Fennel *Foeniculum vulgare* | lactogenic (promotes milk), oestrogen-like (insufficient milk) |
| Geranium *Pelargonium graveolens* | decongestant (breast congestion – for too much milk) |
| Peppermint *Mentha x piperita* | antilactogenic (prevents milk forming) |
| **cracked nipples or mastitis** | |
| Chamomile (German) *Matricaria recutica* | cicatrizant (infected wounds, ulcers) |
| Geranium *Pelargonium graveolens* | cicatrizant (burns, cuts, ulcers, wounds) |
| Lavender *Lavandula angustifolia* | cicatrizant (burns, scars, varicose veins, wounds) |
| **nappy rash** | |
| Patchouli *Pogostemon patchouli* | anti-inflammatory, cicatrizant (cracked skin, scar tissue) |
| Peppermint *Mentha x piperita* | analgesic, anti-inflammatory, soothing (skin irritation, rashes) |
| **post-natal depression** | |
| Basil *Ocimum basilicum* var. *album* | nervous system regulator (anxiety), neurotonic (convalescence, depression) |
| Chamomile (Roman) *Chamaemelum nobile* | calming (nervous depression, nervous shock) |

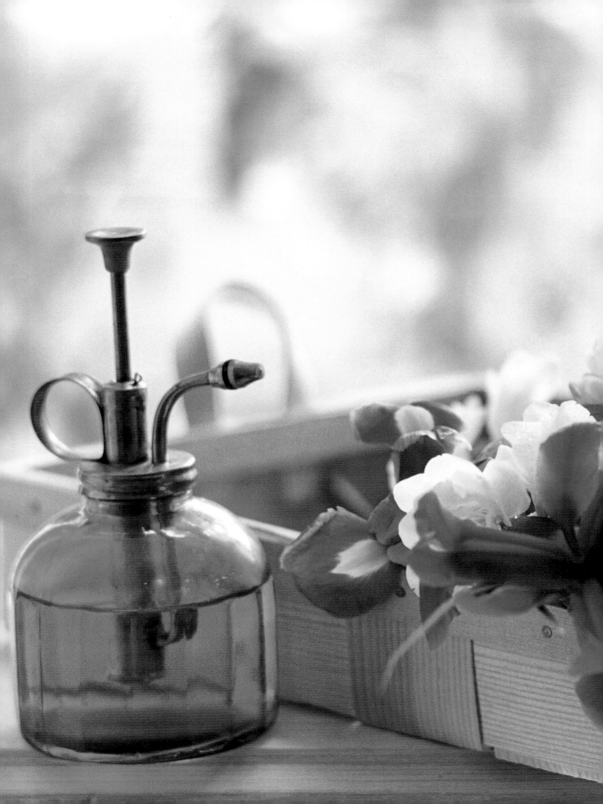

# The Sunset Years

The onset of the menopause can bring with it physical and emotional problems that can be relieved by the use of essential oils. As we continue to age, essential oil treatments can play their part as a safeguard against the onset of more serious concerns of circulatory disorders, arthritis and digestive problems.

# The menopause

The word menopause derives from the Greek words for month, *men*, and halt, *pausis*. It refers to the end of menstruation, when a woman's ovaries no longer produce eggs for fertilization and her periods stop. The accepted average age at which the menopause occurs is 51, with around five per cent of women ceasing their periods before they are 45.

The menopause does not happen overnight. It is a gradual process brought about by growing irregularity in, and gradual reduction of, the reproductive hormones, oestrogen and progesterone. Oestrogen is probably the most important hormone concerned with a woman's health: it helps to lower cholesterol levels, protect against heart attacks and strokes, to preserve bone tissue and regulate mood and behaviour patterns. Instability occurs in the mental and physical body because of these reduced hormone levels. The early stages of the menopause can present similar emotional imbalances to PMS, and physical symptoms, to varying degrees of severity, may also develop.

As with menstruation, different women will be affected in different ways by the menopause. For women who have had a lifetime of period-associated problems, the menopause may come as a welcome relief.

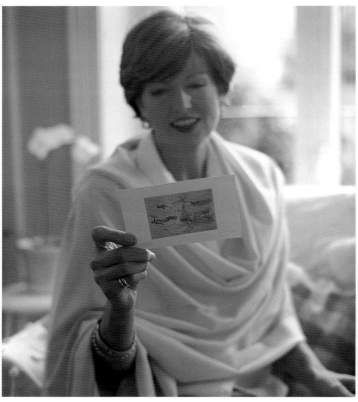

△ **The menopause is a major life transition. How we cope with it will depend to some extent on our mental attitude. Staying in touch with friends and leading an active life can help us to feel positive.**

She is clothed with strength and

dignity and can laugh at years to

come. She speaks with wisdom and

faithful instruction is on her tongue.

*From Proverbs 31:25 The Holy Bible.*

Once a woman's periods have stopped for a year, there is no longer any need to worry about becoming pregnant or, therefore, to practise any form of birth control. Some women experience few or no problems at all with the menopause, yet for others, this can be a difficult time as their bodies adjust to a major life change.

Other physical changes may be noticed, affecting the skin and hair, the activity of the thyroid glands and the distribution of body fat. Some women may experience sudden haemorrhaging, headaches, dizzy spells and sleep disturbances.

## osteoporosis

One of the more serious potential side effects of the menopause is the development of osteoporosis, which is caused by lack of oestrogen production. This is when the bones of the body become increasingly fragile and brittle. The bones fracture easily, particularly at the more vulnerable points such as the wrists, ankles or hip joints in the event of physical stress, such as a fall. Osteoporosis is also responsible for the eventual development of stooping shoulders in older women, often referred to as a "dowager's hump".

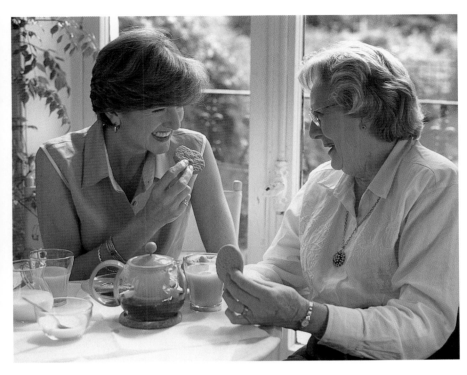

◁ With the children grown up, you are likely to have more time for yourself. Now is a good time to catch up with family and friends.

## Hormone replacement therapy

Advances in medical science now mean that synthetic hormone replacements can offset the symptoms of the menopause. Many women decide to try hormone replacement therapy (HRT) if they find that the discomforts of the menopause are affecting their quality of life. HRT is not suitable for all women, however, and much will depend on the needs and medical background of the individual. Because HRT is still a relatively new treatment, its long-term effects are not yet fully known. Treatments are now available from your doctor which are made with natural progesterone. These are believed to be safer than treatments using synthetic oestrogen, and this will make them popular with many women.

Some menopausal symptoms can also be helped by aromatherapy. Clary sage is one of several oestrogen-like essential oils. It is worth using essential oils on a regular basis to see how your symptoms are affected before deciding on HRT.

▽ Clary sage and cypress can help with night sweats. Prepare a mix and use it at bedtime.

**COMMON SYMPTOMS OF THE MENOPAUSE**

- Hot flushes
- Night sweats
- Depression
- Sweating
- Fatigue
- Water retention
- Vaginal dryness

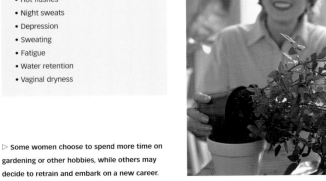

▷ Some women choose to spend more time on gardening or other hobbies, while others may decide to retrain and embark on a new career.

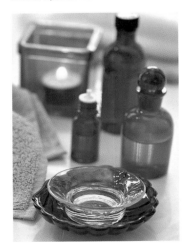

# Common symptoms of menopause

Although a large percentage of women have no problems with the menopause, many do experience some discomfort.

## night sweats

These are best tackled through preventative treatment. Try taking an aromatherapy bath with the relevant oils each night before bedtime. Alternatively, try massaging the oils in a suitable carrier base into the body.

## hot flushes

Put 20 drops of the same blend of essential oils in 1 litre (1¾ pints) of spring water in a screw-topped bottle. Fit the lid, shake well and transfer some into a purse-size spray and some into a small bottle that you can carry around with you. As soon as you feel a flush coming on, drink two mouthfuls of the water and spray your face and neck. Vitamin E is also said to be effective.

## water retention and bloating

To reduce water retention and cellulite, the relevant essential oils should be added to a suitable carrier base and applied daily to the affected areas. The same oils can also be used neat in the bath.

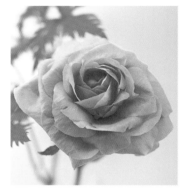

△ **Rose otto can help with haemorrhaging. It is also useful for both loss of libido and dry skin.**

## hair and skin

The condition of the hair and skin can be affected by the hormonal changes of the menopause. Both will become thinner and drier, and it is a good idea to adapt your daily care regime to compensate.

### hair

For hair dryness, use a good conditioner. You may like to add appropriate essential oils to give extra shine. For thinning hair, try a daily scalp massage with essential oils (see Aromatherapy Techniques).

### skin

This not only becomes drier, but is more prone to wrinkles. Try a product containing essential oils or prepare your own mix.

## haemorrhaging

Occasional and sudden bleeding can occur when you least expect it. Although essential oils can reduce the amount of blood loss, as far as we know, they do not seem to stop it happening. As a preventative measure, try using styptic and/or astringent essential oils if you are prone to haemorrhaging.

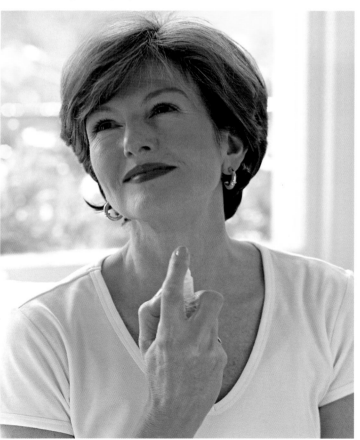

◁ **Peppermint and cypress are useful for hot flushes. Make up a mix and use it in an atomizer.**

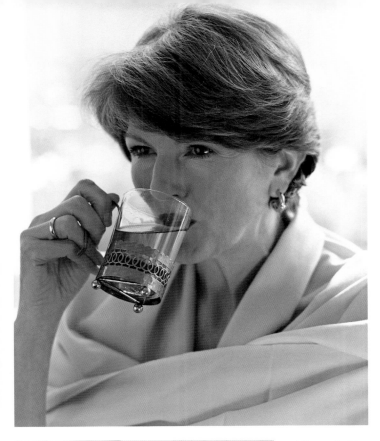

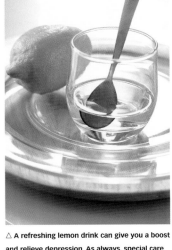

△ A refreshing lemon drink can give you a boost and relieve depression. As always, special care should be taken with oils for internal use.

△ If you are having difficulties sleeping, a soothing cup of sweet marjoram and chamomile tea in the evening can help.

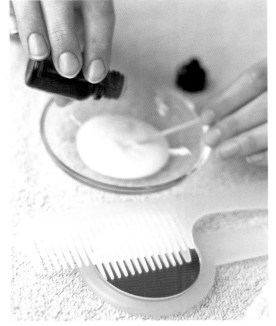

◁ Make your own beauty products by adding combinations of your favourite oils to quality base creams and lotions.

## heart and circulation problems

In developed countries, arterial disease is the commonest cause of death for women over 50, killing one in four. This is almost twice as high as the death-rate from cancer.

There are as yet no essential oils known to treat problems with the heart, and it is advisable to check with your doctor and your family history to see if you are at risk. In the meantime, you can help to prevent heart and blood-pressure problems by giving up smoking, avoiding fatty foods and drinks high in caffeine, eating a low-cholesterol diet and taking enough regular exercise. There are also some carrier oils reputed to reduce cholesterol levels.

## vaginal dryness

This can cause both emotional and physical discomfort. There are no known essential oils to increase vaginal fluid. Vitamin E is reputed to improve vaginal secretion, and daily application of sunflower oil all round the vaginal opening may also help.

# Emotions during menopause

For many women the menopause will coincide with their children leaving home. It can represent a new lease of life as a woman suddenly finds that she has more time for herself. However, as with any major life change, the menopause is often accompanied by mixed feelings, and a woman's new-found freedom may be marred not only by physical symptoms but also by emotional disturbances.

## stress-related headaches and sleep disturbances

These disturbances are not necessarily linked to the menopause, and may be stress-related. However, should either of them bother you, inhalation and application of the appropriate essential oils can help.

## weight and diet

Appearance is often important to a woman throughout her life. It is not surprising, then, that poor self-esteem and a lack of confidence can be triggered by the physical changes happening in her body at this time.

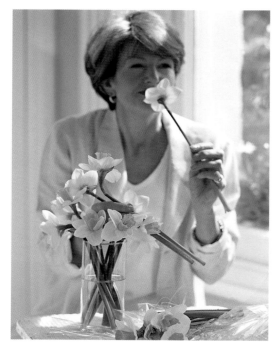

◁ During the menopause, you may experience strong mood swings. Try to keep things in proportion and take pleasure from the simple things in life.

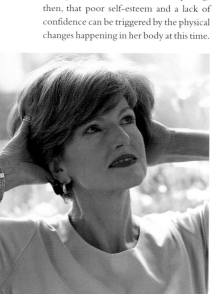

△ When you are feeling tired and irritable, a head massage can help you to relax and unwind.

Water retention can lead to bloating and weight-gain which, in turn, will exacerbate any feelings of low self-esteem. Tackle this with a positive frame of mind and healthy eating habits – these two things combined will improve self-confidence. Essential oils used for low spirits may help weight loss by stimulating the nervous system.

> **EMOTIONAL DISTURBANCES OF THE MENOPAUSE**
> - Irritability
> - Lack of confidence
> - Anxiety and depression
> - Poor concentration, forgetfulness and memory problems
> - Decrease in self-esteem: through weight gain, lack of interest in sex, changes in physical appearance

## tips for healthy eating and drinking
- Drink plenty of water.
- Limit alcohol intake to two units a day.
- Cut down on caffeine drinks.
- Cut down on, or avoid, sugary foods and foods high in fat.
- Eat more fish and less meat (especially red meat); eat plenty of fruit and vegetables, especially those rich in Vitamin C.
- Include foods rich in calcium.

## loss of sex drive

For some women, the menopause is marked by a decrease in sex drive (conversely, some women also report an increase in libido). The reduction in vaginal fluid can make intercourse painful, and this can lead to a change in sexual desire.

Several essential oils are reputed to help with sexual problems and to increase desire. These oils relax the mind, relieving it from pressures and tensions and, at the same time, can stimulate the emotions. Use the appropriate oils in a vaporizer for an hour before retiring, in both the living room and the bedroom. Alternatively, sprinkle a few drops of the oils on to your pillow and exchange a gentle back and shoulder aromatherapy massage with your partner.

## relationship difficulties

The physical and emotional difficulties of the menopause can put a strain on your relationship with your partner. If your children are leaving home, now may be a good time to re-define your partnership. It can help to blend stress-relieving essential oils with oils which correspond to your emotions, such as anger, fear or jealousy.

▷ **Emotional upsets are stressful and can lead to muscular tension. Rub oils on to your shoulders and neck to help restore your equilibrium.**

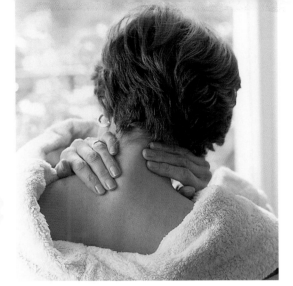

# Useful essential oils

| ESSENTIAL OIL | TREATMENT |
|---|---|
| **hot flushes and sweating** | |
| Clary sage *Salvia sclarea* | antisudorific, oestrogen-like (sweating) |
| Cypress *Cupressus sempervirens* | antisudorific (excessive perspiration) |
| Peppermint *Mentha x piperita* | cooling |
| Pine *Pinus sylvestris* | antisudorific (sweating) |
| **reputed sexual stimulants** | |
| Peppermint *Mentha x piperita* | neurotonic, reproductive tonic |
| Rosemary *Rosmarinus officinalis* | neurotonic, sexual tonic |
| Rose otto *Rosa damascena* | neurotonic, sexual tonic |
| Thyme (sweet) *Thymus vulgaris* | cardiotonic, immunostimulant, neurotonic, sexual tonic |
| Ylang ylang *Cananga odorata* | reproductive tonic |
| **low spirits (depression) and fatigue** | |
| Basil *Ocimum basilicum* var. *album* | neurotonic debility, mental strain, depression |
| Chamomile (Roman) *Chamaemelum nobile* | calming (nervous depression, irritability, nervous shock) |
| Clary sage *Salvia sclarea* | neurotonic (nervous fatigue) |
| Cypress *Cupressus sempervirens* | neurotonic (debility) |
| Frankincense *Boswellia carteri* | antidepressive (nervous depression) |
| Geranium *Pelargonium graveolens* | neurotonic (debility, nervous fatigue) |
| Juniper *Juniperus communis* | neurotonic (debility, fatigue) |
| Marjoram (sweet) *Origanum majorana* | neurotonic (debility, anguish, agitation, nervous depression) |
| Rosemary *Rosmarinus officinalis* | neurotonic (general debility and fatigue) |

| ESSENTIAL OIL | TREATMENT |
|---|---|
| **fluid retention and cellulite** | |
| Cypress *Cupressus sempervirens* | diuretic (oedema, rheumatic swelling) |
| Geranium *Pelargonium graveolens* | decongestant (lymphatic congestion) |
| **headaches and sleep problems** | |
| Chamomile (Roman) *Chamaemelum nobile* | antispasmodic, calming (migraines, insomnia, irritability) |
| Lavender *Lavandula angustifolia* | analgesic, calming (headaches, migraines, insomnia – low dose) |
| Marjoram (sweet) *Origanum majorana* | analgesic, calming (agitation, migraines, insomnia) |
| **headaches and migraines only** | |
| Peppermint *Mentha x piperita* | analgesic (headaches, migraine) |
| Rosemary *Rosmarinus officinalis* | decongestant (headaches, migraine) |
| **irritability** | |
| Chamomile (Roman) *Chamaemelum nobile* | calming (irritability, nervous depression, nervous shock) |
| Cypress *Cupressus sempervirens* | calming (irritability), regulates sympathetic nervous system |
| **haemorrhage** | |
| Cypress *Cupressus sempervirens* | astringent, phlebotonic (broken capillaries, varicose veins) |
| Rose otto *Rosa damascena* | astringent, styptic (wounds) |

# Aging gracefully

Once the menopause is over women enter a new phase of life, sometimes referred to as "the sunset years", before reaching old-age. During these years it is especially important for women to take care of themselves so as to prolong a happy, healthy and active life.

During the aging process, circulation slows down and the body's cells neither receive nourishment nor have harmful toxins eliminated as quickly as before. As a result, circulatory disorders are common: the hands and feet become cold, and wounds take longer to heal, for example. Digestive disorders in the elderly are also quite common. As the digestive processes slow down and the large intestine muscles weaken, constipation may occur. This is made more likely by inadequate roughage and fibre in the diet, and can also be seen as a side effect of other medicines. Eating while anxious or frightened can also bring on a variety of digestive disorders.

All cell renewal takes longer with age, the skin becomes dry and flaky, and the hair often becomes thinner. Because of this

> **An essence of balm (melissa) given in Canary wine every morning will renew youth, strengthen the brain, relieve languishing nature and prevent baldness.**
>
> *From the London Dispensary, 1696.*

slowing down process, every organ of every system in the body is more susceptible to common illnesses, which are more difficult to shake off. Older people are particularly vulnerable to colds and 'flu, which can settle on the chest, causing or exacerbating respiratory problems such as bronchitis and asthma. The joints gradually become less

flexible and the muscles are more prone to inflammation, and conditions such as arthritis or rheumatism may develop or get worse. As it is often first highlighted during the menopause, osteoporosis can become a problem, with the skeletal bones becoming more brittle: falls resulting in broken bones, such as the hip, are much more common in later years.

For many women, the prospect of old age is very frightening and creates tension and anxiety. Many women worry about the possibility of incapacitating illnesses, such as dementia, Parkinson's or Alzheimer's disease. Others suffer frequent headaches, migraines, insomnia and digestive upsets, which may be caused by the side effects of medical drugs that are being taken for other conditions. In fact, the side effects of medication can be responsible for many ailments apparent in older people. This can set up a vicious circle, where new medicines are prescribed to deal with the side effects of the original drug and which, in turn, can eventually lead to even more unpleasant

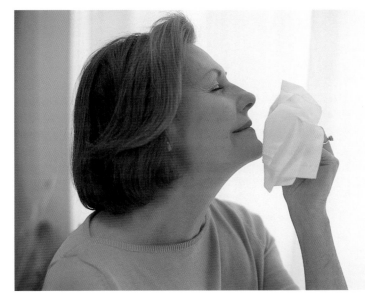

◁ **Extra care should be taken with a cold as it can develop into bronchitis. Use pine and niaouli on a tissue and inhale throughout the day.**

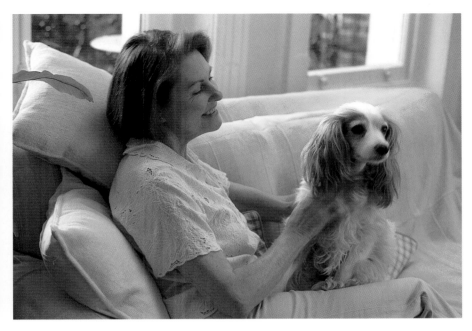

◁ Striking a healthy balance between relaxation and activity is important. Besides keeping you company, a dog will encourage you to take a daily walk.

symptoms. These resulting afflictions are termed iatrogenic because they arise as the side effects of medication taken for the original disease or problem. Aromatherapy is now used in a growing number of hospitals to alleviate the more minor, but unpleasant, effects of iatrogenic disease: insomnia and digestive disorders are the most common, followed by pressure sores for those who are bedridden.

## aromatherapy in later life

For women in their later years the amount of essential oils to be used in any treatment depends on the state of their general health. For those in good mental and physical health, the normal number of drops can be used. For women who are run down, suffering ill-health or are on medication the dosage should be lowered, as follows (*see also* Aromatherapy Techniques).

### dosage

**In the bath:** 4–6 drops of oil dispersed or dissolved first in dairy cream or honey
**For application to the body:** 8–10 drops in 50 ml (3½ tbsp) carrier lotion
**For inhalation:** The number of drops here is not crucial as many of the molecules are carried away by evaporation.

When preparing oils for application, a lotion is the preferred choice for a carrier base: oil bases can cause bottles to become too slippery and messy, often resulting in

oil stains. If you suffer from arthritis, for example, you can add the relevant essential oils to a base hand and/or body lotion, to make the treatment easier to administer.

◁ Holding a cotton pad with a few drops each of sweet marjoram and melissa to your head can relieve a tension headache. If it persists, try adding a few drops of Roman chamomile.

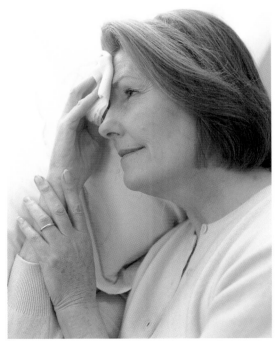

# Strengthening physical health

In our sunset years, we have the time to look after our health. Now is the time to use essential oils as a safeguard against problems starting in the first place.

## circulatory disorders

The regular daily use of hand and/or body lotion containing the appropriate essential oils will maintain a healthy circulation. Used early enough this could delay and, in some cases, prevent, many circulatory problems occurring.

After a stroke, the daily application of a lotion blend to legs and arms, in an upward direction only (to aid blood flow towards the heart), can help to regain movement in affected limbs.

## varicose ulcers

These ulcers can originate from varicose veins, but they can also arise as secondary symptoms of diabetes, sickle-cell anaemia and rheumatoid arthritis. Essential oils dispersed in water and sprayed on to the area is the best method if the ulcers are too raw to touch. A compress is the next step, followed by application with oils in a calendula base as soon as the area can be touched.

## arthritis, rheumatism and osteoarthritis

The main symptoms of arthritis are pain and stiffness, and of rheumatoid arthritis, inflammation and swelling around the joints, especially the knuckles, wrists, knees and ankles. Osteoarthritis is degeneration of the joint cartilage. A common site is the hip and, often, the only cure is to have an artificial hip replacement. Aromatherapy helps to alleviate pain and improve mobility in arthritic joints. The recommended treatment is the twice-daily use of a lotion containing relevant essential oils gently massaged into the affected knees or hips. Use overnight compresses for affected hands and feet.

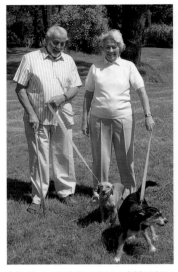

△ Gentle exercise helps to keep arthritis at bay and maintain a healthy circulatory system.

## bronchial asthma and bronchitis

Many of the expectorant essential oils, which ease breathing, come from the conifer and melaleuca families, such as pine and niaouli. Try application of the oils in a carrier lotion, rubbed into the chest at bedtime. If a visit to hospital is necessary for any reason, take the lotion with you as it will help to prevent infections, such as pneumonia, which are often picked up in hospital.

## influenza

Many essential oils are anti-infectious and can be of great help against influenza if they are used early enough: the sooner they are used after the onset of symptoms, the more likely they are to give a positive result. With the onset of a sore throat or fever, add the oils to water and use them as a gargle (see Aromatherapy Techniques). Try inhalations, a room vaporizer, aromatherapy baths, or direct application of the oils on to the body via a carrier lotion.

## Preparing a multi-purpose treatment cream

It can be very useful to have a ready-mixed treatment to hand in case it is needed urgently. Choose an unperfumed base cream and add your choice of appropriate essential oils.

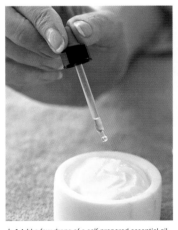

△ 1 Add a few drops of a self-prepared essential oil mix to your base cream. Use 5 drops of essential oil for every 50 ml base cream for a moisturizer.

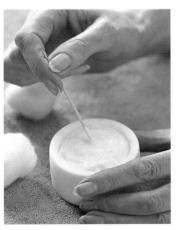

△ 2 Use a toothpick or the handle of a teaspoon to blend the oils into the cream. The prepared cream is ideal for use as a moisturizer or hand cream.

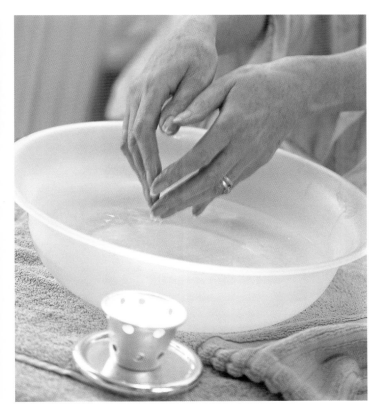

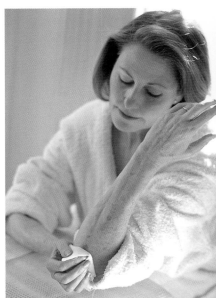

◁ If it is not possible to take a full aromatherapy bath, a hand or foot bath can be as effective for arthritic hands and feet. Add a few drops of your chosen oils to warm water and soak your hands for ten to fifteen minutes.

## incontinence

This upsetting condition can be helped by gentle exercise to strengthen the pelvic floor muscles. Lying on your back, tense and relax your pelvic muscles, by raising your hips 10–20 times a day, at regular intervals. Astringent essential oils can also be useful, taken internally in a tea (*see* Aromatherapy Techniques).

## pressure sores

If a woman becomes bed-bound she is at risk of developing pressure sores, which are notoriously difficult to heal. To prevent these, the patient should be moved every few hours so that she is not left too long in the same position. Rub a mix of essential oils in calendula into the buttock area every day. If weeping sores develop, prepare a mineral water mix (*see* Aromatherapy Techniques) with essential oils, shake well and use to spray on to the affected area.

## digestive problems

There are two ways to treat upsetting digestive problems with aromatherapy. The most effective way to treat digestive disorders with essential oils is by ingestion (*see* Aromatherapy Techniques). Ideally, you should consult a qualified aromatologist. If you do decide to treat yourself, it is imperative to use only genuine essential oils from a reputable supplier and to carefully follow the directions in this book.

Application of recommended essential oils can also give good results. The oils can be mixed in a carrier lotion and rubbed gently on to the abdomen in a clockwise direction, or applied on a compress and left on the abdomen overnight.

### indigestion

This can occur for a number of reasons: eating too much or too quickly, eating foods which are too rich, or through emotional causes such as worry, impatience and frustration. Essential oils are excellent for indigestion. Relevant essential oils can be used in an abdominal massage every 30 minutes before a meal.

### constipation

This may arise as a side-effect of medication or through emotional causes, such as fear and anxiety. Changes in environment and routine can also bring on constipation.

### diarrhoea

This may be due to anxiety, fear, infections, other medication or an overdose of laxatives taken to relieve constipation.

### diverticulitis

Small, harmless, thin-walled sacs can form on the colon in elderly people, through insufficient fibre in the diet. Diverticulitis is when these sacs become inflamed and painful, leading to occasional bleeding and chronic constipation. Switch to a fibre-rich diet, and use essential oils for constipation and other anti-inflammatory conditions.

△ Lavender oil soaked into a warm compress can help to relieve the pain of arthritic joints.

# Strengthening mental health

Physical health problems, minor or major, can become a source of worry and anxiety for an aging person, and can affect their overall mental and emotional health.

## headaches and migraines

The reason for these, especially in the elderly, is not always apparent. It is therefore a good idea to use two or more essential oils, to make best use of their synergy. Put the relevant essential oils into your moisturizing cream and use twice daily. This helps both to relieve and prevent the problem, and will benefit the skin at the same time. If headaches persist throughout the day, try inhalation. If the headaches frequently recur, consider that it may be due to a food allergy, such as caffeine. If home treatment is unsuccessful it may be worth visiting a qualified aromatherapist.

## shock

The emotional impact of shock can be particularly traumatic for an elderly person. Very often the shock is accompanied by fear, especially in the case of someone who lives on their own. Shock-induced trauma can be helped immediately by inhaling or applying essential oils with a sedative effect.

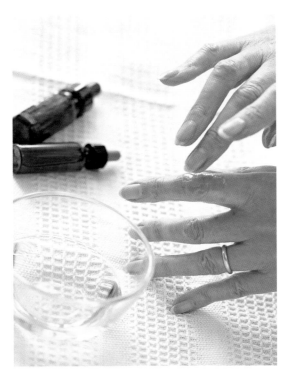

◁ **Oils for fear and anger can be a useful support for cancer patients. Use juniper, lemon and geranium in a base lotion and apply the mix to the hands and body.**

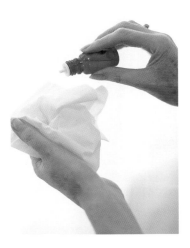

◁ **Lavender and sweet marjoram oils can help with grief and fear. Inhale them from a tissue.**

## insomnia

Insomnia is fairly common amongst older people, and can get worse as age advances. Sometimes, there is no clear explanation for it – older people seem to need less sleep. However, the problem may be caused or exacerbated by anxiety and worry. Cramp in the leg muscles or arthritic pain during the night can also disturb the sleep pattern. The traditional essential oil used to help insomnia is lavender, although care should be taken with the dose, as too much will keep you wide awake. Lavender oil, used alone or in a synergy with two or three oils, has been used successfully by some hospitals to treat insomnia.

## cancer

Aromatherapy cannot cure cancer but it can be used in a supportive role and can greatly improve the quality of life for many cancer patients. Fear of developing cancer can be a big worry for someone who has already lost a relative through the disease, and for cancer patients whose cancer is in remission. Use oils which are good for stress conditions (see Coping with Stress and Emotions), and apply by inhalation, compresses and direct application in a carrier lotion.

## dementia

Some people, more often in old age, suffer deterioration of their mental faculties, and are unable to think clearly or to concentrate for any length of time. The memory can become unreliable and confused, and some

▷ Persistent headaches are debilitating and stressful. Massaging the shoulders with Roman chamomile and lavender will have a sedative and calming effect, while peppermint and rosemary will be energizing and uplifting.

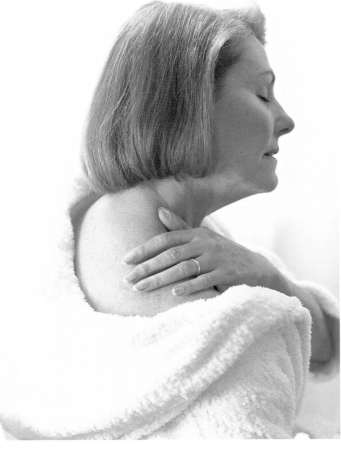

speech difficulties may develop (this is particularly true after a stroke). Alzheimer's disease may develop if the nerve tissue (which cannot regenerate itself) withers and dies in the brain. Try using essential oils which stimulate the mind and improve memory. Some oils are also thought to be able to trigger past experiences, which is helpful for people with Alzheimer's.

## Parkinson's disease

The cause of this debilitating, progressive disease is unknown, but a lack of the chemical substance, dopamine, which is needed for co-ordination of the brain muscles, seems to be responsible for its symptoms. Parkinson's disease is characterized by tremors, muscular rigidity and emaciation, and causes difficulty in speech and movement. Strong drugs are available to replace the dopamine; these help for a while, but they gradually lose efficiency as the body gets used to them. This necessitates a regular increase in dosage levels as the years pass, until, finally, the maximum dose loses its effect, and nothing more can be done to help the patient.

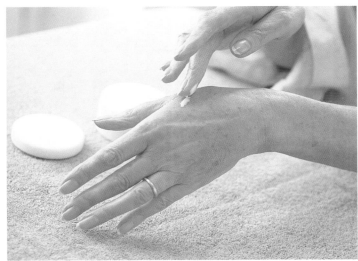

Side effects of the drugs include nausea, insomnia and constipation, all of which can be helped by aromatherapy. One study has also shown that essential oils can alleviate muscular problems, occasionally reducing the degree of slurred speech and tremors. Daily application of a lotion containing essential oils, plus daily aromatherapy baths (where possible) were used in the study. The symptoms which cause the most problems seem to be anxiety, lack of energy, muscular pains and stiffness. Others are constipation, insomnia, cramp, rigidity, tremors and slurred speech. Choose essential oils on the basis of the symptoms causing the trouble.

◁ For sufferers of Parkinson's disease, a hand and body lotion containing clary sage, sweet marjoram and rosemary can help the condition.

# Useful essential oils

| ESSENTIAL OIL | TREATMENT |
|---|---|
| **poor circulation** | |
| Clary sage *Salvia sclarea* | circulatory problems, haemorrhoids, varicose veins, venous aneurism, cholesterol |
| Lemon *Citrus limon* | poor circulation, thrombosis, varicose veins |
| Rosemary *Rosmarinus officinalis* | decongestant, poor circulation, hardening of the arteries |
| **arthritis and rheumatism** | |
| Chamomile (Roman) *Chamaemelum nobile* | anti-inflammatory, stress-relieving |
| Clove bud *Syzygium aromaticum* | analgesic (severe pain), anti-inflammatory, neurotonic (use sparingly - see The Essential Oils) |
| Lavender *Lavandula angustifolia* | analgesic, anti-inflammatory, stress-relieving |
| Marjoram (sweet) *Origanum majorana* | analgesic, stress-relieving |
| Niaouli *Melaleuca viridiflora* | analgesic, anti-inflammatory, neurotonic |
| Rosemary *Rosmarinus officinalis* | analgesic, anti-inflammatory, decongestant, neuromuscular action, neurotonic |
| **bronchial asthma and bronchitis** | |
| Marjoram (sweet) *Origanum majorana* | antispasmodic, anti-infectious, expels mucus, respiratory tonic |
| Niaouli *Melaleuca viridiflora* | anticatarrhal, anti-infectious, anti-inflammatory, expels mucus |
| Peppermint *Mentha x piperita* | anti-inflammatory, breaks down and expels mucus |
| Pine *Pinus sylvestris* | analgesic, anti-infectious, anti-inflammatory, decongestant, breaks down and expels mucus |
| Rosemary *Rosmarinus officinalis* | breaks down mucus, anti-inflammatory, decongestant, expels mucus |
| **headaches** | |
| Chamomile (Roman) *Chamaemelum nobile* | antispasmodic, calming, sedative |
| Lavender *Lavandula angustifolia* | analgesic, calming, sedative |
| Marjoram (sweet) *Origanum majorana* | analgesic, antispasmodic, calming |
| Melissa *Melissa officinalis* | calming, sedative |
| Peppermint *Mentha x piperita* | analgesic, antispasmodic |
| Rosemary *Rosmarinus officinalis* | analgesic, antispasmodic, decongestant |

| ESSENTIAL OIL | TREATMENT |
|---|---|
| **influenza** | |
| Eucalyptus *Eucalyptus smithii* | anti-infectious, antiviral, prophylactic |
| Cypress *Cupressus sempervirens* | anti-infectious |
| Lemon *Citrus limon* | anti-infectious, antiviral |
| Pine *Pinus sylvestris* | anti-infectious |
| **insomnia** | |
| Basil *Ocimum basilicum var. album* | nervous system regulator (nervous insomnia) |
| Chamomile (Roman) *Chamaemelum nobile* | calming |
| Lavender *Lavandula angustifolia* | calming, sedative |
| Lemon *Citrus limon* | calming |
| Marjoram (sweet) *Origanum majorana* | calming |
| Melissa *Melissa officinalis* | calming, sedative |
| **shock** | |
| Bergamot *Citrus bergamia* | balancing, calming, sedative, tonic to central nervous system |
| Chamomile (Roman) *Chamaemelum nobile* | calming, sedative |
| Lavender *Lavandula angustifolia* | balancing, calming, sedative, tonic |
| Melissa *Melissa officinalis* | calming, sedative |
| **incontinence** | |
| Cypress *Cupressus sempervirens* | astringent |
| Lemon *Citrus limon* | astringent |
| **pressure sores** | |
| Chamomile (German) *Matricaria recutica* | cicatrizant (infected wounds, ulcers) |
| Chamomile (Roman) *Chamaemelum nobile* | vulnerary (boils, burns wounds). |
| Frankincense *Boswellia carteri* | cicatrizant (scars, ulcers, wounds) |
| Geranium *Pelargonium graveolens* | cicatrizant (burns, cuts, ulcers, wounds) |
| Lavender *Lavandula angustifolia* | cicatrizant (burns, scars, varicose veins, wounds) |
| **constipation and diverticulitis** | |
| Ginger *Zingiber officinale* | analgesic, digestive stimulant, general tonic |
| Mandarin *Citrus reticulata* | antispasmodic, calming, digestive. |
| Orange (bitter) *Citrus aurantium var. amara* | calming, digestive |

| ESSENTIAL OIL | TREATMENT |
|---|---|
| Rosemary *Rosmarinus officinalis* | analgesic, anti-inflammatory, digestive (constipation, sluggish or painful digestion) |

## diarrhoea

| ESSENTIAL OIL | TREATMENT |
|---|---|
| Geranium *Pelargonium graveolens* | anti-inflammatory (colitis), anti-spasmodic (colic, gastroenteritis), astringent |
| Lemon *Citrus limon* | antispasmodic, astringent, stomachic (gastritis, stomach ulcers). |
| Marjoram (sweet) *Origanum majorana* | analgesic, anti-infectious, anti-spasmodic (colic), stomachic (enteritis) |
| Niaouli *Melaleuca viridiflora* | anti-infectious, anti-inflammatory, antiviral (viral enteritis), digestive (gastritis) |
| Peppermint *Mentha x piperita* | anti-infectious, anti-inflammatory (colitis, enteritis, gastritis), antispasmodic (gastric spasm), digestive |

## indigestion (dyspepsia)

| ESSENTIAL OIL | TREATMENT |
|---|---|
| Basil *Ocimum basilicum* var. *album* | analgesic, carminative (flat-ulence, sluggish digestion) |
| Lemon *Citrus limon* | digestive (nausea, painful digestion, flatulence, appetite loss) |
| Marjoram (sweet) *Origanum majorana* | analgesic, calming, digestive - (flatulence, indigestion) |
| Orange (bitter) *Citrus aurantium* var. *amara* | calming, digestive |
| Peppermint *Mentha x piperita* | analgesic, carminative (flatulence), digestive (nausea, painful digestion) |
| Rosemary *Rosmarinus officinalis* | analgesic (painful digestion), carminative (flatulence) |

## dementia and Alzheimer's disease

| ESSENTIAL OIL | TREATMENT |
|---|---|
| Basil *Ocimum basilicum* var. *album* | neurotonic (mental strain) |
| Clove bud *Syzygium aromaticum* | mental stimulant (memory loss, mental fatigue), neurotonic |
| Marjoram (sweet) *Origanum majorana* | neurotonic (mental instability) |
| Peppermint *Mentha x piperita* | mental stimulant (concentration), neurotonic |
| Rosemary *Rosmarinus officinalis* | neurotonic (loss of memory, concentration) |

## Parkinson's disease

| ESSENTIAL OIL | TREATMENT |
|---|---|
| Clary sage *Salvia sclarea* | antispasmodic, calming, regenerative (cellular aging), neurotonic |
| Lavender *Lavandula angustifolia* | analgesic, antispasmodic, calming, sedative (anxiety, headaches, insomnia), neurotonic |
| Marjoram (sweet) *Origanum majorana* | analgesic, antispasmodic, digestive tonic, calming (anxiety, insomnia), |
| Rosemary *Rosmarinus officinalis* | analgesic, antispasmodic, digestive (constipation, sluggish digestion), neurotonic |

…'Tis the hour

That scatters spells on herb and flower

And garlands might be gathered now

That turn'd around the sleeper's brow.

*From Light of the Haram, Thomas Moore, 1779–1852.*

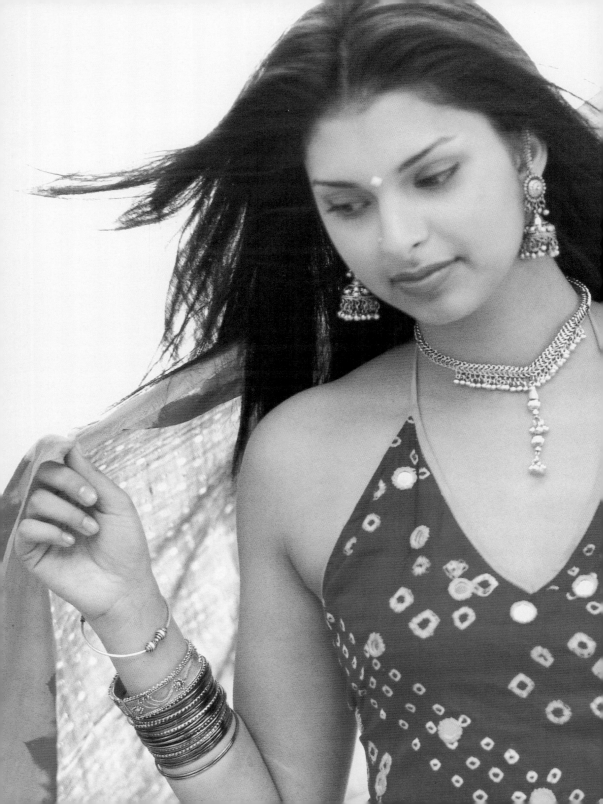

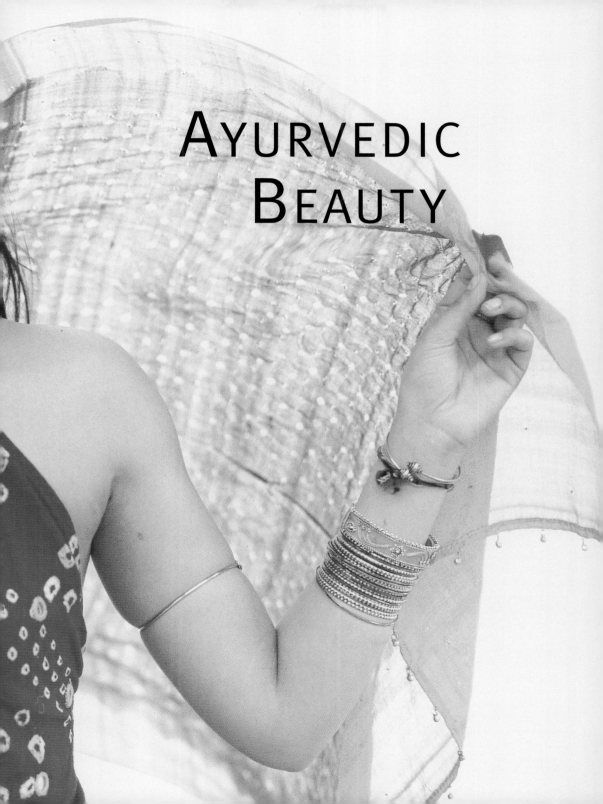

# AYURVEDIC BEAUTY

# A tradition of beauty

Ayurveda, the "science of life", is a philosophy that covers every aspect of being: health, food, spirit, sex, occupation and relationships. It teaches how to live in harmony with your inner self and with the world around you. At one extreme of this far-reaching philosophy are the practices of religious ascetics, who subject themselves to fasts and other rigours to try to transcend the physical. At the other extreme are the sensual paintings, sculptures and writings that reveal a people at ease with their bodies and appreciative of the pleasures of life.

## beauty of body and soul

For both men and women, beauty is seen as a blessing in India: gods and goddesses, heroes and heroines are depicted as handsome and graceful, with arched eyebrows and delicate features, and images of women's beauty and vigour appear in the earliest sacred texts. Traditionally, Indian women have adorned themselves with jewellery, make-up and body art. They have perfumed their hair and dressed it with flowers and gems. They have worn garments in dazzling colours, choosing fitted blouses that emphasize body shape, or swirling saris that draw attention to graceful movement.

Both sexes have traditionally groomed themselves to make the most of their looks. Since the earliest times, Ayurvedic remedies have included techniques to brighten eyes, clear skin and enhance the lustre of hair. Anti-aging treatments are among the most popular, aimed at restoring not only physical vigour but also a youthful appearance.

Because the philosophy of Ayurveda treats body, mind and soul as interrelated, beauty is not limited to the physical dimension, but reflects the vitality and health of the whole person, and adornment plays only a minor part. Jewels are valued not only for their beauty but also because they are considered to possess health-enhancing properties. Herbal remedies and treatments aim to cleanse the body from the

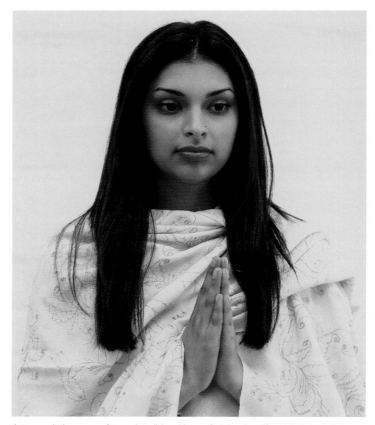

△ **Harmony is the essence of Ayurveda. India's goddesses of wisdom, love, life and death teach their followers to blend action with reflection, courage with compassion, so beauty grows from inner radiance.**

inside, while meditative practices prevent stress leaving its mark, and a fitness regime ensures agelessly youthful physical grace.

## Ayurvedic medicine

Some of the basic principles of Ayurveda were set out more than 3,000 years ago in the Vedas, the sacred texts of Hinduism, and its teachings are believed to have been passed on by word of mouth for many centuries before that. The earliest medical textbooks, the *Susruta Samhita* and the *Charaka Samhita* (written before 500 BC and still consulted

today), list more than 700 herbal medicines, 125 surgical instruments and a range of procedures including cosmetic surgery and kidney-stone removal. Human bones excavated from the city of Harappa, dating from before 1500 BC, bear evidence of surgical repairs.

In the ancient world, Ayurveda's influence spread as far as Egypt, China and Greece. Since Western medicine developed from that of the ancient Greeks, a trace of Ayurveda survives in modern medical training, for example in kidney operations and the diagnosis of eye disease. In most ways, modern medicine has diverged from older traditions, focusing on symptoms and specific diseases, but now, when the healing power of antibiotics is waning because of overuse, and other wonder drugs have revealed harmful side-effects, the ancient wisdom of traditional holistic healing systems is again being sought. Western medicine is starting to open its mind, admitting that some treatments work in ways that no one understands and that mind and body can work together to heal illness.

Meanwhile, Ayurvedic researchers are publishing impressive results in mainstream medical journals. In one study, a remedy called gugalipid, made of resin from the myrrh tree, was found to lower cholesterol levels by an average of 20 per cent. In another, doctors reported that the skin condition of patients using an Ayurvedic remedy improved noticeably, while a placebo had no such results.

## balance and harmony

The principle of Ayurveda is that good health stems from a correct balance of different energies and harmony with the outside world. As a medical system it is holistic, and though remedies exist for specific problems, they are varied according to the person.

▽ A traditional exercise regime and an active lifestyle can allow every woman to achieve the natural grace of a classical dancer.

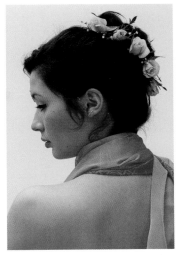

△ Jewellery and ornament symbolize some of the links between the worlds of body and spirit.

Ayurveda also works on levels other than the physical, and this is where it differs most radically from Western medicine. It is part of a world-view that accepts the existence of the unseen, both as part of a human being (a non-physical body that overlaps with the physical one) and as external energies that can affect us. Ayurveda makes no division between science and religion, so its medical system places at least as much emphasis on the psychological and spiritual as on the physical. Most treatments are intended to bring disturbed energies back into balance, allowing the body to heal itself.

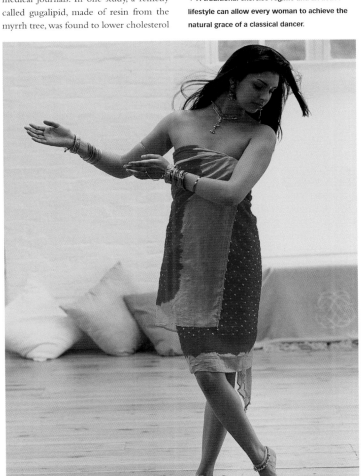

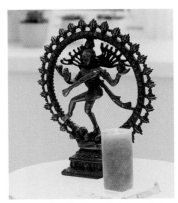

△ Prayer and meditation may help as much as herbal remedies when health disorders indicate that vital energies have been disturbed.

# Living energies, healing powers

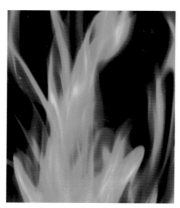

△ **Fire is one of the five elemental forces present in the whole of creation, including ourselves.**

According to Ayurveda, five *mahabhutas* or "great elements" – air, fire, water, earth, and ether (or space) – constitute the world with everything in it, including ourselves, and they affect us through three primary forces called *doshas* (meaning "flaws"): *vata*, *pitta* and *kapha*. Each dosha owes its character to the elements associated with it:

• Vata, linked with the elements air and ether, is dry. It governs movement of every kind, both mental and physical.

• Pitta, linked with fire and water, is hot. It governs all the processes of change and transformation, such as digestion.

• Kapha, linked with earth and water, is heavy. It governs structure and stability.

## channels of energy

The doshas are not the only forces that affect us, because our non-physical body has its own detailed anatomy. Just as the blood carries oxygen around the body, another equally essential life force called *prana* circulates in channels of its own. At any junction – for example where two kinds of tissue meet, such as bone and tendon, or where the influences of two energies meet – there are *marma points*, where energy sometimes gets blocked. One of the major

energy channels follows the line of the backbone and is studded with seven important points called *chakras*.

The physical and non-physical constantly overlap. For example, *ama*, a toxin formed in the body, can be created by poorly digested food or by an experience you can't assimilate – or swallow. *Ojas*, the subtle energy that connects body, mind and spirit, both creates our aura and underpins the immune system. It is formed from the seven kinds of body tissue, and is also influenced by meditation.

## imbalance

We are born in a state called *prakruti*, with all three doshas in balance though not in equal amounts. Each of us is governed by one more than the others, and our individual natures mean that even with the energies comfortably in balance, we'll show the attributes of the dominant dosha. Problems begin when one dosha becomes excessively powerful, pushing us to extremes of behaviour or creating ill-health. Excessive vata might cause anxiety or a hacking cough. Too much fiery pitta could trigger an attack of road rage or heartburn.

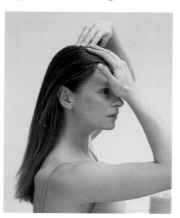

△ **To locate the crown marma point, rest one hand on the bridge of your nose and measure three fingerwidths back from your fingertips.**

Stolid kapha could bring everything to a standstill, resulting in anything from lethargy to blocked sinuses. To prevent or remedy such problems, Ayurveda aims to maintain balance in all things. That includes keeping people in harmony with their surroundings and with each other, keeping bodily processes working effectively, and keeping body, mind and spirit integrated.

Sometimes imbalance results from an excess of one of the doshas, perhaps because we're eating the wrong kinds of food. Or we could be affected by something we've come into contact with, since everything has one of three *gunas*, or inner qualities: harmonious *sattva*, aggressive *rajas* or dull *tamas*. Anything from foods to colours to thoughts will do us good if it's sattvic, but is likely to cause irritation if it's rajasic or heaviness if it's tamasic. The problem could even be caused by karma: the result of misdeeds in this life or a previous one.

## Ayurvedic therapies

All Ayurvedic treatment is aimed at restoring balance, in order to keep us strong enough – both in spirit and in immune system – to withstand disease, so it is used for

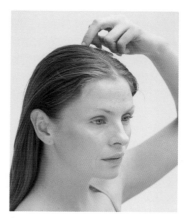

△ **Massage this point to get blocked energy moving on if you are suffering from a feeling of confusion.**

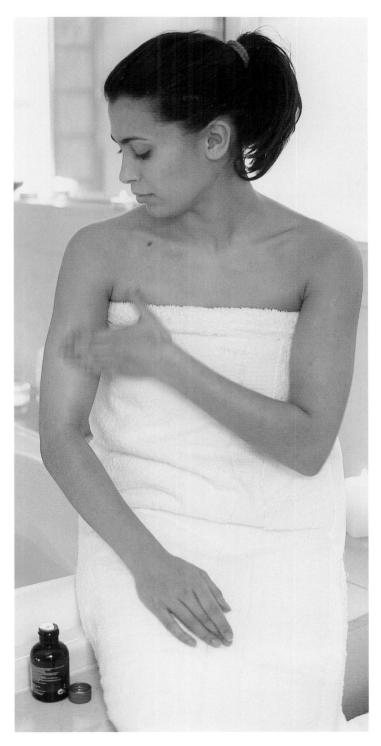

▷ Ayurveda recommends regular detoxifying
treatments, starting with steam baths and
herbal oil massage. Spring is a good time to
initiate these cleansing practices.

prevention as well as for cure. Massage, yoga
and meditation form part of Ayurveda's
recommended daily routine, but can also be
used to treat certain health problems.

Nutrition is one of Ayurveda's central
elements, with the emphasis not only on
wholesome ingredients but also on the right
foods for you as an individual. Each dosha
can be aggravated by certain foods, so if
you're suffering from an imbalance, you'll
be urged to avoid those foods and eat others
that have a calming effect.

Detoxification, or *shodhana*, begins with
*purvakarma*: cleansing steam baths and
herbal oil massages. Then comes
*panchakarma*, a more rigorous detox that
may include enemas, laxatives, and nasal
washes with herbs or oils. In case blocked
energy is causing congestion, the marma
points may be stimulated to encourage the
flow. This is usually done with finger
pressure, though needles may also be used.

The next step, *rasayana*, aims to restore
long-term health and slow down the aging
process through lifestyle changes,
meditation and exercises, with herbal
remedies if necessary. A course of treatment
may last for up to six months.

Though some of Ayurveda's practices
seem strenuous, it's a compassionate
philosophy that understands human desires
and aims to increase the quality of life,
promoting vitality and inner harmony.

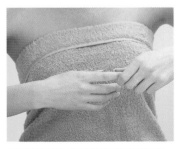

△ Hand massage stimulates the marma points
that are clustered in this area, and it is easy to
do it for yourself.

# Dosha analysis

If you consult an Ayurvedic doctor you may be asked to complete a questionnaire to find out your *prakruti* – your constitution, determined at the time of your birth – and your current imbalance, or *vikruti*. The questionnaire is part of a package of diagnostic tools; others include checking your pulses (subtle energy flows) and examining the condition of your tongue. Answering a questionnaire at home can give you an idea of your vikruti, as your answers will usually be based on your current condition, but it does not replace a full consultation with a practitioner.

You may find that more than one description applies to you. In this case, tick all that are relevant. In the skin and hair sections, respond only to the descriptions that apply to you. Give yourself plenty of time to think before answering, so your answers will be as accurate as possible.

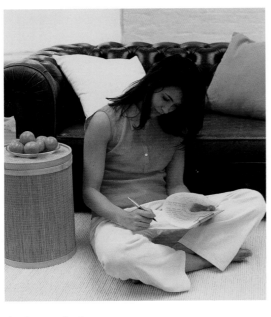

◁ **Completing a questionnaire can give some insight into your current needs, so make sure your answers reflect the way you're feeling right now.**

▷ **To discover your true constitution – the state in which you were born – you'll need to consult an Ayurvedic practitioner. The results may surprise you.**

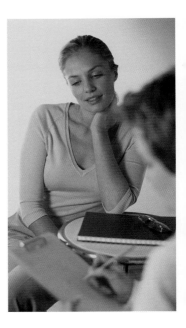

## dosha analysis

| PHYSICAL TRAITS | VATA | PITTA | KAPHA |
|---|---|---|---|
| Body frame | Thin | Medium | Large |
| Fingernails | Thin/cracking | Pink/soft/medium | Thick/wide/pale |
| Weight | Low/bony | Medium/muscular | Gains easily |
| Stool/bowel movement | Small/hard/wind | Loose/burning | Moderate/solid |
| Forehead size | Small | Medium | Large |
| Appetite | Variable | Strong | Constant |
| Eyes | Small/unsteady | Reddish/focused | Wide/white |
| Voice | Low or weak | High or sharp | Slow or quiet |
| Lips | Cracking, thin, dry | Medium or soft | Large or smooth |
| Speech | Quick or talkative | Moderate or argumentative | Deep or melodious |
| Weather: what bothers you? | Cold and dry | Heat and sun | Cold and damp |
| Sleep patterns | Light | Moderate | Deep/heavy |
| Which do you like best? | Travel or nature | Sports or politics | Water or flowers |

| MENTAL TRAITS | VATA | PITTA | KAPHA |
|---|---|---|---|
| Temperament | Nervous or fearful | Irritable or impatient | Easy-going |
| Memory | Quickly grasps, but forgets | Sharp or clear | Slow to learn, never forgets |
| Faith | Radical or changing | Leader- or goal-oriented | Loyal or constant |
| Dreams | Flying or anxious | Fighting or in colour | Few or romantic |
| Emotions | Enthusiastic or worried | Warm or angry | Calm or attached |
| Mind | Quick or adaptable | Penetrating or critical | Slow and steady |

| SKIN TENDENCIES | VATA | PITTA | KAPHA |
|---|---|---|---|
| | Lack of tone or lustre | Rashes, inflammation, itching | Dull, sluggish, congested |
| | Rough patches | Oily T-zone | Enlarged pores |
| | Chapping and cracking | Premature wrinkling | Large pustules |
| | Dry eczema | Blackheads | Cystic formations |
| | General dryness | General excessive oiliness | Thick, oily secretions |
| | Dandruff/dry scalp | Discoloration | Oily scalp |
| | Fine, porcelain | Warm, smooth | Strong, flawless |

| HAIR | VATA | PITTA | KAPHA |
|---|---|---|---|
| | Dry and dull | Oily | Thick |
| | Frizzy | Balding | Glossy |
| | Scaly scalp | Excessive hair loss | Shiny |
| | Split ends | Thinning | Grows easily |

▽ Vata is a fine, light, speedy energy that can cause problems with dryness of skin and hair.

▽ If pitta's fiery warmth slips out of balance, it may express itself in rashes and discoloration.

▽ Kapha's strong skin and thick hair age slowly; excess oiliness is the main beauty pitfall.

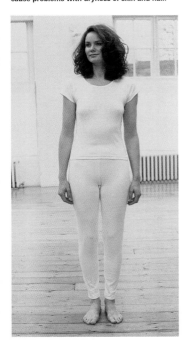

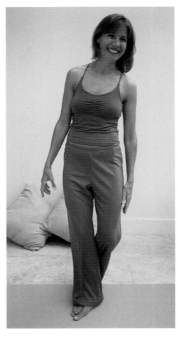

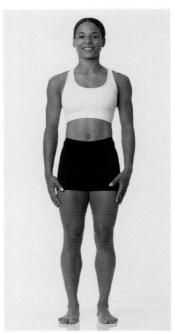

# Your dosha and you

Few people are ruled by a single dosha. Most of us are governed by dual doshas, one of which is more powerful than the other. A very few are ruled equally by all three.

If your score in the questionnaire is highest in pitta but still quite high in kapha, for example, that makes you a pitta-kapha combination. Scores reversed for pitta and kapha would make you a kapha-pitta. The pitta-kapha person is more likely to suffer from a pitta imbalance than anything else. But a combination of factors that aggravate kapha – such as eating a lot of heavy food during a cold, damp spring – could produce an excess of kapha energy.

## self-analysis

The results of the questionnaire can be enlightening. If they are puzzling because they seem unlike you, your answers to the questions may not have been completely accurate: perhaps you overstated your faults or gave answers you felt ought to be true. You may be used to thinking of yourself in a way that is no longer relevant.

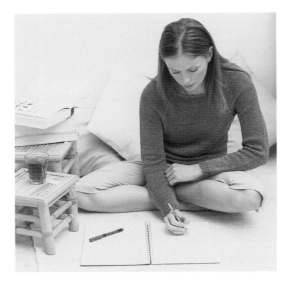

◁ Vata dominates the afternoon hours, making this a good time for thought and intellectual activity, rather than physical work.

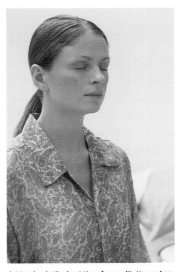

△ Morning is the best time for meditation, when peaceful kapha energy helps to still your mind.

Comparisons should be made with other people of your own ethnic background, not against some kind of world average. Kapha, for example, tends to go with fair skin and vata with dark skin. But a typical kapha person from Sri Lanka would be darker than, say, a typical vata from Sweden.

Remember too that your mind and body may be ruled by different doshas, so you might have a fiery pitta temperament in a curvy kapha body. All kinds of external factors can affect you: even the season or weather could influence your answers. So don't feel ruled by the results you obtain. They are meant to offer guidance, not lay down the law.

In order to discover your prakruti, or constitutional dosha, an Ayurvedic practitioner will carry out a pulse analysis, taking the pulses of the subtle energy flows at 21 points. The difference between your prakruti and your vikruti can be revealing. Prakruti is your ideal state, with everything in the best balance for your personality – if there's a big difference it could mean you're living in a way that doesn't suit you.

## what is an imbalance?

We all have one or two doshas that dominate. It's natural for each of us to show some characteristics of these, whether they are most noticeable in our looks, behaviour or tastes. The doshas also give us warning of what needs to be tackled if something goes wrong with our well-being.

When a dominant dosha becomes excessively strong, its characteristics are exaggerated. As a pitta type you will be naturally ambitious and competitive, for example, but if pitta grows too strong you may become irritable and critical, and have trouble sleeping. This is known as a pitta imbalance. If you don't tackle an imbalance

### THE DOSHAS THROUGH THE DAY

| | |
|---|---|
| 6am–10am | Kapha |
| 10am–2pm | Pitta |
| 2pm–6pm | Vata |
| 6pm–10pm | Kapha |
| 10pm–2am | Pitta |
| 2am–6am | Vata |

early on, it can eventually manifest itself in sickness, so you need to reduce your dominant dosha. In this case, that means cutting down on things like spicy food and dance music, which fuel pitta.

## a time for everything

According to Ayurvedic teaching, each period of the day is ruled by a different energy, which can reinforce or counteract the influence of your dominant dosha.

Tranquil kapha governs early morning, the time for meditation. Later in the morning is the time to exercise, combining kapha strength with pitta energy. Pitta, which aids digestion, rules midday, making that the best time to eat. Vata dominates the afternoon – an ideal time for mental work, as vata promotes intelligence. Then come the quiet kapha hours again, making this the best time to get to sleep. Pitta takes over again after 10pm, when its fiery energy is meant to stop your temperature dropping too low while you sleep. If you go to bed after 10pm, you may find that a new rush of pitta-fuelled energy stops you dropping off.

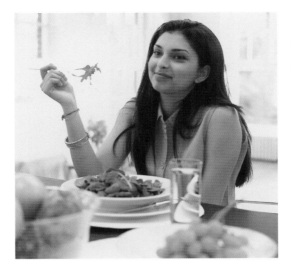

◁ **Pitta energy, which aids digestion, is in full force around lunchtime, making this the best time to enjoy your main meal of the day.**

▽ **Ayurveda advocates "early to bed, early to rise". Before 10pm, kapha helps you to get to sleep – after that, pitta could keep you awake.**

The seasons follow the same rhythm as the hours of the day, with kapha ruling the weeks from spring to early summer, pitta ruling high summer and autumn, and vata rising when the leaves have fallen to dominate the winter.

Since an excess of any dosha brings out its harmful side, watch out for signs of an imbalance, especially during the times or seasons that correspond with your own dominant dosha. You might find it hard to drag yourself out of bed in the kapha-ruled morning, or that pitta's summer heat brings you out in a rash, or that you're getting stressed under vata's influence during the winter months. Medical researchers have found that seasonal affective disorder, or "winter blues", actually affects most people during spring, when depressive kapha is coming into force.

Even our own lives follow these phases. As children we are ruled by kapha, as adults pitta takes over and with the onset of wise old age we come into our vata time.

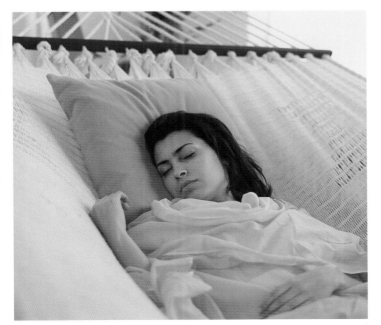

### ESSENTIAL FLAWS

Why are the forces of vata, pitta and kapha called doshas, or "flaws"? Ayurveda takes the very practical view that, though everything ought to exist in perfect balance, it usually doesn't. Our individual natures dictate that one dosha will generally be dominant, and this is fine when it is just enough to express your individual personality, but when it becomes too strong and overrules the others, it throws your constitution out of balance, which leads to ill health. So a healthy life is one in which we manage to keep the balance steady.

# Vata movement and life force

Slender, willowy and long-legged, the classic vata woman looks good on a catwalk. She's more likely to be either tall or petite than of medium height. Her cool, porcelain skin is rarely bothered by spots or oily patches. Her rather small eyes sparkle with life and intelligence, and her fine hair complements her delicate bone structure.

She never thinks about her weight – she's naturally light. Her active lifestyle keeps her in shape, and she doesn't tend to eat a lot. She'd rather be in a club, dancing until dawn, than wasting time in a restaurant where you can't move to the music. Though a born athlete, she rarely builds a lot of muscle, but remains slim and slightly ethereal-looking.

## as free as the air

Vata women love change, travel and movement. They're fast – whether they're running for the sheer joy of it or tackling some new concept in a physics class. They talk rapidly and their quick intellects mean they're full of ideas, plans and theories.

At work, vatas are the ones with all the ideas who'll get any project under way with the force of their enthusiasm, though they may not be so good at seeing it through: while someone with a steadier dosha takes over, they'll be hatching a dozen new plans. They're highly creative and often artistic, so no one really expects them to be utterly practical. They'd be exhausting company if they weren't so stimulating, but they rarely stay long enough to wear out their welcome.

## vata imbalance

No one can keep up that pace for ever. Vatas are smart enough to know this, but often don't slow down until they've built up a massive vata imbalance by doing all the things that aggravate this ethereal dosha. These include skipping meals, not getting enough sleep and generally running themselves into the ground.

When vatas finally crash they may have trouble getting up again. Then they suffer

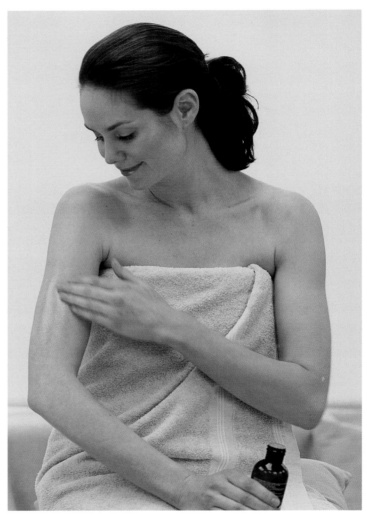

△ **Soothing oils do more than just nourish dry skin: they can help pacify excess vata energy.**

from stress and exhaustion, probably compounded by insomnia. Living on their nerves, they can forget to eat or may feel too anxious to swallow anything. Their rapid intellect can spin off into confusion. Tension can lead to muscle pain, cramps and irritable bowel syndrome. Excessive weight loss can also lead to serious health problems such as osteoporosis.

Dryness is the essential vata attribute, so an excess of vata causes dehydration in everything: hair and fingernails become brittle, lips crack, the tongue feels like felt, the eyes are sore. Dry skin conditions such as

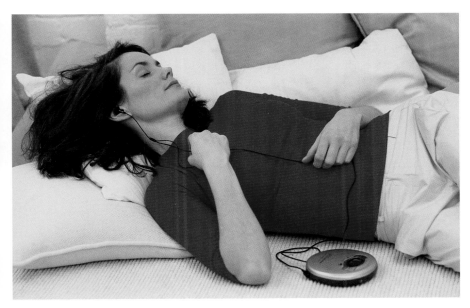

◁ Listening to classical music with a slow, rhythmic beat can help to calm a vata imbalance, easing away feelings of tension and anxiety.

eczema can be a problem. A dry cough adds to the feeling of debility. Internal dryness can cause arthritis and constipation and even thicken the blood – add this to vata's raised stress levels, and it's not surprising that high blood pressure and heart palpitations are vata complaints.

## pacifying vata

This dosha needs help to become more grounded. Pacifying influences are warm, moist, slow and contained. If you're vata, you're drawn towards speed, lightness, novelty. Try to balance these with activities that slow and centre you. Take a relaxing spa break instead of a strenuous activity holiday and discover the steam room and the jacuzzi. Listen to peaceful New Age or classical music. Find a course in meditation, then practise it at home some mornings instead of heading for the gym for your normal workout.

You like being with people, but this doesn't have to be in a crowded club. Invite friends around for supper instead. Take your time selecting wonderful ingredients, cooking the meal to perfection and eating it with people who care about you. Relax and enjoy the warmth of their company.

Cold, dry, windy weather makes you tense, so cocoon yourself away from it when you can, and take your holidays on a tropical beach. Even the scents you use can fuel or calm your dosha: jasmine, sandalwood and rose all help to keep vata in balance.

## your beauty needs

Dry skin is the classic vata complaint. The fine texture of your skin looks good when vata is in balance, but an imbalance makes it dull and lifeless. This kind of skin ages easily, so moisturizing is vital: the Ayurvedic way is to drink lots of water and eat plenty of the juicy fruits that help to pacify vata. Putting on weight isn't a problem for this dosha, so

you should never really need to count any calories, but you do need to beware of letting your weight fall too low.

Vata's flyaway hair is prone to dandruff, so a weekly sesame oil massage will relieve your dry scalp as well as easing tension. Teeth are a weak spot, exacerbated by the vata tendency to graze instead of eating meals, leaving teeth constantly coated in acid. If you can't cut out the snacks, rinse your mouth with water after every one.

▽ As a vata, you love company, and a leisurely meal with a friend will help you relax.

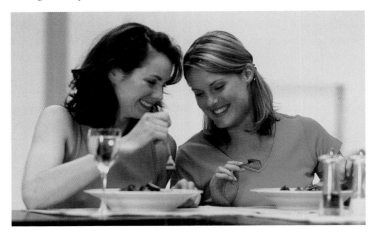

# Pitta fire and transformation

Pitta woman is a dazzler. Fire is her dominant element, and it shows. Women of this dosha radiate energy like the sun, and their skin reflects their emotions with a surge of colour. Yet pitta also includes an element of water, which can stop this dosha burning out.

Despite a healthy appetite, pittas rarely become overweight. You're likely to spot them at the gym, where their powerful workouts result in toned muscles that curve rather than bulking up. They are usually blessed with soft hair, neat noses and small chins, and may have numerous beauty spots in the form of moles and freckles.

Though they're likely to have combination skin – with an oilier T-zone of forehead, nose and mouth – as long as pitta remains in balance the skin should be neither too dry nor too oily, but smooth and warm to the touch. Pittas often have warm, coppery skin tones.

## fiery energies

The heat extends to the pitta character. Passionate and ambitious, pitta women know what they want and will strive to achieve it. They may fly off the handle, but

they're not the sort to hide a simmering grievance behind a mask of friendliness. Don't be fooled by this fiery image, though. As long as pitta remains in balance, they are intelligent, calm and rational. Born leaders, their qualities reward those who are drawn to their fire.

At work, they're high-fliers, strong-minded and focused: if they're enthusiastic about a project they'll see it through. They aim for the heights of success and often reach them, thanks to the single-minded work they put into getting there.

## pitta imbalance

When pitta energy boils over, the heat is on. Rashes, inflammation, sweating, fevers and heartburn are all signs of a pitta imbalance, as are acne eruptions and hot flushes, which characterize the beginning and end of the fertile life period ruled by this fiery dosha.

A pitta imbalance will often reveal itself through the skin, in blotching or changes in pigmentation, or the flushing caused by indigestion. More serious ailments may be signalled by a yellowish complexion: this could be caused by liver dysfunction, which needs medical attention.

Fiery mood swings may be caused by another of pitta's problems – hormone imbalances. An excess of pitta can make someone overambitious, temperamental, jealous, aggressive and likely to trample on anyone in their path.

## pacifying pitta

Your inner fire provides all the heat you need. Sultry weather and overheated buildings can provoke a pitta imbalance. When you go to the gym, head for the swimming pool rather than the sauna or hot tub. On holiday, go for the snow. In the summer, slow down to keep cool. The

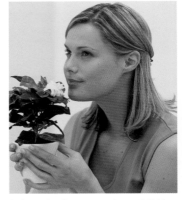

△ **If excessive pitta energy makes you irritable, soothe yourself with gentle influences: the scent of a gardenia, the sound of trickling water.**

influences that pacify excess pitta are cool, soft, kind and generally calming. The smell of gardenias is meant to cool pitta energy.

Give yourself time to eat breakfast and lunch sitting down, instead of skipping meals and overdosing on food in the evening. This can help you to avoid the pitta pitfalls of insomnia and indigestion, which add to your stress.

Avoid harsh or aggressive music, or anything with a driving beat or lots of drumming. Try soothing music with a slowish beat and gentle, minor chords.

Since high-tech equipment also increases pitta energy, an overheated office can cause problems. Freelance work can be one solution, keeping you away from office politics. On the other hand, being part of a team could help control your tendency to overwork. Whichever you choose, keep an eye on your stress levels and remember there's a world outside work. Cultivate friends who help you relax rather than contacts who can advance your career. Use some of your abundant creativity to express your artistic gifts, and divert some energy into working for a good cause that gives you a feelgood buzz.

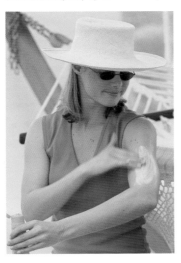

◁ **Use sunscreen at all times to protect yourself from the sun (and be sure to avoid sunbeds), especially if you have moles or freckles.**

## your beauty needs

Ruled by fire, your skin reacts readily to inner or outer heat. You flush when you are angry and blush with embarrassment. Indigestion may give you an unwanted glow, and hot conditions make you look and feel uncomfortable. Colour-reducing foundation creams were made for you.

Your skin is sensitive, and a pitta imbalance can bring you out in rashes, rosacea, acne or – in later life – blotchy liver spots. Dark-skinned pittas sometimes suffer from pigmented patches. Your most important beauty rule is to keep cool. A mineral-water spray lives in your handbag or desk drawer; at home, cucumber makes an instant skin-cooling mask. Treat your skin kindly, avoiding harsh treatments that could bring it out in a rash.

Your skin isn't dry and shouldn't age too fast, as long as you protect it from the sun. It's lucky that pitta's sensitive skin and dislike of heat tend to stop you sunbathing, because you're more prone than anyone else to skin cancer. Keep an eye on all those moles, reporting any changes to your doctor.

A pitta imbalance can also affect your hair, making it prematurely thin and grey. Ayurvedic hair care aims at keeping the scalp healthy and strengthening growth.

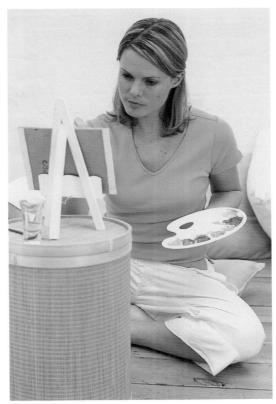

◁ To keep your life in balance, put some of your abundant pitta energy into expressing your natural creativity.

▽ Calm pitta heat with a refreshing spray of cool water – it's good for your skin, and for your equilibrium – or, even better, go for a swim.

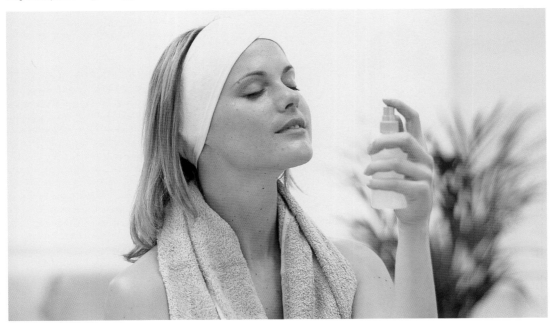

# Kapha growth and protection

A classic kapha type has perfect teeth, full lips and a flawless complexion, surrounded by masses of shining hair. But her greatest beauty shines out through her eyes, which are large, deep and thickly fringed with long eyelashes. The inner quality they reveal is one of peace and serenity. Kapha's very presence is calming, and the stress that aggravates vata's dizziness and pitta's temper seems to dissipate when a kapha person takes over. This is a peaceful, stable energy, combining earth's strength with water's deep stillness. Kapha people relax easily and rarely experience a troubled night.

▷ Sensual kaphas appreciate the pleasures of food, but this can lead to weight gain. Spicy soups and curries will satisfy your tastebuds and pacify excess kapha energy.

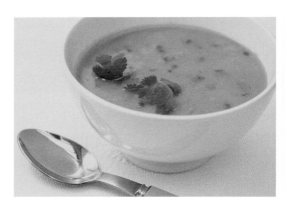

## peace from earth

Calm and tolerant, kaphas are natural peace-makers. They make friends easily, love deeply and are wise enough to forgive things that would offend others. They happily nurture those they love, and frequently all those around them too, maintaining deep, rewarding relationships of all kinds. They are outstanding homemakers, and will go to great lengths to avoid change or upheaval.

At work they defuse tense situations with their down-to-earth good humour. In fact, tension is less likely to develop when there are kapha people around to carry a burden, because they are both physically and psychologically strong, with legendary powers of endurance. On a practical level, they'll finish the work that airy vatas started and lost interest in — and they won't be drawn into arguments with a bossy pitta. Good memory, aided by their natural patience, helps them stay on course and get the details right.

All sorts of people are drawn towards kapha's sweetness and warmth. Kaphas are too kind to reject anyone, but they have to beware of a tendency to let more demanding types take advantage.

## kapha imbalance

In excess, grounded kapha energy can become heavy and stagnant. Kapha people relax very easily, and have to battle with their lazy tendencies. When kapha starts to overrule everything else, it's hard to get them off the sofa.

Exercise is vital to keep kapha energy at a healthy level, but lethargy may be a sign of another characteristic problem: depression. A kapha person in low spirits will tend to stay at home eating chocolate in front of the television: negative traits combining to increase the imbalance.

Groundedness can also distort into materialism, and when that happens, greed

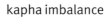

◁ Lethargy can be a problem for kaphas, especially when they are bored or lonely.

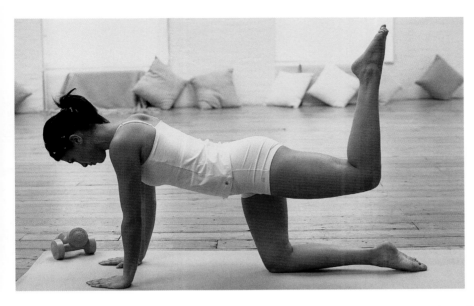

◁ **Kaphas have to push themselves to exercise, but the ease with which they develop muscles is encouraging. They also need to work on flexibility and lightness.**

and envy are kapha's less appealing traits, along with a possessive attachment to material things. A kapha overdose has a blunting, dulling effect on mental faculties, leading to obstinacy and narrow-mindedness. Physically, it is associated with sluggish digestion, constipation, respiratory congestion, diabetes, coronary artery disease, slowed metabolism and obesity.

## pacifying kapha

You probably love rich food, sweet or savoury, and plenty of it. But that increases kapha energy as well as your hip measurement. If you're becoming greedy or sluggish, try some hot, spicy food for a change, and eat a bit less. Brisk scents such as cedar or camphor can sometimes help, as does anything that has a tendency to lighten, warm or invigorate.

Kapha people need to get up early and take daily exercise. If you're sleeping more than eight hours a night (nine in your teens), get your doctor to check for an underactive thyroid gland. Depression can also make you oversleep; to break the cycle, find an activity you can enjoy in company: team sports, walking or aerobics classes with a friend.

You need to stay stimulated, so seek new experiences and motivate yourself to go out to evening classes or art galleries. Put aside your cookbook and read a history of your

area, a thriller (make sure you solve the mystery before it's all revealed), or a biography of someone you admire.

Coldness increases kapha, so work up a sweat in the gym and enjoy the sauna too – not the steam room, because you need dry heat. Slap on the sunscreen and go out on sunny days. Take an outdoor holiday visiting archaeological sites in the North African

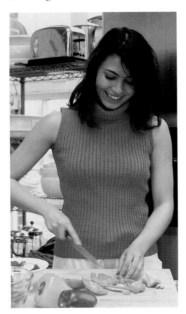

desert or exploring the Australian outback. Let your nurturing tendencies do yourself some good and adopt an unwanted dog: you're too kind-hearted to neglect the long walks it'll need.

## your beauty needs

Kaphas have the sort of strong, smooth skin that shrugs off most blemishes and goes on to age well. Your idea of a bad-hair day would win no sympathy from anyone else.

What you have to watch out for is your weight. You're naturally strong and fit, so the health benefits of exercise aren't much of a draw. You enjoy life's little indulgences, such as good food, warmth and relaxation. A run down to the gym on a cold night sounds as much fun to you as drilling your own teeth.

The strongest of the doshas, you build muscle easily, so you'll see easy gains when you start working out. You'll need to cut down your fuel intake as well. But if you eat at the right time – just long enough before exercise to give you the energy you need without risking indigestion – you'll find working out doesn't make you overeat in compensation. Then your honed physique will start to offer its own rewards.

◁ **Generous kaphas are the world's best cooks and decorators, with large circles of friends. They make wonderful party hosts.**

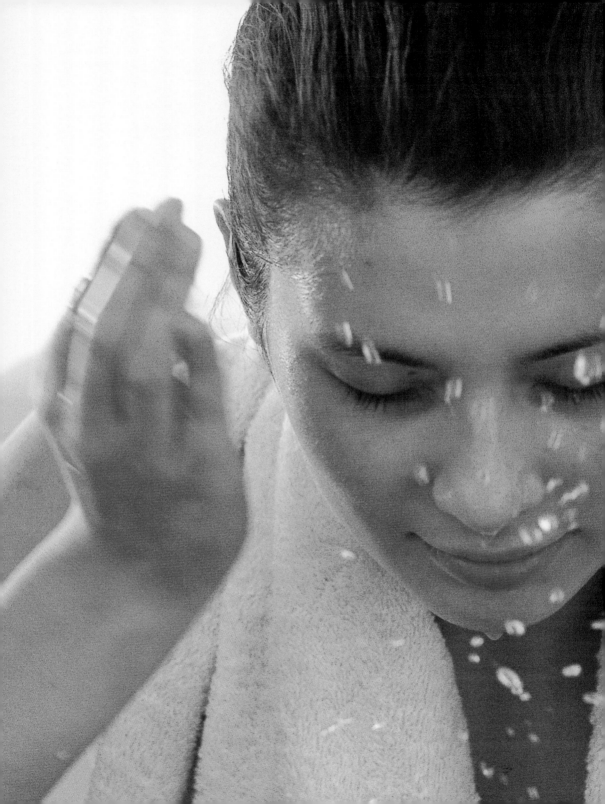

# Cleansing the Body, Clearing the Mind

Ayurveda aims to promote natural beauty and lifelong youthfulness by keeping all the systems in balance. The first essential is to clear the systems of anything that hinders this aim. In physical terms, it includes cleansing treatments such as massage, steam therapy and fasting. For the mind and spirit it means discarding old habits of thought that clutter up the consciousness.

# Healing hands

Massage plays a central role in Ayurvedic treatments, stimulating circulation and promoting the elimination of waste. Different versions are used to treat illness, heal injuries, aid detoxification, calm the mind, beautify the skin and rejuvenate the body. These treatments can now be found at Ayurvedic centres worldwide.

**Abhyanga** is the classic full-body massage, carried out by one or two therapists. As well as stroking and kneading movements, the therapists apply finger or hand pressure to some of the body's 107 marma points.

**Champissage** is a specialized head massage that stimulates marma points across the head, aiming to tone up all the body's systems. It helps to improve circulation, boost the immune system and slow down the aging process.

**Shirodhara** consists of pouring warm oil slowly on to your forehead while a therapist massages it gently into your scalp.

**Pottali** or **Navrakhizi** is a massage with hot poultices of rice, oil, milk and herbs. The resulting paste is washed off and more oil is massaged in. Traditionally used to treat vata conditions, it's as beneficial for stress and anxiety as for bodily aches.

**Sarvangadhara** or **Pizhichil** requires three therapists. One keeps a constant supply of oil warmed while two others dip linen cloths into the oil and squeeze it over the entire body, massaging it in lightly. This is a rejuvenating treatment that also aims to build up the immune system.

## oil essentials

In Ayurvedic practice, oil is believed to help clear toxic ama out of the body. It also reduces excess dosha, which is considered to stick like a solid substance until softened and flushed out in the form of bodily secretions. Oil should be washed off after a treatment, so any waste products released into it don't re-enter the body.

### MASSAGE FOR YOUR DOSHA

All dosha types benefit from massage. Vata people, and others who have dry skin, should always use oil for massage. The pitta dosha can be over-stimulated if too much oil is used, so just enough should be applied to avoid dragging the skin. Any kind of massage helps to provide the stimulation a kapha body requires, but deep-tissue massage is especially useful in aiding waste disposal via the lymph system.

You can choose an oil purely because it is suitable for your skin type. But if you feel that you are suffering from an excess of one of your energies – light-headed vata, for example, or impatient pitta – choose an appropriate oil for your dosha. Take outside influences into account: if it's a damp evening in spring, for example, kapha energy will already be high.

## Full body self-massage

Ayurveda recommends self-massage each morning. As you do it, vary your touch so that you're sometimes moving your hands lightly over the skin, and at other times pressing firmly enough to move the skin over the bone. Use the fingertips for static pressure, but the softer pads of the fingers for kneading or circling movements. Avoid putting pressure on any joints. Unless otherwise stated, any pressure should be upward, towards the head. Always warm the oil, and make sure the room is pleasantly warm. Start by pouring a little oil into one palm and rubbing your hands together. Repeat from time to time as the oil wears off your hands. If you prefer not to get oil in your hair, you can do the head massage without it.

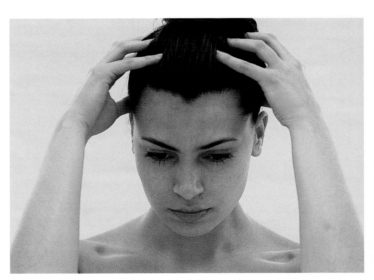

△ **1** Press your hands against your scalp and move the skin in large circles. Run your fingers through your hair and gently tug and rotate small sections of it to stimulate the scalp. With the tips of your fingers and thumbs, make little circles all over your head.

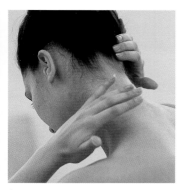

△ **2** Smooth oil into your neck and work it up over the back of your head. Cup the base of the skull in your palms and press gently upwards.

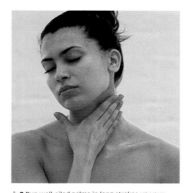

△ **3** Run well-oiled palms in long strokes up your throat from the collarbones, covering the front and the sides; repeat several times.

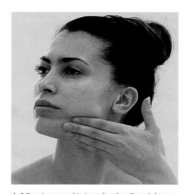

△ **4** Cupping your chin in each palm alternately, run the fingers up along the jawline to the ears several times, using firm pressure without dragging the skin.

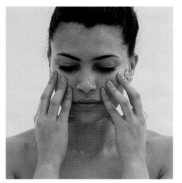

△ **5** Place your thumbs on your temples and massage the forehead in small circles with your fingertips. Use light pressure, and keep the movement upward and outward. Massage the cheeks in the same way.

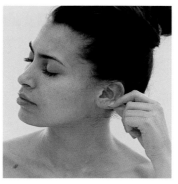

△ **6** Continue massaging in small circles all over the scalp and along the base of the skull. Gently pull and twist sections of the hair to stimulate the scalp. Then rub and squeeze the ears and massage all around them.

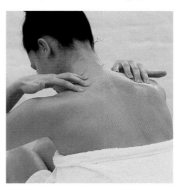

△ **7** Relax your head and shoulders and let your head sink forwards, keeping your shoulders down. Place your oiled palms on the back of your neck and rub firmly from the spine out to the sides.

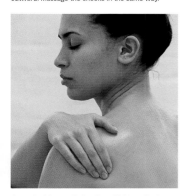

△ **8** Rub oil into each shoulder with large circular motions, using your whole palm and fingers. If you have any stiffness, cup your hand around the joint and rotate it as far as you find comfortable.

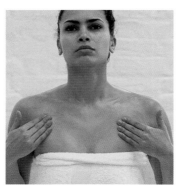

△ **9** Stroke oil outwards across your chest from your breastbone. Pull the fingers outwards in a semicircular movement, from the nipples towards the armpits, both above and below the breasts.

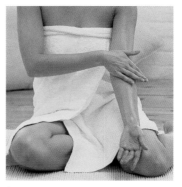

△ **10** Extend one arm, thumb upwards, and stroke lightly down the outside of the arm with your palm. Then reverse the movement and rub more firmly back up the inside of the arm.

*continued over page* ▷

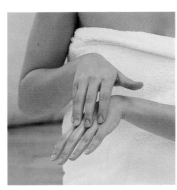

**11** Grip your left arm just below the shoulder (▷), squeezing it between your fingers and the heel of your right hand. Move your hand a couple of fingers' width down your arm and repeat, working your way down to the hand. With the left hand extended, palm down, massage the wrist and the back of the hand (△) with the right hand. Grip and release the side of the wrist (▽). Repeat, working down the side of the hand to the fingertips.

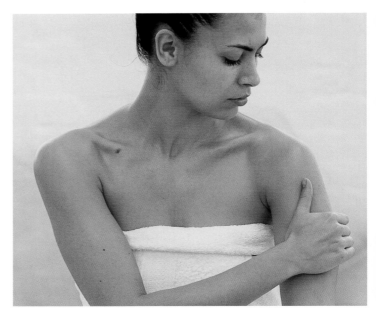

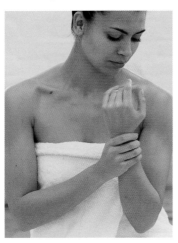

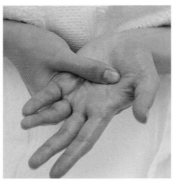

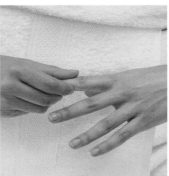

△ **12** Hold the left hand and massage the palm with your right thumb (above left). Now squeeze and massage each finger, finishing by pulling it gently (above right). Interlace your fingers and stretch the arms out in front of you, palms facing outwards. Keep your shoulders relaxed and low. Release your grip. Turning your left palm down, rub briskly up from the back of your hand to the shoulder. Repeat the arm and hand massage on the right.

**CURING OIL**

Oil for Ayurvedic massage is traditionally "cured" before use. To cure oil, pour it into an enamelled or non-metallic pan, add a drop of water and place over a gentle heat until the water pops, then remove from the stove. When cool, pour the oil into a glass bottle and store away from light. Just before a massage, warm a little of the oil to a comfortable temperature.

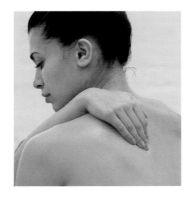

◁ **13** Reach over each shoulder with your fingers pointing downwards. Rub as far as you can stretch down and across your back, and press your fingers in as you pull back up, feeling that you are stretching the muscles upwards.

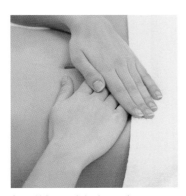

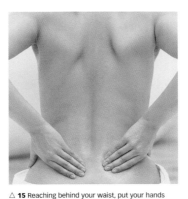

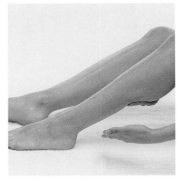

△ **14** With fingers pointing downwards, massage your abdomen with the flat of your hands in large clockwise movements, above and below the navel. If you suffer from poor digestion, you may massage with your fist, slowly circling down on the left and up on the right. Finish by stroking outwards from the centre.

△ **15** Reaching behind your waist, put your hands flat on your lower back, with fingertips on the spine, and draw them out to the sides, pressing firmly. Massage your hips and buttocks briskly with kneading, pummelling and large circular stroking movements, being careful to avoid direct pressure on your hip joints.

△ **16** Lightly rub oil down your legs, then massage up the calf muscles. Grip and release, or rub firmly in circles with fists spiralling upwards, or simply stroke firmly up towards the knees. If you have varicose or visible veins, stroke gently without any pressure.

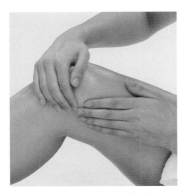

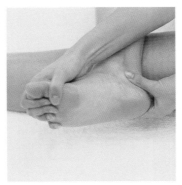

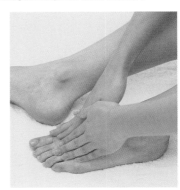

△ **17** Work gently over each knee, rubbing the kneecap, sides and back of the leg in circles using plenty of oil. Then stroke vigorously up the insides of the thighs, with brisk overlapping movements, into the groin.

**18** Massage your feet one at a time. To begin, cup the heel in one hand and, with the other hand, grasp the toes and gently rotate the foot (△ above left) in both directions. Massage lightly over the ankle and top of the foot in circles, using more pressure on the sole to avoid tickling. Gently rotate each toe (△ above right). Finish by stroking firmly down from the ankle several times as if brushing something off the ends of the toes (▽).

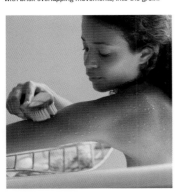

**A TOUCH OF SILK**
The full-body massage can be done without oil, using a glove made of raw silk instead. Pitta and kapha types should try this as a change from oil. Body-brushing, using a natural bristle brush or a textured mitt, also stimulates lymph circulation, which helps the body rid itself of waste products.

◁ **Use a natural bristle brush for a stimulating body massage while you are bathing.**

# Painless detoxification

Spring is traditionally the time for detoxifying. *Swedana*, or sweat therapy, adds to the benefits of massage by helping the body cleanse itself through the pores, while a cleansing diet eases the pressure on digestion, promoting radiantly clear skin and boundless vitality.

## steaming

For deep cleaning the skin, steam baths offer an easy solution and the benefits are instantly noticeable. The moist heat allows the pores to open and sweat flushes out impurities. Steam softens the outer layer of skin, encourages renewal by increasing circulation, and helps shed the dead cells – traditionally removed with a metal scraper. For those who can't stand damp heat, or who suffer from an excess of kapha dosha, a sauna may be an effective alternative.

Start with a shower, then oil your skin while still damp, before entering the steam room, to nourish the skin and bring your dosha back into balance. Shower again after steaming, and finish the treatment with a refreshing cool splash: the combination of hot steam and cold pool or shower is profoundly revitalizing.

At home, enjoy the benefits of steam by running a very hot bath and oiling your skin while you relax beside the bath and wait for it to cool. Throw a bag of herbs into the water, choosing a blend to suit your skin or your dosha. When the bath is a comfortable temperature, massage the oil off with an *ubtan*, or herbal powder, then bathe off the residues and finish with a cool shower.

## a cleansing diet

Rigorous fasts can cause health problems, including a serious vata or pitta imbalance, but semi-fasting for a few days can help clear accumulated waste. Choose vegetables, fruits and grains that suit your dosha.

• Start the day by drinking a cup of hot water with a dash of fresh lemon juice, and add some honey if you wish.

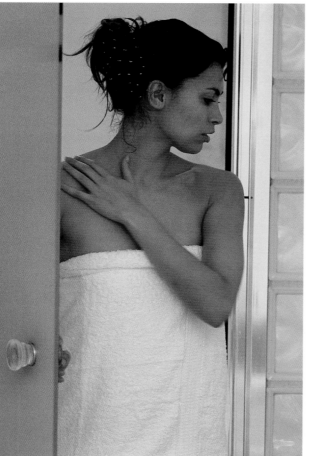

◁ Oil your skin before a steam bath and shower afterwards, using a massage mitt or sponge to slough off dead skin and leave yourself glowing.

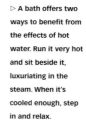

▷ A bath offers two ways to benefit from the effects of hot water. Run it very hot and sit beside it, luxuriating in the steam. When it's cooled enough, step in and relax.

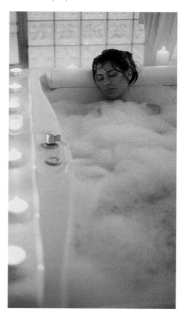

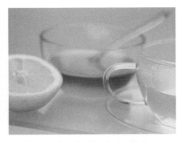

△ Wake up to the refreshing taste of hot water with a splash of lemon and a trickle of honey.

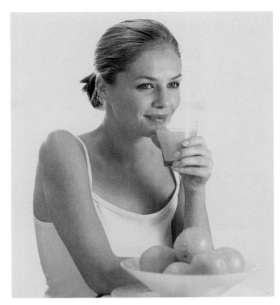

• For breakfast, at least half an hour later, squeeze some fresh fruit juice.
• A light lunch should be your main meal, consisting of boiled or steamed vegetables and grains. Eat slowly, so you notice when you're comfortably full.
• In the early evening, drink some fresh vegetable soup or vegetable juice.
• Throughout the day, except within about an hour of your lunch or supper, drink plain hot water or diluted vegetable juice whenever you wish.

If you're following this regime for less than four days, you can cut out the midday grains. Otherwise you can continue for up to 10 days, but no longer, because the diet does not provide all the nutrients you need in the long term.

## the secret of eternal youth

Rasayana is Ayurveda's method of staying young. It includes taking herbal remedies selected by a practitioner, practising yoga asanas, and doing *pranayama*, or breathing exercises. Since toxins accelerate the aging process, it also means keeping your intake of these to a minimum.

Eating well becomes more than a question of balancing nutrients: food actually reduces your life force if it's stale, overprocessed, laden with chemicals or irradiated. Alcohol is doubly toxic, through its befuddling influence on the brain as well as its physical effects on the liver.

## mental discipline

Ayurveda believes that your health and vitality are strongly influenced by factors such as the environment and your own outlook. Rasayana may require changing your whole lifestyle. How much do you want to keep your energy and your wrinkle-free complexion?

You need to check whether you're producing toxic thoughts. Anger, envy, dishonesty, resentment, greed, callousness and even anxiety can all sap your life force. Just let such feelings go if you can; otherwise seek a practical short-term form of therapy to help root them out. If you spend too much time delving into the reasons for these unworthy thoughts, you're giving them undue attention.

What about your relations with the people around you? Ayurveda values harmony and teaches that you should seek to create it in all areas. If your efforts to free your mind of toxic thoughts are sabotaged by someone who drives you mad, either come to terms with them or keep out of the way. If it's a family member, listen to their grievances and try to understand them.

## outside influences

Ensure that your environment isn't dragging you down. Bad air and water are obvious dangers. But do you live in an ugly environment? Can you often hear noisy neighbours or angry car drivers? If you're in the country, are you affected by chemical sprays? Are your surroundings more demoralizing than invigorating? You can build up resistance to outside factors, but it all uses energy that could be better spent.

Your occupation and daily life should tend towards harmony, with the natural world as well as with other people. Is your job worth doing, or does it cause harm? Do you live a wasteful, high-consumption life? Consider whether you need to move house, change jobs or rethink your way of life.

▽ Oiling the skin is an essential element of Indian beauty, and is also believed to help clear the body of ama, or toxic residues.

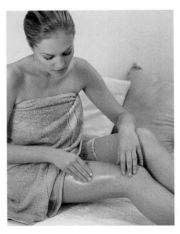

# Bringing meditation into your life

Meditation is part of the detoxifying process, helping to clear waste products from the mind. By counteracting stress and promoting a balanced lifestyle, it creates health benefits that show on your face and body. It's simply a way of focusing the mind, freeing up mental energy by stilling the chatter that runs endlessly through our heads. Each time you meditate successfully, your heart slows down, your blood pressure drops and and you move into the relaxed but alert "alpha" state – thinking clearly and living in the moment.

Meditation can increase concentration, aid healing, ease the symptoms of many health conditions, break the habit of worrying and slow the aging process. In rare cases, it can trigger psychological problems – go to your doctor if this happens, since it may have revealed a disorder needing treatment. Also check with your doctor before starting meditation if you have any medical condition, especially one that affects your heart or blood pressure.

## beginning meditation

It's easiest to get into the habit of meditation if you do it at the same time and place every day. Choose one form of meditation (for example, counting breaths) and stick to it for at least a week. Set a timer for 10 minutes once a day and you may notice improvements before the end of the week.

Sit on a comfortable straight-backed chair with your feet on the floor and close your eyes. Straight away, your mind will be filled with chatter. You can't relax, you have a brilliant idea, you've remembered something important. Don't do battle with these distractions. As thoughts enter your mind just let them drift on out. When, inevitably, you realise your mind has wandered, calmly bring it back to the meditation without criticism.

Always keep your back straight to let energy move freely. Keep your breathing steady and remain aware of it throughout.

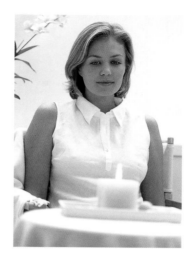

△ A candle flame can be an aid to meditation – a simple, calming point on which to focus while your mind comes gently to rest.

## counting breaths

Let your breathing slow down, then count each breath just before you take a new one. In-out, one. In-out, two. In-out, three. Count up to 10, then start again. Before long your breath becomes steady and it becomes easier to bring your focus back after each detour. You stop fidgeting and begin to feel a sense of peace.

## mantra meditation

A classic form of ayurvedic meditation is repeating a sacred sound, or mantra, over and over again, keeping your attention on the sound. Or you can repeat a word of phrase you find helpful, such as "Om" or "Stillness" or "I am calm". Try to feel nothing but that quality filling you.

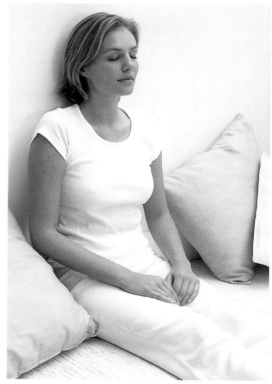

▷ In the Western world, we feel we have to keep busy. Ayurveda, with its concept of balance in all things, reminds us of the value of stillness too.

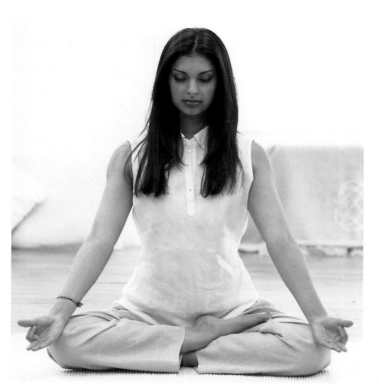

sound and movement, you may be motivated by chanting mantras and walking meditation. If your dosha is aggravated, choose a slow and soothing method. Do try to practise seated meditation, because this is a powerful calming and centring force.

Pitta dosha gives you the drive to succeed at whatever you take up. You can benefit from all kinds of meditation, working on emptying your mind. Any obsessive thoughts soon make themselves obvious by clinging on there. Don't give them attention at all – just quietly waft them away. Mindfulness meditation is also ideal, giving you something else to occupy that space. Since you love beauty and colour, you could try meditating on a mandala, a flame or a favourite flower.

Since kapha people are naturally quiet and calm, you don't need to work on stillness. Instead, try working on keeping the mind focused. Physical activity is always useful for kapha dosha, so you may get more benefit from a moving meditation. Try the livelier forms, such as dancing.

▽ Just one session of meditation can leave you feeling better, and long-term practice can transform your life.

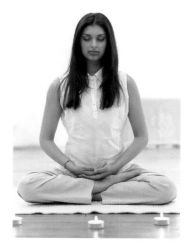

## mandala meditation

Gaze at one of these beautiful, complex paintings and let yourself feel the devotion that went into creating it. Keep your focus on the mandala itself, letting any thoughts it inspires drift away. Go on blinking naturally.

## candle meditation

This peaceful method is ideal for times when you feel upset. Focus on the beautiful flame, without letting your imagination take over. Just be in this moment, looking at this flame. Remember to blink frequently so your eyes don't become sore.

## moving meditation

Movement prevents the restlessness that stops some people meditating. A simple method is walking slowly, regulating your steps to the slow rhythm of your breath. Meditative exercises such as yoga and t'ai chi are also effective.

Experienced meditators can bring the same mental focus to their activities. The key is to do something just complex enough to engage your mind without taking an effort of concentration, while remaining aware of your steady breathing. A steady, rhythmic movement is most helpful, as in swimming. Dancing is uplifting – even though your breathing speeds up, the music and joyful movements can successfully flip you into the alpha state.

## mindfulness

A different route to the alpha state is mindfulness meditation, when instead of trying to switch off you focus fully on what you're doing. When you're massaging yourself, for example, instead of planning or day-dreaming, just be totally aware of the fragrance of the oil, the feel of your skin on different parts of the body, the nurturing movements of your hands.

## meditation for your dosha

Vata energy is rather speedy, so if you have a predominance of this you'll gain a lot from the calming effects of meditation. Being sensitive to subtle energy and attracted to

# The colour of energy

cleansing the body, clearing the mind

According to Ayurvedic philosophy, colours have healing or harmful properties that can affect our bodies as well as our moods. Each shade contains different wavelengths of light energy, and generates different vibrations that subtly affect our own energies. The body's seven important energy centres, the chakras, are depicted in the form of many-petalled lotuses or whirling wheels of colour. These centres draw in energy from the universe and supply it to our physical and non-physical bodies. The energy channel that connects all the chakras follows the course of the spine.

## using colour

The effect of colour is recognized by many people who don't care about the theories but just do what works: they paint fast-food eateries bright red – to make us eat up and leave quickly – and hospitals in healing blues and greens. We are acknowledging the power of colour when we see red, feel blue, lapse into a brown study or walk around under our own personal grey cloud.

Like everything else, shades of colour have *gunas*, or inner qualities. You can train your eye to pick out those that are sattvic: their clear tones promote harmony and

▷ Green is an ideal colour to use for a workplace, as it balances *tejas* – the mental fire that fuels intellectual efforts – and promotes a feeling of calm alertness.

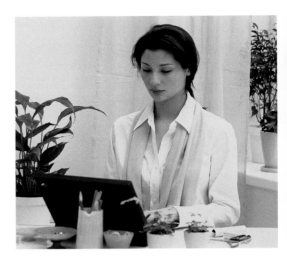

enlightenment. Harsh, over-bright rajasic hues put your nerves on edge, and muddy tamasic shades dull the senses.

Though we can't always control the colours that surround us, we can choose what to wear and how to decorate our

▽ If you're run down or lethargic, surround yourself with energizing colours and feel them gently raise your spirits.

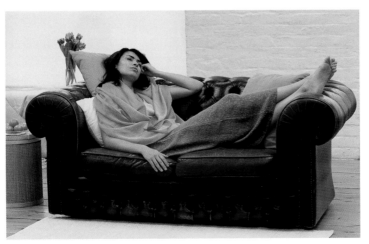

homes. An insomniac whose bedroom is red or orange, for example, would be well advised to redecorate in a gentle shade of blue. If you sometimes feel out of touch with reality, repaint any white walls with warm pastels. Sombre colours (including certain cold shades of blue) can deepen depression. A clear violet will help you to pray or meditate, and green will keep your judgement unclouded while you work.

### COLOURS FOR BALANCE

When your dominant dosha is aggravated, you can choose colours that help bring it back into balance.

**Vata** needs warming and grounding with colours such as red, orange or yellow. Avoid violet or purple, which can make vata types light-headed. Pastel shades such as pink are often helpful.

**Pitta** needs cooling colours such as blue, violet or white. Avoid red, orange, yellow, black, and rajasic shades of any colour.

**Kapha** needs warm, bright, energizing colours such as red, orange, yellow or violet. Avoid brown or grey.

▷ Warm colours have a nourishing, grounding effect on light-headed vata, and can help create a state of relaxed alertness. These rich shades ease feelings of coldness and dryness.

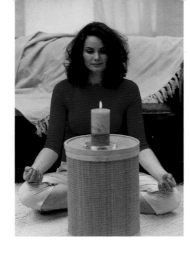

## the chakras

Ayurveda teaches that each chakra governs a different part of the body and supplies a distinctive kind of energy. A blockage in one of the chakras will cause specific diseases or emotional disorders. If you feel that you have a problem in one of these areas, try visualizing the chakra bathed in light of its own colour while meditating.

**Muladhara, the root chakra:** The first chakra is situated just behind the genitals. Its colour is red, and it is the source of strength and stability. The first chakra governs the body's eliminatory systems and its influence makes you practical and grounded. When it

is blocked or damaged in some way you may suffer from lower back pain, or become angry or disorganized.

**Svadisthana, the sacral chakra:** The second chakra is orange and lies just below the navel. It inspires passion, sexuality and creativity. It governs the reproductive system. Potential problems include sexual problems, self-pity and cystitis.

**Manipura, the solar plexus chakra:** The third chakra is yellow and provides willpower. It rules the digestive system and many internal organs. Problems include fear, low self-esteem and digestive disorders.

**Anahata, the heart chakra:** The fourth chakra is green and it is the source of compassion and equilibrium. Its area of influence is the heart and blood circulation. Problems include despair, unbalanced judgement, heart and lung disorders.

**Vishudda, the throat chakra:** The fifth chakra is blue. It rules the mouth and the thyroid gland, and the ability to learn. Problems include sore throats and difficulty in speaking out.

**Ajna, the brow chakra:** The sixth chakra, or third eye, is indigo. Situated in the middle of the forehead, it is the source of intuition and governs the nervous system and pituitary gland. It is the spot we instinctively touch when trying to think. Problems are nightmares, lack of concentration or detachment from reality.

**Sahasrara, the crown chakra:** The seventh chakra rules the pineal gland and is the source of enlightenment. It is shown coloured either violet or white – which contains all colours. If the crown chakra is blocked you may feel confused, or behave selfishly and unethically.

▽ Tranquil shades of blue and clean, clear white help keep pitta cool on even the hottest days.

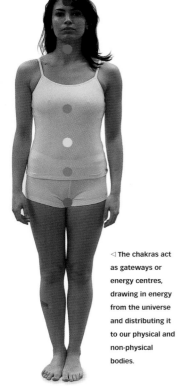

◁ The chakras act as gateways or energy centres, drawing in energy from the universe and distributing it to our physical and non-physical bodies.

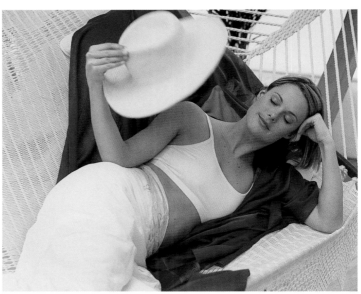

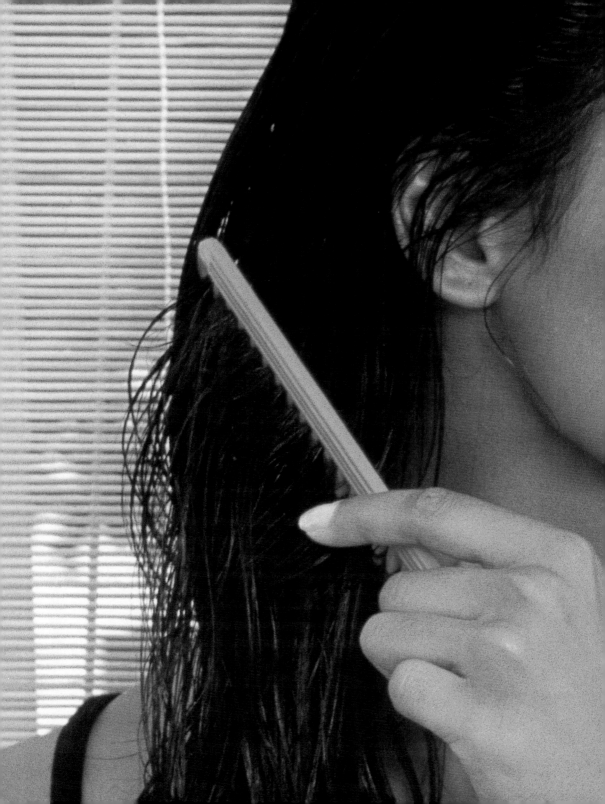

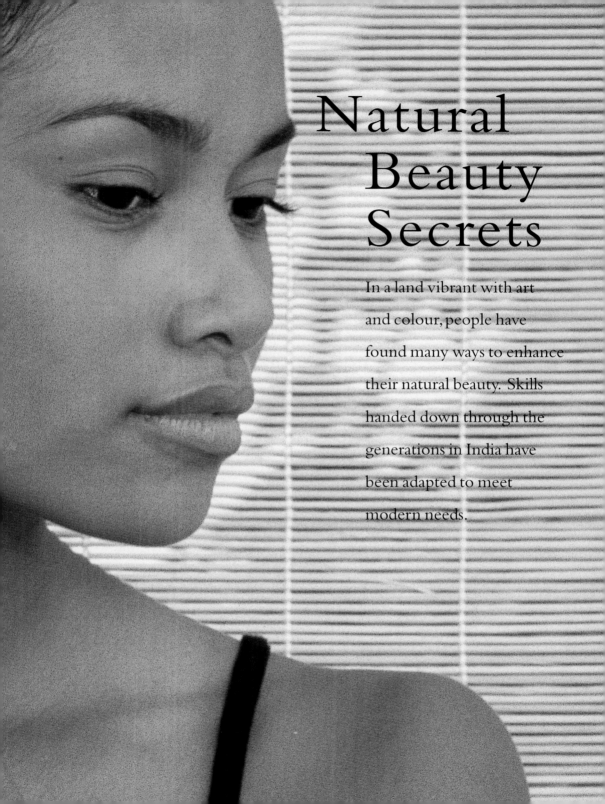

# Natural Beauty Secrets

In a land vibrant with art and colour, people have found many ways to enhance their natural beauty. Skills handed down through the generations in India have been adapted to meet modern needs.

# A home facial

Ayurvedic beauty treatments don't just improve skin quality: they're also an antidote to stress. The full routine for a facial treatment takes about an hour, so dedicate one evening every week or month to treat yourself luxuriously, but you can use the cleansing, toning and (for dry skins) moisturizing steps of this facial every day. Commercially made Ayurvedic beauty products are internationally available, but for those who like to make their own, recipes for each stage of the treatment are given on the following pages.

## cleansing with oil

Oil is a good make-up remover for all skin types, and is ideal for cleansing off city grime or dust. You can make up your own blend, using a suitable base oil for your skin type, or use a base oil alone. Apply oil with your fingertips in a circular motion. Instead of washing the oil off, Indian women traditionally blot it up with a herbal powder called an *ubtan*.

## ubtans

These powders clean and stimulate the skin, and can be used as a cleanser alone or after applying oil. The simplest ubtan is a mix of plain besan (chickpea or gram flour) made into a paste with a few drops of liquid: use lemon juice for oily skin or warm milk for dry skin. The paste should be firm and not too liquid. Apply to the skin with the fingertips using circular or upward movements, and when it feels dry massage it off with warm water.

More complex mixtures, containing herbs and grains, are used as exfoliants, usually after a herbal heat treatment. For skin that's not blemished or sensitive, it's a good idea to use a slightly coarser formulation every few weeks, always avoiding the delicate eye area. If your skin is sensitive, though, ensure the ubtan is finely ground – and resist that enthusiastic pitta tendency to scrub too hard.

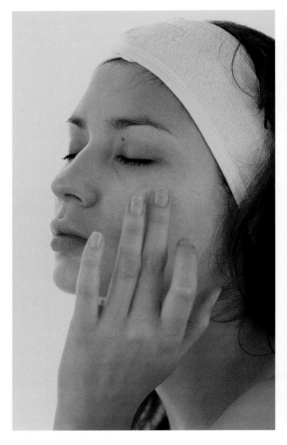

▷ Oil is excellent for removing make-up and nourishing all types of skin. It enters the finest pores without causing harm. Almond oil, rich in Vitamin E, is the traditional favourite.

## herbal heat treatment

A weekly heat treatment suits most skin types, though once a month is enough for dry and mature skins. Damp heat opens the pores, encourages sweat to flush out ingrained dirt and brings oxygen-rich blood to renew the skin. You may choose to put oil on your skin first, since the heat helps the oil penetrate more deeply. But don't leave cleansing oil on, or you'll be drawing dirt back into the skin.

**Herbal steam:** Sit with your head forward over a bowl of hot, herb-infused water, draped in a towel to stop the steam escaping, for about 5 minutes. Stop immediately if you feel dizzy or overheated.

**Herbal compress:** Soak several face cloths in hot, herb-infused water, and wring out. Sitting with your head back and supported, put the cloths over your face and relax for 5 minutes. As the cloths cool down, wring them out in the hot water again.

**Herbal bath:** Infuse a bag of herbs in your bath and let the heat open your pores.

Finish by patting your face with a clean cloth wrung out in cool water. Give your face a cooling splash of toner or water, then rest for a few minutes to cool down.

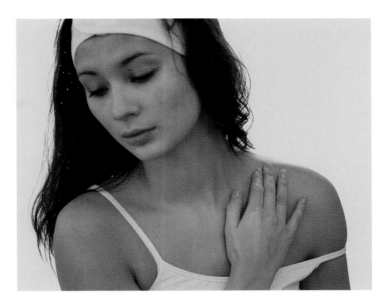

## oil massage

This is a traditional Indian technique. Oils are highly prized in Ayurveda, and considered essential to the healthy functioning of the body, but moisturizer can be used instead of oil if you prefer.

Warm some oil and pour a little into your hands. Starting just below your collarbones, smooth it into your skin using long strokes upwards and outwards, or clockwise circular movements. Continue for up to 10 minutes, covering your throat and face. Your touch should be just firm enough to move the skin slightly, without dragging it. Be especially careful not to drag dry or mature skin. Those with kapha skin should wipe off the oil before continuing.

## facepack or mask

Few treatments give your skin such a quick lift as a facepack. These simple treatments, based on fruit or vegetables, can be left on for up to an hour, while you have a massage or meditate (you may need to be lying down if the mask is runny; try the Corpse yoga

pose). A mask is a stronger version of a facepack, using a powder such as flour or clay to penetrate the pores more deeply. It should be left on for 10–20 minutes.

To remove the facepack or mask, dab it with water (for oily skin) or milk (for dry skin) to soften it, then gently massage and rinse the mix off your skin.

## toning

Remove any residues and soothe the skin with a splash of cool flower water or, for oily skin, witch hazel and flower water. Skin that

is very oily or has darker patches can be rubbed with a slice of lemon and left for a few minutes before rinsing off.

## moisturizing

Only moisturize skin that feels dry. If you have oily skin or acne and follow the Ayurvedic process, you needn't use a moisturizer – none of the cleansing recipes will strip the skin of oil.

▽ A slice of lemon helps lighten darker patches, but don't use this on dry or sensitive skin.

▽ Take a break while the mask does its work – use the time for some other pampering treat.

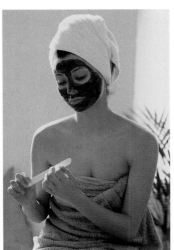

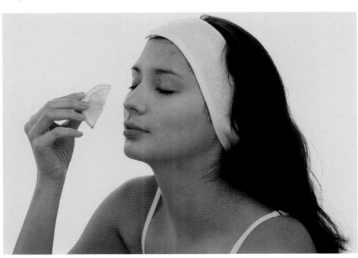

# First step: cleansing

Traditional wisdom is a dynamic resource, adapting to new conditions as it passes down through the generations. Indian families who move to other countries often modify their age-old recipes to suit what they have to hand, replacing ingredients that are hard to find outside India with others that are easily obtainable, including essential oils.

You can turn your kitchen cupboard into a beauty treasure-trove, as practically all the ingredients needed for the following recipes are used in everyday Indian cookery. All are available from Asian stores, and most can be found in supermarkets.

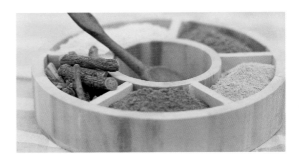
▷ Ingredients for an ubtan (clockwise from front): ground coriander, liquorice sticks, besan, ground cumin and ground fenugreek.

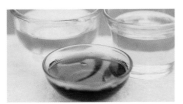
△ Oils to suit your skin, from left: almond for all complexions, sesame for dry, sunflower for oily.

## cleansing cream

The best oils for cleansing are almond, sesame and sunflower. Alternatively, you can use this light cream cleanser.

### ingredients

• 7.5 ml/1/2 tbsp beeswax
• 30 ml/2 tbsp coconut oil
• 30 ml/2 tbsp almond oil
• 60 ml/4 tbsp cucumber juice (or water)
• 1.5 ml/1/4 tsp borax
• 15 ml/1 tbsp witch hazel
• few drops rose water

> **ALLERGY ALERT**
> Before applying any cosmetic to your face, test it on your inner arm, leaving it for as long as you intend to leave it on your face. If any redness or irritation develops, wash off the mixture at once and discard it.

Melt the beeswax in a non-metallic bowl over a pan of hot water, and add the oils. In a separate bowl, heat the cucumber juice and borax (a good natural emulsifier) until the borax is completely dissolved. Add the witch hazel and remove from the heat. Combine the contents of the two bowls and allow to cool a little, then add the rose water. Beat the mixture until it cools and thickens.

## herbal ubtan

This a traditional Indian cleanser. Many different blends are possible, but all have gentle softening and cleansing effects.

### ingredients

• ground coriander
• ground cumin
• ground fenugreek
• ground liquorice
• besan (chickpea flour)

Mix together equal quantities of all of the ingredients and then store your mixed powder in a clean and airtight container. You will need about a small handful for one treatment. The dry base blend should be mixed to a paste consistency with the appropriate liquid ingredient for immediate use whenever it is needed.

• For oily, combination or blemished skin, mix the base blend to a paste with yogurt or diluted lemon juice.

• For dry or mature skin, mix the ubtan with milk or cream.

• For normal skin, or if the other combinations feel too sticky, mix with water or rose water.

Mix to a smooth, soft paste, then rub it into your skin – gently for dry vata or sensitive pitta complexions – using small circular movements. Massage off with warm, followed by cool, water.

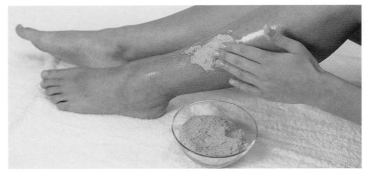
△ If you've made more than you need for a facial, why not give your feet and legs a treat too?

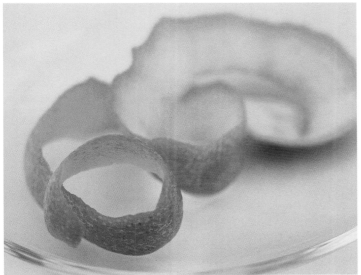

◁ Orange peel contains astringent oils that cleanse away excessive skin secretions and help to remove blemishes caused by blocked pores.

## almond ubtan

This mixture is especially useful for reducing a pitta or vata imbalance, or for dry or sensitive skin.

**ingredients**
- walnuts
- fine oatmeal
- ground almonds

Grind the walnuts to a coarse powder and mix with equal quantities of the oatmeal and ground almonds. Store the mixture in an airtight container. To use, mix a small handful of the powder to a paste using water (for oily skin) or milk (for dry skin).

▽ **Preparing ingredients, such as these walnuts for an ubtan for dry skin, is part of an almost meditative process of self-nourishment.**

## orange peel ubtan

This is useful for people with oily skin or a kapha imbalance, who should use it every second day. It helps remove blackheads gently and leaves skin feeling smooth. Start off by using equal quantities of all the ingredients. Later, you may decide to vary the proportions to suit your own skin.

**ingredients**
- lentils
- wheat
- dried orange peel
- fine oatmeal
- besan (chickpea flour)

Grind the lentils, wheat and dried orange peel to a coarse powder. For sensitive pitta skin, grind the powders more finely. Mix all the ingredients together and store the blend in an airtight container.

To use the ubtan, mix a small handful of the powder to a soft paste using a few drops of water, or lemon juice, or both, depending on your skin type. Use the paste as a facial scrub.

### MILK AND SUGAR

These make the simplest facial. Moisten your face with water, then gently massage clean with a teaspoonful of sugar. Tone with a splash of water. Moisturize with skin from the top of boiled milk that's been left to cool. Leave this on for 2 minutes, then massage off with water.

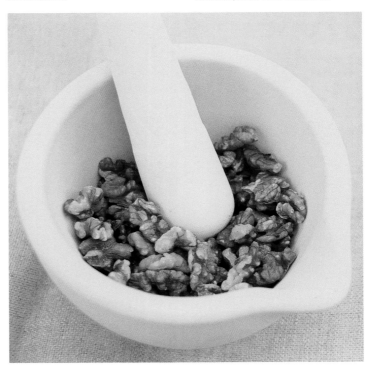

# The next steps: heat and oil

For body massage, Ayurvedic practitioners normally choose an oil that will help to bring the doshas into balance, such as sesame oil to reduce vata or kapha and coconut oil to cool an excess of pitta. For the face and throat, however, they base their choice on skin type and condition – which are often an expression of dosha energy anyway.

In general, vata energy is expressed in dry skin, pitta in sensitive skin and kapha in oily skin. So you may wish to use treatments that suit your skin condition, while eating and following other guidelines to pacify the relevant dosha.

## skin types

Classic vata skin is thin and fine-pored, dry, cool and often dark. This fragile complexion needs very gentle care and moisturizing. It should never be rubbed hard or dragged.

▽ For an easy steam treatment, pour a few drops of herbal oil blend into the bath and relax.

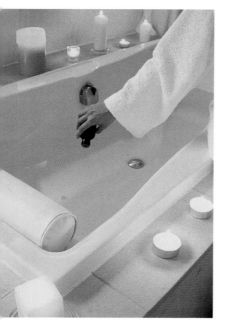

Pitta skin is soft, warm and rosy, but often sensitive. Avoid harsh chemicals or anything that could cause a rash or inflammation. Pittas often have combination skin, with an oily T-zone of forehead, nose and chin but drier skin on the cheeks and beside the mouth. Common problems are acne and patches of pigmentation.

Kapha skin is strong, thick and naturally moist. It's therefore slow to show signs of aging or environmental damage, but it is prone to enlarged pores, blackheads and excessive oiliness.

If, like most people, you are influenced by two doshas, you should note which one seems dominant in your complexion. You may be mainly kapha, but if your skin is sensitive to heat and chemicals, and is much drier on your cheeks and beside your mouth, it's expressing pitta energy and needs to be treated for this. Your skin condition will also vary with external factors such as the weather: the cold dryness of winter increases vata energy, for example, and may affect your skin accordingly.

## herbal steam treatment

Add a scented mixture of herbs and spices to hot water for a gentle heat treatment. Test the steam with your inner arm before allowing it near your face.

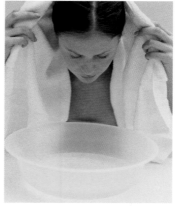

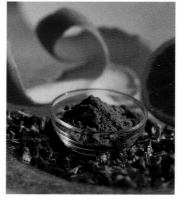

△ Fresh ingredients boiled in water release their fragrance and healing powers in steam.

**ingredients**
- half a lemon
- strips of orange peel
- pinch of pure sandalwood powder
- dried rose petals

Possible added ingredients you could use:
- For oily skin: liquorice root, lavender, fennel seeds, rosemary.
- For mature skin: liquorice root, fennel seeds, clove, grated ginger, mint.
- For dry skin: liquorice root, bay leaf, chamomile.
- For blemished skin: liquorice root, lemon grass, lavender, dandelion root.
- For normal skin: liquorice root, thyme, chamomile, fennel seeds, lavender.

Put at least 1.2 litres/2 pints/5 cups water in an enamelled or non-metallic pan and add the lemon and about two handfuls of a mixture of the remaining ingredients. Cover and bring to the boil, stirring occasionally, then remove from the heat. Leave covered and allow to cool until the steam is a comfortable temperature.

◁ If you're short of time – or herbs – even plain hot water can be used to steam oiled skin.

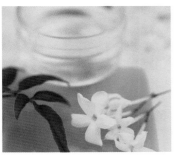

△ **Sesame or almond oil, infused with jasmine, makes a soothing massage oil for dry skin.**

## facial massage oils

The base oils can be used alone, but do try making a herbal oil for face or body massage: two methods are given below. Some infused oils can be bought ready-made, or you could add a drop of essential oil. (A few essential oils should be avoided in pregnancy; check with an expert before using.)

## simple herbal oil

**ingredients**

- handful of fresh herb (see box)
- 250 ml / 8 fl oz / 1 cup base oil (see box)

Crush the herb leaves using a pestle and mortar, then add a small amount of your

### HERBAL OILS FOR YOUR SKIN TYPE

- Normal skin: almond oil with lavender or geranium.
- Skin infections: almond oil with neem, sandalwood or triphala.
- Rough or dehydrated skin: almond oil with rose, manjishtha or arjun.
- Dry skin: almond or sesame oil with rose or jasmine.
- Mature skin: almond or sesame oil with lavender or frankincense.
- Oily skin: almond, sunflower or jojoba oil with lemon or bergamot.
- Blemished skin: almond, sunflower or jojoba oil with lavender or tea tree.
- Cellulite: almond oil with lemon or orange.

chosen base oil and blend thoroughly. Now add this blend to the rest of the oil, pour into a screw-top jar and shake well. Keep in a cool, dark place and shake several times a day for three days before using.

## herbal oil infusion

**ingredients**

- 4 parts base oil (see box)
- 16 parts water
- 1 part ground or powdered herb (see box)

Measure the oil into an enamelled or non-metallic pan and add the water and your chosen herb. Bring to the boil over a medium heat, stirring briskly, then reduce the heat and leave to simmer gently, stirring occasionally, until all of the water has evaporated. Depending on the amount of infused oil you are making, this may take an hour or more. You could leave the pan on the back burner while you are preparing food, unless you are cooking something with a strong smell that could affect the oil.

▽ **Rosemary adds a clean, sharp tang to a herbal steam for oily or teenage skin.**

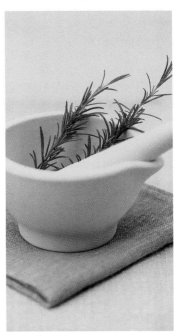

### RULES OF THUMB

Traditionally, people learnt these recipes by watching their mothers and aunts preparing them. They were tailored to each person's needs, so would vary according to their individual constitution, their current state of health and the season. Ingredients would be measured in handfuls, and the proportions given here are guides rather than rules: experiment to find, or create, a formulation that suits you.

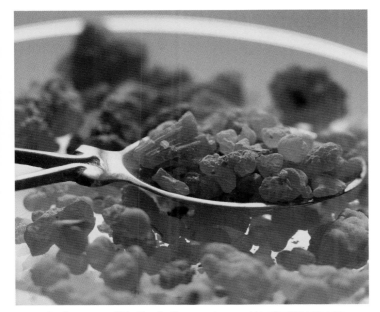

△ **So precious it was once a gift for kings, frankincense makes a nourishing blend for mature skin.**

# Deep-cleansing facepacks and masks

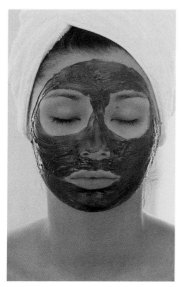

△ **Masks contain earth or flour, so don't apply near the delicate eye area or leave them on for more than 20 minutes, as they can be drying.**

Applying the very simplest cleansing and nourishing facepacks involves little more than squashing ripe fruit on to your face. Most fruits and vegetables can be used in this way, though harder types need to be grated or puréed: experiment with the suggestions given here to find what produces the best result on your skin. Smooth the facepack on with your fingers – or, if you find it easier, paint it on with a pastry brush kept for this purpose – and leave it on your face for up to 20 minutes (unless stated otherwise) while you relax. At the end of that time, massage the facepack off your skin and then finish by rinsing with water.

Clay, oatmeal or besan (chickpea or gram flour) can be added to any of the facepack recipes to make a mask that aids the cleansing process by drawing out dirt from deep in the pores. Oat flour is very soothing for eczema, while chickpea flour can leave skin feeling very taut, so is best combined with other dry ingredients. Mix the mask to a consistency that won't slide straight off your face – experiment on the back of your hand – and leave for up to 20 minutes before massaging and rinsing it off.

## simple facepack

**ingredients**
- selection of fruit and/or vegetables (see box)
- 5 ml/1 tsp yogurt or almond oil

In a non-metallic bowl, chop, grate or mash the fruit and vegetables to a pulp. Strain off the excess juice for a healthy drink, and add the yogurt (for oily skin) or oil (for dry skin) to the pulp. Spread or brush the mixture over your face and neck, avoiding the delicate skin around the eyes. Lie down for at least 10 minutes while it takes effect, then massage and rinse off with cool water.

## skin rejuvenator

This is kind to mature skin and can help reduce the appearance of wrinkles.

**ingredients**
- handful of fresh scented geranium (*Pelargonium graveolens*) leaves
- rose water to cover

Soak the geranium leaves in rose water for a few hours until softened, then spread on your face and lie down for 15–30 minutes.

## avocado facepack

Egg white and lemon juice usually suit oily complexions, but the addition of avocado, rich in natural oils, makes this a great soother for dry skin too.

**ingredients**
- 1 avocado
- 5 ml/1 tsp lemon juice
- 1 egg white

Mash the avocado, mix in the other ingredients and apply to the face.

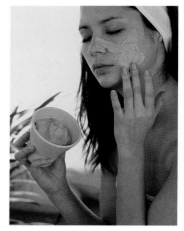

△ **Experiment to find what suits you: the richness of avocado makes a soothing facepack.**

## apple facepack

This suits all skin types. If you have very oily skin, you may wish to use jojoba oil instead of almond.

**FACEPACK INGREDIENTS FOR YOUR SKIN TYPE**

Sharp-tasting fruits, such as grape, lemon, tomato or peach, should be combined with a more soothing, starchy fruit or vegetable, such as banana. Be careful if you include grape in a mixture, as it has a peeling effect on the skin; don't use it at all if your skin is dry or sensitive.
- Normal skin: avocado, banana, courgette, grape, peach.
- Dry skin: avocado, banana, carrot, melon, pear.
- Oily or combination skin: cabbage, cucumber, lemon, pear, strawberries, tomatoes, tangerine.
- Mature skin: apple, avocado, banana.
- Blemished skin: apple, cabbage, plums (boiled and allowed to cool), tomato.
- In hot weather: cucumber, strawberries.

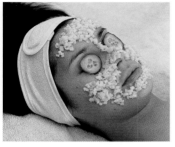

△ **Relax while an apple facepack rebalances your skin and cucumber reduces any puffiness.**

**ingredients**
- ¹/₂ small apple, peeled and grated
- 15 ml/1 tbsp honey
- 1 egg yolk
- 15 ml/1 tbsp cider or wine vinegar
- 45 ml/3 tbsp almond oil

Mix together all ingredients.

## spot remedy facepack
**ingredients**
- 1 egg white
- 5 ml/1 tsp honey
- 5 ml/1 tsp carrot juice
- 5 ml/1 tsp crushed garlic

Beat the egg white until stiff. Mix in the other ingredients and apply for 20 minutes to help heal spots and blemishes.

## honey and egg facepack
This instantly rejuvenates dry skin.

**ingredients**
- 2.5 ml/¹/₂ tsp honey
- 1 egg yolk
- 15 ml/1 tbsp dried skimmed milk

Mix to a paste and leave on for 20 minutes.

## juicy mask
Yogurt cleanses the skin, while the juices feed it with vitamins and minerals.

**ingredients**
- 15 ml/1 tbsp powdered brewer's yeast
- 2.5 ml/¹/₂ tsp yogurt
- 5 ml/1 tsp orange juice
- 5 ml/1 tsp carrot juice
- 5 ml/1 tsp almond oil

Mix all the ingredients into a paste. If you have oily skin or darker patches, add 5 ml/1 tsp lemon juice; for very dry skin, double the oil content.

## clarifying mask
**ingredients**
- 10 ml/2 tsp ground almonds
- 5 ml/1 tsp rose water
- 2.5 ml/¹/₂ tsp honey

Mix into a paste and apply as a thin layer. Rinse off with cool rose water.

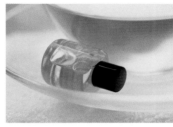

△ **Add a little light oil, such as almond or jojoba, to counteract the drying effect of face masks on delicate vata skin.**

## oatmeal mask
Use yogurt to bind the dry ingredients if you have oily skin, or almond oil for dry skin. For other skin types, choose whichever you prefer – try one version on each cheek and see which feels better.

**ingredients**
- 10 ml/2 tsp fine oatmeal
- 30 ml/2 tbsp powdered orange peel
- yogurt or almond oil

Mix the oatmeal and powdered orange peel together and add enough yogurt or almond oil to make a paste.

## potato mask
Rich in Vitamin C, potatoes also tighten the skin, making this a good choice for tired or mature complexions.

**ingredients**
- 15 ml/1 tbsp potato juice
- 15 ml/1 tbsp multani mitti (fuller's earth)

Mix together thoroughly to make a paste and spread on the skin.

377

---

**BESAN (CHICKPEA FLOUR) MASKS**
- For oily skin: mix besan with some olive oil and lemon juice.
- For dry or normal skin: mix besan with some olive oil and yogurt.

## spot remedy mask
This is effective against spots and blemishes.

**ingredients**
- 1 egg yolk
- 15 ml/1 tbsp powdered brewer's yeast
- 15 ml/1 tbsp sunflower oil

Mix to a paste and apply to the face. After 15 minutes rinse off with milk.

## orange mask
This is suitable for dry skin.

**ingredients**
- 5 ml/1 tsp freshly squeezed orange juice
- 15 ml/1 tbsp multani mitti (fuller's earth)
- 15 ml/1 tbsp rose water
- 15 ml/1 tbsp liquid honey

Mix all the ingredients together to make a paste and smooth lightly on to the skin.

---

**EGG ON YOUR FACE**
When you need to look good and haven't time for a full treatment, just try an egg. For oily skin, beat an egg white and spread on to your face. Leave to dry and then wash off thoroughly. This tightens skin for a temporary face-lifting effect. If you have dry skin, use the whole egg, beaten. You can also use egg white or whole egg, depending on your skin type, as a substitute for oil or yogurt in herbal ubtans and facepacks.

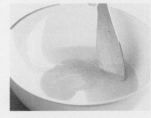

△ **Egg feeds the skin and binds powders.**

# toning and moisturizing

A splash of cool filtered or spring water refreshes skin after any treatment. Flower waters add their own natural benefits, and gently close pores without the harshness of alcohol-based toners. For oily skin, try water with a dash of vinegar, or rose water with a dash of witch hazel.

## flower waters

Rose water is perfect for skin care. Mildly astringent, it soothes and rehydrates skin. It's cooling in a hot climate, reduces inflammation, and the subtle fragrance is said to have antidepressant and aphrodisiac qualities. Buy the highest quality you can find, or make your own.

Rose water makes a refreshing spray, especially in the dryness of air-conditioned rooms or the stuffy heat of a plane, and also helps to set make-up. A cloth or cotton pads wrung out in rose water and placed over closed eyes is the kindest treatment when your eyes are sore.

Other flowers can be used in the same way. Lavender water has long been prized for its cleansing, deodorant properties and refreshing scent. In hot weather it is ideal to use over the entire body – and also for spraying on clothes and bedlinen.

▽ **Simple pleasure: a splash of plain water revitalizes your mind and refreshes your skin.**

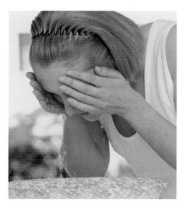

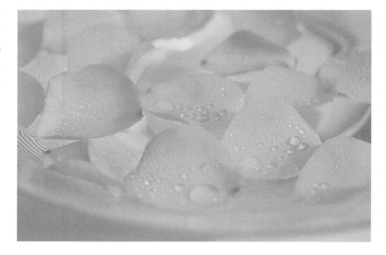

## rose water

Use equal quantities, by volume, of rose petals and pure water to give a delicately scented result. Increase the water's strength by using more petals, as long as the water still covers them. For an even stronger scent, use dried rose petals: simply shake fresh petals into a paper bag, loosely close the top, hang up and leave to dry.

### ingredients

- 1 cup fresh scented rose petals, tightly packed
- 1 cup spring or filtered water

Put the petals in a heatproof, non-metallic container. Boil the water and pour it over the petals. Cover and leave to cool. Decant into a screwtop bottle or jar and store in the fridge.

## rose water astringent

For oily or blemished skin.

### ingredients

- 1 part rose water
- 1 part witch hazel

Pour both ingredients into a screwtop jar or bottle and shake to mix.

△ **The fragrance of rose water has been treasured throughout history.**

## rose water soother

A treat for a dry complexion and tired skin under the eyes.

### ingredients

- 250 ml/8 fl oz/1 cup rose water
- 1 drop sandalwood oil
- 1 drop rose, tea rose or rose geranium essential oil

Pour all ingredients into a screwtop jar or bottle and shake to mix.

## lavender water

### ingredients

- handful of fresh lavender heads, stems removed
- 475 ml/16 fl oz/2 cups filtered or spring water

Put the flowers into a jar with a screw top and pour the water over them. Leave for a day, shaking occasionally. For a stronger scent, leave it for up to three weeks, taking the top off every few days to check the scent. Strain off the water into a clean jar or bottle and keep in the refrigerator.

# flower water refresher

**ingredients**

- 1 part water
- 1 part rose water or lavender water
- 2 slices cucumber
- few drops lemon juice (optional, for oily skin)

Combine the water and flower water and refrigerate for 5 minutes. Dip the cucumber slices in the liquid and put over closed eyes while you rest. Pour the remaining liquid into a spray bottle, adding a few drops of lemon juice if you have oily skin. Use as a refreshing spritz for face and throat.

## moisturizing cream

Adjust the measurements given to find a consistency that suits your skin, and choose a herbal powder to balance your dosha: white sandalwood or jasmine for pitta, manjishtha for vata, or neem for kapha.

**ingredients**

- 30 ml/2 tbsp beeswax
- 175 ml/6 fl oz/³⁄₄ cup almond oil
- pinch of herbal powder (see above) or a few drops rose or jasmine essential oil

Melt the beeswax gently in a non-metallic bowl over hot water. Stir in the oil. Add the herbal powder or essential oil, and whisk until the mixture is soft. Allow to cool.

▷ **For a subtle and unique fragrance, look around your garden and pick your favourite blooms to create flower water recipes of your own.**

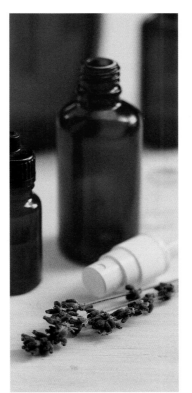

◁ **Keep some screwtop jars for mixing and spray bottles for spritzing. Remember to store all natural cosmetics – and even bottled water, once it's opened – in the refrigerator for safety.**

### SAFE STORAGE

Traditionally, women grew their own plants or bought them freshly picked. They ground their own spices, grains and other powders, and used them immediately, whether in cooking or on their skin. Not many of us have a chance to do the same now, so we need to store ingredients safely.

Dry ingredients should be kept in clean, airtight containers. Stored in a dark cupboard, they should keep their fragrance and potency for weeks or months. Anything moist should be refrigerated to prevent the growth of moulds or bacteria. Since home-made cosmetics don't contain strong preservatives, mix them as you need them and don't keep the leftovers for more than a few days.

### TAKE CARE OF YOURSELF

Don't hurry while giving yourself a facial. If time is short, it's better to leave out some of the steps than to rush through them. As far as possible, ensure that your surroundings are quiet and you're not interrupted. The results can be seen as stress dissolves from your face.

Preparation, too, should be a meditative process. Focus, one by one, on the colours of the ingredients, their textures as they are mixed together, the different scents as they develop, the small sounds of the spoon against the bowl and the feel of the various mixtures on your skin.

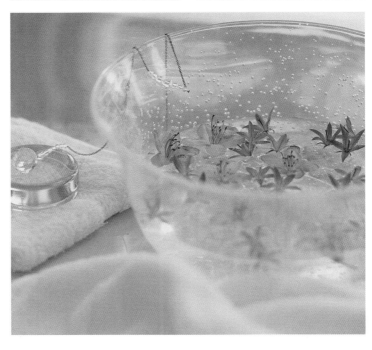

# An Ayurvedic facelift

Your skin type, build and dosha will determine whether lines or sagging will be more of a problem as your skin ages. Generally, if you're thin and have dry skin you're more likely to develop wrinkles, a problem that besets many vata people. Kaphas are more likely to have oily skin and put on weight. This can bring beauty benefits, but the downside is that extra flesh starts to sag, causing a jowly effect. Anyone ruled by pitta or (like most of us) by more than one dosha could encounter any of these problems. So the best treatment aims to keep them all at bay.

## Marma-point facial massage

**A 30-minute daily marma-point massage will slow down the effects of time on your face. In Ayurvedic terms you're encouraging the movement of prana, the life force; Western science explains it as releasing muscle stiffness and increasing blood circulation. Sit with your back straight but not arched. It's useful to have a table to lean your elbows on, and to use a mirror to check the positions of your fingers, but close your eyes when you don't need to look. Before starting, massage your shoulders, neck and head for a few minutes: tension in these neighbouring muscles creates tension in your face.**

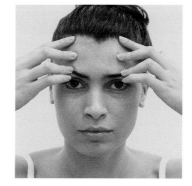

**VARYING PRESSURE**

Throughout the massage you can either continue the 7–5–7–5–7–5 pressure used in step 1, or simply press once for a count of 7. Either way, press slowly and firmly, pressing inwards against the bone, not upwards or downwards unless specified. You can also vary the direct touch with small circling movements, maintaining the pressure and moving the skin over the bone.

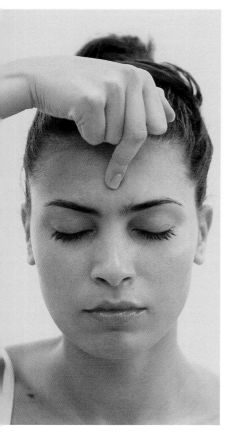

◁ **1** Begin by working on the Third Eye point, slightly above the bridge of your nose. Feel for a slight indentation, which is often the sign of an important marma point. Apply firm pressure for a count of 7 as you breathe out, then reduce to light pressure for 5, breathing in. Repeat 3 times.

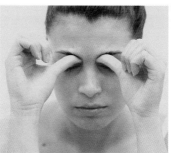

◁ **2** Find the point in each eyebrow directly above the centre of the eye, and visualize a line from there up into your hair. Following this line, press your ring finger into the eyebrow point, the index finger into the hairline, and the middle finger between them.

△ **3** Feel for the upper edges of the eye sockets and press firmly with the thumbs. Be careful to press the bone, without letting your thumbs slip into your eyes or eye sockets. Lift your thumbs, move them just above the eye sockets and press again, pushing upwards so that your forehead furrows.

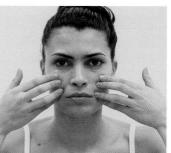

△ **4** Place the tips of your index fingers on your cheek bones, with your other fingertips vertically below them under the centre of each eye, and apply firm pressure.

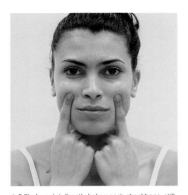

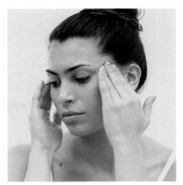

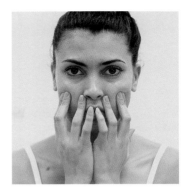

△ **5** Find a point directly below each cheekbone, still in line with the centre of your eyes. Press inwards and upwards into the bottom of the cheekbone.

△ **6** Put the flat of each ring finger on the outer edge of each eye socket, and spread the other fingers out along a diagonal line to the edge of the ear. Press the fingers firmly.

△ **7** Find a point at the outer edge of each nostril and press diagonally inwards with your third fingers, while your index and middle fingers press inwards and upwards below the cheekbones.

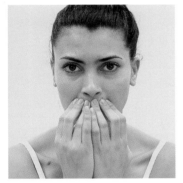

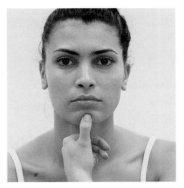

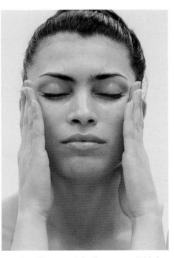

△ **8** Bunch all fingertips close together and press along the space between your top lip and your nose – an area containing numerous marma points. Do the same below your lower lip.

△ **9** Press one thumbtip into the centre of your chin.

△ **10** If you like, pour a little oil or cream suitable for your skin type onto your hands. Bring your hands down the centre of your face, barely touching it, until the heels of your hands are under your chin. Now lightly stroke your fingertips out to the side across the cheekbones, without rubbing the fine skin directly beneath the eyes. Then bring the hands, with a firmer stroke, up the sides of the face. Repeat two or three times. Cup your hands over your closed eyes for several breaths.

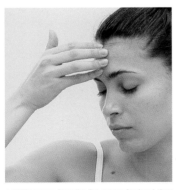

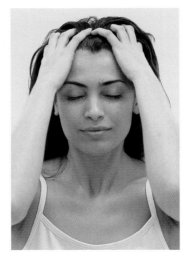

△ **11** Place your fingertips flat on your forehead, then stroke lightly towards the right ear. Repeat on the left. Stroke in both directions several times. If there's any feeling of drag, apply more oil to your skin. Continue the movement into your hair.

◁**12** Massage your head. Lightly pull sections of hair, making your scalp move in circles over your skull. Finish by combing with your fingers in long movements to the ends of the hair.

# Body care

When you see the difference a facepack makes to your complexion, why stop there? Indian women have long enjoyed the benefits of herbal pastes, using them to enhance skin quality over the entire body.

Herbal baths are the easiest skincare treatment of all. Simply relax in a warm bath and let the ingredients nourish your skin while the heat eases away tension. Liquid ingredients can be poured straight into the water. Put other ingredients in a muslin bag, swish it around in the bath and leave it in while you soak.

## body mask for oily or blemished skin

This mask is designed to detoxify, balance, remove impurities and polish the skin surface, leaving it silky smooth.

### ingredients

- 115 g/4 oz/1 cup besan (chickpea flour)
- 5–10 ml/1–2 tsp turmeric
- 30 ml/2 tbsp white sandalwood powder
- 15 ml/1 tbsp red sandalwood powder
- 30 ml/2 tbsp neem leaf powder
- 30 ml/2 tbsp powdered orange peel
- water
- yogurt (optional)

Mix all the dry ingredients together and add water, or a combination of water and yogurt, to make a thin paste. Brush over the skin and leave for about 30 minutes, until dry. Wet the mask with water or milk, then massage off with fairly firm pressure. Rinse with water.

## body mask for dry skin

### ingredients

- 115 g/4 oz/1 cup besan (chickpea flour)
- 15 ml/1 tbsp white sandalwood powder
- 15 ml/1 tbsp red sandalwood powder
- 15 ml/1 tbsp Indian madder
- 15 ml/1 tbsp arjuna
- 15 ml/1 tbsp brahmi
- 15 ml/1 tbsp shatavari
- unhomogenized milk to mix

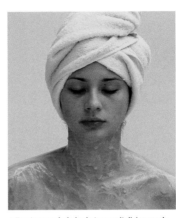

△ **Treat your whole body to a revitalizing mask that sloughs off dead cells, letting skin shine.**

Mix the dry ingredients then add the milk, warmed to body temperature, to make a paste. Brush this on to the skin and leave until it is dry. Remove with more of the warm milk.

## bridal body mask

This is traditionally used by brides-to-be every day for 10 days before the wedding. It leaves the skin feeling soft and clean. A very simple form can be made using just turmeric and oil.

### ingredients

- 15 ml/1 tbsp powdered orange peel
- 15 ml/1 tbsp powdered lemon peel
- 30 ml/2 tbsp ground almonds
- pinch of salt
- 25 g/1 oz/4 tbsp finely ground wheatgerm
- 15 ml/1 tbsp ground thyme
- 7.5 ml/$^1$/$_2$ tbsp turmeric
- almond oil to mix
- few drops jasmine or rose essential oil

Mix all the dry ingredients and add enough almond oil to make a paste. Add the jasmine or rose oil. Spread over the body and leave for 15–20 minutes. Rub off firmly, as though you are gently "sanding" the skin.

**QUICK BEAUTY TIP**
For the simplest body scrub of all, massage sea salt on to damp skin and shower off.

## soothing bath mix

Add to the bath water to calm irritated skin, but don't use this on broken skin.

### ingredients

- 120 ml/4 fl oz/$^1$/$_2$ cup cider or wine vinegar
- 30 ml/2 tbsp honey
- 120 ml/4 fl oz/$^1$/$_2$ cup lemon juice
  (or 115 g/4 oz/1 cup oatmeal)

If the sensitivity is intense, leave out the lemon juice as it will sting, and substitute a muslin bag of oatmeal.

▽ **A bath treatment to soften your skin can be as simple as a bagful of plain oatmeal swirled in the water.**

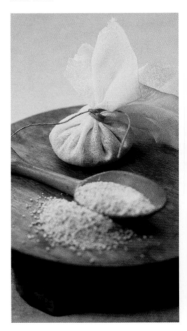

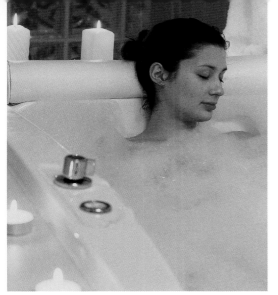

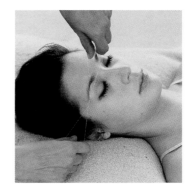

▷ Having your eyebrows professionally threaded gives long-lasting shape and definition, and you can learn to do it yourself.

◁ Time to relax and let the tension drift out of tired muscles. Finishing with a cool shower gives skin a healthy glow.

## skin softening bath mix

A very nourishing, soothing combination.

**ingredients**

- 45 ml/3 tbsp oatmeal
- 15 ml/1 tbsp bran
- 15 ml/1 tbsp ground almonds
- 15 ml/1 tbsp wheat flour
- few drops rose water

Put all the dry ingredients together into a muslin bag and add to the bathwater with the rose water.

## milk bath

The classic: just add a few handfuls of powdered milk to the warm water and bathe like Cleopatra.

## breast oil

Use this massage blend to tone and firm the breasts: the mustard oil makes the skin softer, while the powdered pomegranate rind has a firming effect.

**ingredients**

- 4 parts mustard oil
- 1 part dried pomegranate rind

Grind the pomegranate rind to a powder. Warm the mustard oil in a bowl over a pan of hot water. Mix the ingredients and leave to cool. Use the blend to massage the breasts with upward, circular motions, working outward from the nipples. Leave the oil on for at least 20 minutes, then rinse off with warm water and finish by splashing your breasts with cold water.

## nail care

Whenever you're using oil, take a moment to rub some of it into your nails. Vata types often have pale, irregular nails that break easily. Pitta is linked with pink, oval nails that may be quite soft. Kapha nails are square and strong. All types can benefit from a hand cream of almond oil and honey.

## hair removal

Women across Asia remove unwanted hair using the technique called threading. They hold one end of a cotton thread between their teeth, making a loop to lasso each hair, and tweak it out. This can be done professionally by beauty therapists. Easier to learn, and suitable for larger areas, is sugaring, using a mixture that is traditionally made at home. This can be made in large batches and kept in a jar. Sit the jar in hot water to soften it before use. It should last for a few months, as lemon is a natural preservative. You'll also need some strips of thick cotton, about 5–7.5 cm/2–3 in wide and 25 cm/10 in long.

**ingredients**

- 50 g/2 oz/4 tbsp sugar
- 30 ml/2 tbsp lemon juice

Simmer the lemon and sugar very slowly over a very low heat for a few minutes, stirring constantly, until they form a honey-coloured substance like sticky toffee. Experiment to get the consistency right: if it is too thin, add less lemon juice next time.

Allow to cool a little, then patch test to see if the temperature is tolerable. While still warm, spread on to the skin using a spatula. Place a cotton strip on the sugared area, press it down so that the warmth of your hands helps it to stick, and then pull off. On soft areas such as the calf, hold the muscle taut to prevent bruising.

▽ Practice makes perfect with sugaring, but the reward for your patience is silky smooth skin.

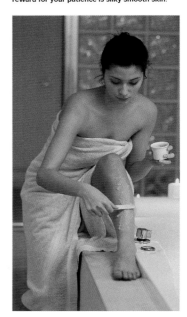

# Shimmering tresses

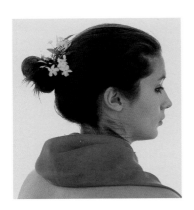

◁ **The fragrance of jasmine and its delicate, waxy flowers complement the gleam of sleek, shining hair.**

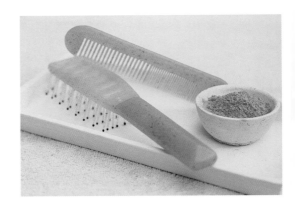

△ **Neem has many healing properties, and is available in the form of powder, oil or leaves. It has long been used to improve hair condition.**

Historically, perhaps no part of a woman's body has aroused more adulation than her hair. Throughout the ages flowing tresses have been praised in poetry and celebrated in art. In some cultures hair is still hidden to avoid tempting men or angels. The fifth-century Sanskrit poet Bhartrhari described a woman's hair as a forest, enticing the explorer into unknown territory where love waits like a bandit to ambush him.

Indian women have always been proud of their shining hair. The ancient carvings of Mohenjo-Daro and Harappa show women with their hair magnificently styled and jewelled. Traders carried perfumes from one continent to another for noblewomen to scent their tresses, jewellers created gold clips to hold their hair in place, and village carvers made combs of wood or bone for themselves and their daughters.

Lustrous hair is one beauty available to most women. The rich anointed their heads with priceless unguents and twined strings of gems through their artfully arranged curls. But any woman can scent and enhance her hair with a simple flower-sprig.

## hair treatments

Traditionally, people massaged their hair with oil to keep it healthy and counteract the drying effects of heat. Fragments of a dried tree resin called sambraani would be burned and the hair allowed to dry in its fragrant smoke after washing. Harsh shampoos and chemical treatments were unknown. Despite the range of hair products now available, many people are turning back to tried and tested formulas, some of which blend traditional knowledge with modern convenience. Instead of crushing leaves from the neem tree to enhance hair condition, for example, you can now pick up a bottle of neem shampoo or conditioner.

Hair and scalp problems may suggest a dosha imbalance, though they may also be

▽ **Use your fingers to comb the mixture through your hair down to the tips before rinsing out.**

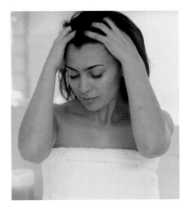

aggravated by stress, harsh shampoos, excessive heating or air conditioning. Dandruff, with a dry and flaky scalp, is frequently caused by the drying effects of aggravated vata dosha. But if the hair is dull and the scalp red and inflamed, the imbalance is more likely to be pitta – which is the commonest cause of hair problems. An Ayurvedic practitioner may suggest herbal remedies and massage with particular oils to calm the aggravated dosha. Changes to the diet are likely to include more green leafy vegetables, salads, milk, fruits and sprouts, buttermilk, yeast, wheat germ, soy beans, whole grains and nuts.

## blends to combat dandruff

These blends can be made in a screwtop glass jar and shaken to mix before using. The mixture should be worked into the scalp and left on overnight if possible; if not, wait at least 3 hours before washing your hair.

• 5 ml/1 tsp camphor added to 120 ml/ 4 fl oz/$^1$/$_2$ cup neem oil.

• 5 ml/1 tsp each castor oil, mustard oil and coconut oil.

• 1 part fresh lemon juice added to 2 parts coconut oil.

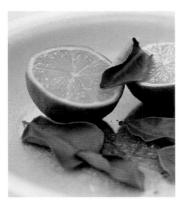

△ Lime juice helps to soothe an irritated scalp and leaves hair with a lustrous shine.

## blends to soothe an itchy scalp

• 5 ml/1 tsp camphor added to 120 ml/ 4 fl oz/¹/₂ cup coconut oil. Massage the mixture into the scalp. Leave for at least three hours before washing off.
• Dried jasmine root, ground into a bowl of lime juice. Wash the hair and scalp with this mixture and rinse with lukewarm water.

## rinses to add shine to the hair

• Squeeze a little lemon juice into a bowl of warm water and use as a final rinse.
• Add a little lime juice to a cup of rose water, add a cup or two of warm water and use as a final rinse.

## egg conditioner

For dry hair, massage a beaten egg into the hair after washing and rinsing. Rinse out thoroughly.

## rinse to prevent hair loss

Boil some neem leaves in water and leave to cool before straining off.

## hot-weather conditioner

### ingredients

• 1 egg
• 30 ml/2 tbsp castor oil
• 5 ml/1 tsp cider vinegar or wine vinegar
• 5 ml/1 tsp glycerine

To bring limp hair to life, mix the ingredients and beat well. Massage into the hair, leave as long as you like and wash out.

### WHAT IS YOUR HAIR TYPE?

Like the rest of our bodies, our hair can show signs of our predominant doshas. If you're a dual-dosha person, you may feel that your hair seems to be out of line with your personality. How can a calm kapha have such dry, brittle hair? The answer is that your hair is reflecting your vata side while your inner self reflects kapha.

• If your constitution is mainly vata, you're likely to have dark, dry, coarse or frizzy hair that's prone to tangling, split ends and dandruff.

• Pittas are often blondes or redheads. They have enviable hair – fine and silky – but it needs looking after to prevent a tendency to go thin and grey before its time. It tends to be oily, but harsh shampoos make matters worse and can accelerate aging.

• People of kapha constitution may complain about their oiliness, but they have the least to worry about with hair that's naturally thick, glossy and wavy.

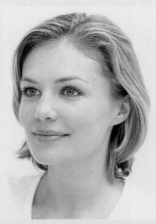

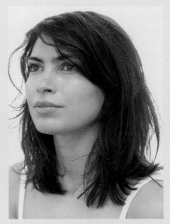

△ Pitta hair rewards gentle treatment with silky sleekness. Don't be tempted to use harsh products that may cause thinning.

△ Kapha's fabulous mane grows long and thick at any age. If it shakes off efforts to control it, just revel in its exuberance.

▷ The traditional oil-based hair treatments used in India are particularly valuable for vata's dry hair, which is prone to tangling and splitting.

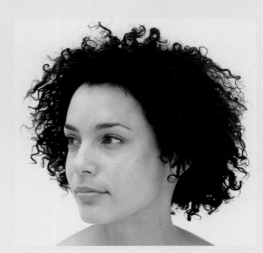

# Enriching oil treatments

Traditionally, Indian women regularly treat their hair with oil, using vigorous circular motions of the palms and fingertips to work it well into the scalp and down the length of the hair. They leave the oil in until they next wash their hair and then oil the hair again as soon as it dries. It's an intense massage treatment that stimulates the scalp as well as coating the hair shaft.

The lustrous, gleaming effect used to be admired in Western countries too. These days, we tend to prefer a just-washed look, replacing the hair's natural oils with conditioner. But for a change, why not try a pre-wash oil massage instead? After the massage, wrap a towel round your head, and leave it on for a few hours or overnight. You may need to vary the amount of shampoo you use. Why not also try leaving off conditioner for a while, to see whether you really need it?

## warming and cooling oils

Oil is used to strengthen and nourish all kinds of hair, but like most Ayurvedic treatments it should be tailored to suit the person. Your choice should also be influenced by external conditions such as the weather or the time of year. Coconut oil is popular for head massage, as it is renowned for its nourishing and strengthening powers. But it also has a cooling effect, which means it's best used in hot weather. The same goes for oil infused with brahmi – a valuable herb that's believed to stimulate the brain as well as the body.

In the winter, use a warming oil such as mustard or olive. Mustard is very nourishing and has a strong heating effect, though it smells rather strong. Almond is more neutral but has a slightly warming effect.

Choosing the right oil for the time of year is part of the Ayurvedic rhythm. But if you're feeling out of sorts, your need to balance your dosha by using particular oils may override this consideration. If you use a cooling oil in winter, stay in a warm room and don't go out till you've showered the oil off and dried your hair. If you use a warming oil in hot weather, rest until you feel more comfortable with the temperature.

## hair oil and your dosha

Vata's typically dry hair will revel in the luxury of black sesame oil, showing its benefits in a rich lustre. Pitta needs very gentle massage with brahmi oil or coconut oil, to stimulate the scalp without damaging the follicles. These two oils are good for all hair types.

If you're kapha, good hair is your birthright and the only thing that's likely to go wrong is an excess of oil – possibly because you scrub your scalp too vigorously or use harsh shampoos. Use sesame or mustard oil, but leave it on for only 30–60 minutes before showering it off. Avoid stimulating the scalp with intense massage or when washing your hair.

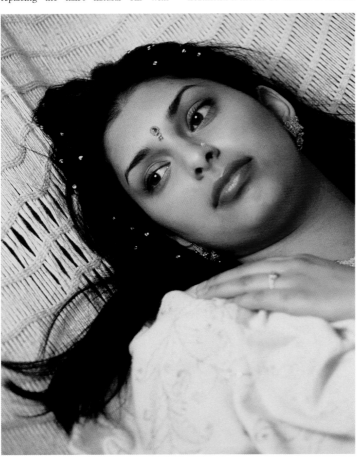

◁ **Luxuriant hair seems to come naturally to Indian women, whatever their dosha. Use of oil is one of their most effective beauty secrets.**

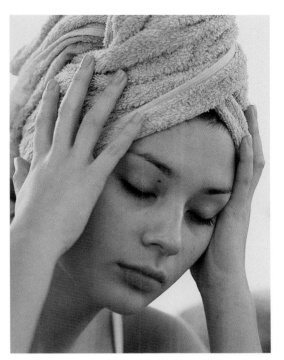

◁ **If you don't want to leave oil on your hair for long, wrap your head in a warm, damp towel after applying it, in order to aid penetration.**

## warmth and penetration

Warming the oil before you use it on your hair can help it penetrate the hair shaft more effectively. Heat it very slightly in a non-metallic bowl over a pan of water. It should be no more than comfortably warm. Alternatively, wring out a towel in hot water and wrap it around your head – again ensuring that the heat is not uncomfortable – when you have applied the oil and again after massaging it in.

If you use a sauna or steam room, oil your hair before you go in and wrap it in a towel. This not only gives the oil a chance to penetrate more deeply, but it also protects the hair from the long-term drying effects of steam and heat.

## hair and head massage

Why not combine an oil treatment for the scalp with a head massage, which Ayurveda recommends as part of your regular self-care routine? The series of movements aims to stimulate the body's systems, including glands, nerves and circulation, with anti-aging effects.

▽ **Gentle treatment brings out the best in fine flyway hair, so nurture it with the softest oil massage to help bring it back into balance.**

## hair strengthening

If your hair is thinning or breaks easily, massage it with a strengthening herb-infused oil. This treatment is particularly recommended during pregnancy, to avoid the hair loss that plagues many women after childbirth.

### ingredients

- 120 ml/4 fl oz/1/2 cup castor oil
- 550 ml/18 fl oz/2 1/2 cups sesame or coconut oil
- 120 ml/4 fl oz/1/2 cup brahmi
- 120 ml/4 fl oz/1/2 cup amla
- 750 ml–1 litre/1 1/4–1 3/4 pints/3–4 cups water

Mix the castor oil with the sesame oil (for vata-type hair) or coconut oil (for pitta) and add the brahmi and amla. Stir with a wooden spoon until the herbs have blended into the oil (you can warm the oil a little to expedite the process). Leave overnight, then pour the herb-infused oil, with the water, into an enamelled or non-metallic pan. Bring to the boil and simmer until all the water has evaporated. Remove from the heat and allow to cool, then strain through muslin or cheesecloth.

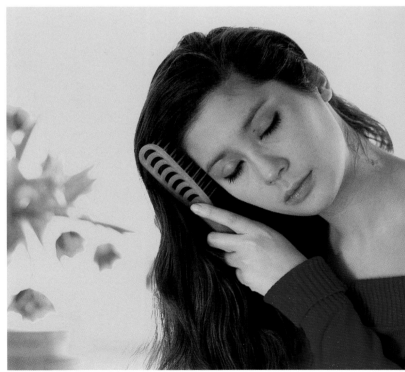

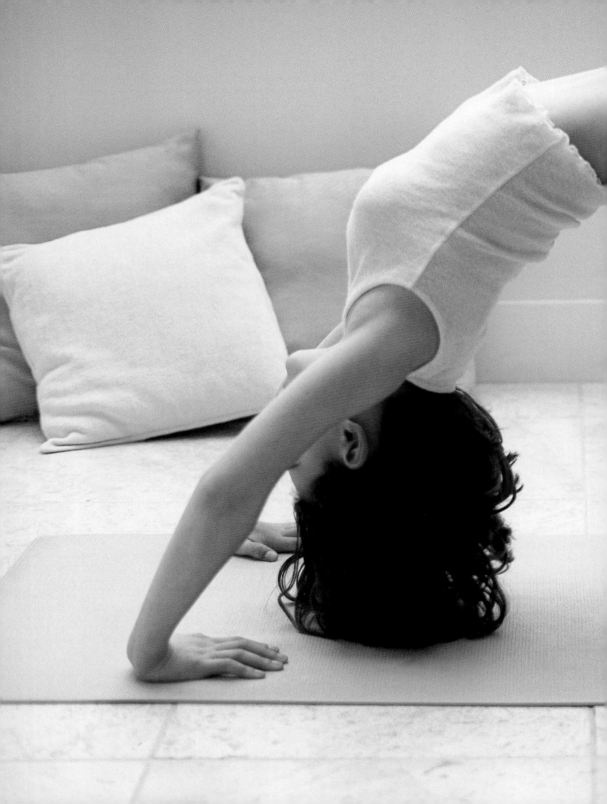

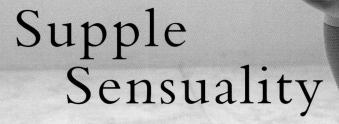

# Supple
# Sensuality

Indian women move with a natural grace
that makes them look like dancers. From
the steady tread of a country woman
carrying a basket home from market on
her head, to the curving hand and head
movements of a classical dance artist, every
movement reflects inner harmony. This
gracefulness can be within everyone's reach.

India's own form of exercise can shape your body,
clarify your skin and endow you with perfect poise.

# Natural grace through yoga

As young children we all moved with unselfconscious grace, but from hunching over a school desk to slumping in front of a computer or television, many of us spend much of our lives with rounded shoulders and crumpled spines, and the heavy bags we carry often twist us to one side, too.

Most forms of exercise will help us look and feel better, but poor posture can sabotage a fitness regime, making exercise harder and leaving well-toned muscles further out of alignment than before. There is no such danger with yoga, and it is excellent for strengthening muscles and improving flexibility. In addition, its emphasis on lengthening and straightening the spine makes for perfect posture, creating an appearance of height and slenderness. Its regulated pattern of breathing lowers stress levels and eases tension from our faces as well as our bodies.

Yoga has become so popular in the West during the past few decades that we don't always remember where it came from. We

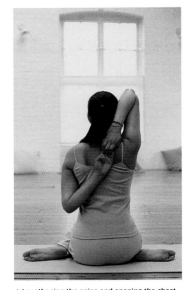

△ **Lengthening the spine and opening the chest is necessary if we are to help our cramped bodies regain a feeling of life.**

usually regard it as a set of flexibility exercises, or add it to a standard fitness regime as a stretch component. True, it is one of the best ways to build suppleness and delay the onset of old age. But yoga is far more than that, and in India it has always been closely linked with Ayurvedic medicine. Its name is Sanskrit for "union" or "connection": linking body, mind and the other non-physical levels to the universal mind. It has several elements, but the exercises generally practised in the West are what's called *hatha*, or physical, yoga.

Awareness of breathing is a central part of hatha yoga, and breath is synchronized with movement. Despite the effort you're putting in, this leads to a very calming, almost meditative rhythm that helps you push on through difficult parts. Pranayama – breathing exercises – form part of a standard yoga practice.

▽ **Working with a partner can help you keep your balance and move more confidently.**

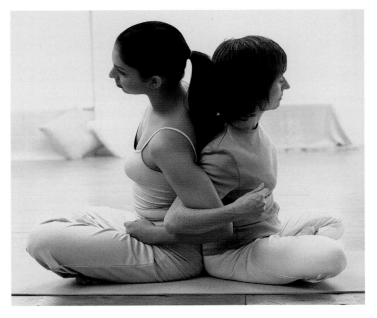

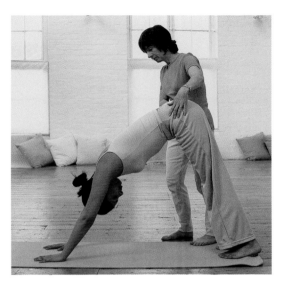

◁ A good teacher will ask about any injuries or health problems, ensure you are holding the poses correctly and also help you come out of them safely.

## styles of hatha yoga

Yoga's dynamic strength allows it to adapt while retaining its essential meaning. In recent years it has changed from a faintly exotic pastime to an everyday event. It is offered in many new forms, some of which are rediscoveries of ancient techniques.

**Ashtanga** is a vigorous form that builds up intense heat, intended to purify the muscles and organs, expel impurities and release hormones to nourish the skin. The fast sequences originally kept warriors fit, and they're an all-round exercise for flexibility, strength and cardiovascular fitness. It is aimed at people who are already very fit.

**Bikram** yoga quickly attracted dancers and celebrities to its creator's Beverly Hills studio. The idea is that practising a stripped-down core of movements in a room heated to above body temperature allows the muscles to stretch more, while impurities are washed out on a tide of perspiration.

**Contact** yoga is practised with a partner, requiring good co-operation and balance. Advanced practitioners may be able to do a headstand on their partner's head, but most stick to supporting each other's back bends or aiding a little more stretch.

**Dru** yoga is a very gentle, peaceful form that includes relaxation and working as a group.

**Iyengar** yoga is the best known form outside India. Detailed poses, or *asanas*, are

▽ Your teacher can help you to increase your stretch while staying within safe limits.

carried out with great attention to technique. It can feel strenuous, but it is done in a slow, controlled manner that should allow you to stop if you feel you're pushing your muscles too far.

**Jivamukti** is fast-paced and rigorous, but also includes chanting and meditation to help maintain the balance between physical and spiritual.

**Kundalini** yoga is an esoteric form that aims for enlightenment through the release of energy up the spine. This is achieved through stretching, breathing exercises, chanting and meditation.

**Sivananda** yoga, one of the least strenuous forms, considers the physical exercises to be part of a holistic lifestyle. It includes meditation and promotes a feeling of peace.

**Vini** yoga emphasizes safe movements and individual tuition, letting you adapt poses to meet your ability rather than trying to force yourself into them.

**Yoga Vanda Scaravelli** is a gentle adaptation of Iyengar, focusing on the spine. It uses gravity and the breath to undo tension in the body and awaken the spine.

▽ Keep the neck long as you look up, visualizing space between the vertebrae. Letting your head slump back could harm your spine.

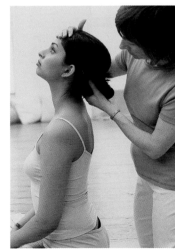

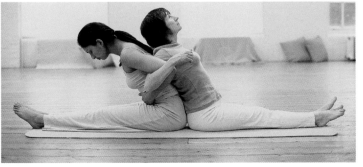

# Find your fitness style

You don't need to read again that exercise is a vital component in any beauty regime. You may even be flipping guiltily past these pages, because you've come to see yourself as a hopeless fitness dropout. The Pilates class your friends rave about leaves you cold, and the last time you lifted a weight you felt like dropping it on the floor and running out of the gym. But don't despair: you could simply be following the wrong path for your dosha.

We all need to improve our cardiovascular fitness, increase flexibility, and build strength through weight-bearing exercise. But finding the right balance, and the right form of exercise, could be as simple as finding your true style. Even if you're perfectly content with your fitness routine – or lack of it – it's still worth considering whether you could make changes. When our energies are out of balance, we tend to slip further into the things that are causing the imbalance.

## achieving balance

An energetic vata person may love running – an excellent and invigorating form of exercise. But when vata energy starts racing

out of control, it's time to take another direction. Instead of arousing it further, turn to something slower and steadier, that will bring you safely back to earth.

A competitive pitta sportswoman may be way ahead of the field, but strangely unsatisfied by her achievement. Working up a daily sweat is just pouring fuel on her fiery nature. And it can be hard to persuade a relaxed kapha that exercise is a good thing when she feels fine without it.

It would be crazy to give up a form of exercise that you enjoy – it's hard enough for most of us to stick to a fitness programme. But Ayurveda suggests bringing more balance into your life, especially when your usual behaviour and routines are exacerbating any imbalances.

Sometimes our bodies instinctively know what's right for us at that moment, but sometimes we become set in ways that aren't the best. As you learn to know yourself better, you start to recognize the difference.

## vata

You probably love lively exercise like dancing and running, but a typically speedy vata lifestyle can leave you feeling

ungrounded. You also need to protect your joints from injury and build strength. As the most active of people, you're the least likely to need to join an aerobics class.

Bring your energies into balance with a steady, strengthening yoga style such as Vini. Iyengar is another good choice, so long as you're careful to recognize your current limits and don't risk harming vulnerable joints by excessive twisting or staying too long in a difficult weight-bearing pose. Instead of trying to force a stretch, let your muscles relax as you sink into a feeling of unhurried calm.

Walking, t'ai chi and Pilates are other useful exercises for you. Add some form of weight-training: the repetitive movements will leave your ever-active mind free to work out a new theory while you tone your abdominals. If these options sound slow and boring, give them a chance. As you become accustomed to this challenge you should start noticing a new smoothness in your movement as well as in your muscles.

▽ **Muscle-toning exercises such as Pilates are useful for vatas, whose high-speed metabolism makes aerobic exercise less of a necessity.**

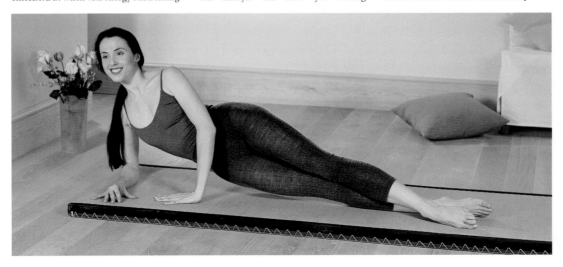

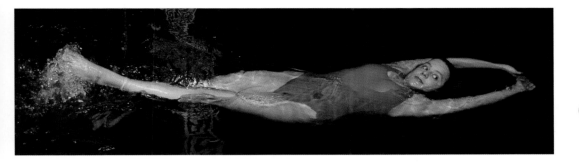

## pitta

Your competitive instincts lead you towards races and sports, but you need to avoid overheating, whether from exertion, a hot room or the midday sun. You could benefit from all yoga styles that increase flexibility without making you sweat. Concentrate on lengthening your muscles or easing gently into a deeper stretch without force or jerky movements, as in the yoga of Vanda Scaravelli. Working with a partner could help develop your co-operative instincts. The gentle routines of Dru or Sivananda yoga will promote feelings of peace that you may not have known for some time.

Swimming is ideal for your hot-blooded nature: the water helps balance your energies while you focus on your own steady progress. Cold-climate holidays give you a chance to enjoy skiing or snowboarding. Day to day, you need a moderate amount of exercise, with long walks providing an easy option.

## kapha

You're naturally strong and healthy, and don't particularly like exercise, but you still need to build up flexibility and cardiovascular fitness. Though you reap the psychological benefits of taking life at a calm, steady pace, you need to build some energetic exercise into your routine.

With yoga, you're most likely to be motivated by a high-speed form that's fun and gets your body pumping out endorphins. Try Ashtanga or Jivamukti, which will also counteract your tendency to gain weight.

Any high-energy exercise class will give you the lively workout you need. Your strength makes you an asset in team sports, or you could take a salsa course.

△ Swimming is the perfect exercise for pittas: it's a rhythmic, calming motion that lets them work off plenty of energy without overheating.

▽ Anyone with kapha tendencies can have fun getting their exercise, and their stamina keeps them on the dance floor when others flag.

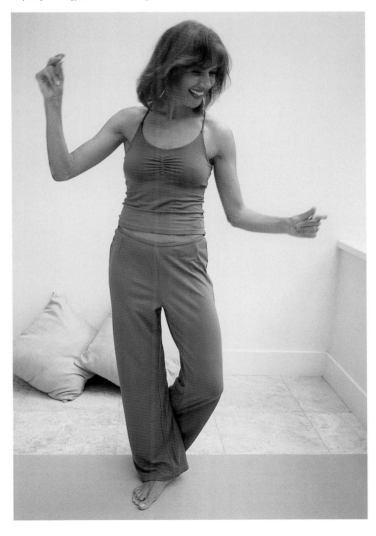

# Move like a dancer

For most of us, brief bouts of exercise are interspersed with long hours of sedentary work, slumped in a chair and barely turning our heads. The effects show in our skin, our tired eyes and even our speech, from throats too constricted to allow our voices to be full and resonant.

All forms of yoga increase suppleness, allowing us to move more freely with a natural sensuality. Once we start practising yoga, the effects spread far beyond the hour spent twisting and stretching in the class. Straightening and lengthening the spine becomes a beneficial habit, changing the way we sit, stand, walk and talk. We hold our head level, as if suspended from the ceiling by a string, and the chin neither sags nor juts.

The asanas described on these pages are suitable for all doshas and are especially valuable for improving posture. In all cases you're aiming to lengthen and straighten your spine and limbs to rediscover a naturally upright stance.

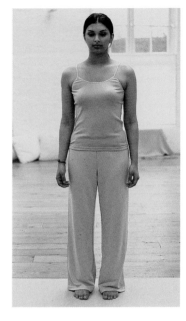

## the Mountain (Tadasana)

◁ **1** Stand with feet parallel and a little apart, arms by your sides. Lift and spread your toes, then plant them firmly on the floor. Keep your legs strong by feeling the front thigh muscles pulling up towards your groin. Tuck in your tailbone so that the front of your pelvis feels slightly higher than the back.

**2** Lengthen your spine upwards while letting your shoulders and arms relax backwards and down. Imagine your head supported by a string from the centre of your scalp; your chin is level, leaving your throat comfortably open without compressing the back of your neck. Let your face relax.

**3** Open your chest, without forcing your shoulders rigidly back. Let your stomach gently swell as breath fills your lungs, then tighten the abdominal muscles and expel all the stale air.

## Standing Side Stretch (Ardha Chandrasana)

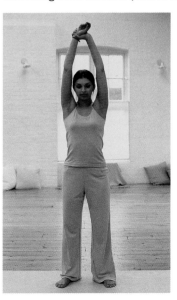

◁ **1** Starting in Mountain pose, take your feet a little further apart and slowly raise your arms above your head as you breathe in. Grasp your right wrist with your left hand as you breathe out.

▷ **2** On the next inbreath, lean to the left, facing forwards and bending sideways from the waist. Don't let your head, arms or torso flop; hold the position strongly and feel strength radiating from your fingers. Return to the centre on an outbreath and repeat on the other side, holding your left wrist.

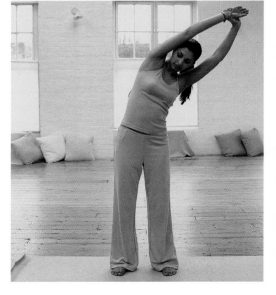

# the Tree (Vrksasana)

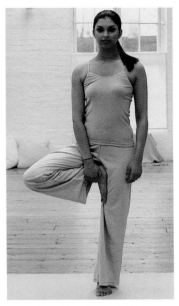

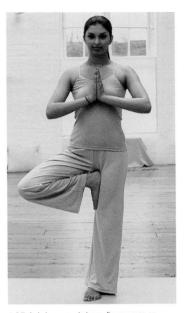

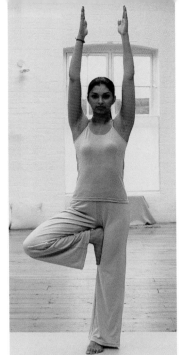

△ **1** Standing straight and looking straight ahead, take a moment to feel balanced and firmly rooted. Bending your right leg, place your foot as close to the top of your inside left thigh as you can comfortably reach, lifting it into position with your right hand if you wish. Stretch your right knee out to the side.

△ **2** To help keep your balance, fix your gaze on something motionless at about eye level. Spread out the toes of your left foot to grip the floor firmly. Breathing in, put your palms together with fingers pointing upwards as if making the Indian greeting *Namaste*. Try to hold this position for about 5 seconds, breathing naturally.

△ **3** On an inbreath stretch your arms straight above your head and turn your palms inwards. Feel the stretch from your raised hands to your feet, and the energy travelling the length of your body. Aim to hold for up to 20 seconds, breathing naturally. On an outbreath, bring your hands down, first to Namaste level, then down by your sides. Return your right foot to the floor and stand for a moment feeling grounded. Then repeat the exercise on the other side.

# the Cow (Gomukhasana)

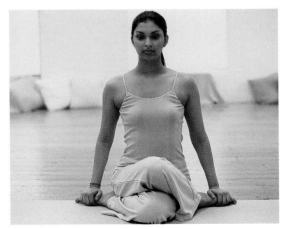

△ **1** Tuck your left heel beside your right buttock, trying to keep the knee on the floor. Cross the right knee over that leg and bring the right foot round beside you. If you find this difficult, sit with legs crossed and concentrate on the arm movements.

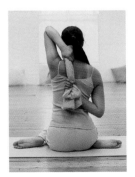

△ **2** Relax your right arm by your side then, on an inbreath, bring the right hand up between your shoulderblades. On the next inbreath, raise the left arm as if reaching for the ceiling. On the outbreath, bring your left hand down and try to grasp the right hand. If (like most of us) you can't reach at first, hold each end of a scarf. Hold the posture for around 10 seconds, breathing naturally, then on an inbreath raise the left hand again and bring both hands down beside you as you breathe out. Uncross your legs and stretch them out. Repeat on the other side.

# Beauty from within

Why does your skin glow so beautifully when you surface from a swimming pool or return from a brisk walk? Any exercise that stimulates the circulation brings fresh oxygenated blood to the face, instantly enlivening the complexion. The long-term effects of regular exercise are just as clear – keeping the complexion fresh and strengthening the muscles that support the skin. The high-energy forms of yoga give your complexion a healthy boost that lasts long after you've showered and cooled down, but yoga's range of asanas includes several that stimulate circulation to the head without working up a sweat. Hold each of the poses for around 30 seconds, or as long as feels comfortable, and come out of them by retracing the steps described.

## Downward-facing Dog (Adho Mukha Shvanasana)

In this position you should feel a stretch in your back and the backs of your legs, but don't force it, and don't try it without an instructor if you have trouble with your knees or lower back. If you're not very fit you may feel dizzy when you put your head down, so adapt the pose until you feel comfortable. (If the dizziness persists whenever you try this kind of exercise, get your doctor to check your heart and blood pressure.)

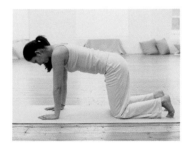

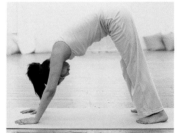

△ **1** Kneel on all fours, with hips directly above knees and shoulders above wrists. Take time to feel well grounded, with toes tucked in below heels and fingers spread out, firmly gripping the floor.

◁ **2** As you breathe out, try to straighten your legs by lifting your hips up and back. Keep your shoulders relaxed and breathe naturally. Your head should remain in line with your spine, not flopping down or pushed back. If you can straighten your legs without forcing your knees uncomfortably, increase the stretch by lowering your heels towards the floor. On an outbreath, try to lengthen your spine by bringing your hips further up and back.

## the Lion (Simhasana)

This is a wonderful way of exercising your face, improving both circulation and muscle support. It firms the muscles of the face and neck, keeping wrinkles at bay.

▷ Sit with your legs crossed or kneel in a comfortable upright position. Rest your hands on your knees. As you breathe out spread your fingers wide apart, open your eyes as wide as you can and look up towards the centre of your forehead. Stick your tongue out and down as far as possible. Breathe out hard, making a loud, forceful "hah" sound. As you breathe in, draw in your tongue and relax your eyes and hands.

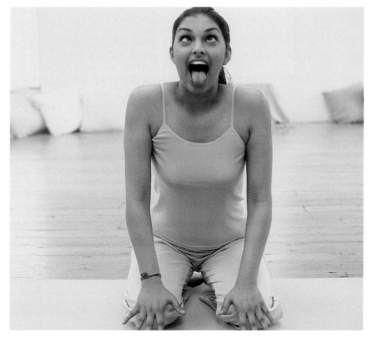

# Standing Forward Bend (Uttanasana)

**This useful asana revitalizes the complexion, tones the leg muscles, calms nerves and reduces vata energy.**

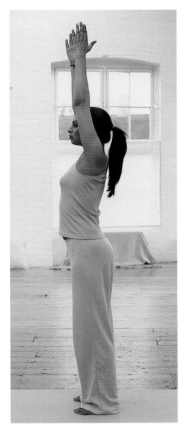

◁ **1** Stand in Mountain pose, then move your feet shoulder-width apart. Breathe in and raise both arms above your head with palms facing in, feeling the spine stretch upwards.

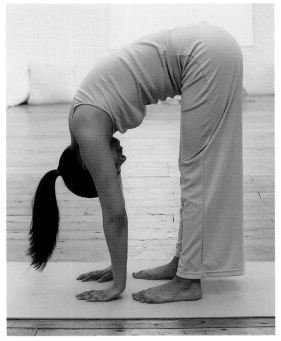

△ **2** Breathe out as you bring your torso and arms slowly forward in a straight line, hinging from the hips and (to keep your back flat) leading with the chest. Go down as far as you can without straining your back. Keep the movement controlled to avoid harming your back, and bend your knees if necessary. Stay down as long as you feel comfortable, up to 30 seconds, breathing naturally, then, on an inbreath, bend your knees and unroll your spine vertebra by vertebra to come slowly up.

# the Child (Murha Janusasana)

**As well as improving circulation to the face and head, this is a very relaxing pose that eases the spine, making it ideal to follow more strenuous asanas.**

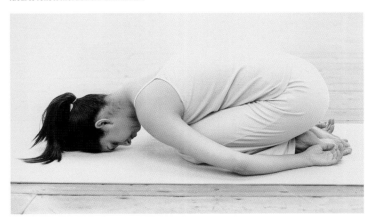

**1** Kneel on the floor, sitting on your heels with legs together, arms relaxed by your sides and spine erect. As you breathe in, stretch your spine upwards as if pulled by a string from the top of your head and feel your chest and diaphragm expanding.

◁ **2** Breathing out, bring your body forwards face first, hinging from the hips without hunching the back. Bring your head down on to your knees or the floor in front. Rest your arms beside your body, palms up, on top of your feet if you can reach that far. Breathe naturally and feel your spine relax. This is a relaxation pose that you can hold for a couple of minutes, as long as you feel comfortable, before coming slowly up.

# Body shaping

A sensuous shape relies on well-toned muscles. That means some kind of strength-building work, but many forms of strengthening exercise, such as weight-training, can create rather chunky muscles. Adding some stretch exercise is vital if you want to firm up without adding bulk, as fitness instructors always warn. The stretching element is built into yoga.

## the Cat (Chakravakasana)

**This tones muscles in the back, arms and buttocks and stretches the hamstrings.**

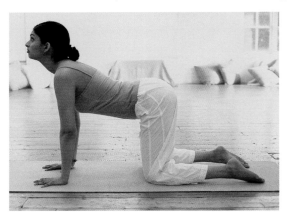

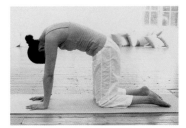

◁ **1** Kneel on all fours with shoulders above wrists, hips above knees and soles facing upwards. As you breathe in, arch your back downwards so that your waist sinks lower than your hips and shoulders. Lift your head, without tipping it back – the length of your neck should be maintained.

△ **2** As you breathe out, come back to a central position. Continuing the outbreath, arch your back upwards and tuck your chin in towards your chest. Breathe in as you return to the central position and on to arch your back downwards. Repeat this movement slowly several times.

## the Cobra (Bhujangasana)

**This tones buttock muscles and pectorals. Don't risk damaging your neck by tipping your head too far back in this or any other backwards bend.**

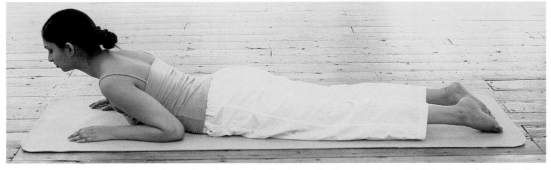

△ **1** Lie on your stomach with your head on one side resting on the floor, legs stretched out, with the soles of the feet pointing upwards, and arms by your side with palms upwards. Bend your arms and bring your hands beside your shoulders and, as you breathe in, slowly raise your chest. Keep your elbows beside your body, shoulders down and chest moving forwards. On an outbreath, push your palms down and raise your upper body as far as possible while keeping your pubic bone in contact with the floor. Look straight ahead, feeling the front of your body opening and expanding.

**2** As you breathe in, raise your head slightly and direct your gaze upwards, but without tipping your head backwards. Relax the muscles in your back and buttocks, and feel your spine lengthen. Breathe naturally. Lower your gaze and look straight ahead again, then slowly lower your upper body to the starting position.

## the Bridge (Setu Bandha)

**In this asana, you're working on your hips and thighs.**

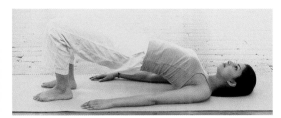

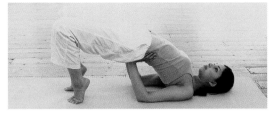

△ **1** Lie on your back, arms by your sides with palms facing downwards. Bring your heels towards your torso, hip-width apart. As you breathe in, raise your buttocks as high as possible, pushing upwards with your pelvis till you are resting on your feet and shoulders. Tuck your chin in and let your head rest on the floor.

△ **2** If this is very easy, try an advanced version: with upper arms on the floor, bend your elbows and as you breathe out put your hands under your waist for support. Do not flop down on to your hands or push your spine up too high. If it's hard to keep your back raised, come down gently.

## Lying-down Twist (Jathara Parivartanasana)

**This works on trimming the waist while releasing tension from muscles in the back.**

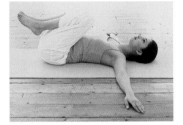

▷ **2** On an outbreath, lower your knees to the floor on one side and turn your head to the other. Hold for as long as is comfortable, then slowly come back to the centre on an outbreath, pause for a moment and repeat on the other side.

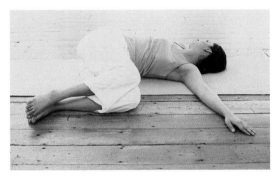

△ **1** Lie on the floor with arms outstretched, palms down. Bend your knees and raise them to your chest. Keep your neck and spine in a straight line.

## the Warrior (Virabhadrasana) I, with arms raised

**This pose tones the thighs, calves and chest.**

**1** Stand in Mountain pose, then move your feet sideways until they are about twice hip-width apart. Breathe in and turn your right foot through a quarter-circle to the right, placing your right heel in line with the left instep. Breathe out and rotate your body from the hips to face right.

▷ **2** Bend your right leg so that your knee forms a right angle, keeping the knee directly above the heel. Breathe in and raise your arms above your head until your hands are shoulder-width apart with palms facing in. Push your feet firmly into the floor and stretch up. Breathe out and lift your head slightly, without tipping it back, to look upwards. Breathe naturally and hold for a few seconds.

**3** On an inbreath, lower your head again so that you are looking ahead. As you breathe out, bring your arms down by your sides, straighten your right leg and turn

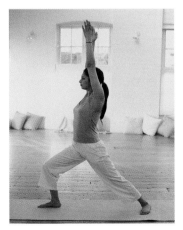

your body to face the front again, with both feet pointing forwards. Keeping your legs wide apart, repeat the movements on the other side.

## the Warrior II, with arms outstretched

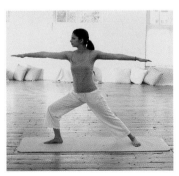

△ Follow the instructions for Warrior I (left) for the leg movements for this version, but do not turn your body to the right or raise your arms above your head. Instead, trying to keep hips facing squarely forwards, stretch both arms out with palms facing down. Turn your head only, to look along your outstretched right arm.

# Dynamic vitality

Different asanas can help you relax or feel more energetic, improve concentration or calm your mind. Calming poses include those where the body closes in on itself, such as the Forward Bends and the Child. For a surge of energy, you should work through dynamic positions such as the Lightning Bolt and the Warrior. Balancing asanas such as the Tree and the Eagle aid concentration and the Warrior poses promote inner strength. Any of the poses that release

tension, such as the Lying-down Twist or the Dog, can aid relaxation. But the classic relaxer is the Corpse.

The way you breathe is almost as important in yoga as the way you move. Keep your respiration steady and match your movements to the flow of breath, breathing in with an upward or outward movement, out as you go down or sink deeper into a stretch. You soon start to notice how it helps you keep a rhythm

to your movements. Aim to breathe out slightly more than you breathe in.

Breathing exercises, or pranayama ("controlling the life force"), form part of a yoga routine. In the Ayurvedic view, the breath carries the prana, or life force, around the body in thousands of channels; pranayama helps keep this flow steady and unobstructed. Because one of the main channels runs down the spine, good posture helps keep it clear.

## Seated Forward Bend (Paschimottanasana)

▷ Sit upright on your tailbone with your legs together and straight out in front of you, toes up. On an outbreath, fold forwards from the hips to hold your ankles or your toes, without hunching your back. Ideally, keep your legs straight and bring your head down towards your knees, but let your knees bend if your back hurts, and don't force yourself to reach further than is comfortable. Hold for up to 30 seconds, then slowly return, on an inbreath, to an upright sitting position.

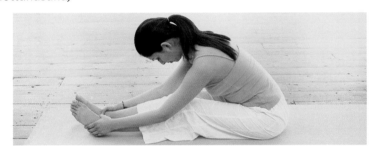

## the Lightning Bolt (Utkatasana)

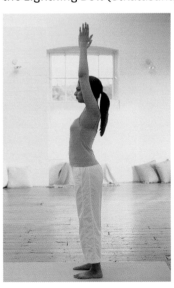

◁ **1** Start in Mountain pose, then breathe in as you raise your arms above your head. Breathe out and bend your knees. They should be no further forward than directly above your toes. Let your body slant naturally forwards, without rounding your back.

▷ **2** Be careful not to let your knees buckle inwards. Extend the arms in line with your torso. Breathe deeply three or four times, feeling the energy of the lightning bolt that your body forms from fingertips to toes. On an inbreath, return to Mountain pose.

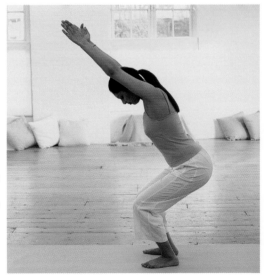

# the Eagle (Garudasana)

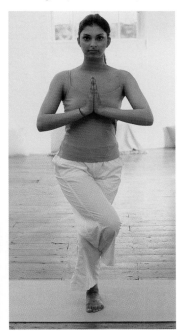

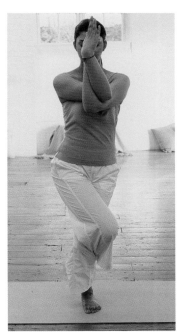

△ **1** Stand in Mountain pose and bring your hands into Namaste position. On an inbreath, bend your knees and wrap the right leg around the left, trying to hook your foot behind the ankle. To aid balance, focus your gaze on something still at eye level. Beginners can stay in Mountain pose and do the arm movements only.

△ **2** Keeping your shoulders relaxed, raise your arms in front of your shoulders on the next inbreath and cross the right elbow over the left. With thumbs at eye level, bring the palms together. Remain still, gazing at the thumbs and breathing normally. Be aware of the feeling of opening and stretching across your upper back; this is also excellent for relieving stiff shoulders.

# the Corpse (Savasana)

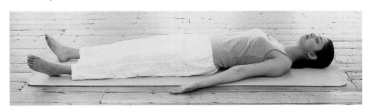

△ Just as it sounds: lie on your back, arms by your sides with palms upwards and legs outstretched. Relax and let your feet roll outwards as your head seems to sink into the floor. If this makes your lower back ache, bend your knees upwards.

**OVERBREATHING**

If you become dizzy you've been breathing in too deeply. Give a long outward breath, then breathe in and out of a paper bag a few times to re-establish the correct levels of oxygen and carbon dioxide.

# cleansing breath (kapalabhati)

**This cleanses the entire respiratory system and freshens the skin. It also strengthens the muscles of the abdomen and aids digestion. It is considered so cleansing that its Sanskrit name means "making your skull shine". If you practise it every day your face should shine with health.**

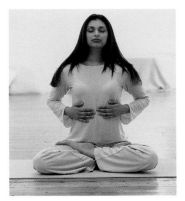

△ Sit with your back straight and breathe out hard in a series of short sharp exhalations through the nose. Tighten your stomach muscles as you breathe out, squeezing air out of your lungs. You won't need to make any effort to breathe in: when you relax the stomach muscles air will flow into the lungs naturally. After the tenth inbreath, breathe out for as long as you can and try to empty the lungs. Take a few normal breaths before doing another set.

# bee breath (brahmari)

**This is a relaxing technique that can send even insomniacs to sleep. It can also give you a deliciously sexy voice, releasing tension in the throat that causes harshness or squeakiness.**

Sit upright, close your eyes and let a long outbreath lead naturally to a long inhalation. Breathing through your nose, make a continuous humming sound each time you breathe out. Relax and let it become a deep, rich sound. Focus your mind on this sound, which should continue the whole time you're breathing out.

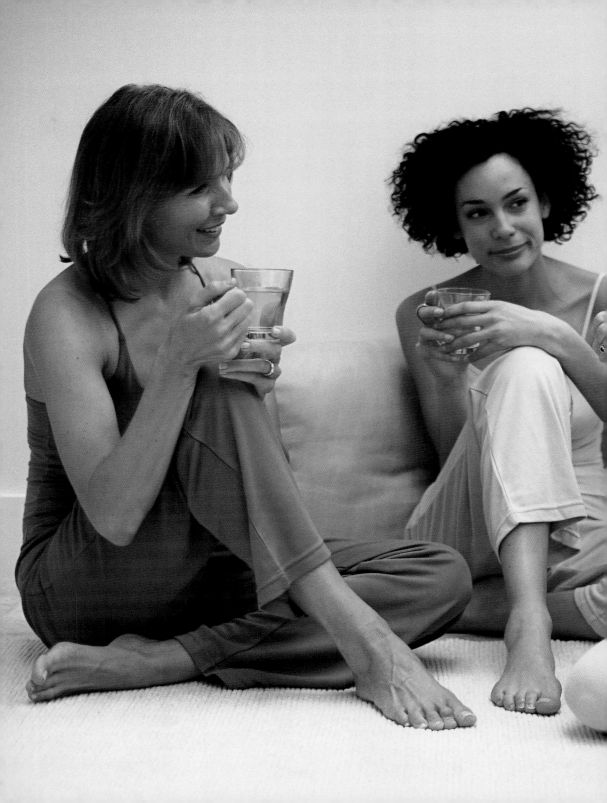

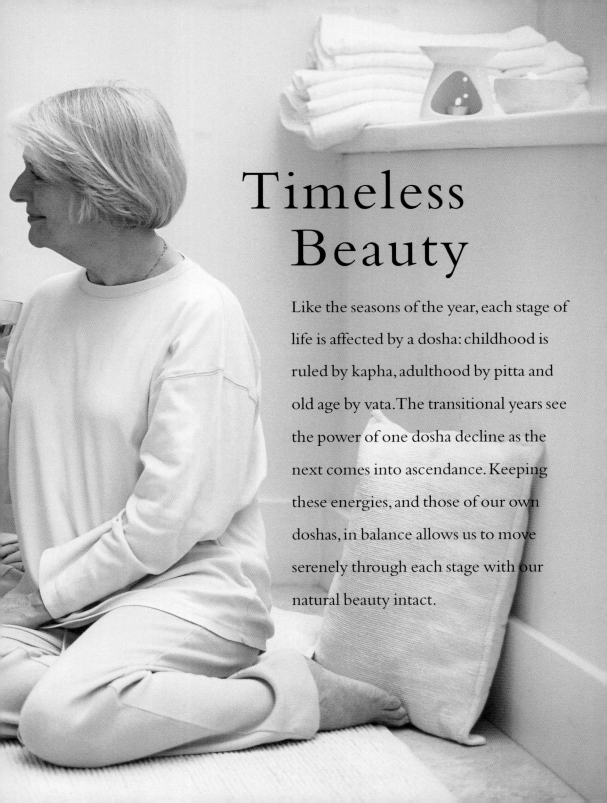

# Timeless Beauty

Like the seasons of the year, each stage of life is affected by a dosha: childhood is ruled by kapha, adulthood by pitta and old age by vata. The transitional years see the power of one dosha decline as the next comes into ascendance. Keeping these energies, and those of our own doshas, in balance allows us to move serenely through each stage with our natural beauty intact.

# The teenage transition

timeless beauty

As children we had kapha's perfect skin, placid outlook and natural grace – not that we cared. Within a few years we're wondering what happened to those desirable attributes and wishing we could get them back. But by then we're already moving on into the pitta stage, which will last until the menopause.

Transitions are always a challenge, and – after birth – adolescence is the first big one. With depressive kapha and fiery pitta energies in conflict, our moods lurch from rage to despair. Since blood is a pitta element, the start of a period banishes premenstrual syndrome by reducing excessive pitta energy – but then hormonal changes make the skin erupt with acne and the hair turn lank. In Ayurvedic terms, the last burst of kapha energy turns skin into an oil well, ready to be ignited by pitta's fire. The body's toxic load of ama builds up too, and can find no way out except into the skin.

We slouch to disguise our embarrassing new height and breast shape (or lack of it), and loss of self-confidence can lead to problems such as eating disorders. Yet this is also a time of excitement and discoveries, as we move towards independence. Ayurveda's holistic teachings show us how to be our best now, and at every stage of life. The earlier we start, the more radiant health and confidence we gain to carry us through challenging stages.

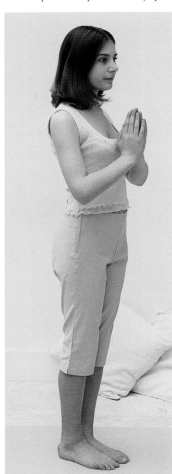

## Yoga routine

**Carrying out this set of asanas every day should help clear your skin, keep your weight steady and give your body image a healthy boost. When you have time and energy, do all the positions instead of making choices. Keep your movements strong, feeling the energy coursing through your body and out to the tips of your fingers and toes.**

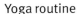 **1** Start in Namaste then move into the Tree, to improve your balance – especially useful for days when you feel clumsy. Or move into the Eagle pose, to improve concentration and stretch the muscles of your back, counteracting the effects of working at a desk. Optional: return to the Mountain pose and do a Standing Side Stretch.

**2** Try the Warrior pose, to shape legs and increase inner strength, helping you cope with mood swings and PMS, or the Lightning Bolt, for more energy.

**3** Perform the Forward Bend, staying down for as long as you feel comfortable – up to 30 seconds – to stretch your hamstrings and bring fresh oxygenated blood to your face to clear skin blemishes.

**4** Lie down and perform the Cobra.

**5** Turn over and move into the Lying-down Twist, to tone your waist and let your hips swing as you walk.

**6** Move into the Corpse. While you're relaxing after your workout, try to let your mind go blank and feel as if you're sinking into the floor.

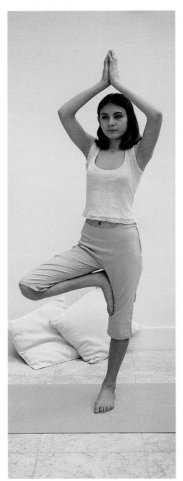

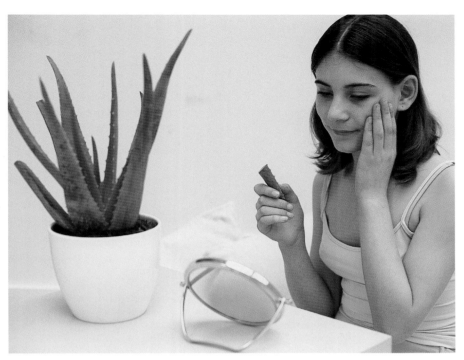

⊲ Soothe spots and inflamed skin with the juicy pulp from an aloe vera leaf. It will leave your face feeling clean and supple.

## feed your face

The skin blemishes that disfigure the teenage years are caused by an excess of kapha and, especially, pitta energies. Kapha increases oiliness, leading to blackheads, while pitta energy causes inflammation and eruptions. These can be counteracted by avoiding the rich, fried and highly spiced foods that aggravate pitta and – to a lesser extent – the sweet or salty foods that do the same to kapha. To reduce ama, eat food as fresh and unprocessed as possible. Junk food breaks most of the laws of Ayurveda and has cruel effects on teenage skin.

## teenage skincare

When skin erupts, it's natural to feel desperate and scrub it with chemicals, but these often make matters worse. Instead, just keep skin normally clean and resist the urge to touch it. Dab spots with cream made from the antiseptic leaves of the neem tree – then leave them alone. For a very simple remedy, keep an aloe vera plant to break tips off, or buy the pure pulp. Fresh air is good for your skin, but don't sunbathe. Strong sunlight slows down oil production temporarily, but it may then go into overdrive to compensate. Skin cancer is a greater risk if you've been sunburnt in your teens.

**SKINCARE RECIPES**

Each of these soothing preparations for troubled skin should be spread over the face and left for 15–30 minutes while you relax. Rinse off thoroughly with warm water and splash with a gentle toner such as rose water.

**FOR OILY SKIN:**

• Beat an egg white until it is fluffy and add 5 ml/1 tsp tangerine juice.

• Mix 2.5 ml/½ tsp honey with 10 ml/2 tsp lemon juice. Mix to a paste with multani mitti (fuller's earth) and a little rose water. This should be removed after 15 minutes.

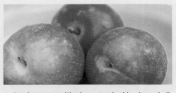

△ **Combat acne with plums mashed in almond oil.**

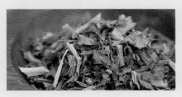

**FOR ACNE:**

• Boil 6 plums until soft, remove the skins and mash the pulp with 5 ml/1 tsp almond oil.

• Mix 5 ml/1 tsp each sandalwood powder and turmeric with enough milk to make a paste.

• Mix 5 ml/1 tsp either nutmeg or ground cumin seeds with water and spread on the affected areas only.

• Make a paste of fenugreek leaves and water, and spread on acne-prone areas. This can help prevent spots appearing.

⊲ **Fenugreek is used as a purifying herb – on the skin as well as in food.**

timeless beauty

Adulthood is pitta, ruled by the fiery dosha whose energetic influence sees us through our many tasks and responsibilities, not the least of which are the bearing and raising of children. At the busiest time of our lives, overwork can trigger a pitta imbalance, manifesting itself as irritability, impatience and heartburn.

## dinacharya

Routines are a central part of Ayurveda, which teaches that living to a rhythm helps to keep us in tune with the energies inside and around us. Establishing an Ayurvedic routine, or *dinacharya*, is the first step to bringing the energies back into balance. It also makes it easier to sleep, exercise and eat healthily, helping to keep your weight steady and your skin clear.

• Wake up early – if not before sunrise, at least an hour before you have to leave home. Take a couple of minutes to visualize the day ahead and see it all going smoothly, then get up within about five minutes of waking.
• Give yourself a brief whole-body massage. If you use oil, leave it on for about 20 minutes before showering.
• Take 10–20 minutes to meditate and do some breathing exercises.
• Wash or shower, and splash your face and eyelids with cold water after cleansing.

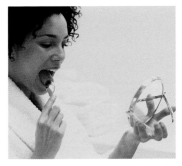

△ Daily cleansing is part of staying healthy, and gently scraping the tongue freshens your mouth.

Clean your tongue with a special scraper, or use the edge of a teaspoon (kept for that purpose only).
• Drink a glass of water, cool or warm but not ice-cold, to aid digestion and help keep skin fresh.
• Do your yoga routine now if possible.
• Don't leave home without eating any breakfast. Clean your teeth and tongue after you have eaten, and try to do the same after every meal.
• Drink water throughout the day so you

never feel thirsty. However, it's best not to drink while you're eating.
• Have a good meal – preferably your main meal – at lunchtime. Eat mindfully, taking time to enjoy your food.
• Get some active exercise and some mental stimulation each day. If you work at a desk, go for a run or attend an exercise class. If you're running after children all day, read a book when you have a moment to yourself.
• If you didn't have time to do yoga in the morning, do it before dinner. Otherwise, meditate then.
• Eat a light evening meal, preferably early.
• Do 10–20 minutes' meditation if you didn't do this before eating.
• Go for a walk after you've eaten.
• Go to bed in time to allow yourself enough sleep. Most people need nine hours a night in their teens, decreasing to eight in their 20s, about seven in the 40s and an hour or so less in old age.

You'll be impressive if you stick to this routine every day – especially with children around. But using it as a basis helps you stay in control of your time and energy.

▷ Balance your mental and physical routine. Read a book if you're always on your feet; go for a run if you do sedentary work.

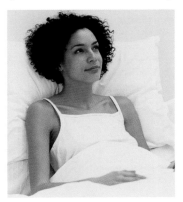

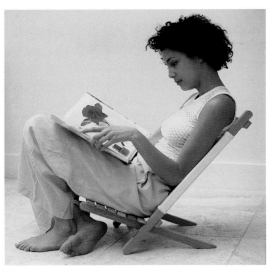

◁ Don't stay in bed long after you've woken in the morning, but take a few moments to plan the day ahead and visualize it all going really well.

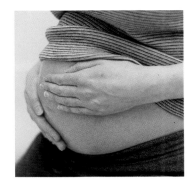

## pregnancy: glowing with new life

For someone used to being independent, pregnancy is a strange time as a new person's needs start encroaching on a woman's own. Some of the bizarre food cravings a pregnant woman experiences may be her body's attempt to balance her own doshas with the baby's.

The beauty benefits of pregnancy are a welcome side effect: glowing skin, voluptuous breasts and a mane of lustrous hair. Ayurveda can help you keep that glow. In India, a pregnant woman would be massaged by her husband and relatives. Gentle foot and ankle massage, with firm upward strokes, helps relieve swelling. After the fourth or fifth month, oil rubbed into the abdomen helps the skin maintain its elasticity, avoiding stretchmarks, and a backrub can wipe away tension from the face as well as the aching back.

Traditionally, pregnant women were encouraged to snack on sugared hibiscus flowers and rest as much as possible – with one exception: they swept the floors in a squatting position, strengthening the pelvic

area to prepare for childbirth. An antenatal yoga class will teach gentle exercises with the same aim.

Be cautious about massaging the back or abdomen during the early months, in case of miscarriage. Ayurveda recommends plain almond oil: if you want to use anything else, check beforehand with a reputable aromatherapist to find out which oils should be avoided during pregnancy.

If you're taking up yoga, make sure your class is run by a suitably qualified teacher. If you already practise yoga, take advice on how to modify your routine. Remember that not all pregnancies are standard, so seek medical advice if you have any concerns.

▽ You and the baby need to rest. If you haven't got a large Indian family to cosset you, seize time for yourself and accept all the help you can get.

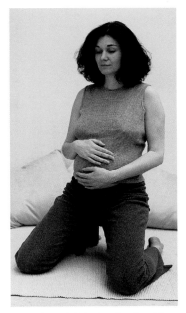

△ Squatting can help to strengthen the pelvic floor, but in the later months of pregnancy it's safer to modify the pose, sitting on a low stool.

## yoga squatting pose

**1** Stand with feet more than shoulder-width apart, toes turned out, and hold the hands in front of you in Namaste position.

**2** On an outbreath, bend your knees and squat, keeping your spine erect. Try to put your heels on the ground if you can, but don't force this. Keep your knees as wide apart as possible.

**3** If you've squatted low enough, bring your elbows down between your knees (fingers still pointing upwards), to encourage them further apart. Support your heels on books if they do not reach the floor, and your buttocks on a low stool or rolled towel if you're not comfortable squatting. Eventually you're aiming to put your heels on the floor.

**TIPS**

• Massage your hair throughout pregnancy and after the birth, to reduce the risk of hair loss caused by hormonal changes.

• Drink hot water with a slice of fresh ginger to relieve morning sickness.

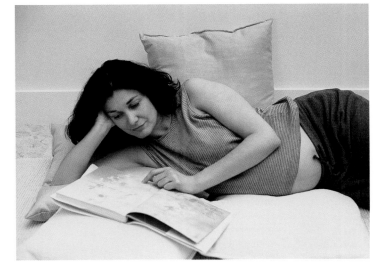

# The middle years

timeless beauty

As pitta dosha starts to subside and vata increases, women reach the second great transition in life: the menopause. Though pitta is waning, it's no longer regularly reduced by the loss of blood during a period, so it may flare up in sweating and irritability. Heavy periods may be a sign that the body is trying to offload excess pitta. Toxic ama tends to build up as periods become irregular. This leads to lower back pain and an increased risk of growths on the reproductive organs.

Meditation helps combat the stress that magnifies some symptoms and triggers others, such as hot flushes. It's especially important to try to meditate in the morning, to leave the mind calm and able to organize the day's tasks.

Insomnia strikes many women as they reach the menopause. A regular bedtime routine helps to train the mind to turn off at the right time. Ayurveda also recommends going to bed during the kapha hours before 10pm. If this makes you wake up even

earlier, don't spend more than 10 minutes trying to return to sleep – get up and meditate instead.

Yoga practice is also important. Keeping a straight back and open chest allows you to breathe more fully, and weight-bearing exercise keeps bones strong. Add some form of exercise that leaves you slightly out of breath, such as brisk walking or low-impact aerobics. As well as keeping weight under control, this improves the skin.

## changing tastes

Choosing the right foods is most important during the menopause, both to bring the doshas into balance and to meet the body's changing needs. Iron, for example, is no longer so necessary, whereas calcium is vital to keep bones strong.

Ayurveda's healthy living rules are made to meet beauty needs as well as promoting long life. The foods that keep the doshas in balance also promote clear skin and a slim, strong physique. Milk and cottage cheese, for example, pacify both vata and pitta while providing calcium and Vitamin D. Base your diet on fresh vegetables and fruit with some dairy foods, nuts, seeds and grains.

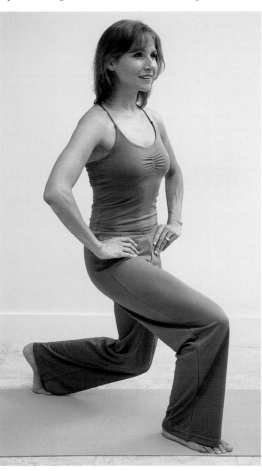

◁ Staying active keeps you in good shape and slows down the effects of aging. It also eases menopausal symptoms by stabilizing your hormones.

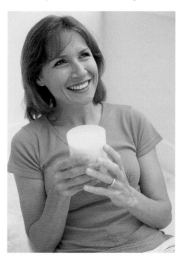

▷ Changes in your body's hormones can make this stage of your life difficult, but an Ayurvedic remedy will help to balance them.

## A REMEDY TO BALANCE THE HORMONES

**ingredients**

- 5 almonds
- 3 black peppercorns
- 2 cardamom pods
- 5 ml/1 tsp anise seeds
- 250 ml/8 fl oz/1 cup milk
- 5 ml/1 tsp honey

Soak the almonds in water overnight. Next morning, peel off the skin and grind to a fine paste. Grind the peppercorns, cardamom and anise seeds and mix with the almond paste. Boil the milk, and add your paste and honey. Drink lukewarm.

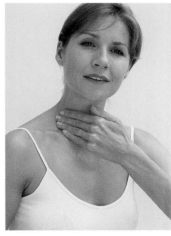

△ Soothe vata with gentle oil massage, brief steaming and a cooling facepack.

## save your skin

As vata dosha increases with age, its drying influence causes lines, wrinkles and thinning of the skin. Milk, honey and yogurt help to lubricate the skin from the inside, keeping it youthful.

Oiling the skin and then steaming reduces excess vata, making this a suitable beauty treatment throughout life. Because fine facial skin can be damaged by too-frequent steaming, it should be done only once or twice a month. Regular use of nourishing facepacks can help to keep the skin properly moisturized, slowing down the aging process.

## seeing clearly

Delay the need for reading glasses with some eye exercises. (If you wear contact lenses, remove them first.) Sit with your spine straight and shoulders relaxed, and look straight ahead. Keep your head still while doing the exercises. Hold each eye position for 3–5 seconds and repeat three times.

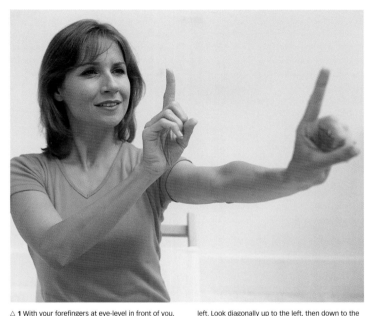

△ **1** With your forefingers at eye-level in front of you, hold one at arm's length and the other half that distance away. Focus on one, then the other.

**2** Look diagonally up to the right, then down to the left. Look diagonally up to the left, then down to the right. Look as far as you can up, down, left and right.

**3** Rub your hands together to warm them, then cup your palms over your eyes for a few minutes.

## NOURISHING MATURE SKIN MASK

**ingredients**

- 30 ml/2 tbsp oatmeal
- 120 ml/4 fl oz/½ cup milk
- 10 ml/2 tsp olive oil

Mix the oatmeal and milk and simmer until soft. Stir in the oil and mix well. When cool, spread on the face and neck. Leave for 20–30 minutes and rinse with cool water.

## TIP

Grate a thumb-sized piece of fresh ginger into a jar of honey and take a teaspoonful a day to slow down the advance of grey hair.

## mula bandha: yogic exercise for the pelvic floor

Many women approaching the menopause find their pelvic floor muscles have weakened, giving little or no warning of the need to urinate. Simple exercises can banish this embarrassing problem. Begin by tightening your anus, then add a squeeze in front as if stopping yourself urinating, and hold both squeezes while trying to lift the pelvic floor. It's a tiny movement. If you lay your forefinger flat along the perineum – the strip of skin between vagina and anus – you should feel a very small lift. Start by doing this three or four times after using the lavatory (don't try to stop the flow of urine as this can cause bladder problems), then practise it for 5 seconds at a time, for example while holding any yoga pose.

# Moving forward

This is a time when many people – whose earlier lives may have been too hectic for regular practice – discover the benefits of yoga. Notice how much more confidence they have than most older people. This confidence is based on a strength and suppleness that makes them far less prone to accidents and falls.

From as early as the 30s, muscles start to stiffen and joints lose their range of movement. As the years pass, even people with good posture start to walk and turn less smoothly. Long-term yoga practice can delay the onset of these restrictions by many years, but taking up yoga in later life can also reverse some of the changes age has made.

By encouraging correct posture and maintaining flexibility in the spine, it helps to delay the effects of aging. Starting each day with a routine lasting 20–30 minutes leaves you in good shape and gives you time to clear your mind for the day.

▽ **Take care of your body, not by reducing activity but by ensuring that all the movements you make are beneficial. Squatting instead of bending, for example, reduces the risk of back pain at any age.**

### TAKE IT EASY

If you have any medical conditions, check with your doctor before starting any kind of exercise and consider taking a remedial yoga class. In particular:

• Don't do inverted poses such as the Standing Forward Bend and the Downward-facing Dog if you have a blood pressure or heart condition. If you feel at all dizzy in any pose, come out of it gently and sit down.

• If you have arthritis or osteoporosis, beware of poses that put weight on your wrists, such as the Downward-facing Dog.

• Don't do the intense straight-legged bends and backward head-rolls that advanced yoga practitioners carry out. These can injure your spine. In any bend it's better to keep your knees soft, even slightly bent, and concentrate on gently rolling your spine down.

• After a yoga session you should be aware of the muscles you've worked, and may even feel a bit stiff over the next day or so when you're new to the practice. But your joints shouldn't hurt and any stiffness should wear off after a couple of days. If you do experience any pain, stop practising and see your doctor.

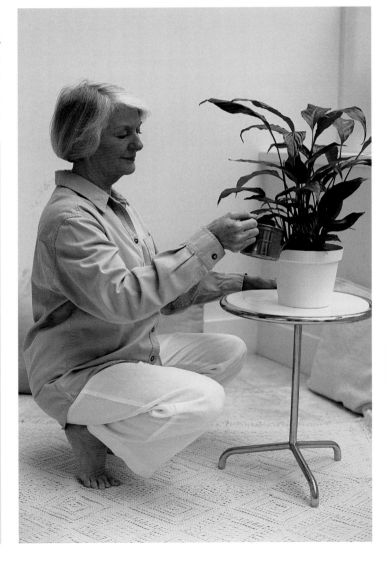

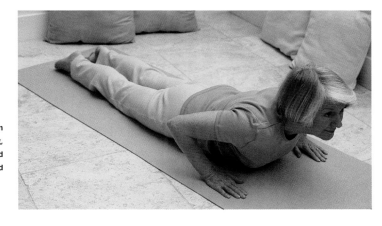

## daily yoga routine

**You should include asanas from each of the main groups, to work all parts of the body: standing, sitting and lying down; back bends, forward bends and twists. The following is a gentle and effective series suitable for older beginners.**

**1** Warm up by performing the Cat movement several times to get your spine working.

**2** Stand up in the Mountain pose, to centre you and help keep your balance steady. As people age their sense of balance starts to fade, and it is this as much as loss of strength that leads to potentially dangerous falls. Keeping a good sense of balance gives you the same confident stride you had when you were young.

**3** Move into the Standing Side Stretch. Check that you are breathing naturally and in rhythm with your movements: in as you lean downwards, out as you come up. Return to the Mountain pose and take a moment to feel centred again.

▽ **4** Now move into the Standing Forward Bend, keeping your knees slightly bent if you are new to this. If you feel any strain on your back, just move forwards enough to put your hands on a support such

as a stable piece of furniture. Concentrate on keeping your back flat and your head in line with your spine.

△ **5** Return to the Mountain pose for a few moments, then lie down on your stomach and move into the Cobra pose. Keep your elbows bent and focus on opening your chest, letting your shoulders sink down and back, away from your ears. When you look upwards, do not to let your head tip back. You're aiming for a natural curve at the neck, without compressing the vertebrae. The same goes for the lower back, don't push yourself up with straight arms and an unnatural arch in your lumbar spine – it's the thoracic vertebrae in your upper spine that need to move.

**6** Lower your chest and come smoothly out of the Cobra, then push your hips back and bend forwards

into the Child pose, relaxing your spine by letting it curve in the other direction.

**7** Move into a kneeling position and into the Dog pose.

**8** Next, go into the Bridge, to increase flexibility in your spine. Keep your heels and your arms on the floor, with your palms facing down. You are aiming for a gentle curve in your spine.

**9** Roll on to your side and sit up, then move into the Cow pose. This is meant to promote long life, because it opens your chest and stops your lower back stiffening. If you find the leg position difficult, simply sit or kneel with your spine straight.

**10** Complete your routine by relaxing for a few minutes in the Corpse pose. Come up by rolling on to your side.

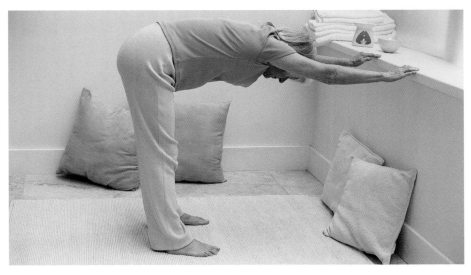

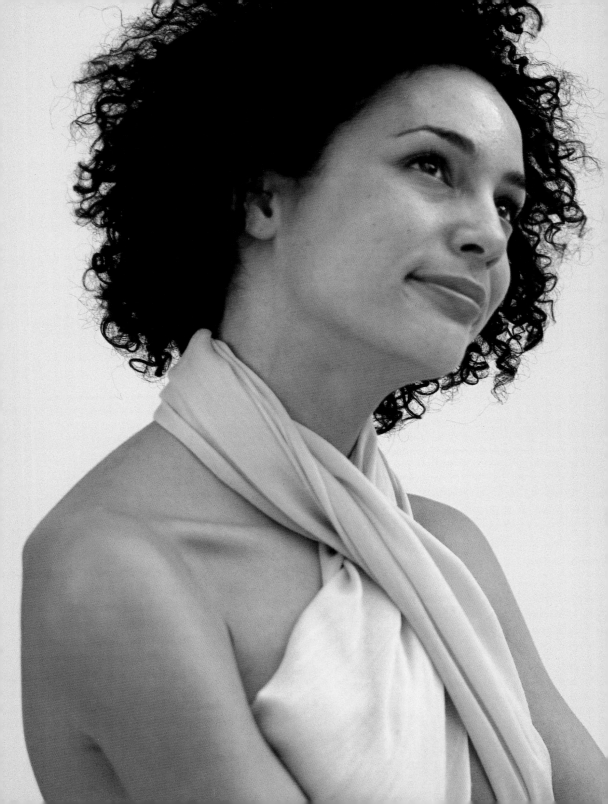

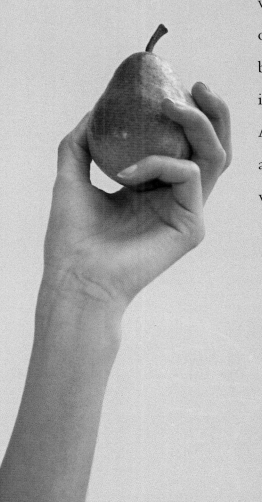

# The Food of Life

A gift from heaven and earth, the food we eat can nourish our spirits as well as our bodies. Eating well enhances beauty and preserves youthful vitality; it's also a sign of healthy self-respect. In Ayurveda, a meal prepared with love is a blessing to those who cook and those who eat.

# Eating well

For many of us, food is at best simply fuel, at worst an enemy. Modern cook books set standards unknown to previous generations, yet most of the food we eat is commercially prepared. Nearly half of us are on a slimming diet at any given time, yet our average weight is rising steadily. No wonder so many of us view food with anxiety.

The Ayurvedic outlook is like a breath of sattvic fresh air. It teaches that eating is a pleasure, and one that does nothing but good. This approach doesn't lead to binge-eating; instead, it means putting a little time and thought into preparing food from fresh ingredients, then savouring it as you eat.

The freshness and quality of the food are important, since unwholesome ingredients create ama, or toxins, in the body. A diet that is based on meat, alcohol, processed foods, dairy products and white sugar and flour produces a lot of ama, leading to disease, bad breath, dull skin and unhealthy hair, while fresh, natural foods give you energy and vitality, and let your natural beauty shine through.

Ayurveda further emphasizes the need to digest food properly, since poor digestion leaves by-products that can also develop into ama. That's why each dosha type needs to eat a slightly different range of foods – those that they're most easily able to digest.

## cooking with love

In today's speedy world we often feel too rushed to cook with fresh ingredients. But the steady rhythm of chopping vegetables and stirring pots can create a calm space in the day. And Ayurveda's simple recipes take little time to prepare.

In a traditional Indian household, the kitchen is an almost sacred place. Since everything in creation is deemed to have a soul, everything is entitled to be treated with respect – especially food, which imparts its life force, or prana, to the eater. Followers of Ayurveda believe that the feelings you experience as you cook enter the food and

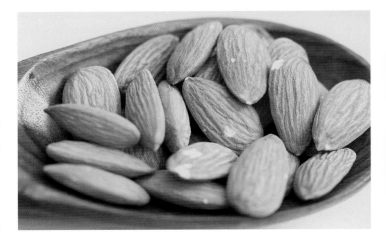

△ To Ayurveda, almonds are full of prana; in Western terms they're rich in Vitamin E, calcium and beneficial fats – either way, a perfect snack.

affect anyone who eats it. So don't resent the time you spend cooking. If you enjoy creating a dish, feel nothing but love for those who are going to eat it (including yourself) and look forward to eating it, you'll be endowing the food with health benefits that can't be bought.

## food basics

The mainstays of your diet should be fresh fruit and cooked vegetables, grains, nuts and seeds. Add salads and certain animal foods, depending on your dosha. Locally grown organic produce in season is the most natural, as long periods in transport or storage reduce nutritional value.

Meat and dairy produce should be organically produced. Factory-farmed animal foods are risky even by Western standards: they may be diseased or contain drug residues. But such foods are doubly harmful by Ayurvedic standards: the miserable lives of the animals produce low-quality prana, and your action in supporting intensive rearing creates bad karma.

Followers of Ayurveda are frequently vegetarian. Plant foods are full of prana and organic choices are best, as their chemical-free growth causes no harm either to them

or to the environment. These are the most physically and spiritually nourishing foods you can find.

## how to eat

• Eat at regular times, leaving at least four hours between meals.

• Don't eat unless you're hungry. If you have no appetite, wait until your next meal time, drinking warm water in between. But don't go without food for more than a day.

• Always sit down to eat, and don't watch television, read or have emotional conversations during the meal.

• Eat slowly and savour food. This stops you over-eating, since it takes a while for your brain to register that you've eaten enough.

• Try doing a mindfulness meditation while eating. Focus your attention on the food: its colours, shapes, smell, texture and taste. You're less likely to overeat when your mind's on your meal.

• Eat raw fruit alone, not as part of a meal.

• Fast on fruit and vegetable juices and water for one day a month.

▷ Fresh organic fruit and vegetables are the mainstay of an Ayurvedic diet, good to eat without harming the earth they came from.

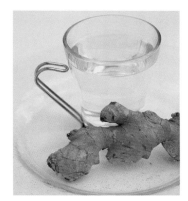

△ Ginger tea is renowned for strengthening the digestion and alleviating feelings of nausea.

## what to drink

• Drink enough water to ensure that your urine is always a pale yellow colour: up to 2 litres/3$^1$/$_2$ pints a day is beneficial. Warm or hot water is best, and Ayurveda doesn't recommend drinking ice-cold water.

• Other healthy drinks are herbal teas, milk (depending on your dosha), fruit juices and vegetable juices.

• Ginger tea strengthens *agni*, the digestive fire. Warm water also aids digestion and should be drunk throughout the day.

• Choose healthy beverages more often than alcohol or stimulants like tea or coffee.

▽ Cranberry and apple juice are both full of vitamins. Dilute fruit juices with water for the best effects on the body.

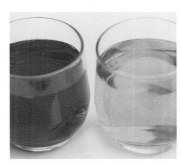

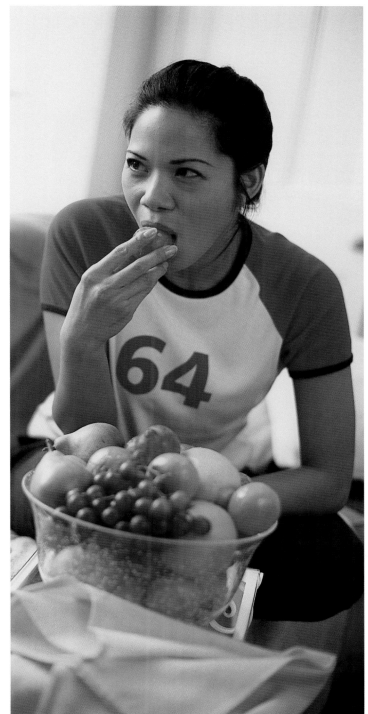

# The inner qualities of food

The gunas, or qualities, of foods are as important as their taste and nutritional value. All aspects of nature contain these inner properties – sattva, rajas and tamas – and therefore affect our own gunas whenever we come into contact with them. Since the food we eat becomes part of us, its guna has a particularly strong effect.

## sattva

Few people attain the sattvic state of enlightenment, but when we approach it we're fully alert, clear-thinking and compassionate. Sattvic foods, the ones closest to that state themselves, help us towards it. They are the lightest and most wholesome ingredients, close to their

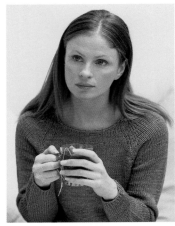

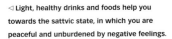

◁ Light, healthy drinks and foods help you towards the sattvic state, in which you are peaceful and unburdened by negative feelings.

natural state, such as fresh fruit and vegetables, honey, nuts and whole grains. The lighter dairy products – milk, yogurt and butter – are also sattvic. In keeping with Ayurveda's non-violent ethic, the most sattvic food causes no harm, so the best diet is based on organic fruit and vegetables, locally grown to reduce the environmental costs of transport, and organic dairy produce from animals kept in humane conditions.

## rajas

The rajasic state is turbulent, always on the go and easily irritated. Rajasic food is the kind that fuels the go-getting Western world, and each time we eat it it adds to that tendency in us. Rajasic food is not bad, because we do need some stimulation, but since Ayurveda values peace more highly than profits, it recommends eating it in smaller quantities. Following that advice will do your body as much good as your soul, since rajasic food is the most likely to cause heartburn. If you have any tendency to be aggressive, cut down on it still further. It's high-protein, high-energy fuel. Rajasic

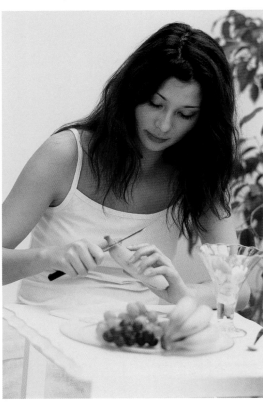

◁ Fruit pacifies vata and pitta doshas and – especially when cooked – makes a healthy substitute for the cakes and sugary foods that can aggravate kapha.

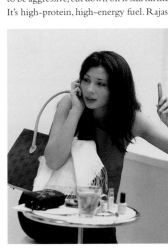

▷ Rajasic foods fuel the Western lifestyle that leads to stress and burnout. Snacking adds to the ill effects, so take time to eat nourishing food.

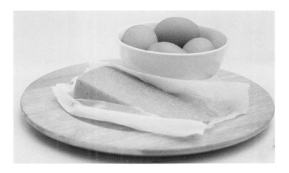

▷ We need high-protein foods to build our physical strength and give us rajasic energy. They only cause harm if, as in the average Western diet, we eat too much of them.

foods include meat, fish, eggs, hard cheese, hot peppers, sugary foods and root vegetables, along with anything that has been fried, pickled or highly spiced.

## tamas

The tamasic state of mind is lethargic, ignorant, selfish and dull. It is fuelled by processed foods, artificial flavours or sweeteners, chemical preservatives, factory-farmed meat and dairy produce, and anything mass-produced without respect or made from low-quality ingredients. Meaty junk food is about as tamasic as food can be. Food that's stale and has lost its life force is tamasic too. For this reason, Ayurveda recommends cooking food fresh every day rather than using leftovers. Alcohol falls into the tamasic group, since although it's a stimulant at first it soon has a dulling effect.

▽ **Mass-produced junk food has tamasic effects, but homemade cakes are a treat: moderation, quality and individual needs are important.**

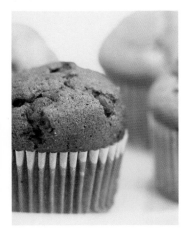

▽ **Alcohol pushes us away from the sattvic state by causing confusion, damaging health and promoting aggression and laziness.**

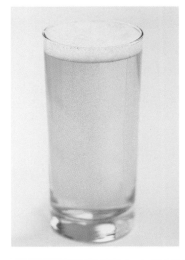

## the six tastes

Ayurveda recognizes six flavours, which affect the balance of doshas. We all need all of them, but in differing amounts. You don't need to give up any of your favourite ingredients completely; if they're in a group that increases your dominant dosha, just eat less of them or prepare them in a way that makes them more suitable, such as tossing salad in a rich dressing to reduce its vata-raising properties.

• **Sweet:** Increases kapha, reduces vata and pitta. Sweet-tasting foods such as honey, cucumber, dried fruit, most fresh fruits, and foods that become sweet when cooked, such as apples and onions. High-protein foods such as meat and nuts. Fats and oils. Butter, ghee and milk. Rice.

• **Sour:** Increases kapha and pitta, reduces vata. Vinegar, pickles and aged food. Yogurt and cheese. Tomatoes. Citrus fruits.

• **Salty:** Increases kapha and pitta, reduces vata. Salt, soy sauce.

• **Pungent (spicy):** Increases vata and pitta, reduces kapha. Chillies, sweet peppers, many herbs and spices.

• **Bitter:** Increases vata and reduces pitta and kapha. Most salad leaves and green leafy vegetables. Fenugreek and a few other bitter herbs. Coffee, chocolate.

• **Astringent:** Increases vata and reduces pitta and kapha. Beans, peas, chickpeas, lentils. Cauliflower, broccoli, fennel, asparagus, chicory, aubergines (eggplant), celery, Savoy cabbage. Tea.

### GHEE

Clarified butter, or ghee, is not only a mainstay of Indian cooking but an important Ayurvedic health product. You can make your own, though it may not taste quite the same as the product bought in Indian shops, which is often made with yogurt. If you have high cholesterol and don't normally eat animal fats, check with your doctor. If you can't use ghee, substitute vegetable oils.

To make ghee, put 1 kg/2¼ lb unsalted organic butter in a heavy pan and heat slowly, stirring constantly, until melted. Turn up the heat and let the butter froth for a few moments, then reduce the heat and simmer gently, uncovered, for about 30 minutes, until transparent. Skim off the froth and any impurities and strain through muslin or cheesecloth, discarding the milky solids. Leave to cool and store in the refrigerator.

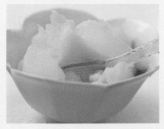

△ **Golden richness with a sweet, nutty taste.**

# Diet and your dosha

Each dosha type is pacified or aggravated by different foods, so the food you eat can help to balance your constitution. Try to eat something from each of the six taste groups every day, with most of your intake coming from the groups that pacify your dosha.

## the vata diet

Vata is pacified by sweet, sour and salty foods, but aggravated by pungent, bitter and astringent tastes. Raw food tends to increase vata. Try to balance your dry, cool, light constitution with foods that are hot, oily and heavy, such as soups and rich stews. Bananas, grapes and all sweet fruits are good, and meat suits your constitution better than most.

Natural foods are particularly important to vata, since it is aggravated by artificial additives. Most dairy foods suit you, but yogurt is best diluted: try mixing it with water, pure rose water and some honey or chopped fruit, or with water and a little salt to make the Indian drink called lassi.

Though many herbs and spices fall into the pungent category, they're only used in small amounts, so enjoy the warming qualities of spicy foods, though chillies are generally not recommended, since they're considered very dry.

▽ If it's a hot day but you need to pacify vata, drink a refreshing glass of sweet or salty lassi.

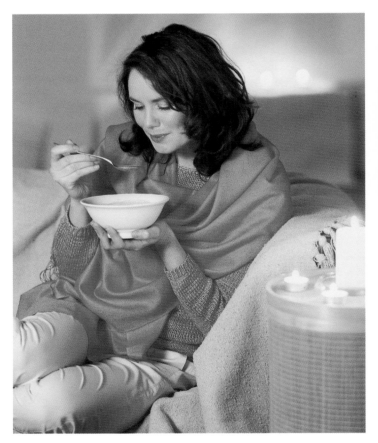

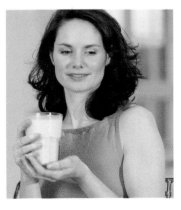

△ Warmth and comfort soothe excess vata: a cosy room, a quiet evening, a bowl of rich soup.

Toss salads in mayonnaise or rich dressings containing oil or coconut milk. You can use cooked ingredients to make a warm salad. If you like vegetables from the bitter and astringent taste-groups, cook them with oil or ghee. Ghee will also aid your digestion, which tends to be irregular. Anything light, dry and cool will increase vata, so you should avoid foods like crisps (potato chips), popcorn, dried fruits and undressed green salads.

Though sweet natural foods are good for vata, white sugar and white bread are too dry and light. Alcohol, tobacco and recreational drugs in general have strong vata-inflaming effects and should be avoided altogether or reduced to a minimum.

### VATAS COULD TRY...

- Porridge with milk and honey.
- Roasted/stir-fried meat and vegetables.
- Stews cooked with ghee or oil.
- Cooked soft fruit with cream.

## the pitta diet

The tastes that help to balance pitta are sweet, bitter and astringent. It is aggravated by those that are pungent, sour or salty. Pitta-pacifying foods are cold, heavy and dry.

Pitta dosha can make you digest your food too quickly, leading to poor absorption. Since Ayurveda teaches that good digestion is the foundation of good health, it is important to strengthen agni, the digestive fire that governs the metabolic processes. Some agni-strengthening foods tend to increase pitta too, but ghee is ideal: it balances pitta while increasing agni. To improve digestion, try to eat slowly in peaceful surroundings at regular times, without overeating. Don't have high-protein food late in the evening. Do take some time to relax after a meal.

Almost all vegetables are good for you, and most fruits that are not sour. Eat plenty of raw food and salad (other than tomatoes). The few vegetables that may not suit you include beetroot, carrots, aubergines (eggplant), garlic, onions and spinach. Chillies, salt and highly spiced food add too much fuel to pitta's fire. Instead, experiment with the cooling tastes of basil, coriander (cilantro), dill, fennel and turmeric, and other mild-tasting herbs. Eat only small amounts of concentrated protein such as red meat, seafood and eggs. Stimulants of all kinds aggravate pitta, so cut down on alcohol and coffee and avoid recreational drugs of any kind.

▽ **Excessive pitta heat is cooled by raw foods such as fruit, mild herbs, and vegetables such as broccoli.**

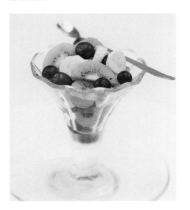

**PITTAS COULD TRY...**

• Cool stewed apple with pumpkin seeds.
• Green salad with fresh asparagus, drizzled with extra virgin olive oil.
• Rice and beans.
• Ice cream with fresh figs or blackberries.

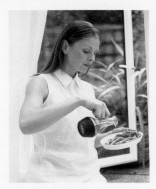

△ **A salad is the ideal pitta lunch.**

## the kapha diet

Kapha is balanced by pungent, bitter and astringent tastes, but aggravated by those that are sweet, sour or salty. Foods should be dry, light and hot.

The kapha constitution tends to be cold, so needs warming foods: freshly cooked, spicy or piquant with chillies. Include plenty of vegetables, cooked and eaten hot. Almost all vegetables are good for you, though sweet potatoes can be a little heavy and cucumber has a cooling effect.

You can improve your sometimes sluggish digestion by strengthening agni, the digestive fire. This can be achieved by eating

▽ **Gourmet kaphas can liven up their cooking with chillies, which provide an invigorating heat.**

cloves, pepper (black or cayenne), mustard, cinnamon and horseradish.

The cold nature of salads makes them less suitable for kapha, especially in winter. But don't rule them out completely: choose warm salads, or leaves with a sharp or mustardy taste, but don't smother them in dressing. You have a free hand with almost all herbs and spices, so use these flavourings instead of oils and fats.

Cut down on heavy foods such as wheat, red meat and cheese; lighter alternatives are barley, poultry and cottage cheese. You may have a taste for sweet or salty foods, but these should play only a minor role. Processed foods are high in fat or sugar, and "lite" versions just substitute artificial sweeteners. So leave them on the supermarket shelves and let your natural kapha cooking skills loose on the huge range of real foods.

**KAPHAS COULD TRY...**

• Cooked buckwheat with cranberries and sunflower seeds.
• Warm salad of raw baby spinach leaves and organic chicken.
• Spicy homemade curries rich with seasonings instead of oil.
• Pears stewed with ginger.

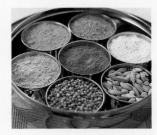

△ **Kaphas can enjoy almost all spices.**

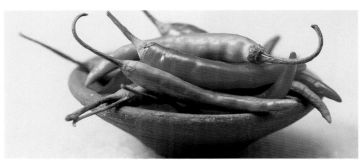

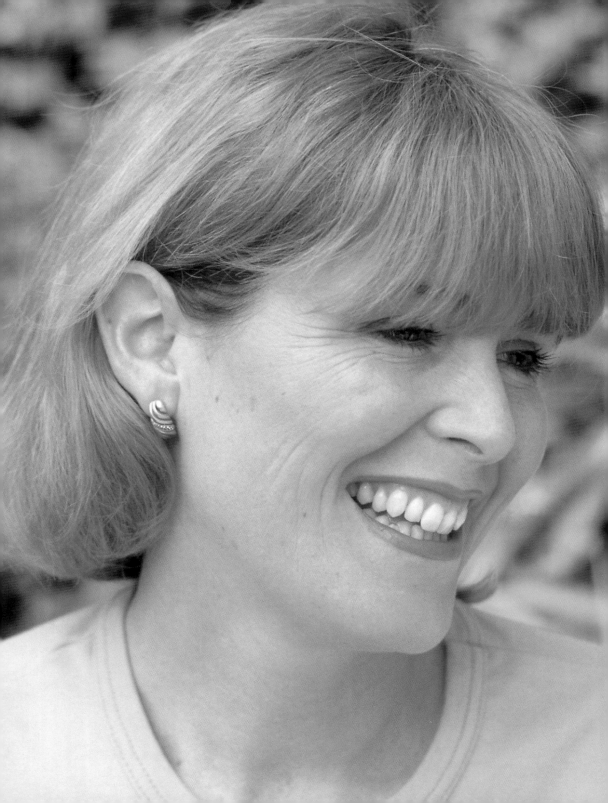

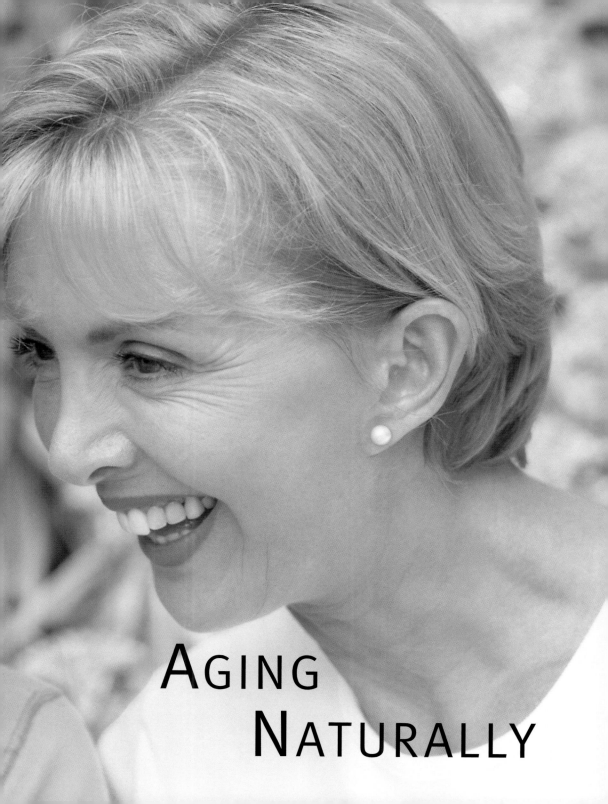

# AGING
# NATURALLY

# The fight against aging

The quest to extend the human life span is nothing new; scientists have long searched for ways to prevent aging and cure life-threatening illnesses such as cancer. Significant progress is being made in the field of gerontology and it is likely that in the future we will be able to slow the aging process down and live actively into old age. For example, in 1999, Italian researchers at the European Institute of Oncology in Milan published findings regarding the existence of a genetic defect in mice that causes them to live a third longer than other mice. The mice ate a normal diet and had a normal body weight but they lacked a gene for a specific protein. The implications of this finding for human life spans is the focus of intensive research.

## taking care for your health

As you grow older it is important to be aware of the changes that take place in your body. You need to know how to prevent problems occurring and how to respond to them when they do. Taking responsibility for your own health and wellbeing gives you a powerful sense of control and self-confidence. However, this does not mean excluding healthcare professionals. For example, tell your doctor if you are taking herbal medicines. Other factors which may help include:

• Listening to your body and responding appropriately.

• Learning about complementary therapies and how they can help you prevent and treat health problems.

• Exercising regularly and concentrating on staying flexible and active rather than "going for the burn".

• Eating plenty of fruit and vegetables.

• Understanding the age-related changes that affect each body system. Learn which changes can be prevented, which ones should be accommodated and which changes may be early warning signs of health problems.

## positive avoidance

Many of the harmful aspects of life have been identified, which means that we can now make a positive effort to avoid the things that cause us harm. For example, stress, cigarette smoking, drinking too much alcohol and long-term exposure to the sun and pollution are five of the major contributors to the aging process. Even if we eat healthy food, exercise regularly and have plenty of sleep, these factors will still have an adverse effect on the body.

Fortunately, it is comparatively easy to avoid cigarette smoking, excessive alcohol consumption and exposure to the sun. It is less easy to avoid pollution and stress; these are things that we need to tackle collectively, and this is now recognized and taken seriously by scientists, employers and governments. Also, even if can we cannot avoid stress and pollution there are ways of mitigating their effects on the body. There is a wide range of complementary therapies that can help us to relax and there is some evidence that taking antioxidant supplements can mitigate the damaging effects of environmental pollution.

## complementary therapies

In the past, remedies for illness were passed down from one generation to the next in a strong tradition of herbal medicine. Although people may not have known how plant remedies worked, they remained tried and trusted ways of treating illness. For example, St John's wort was used as an antidepressant long before science taught us about serotonin, a brain chemical that affects mood. A report in the *British Medical Journal* stated that St John's wort has fewer side effects than imipramine, a widely prescribed antidepressant.

▽ **Acupressure can be particularly helpful for pain control, treatment of common ailments and boosting the immune system to help protect the body from disease.**

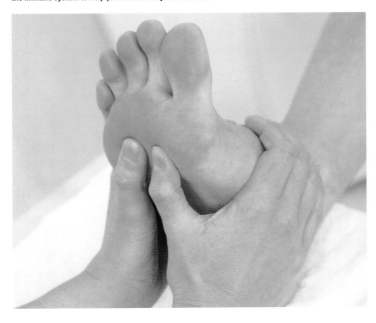

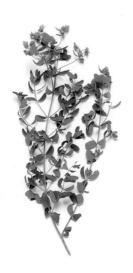

△ **St John's Wort is a natural antidepressant, but prolonged use may cause photosensitivity.**

Although conventional medicine remains the first option for many people during sickness, there is a move towards complementary therapies that treat the body as an interdependent whole rather than a collection of individual parts. It is now thought that many plant remedies are effective because they contain ingredients that work in concert with one another. In contrast, most Western drugs simply isolate the active ingredient in a plant.

Herbalism is just one of many types of complementary therapy available. Other types of recommended treatment include aromatherapy, massage, hypnotherapy, reflexology, dietary medicine and acupuncture. Complementary therapies are now recognized by many doctors and scientists as being valuable aids in assisting the body to fight illness and aging.

▷ **As we age our bodies become less supple and taking the time to undertake gentle stretching exercises each day is a good way of maintaining muscle and joint flexibility.**

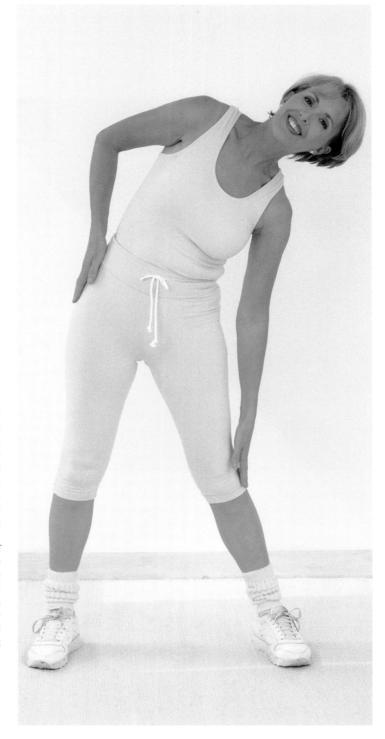

# The harmful effects of free radicals

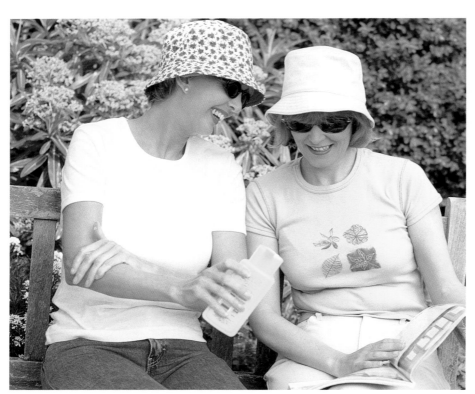

◁ When buying sun tan lotion keep your skin type in mind. Many fair-skinned people begin to suffer skin damage after just 10 minutes in the sun. By buying a factor 10 sunscreen they can multiply this time by 10, and benefit from up to 100 minutes protection, before damage begins to occur.

Although the causes of aging are not entirely understood, we now know that damage to the body by substances known as free radicals plays a critical role. In fact, doctors and nutritionists say that, without doubt, the most important fight against aging should be against free radical damage. Although free radicals have received much press attention, few of us understand exactly what they are or how they affect the body.

## free radicals

Oxygen is essential for life, but it can also be considered a poison. This is because when oxygen is used for essential processes inside the body, it leads to the production of damaging molecules known as free radicals. The most damaging characteristic of free radicals is their chemical structure in that they contain an unpaired electron. This means that they roam around the body "searching" for healthy molecules to pair with. Unfortunately, this pairing process damages the host molecule and irreversibly changes the DNA (material that carries genetic information). If free radicals are allowed to damage body cells in this way over a long period of time, the result is extensive cell damage and aging, as well as diseases such as arthritis, heart disease, cataracts and cancer.

A good way to understand free radical damage to the body is to think of it as continuous internal radiation. Yet free radicals are not just created by normal bodily processes; they are also created by oxidation outside the body. For example, combustion processes, radiation from the sun, cigarette smoking and environmental pollution all give rise to free radicals. Also, some foods and drinks (fried food and alcohol, for example) generate more free radicals than others.

## the fight against free radicals

Although our bodies have evolved their own defences against free radicals, it is essential that we minimize exposure to free radicals where possible. This means giving up cigarette smoking (and avoiding other people's cigarette smoke), not eating burnt food, staying out of direct sunlight, not drinking too much alcohol and minimizing exposure to environmental pollution such as traffic fumes. It is also believed that sleep deprivation can increase free radical damage to the body, so we need to make sure we have sufficient sleep every night.

## the best weapons: antioxidants

By far the best weapons in the war against free radicals are antioxidants, which are found in vitamins A, C and E, in co-enzyme Q10 and betacarotene, as well as in minerals such as selenium and zinc.

When free radicals are roaming around the body, antioxidant molecules can pair with them, preventing them from attacking healthy molecules. When antioxidants pair with (or "mop up") roaming free radicals they can then be eliminated from the body via the excretory systems. This way, no damage is done to the body.

One way to understand the action of antioxidants is to observe what happens when lemon juice is dropped onto the cut surface of an apple. As soon as the apple is cut and exposed to the air it reacts with oxygen and starts to discolour. Yet if lemon juice is squeezed onto the cut surface, the antioxidant action of the vitamin C in the juice will prevent the discoloration. However, this protection is only temporary and the cut surfaces will start to oxidize as the antioxidant function wears down.

The importance of antioxidants in your diet cannot be over-estimated. It is crucial for everyone, especially older people, to eat foods rich in antioxidant vitamins and minerals. Nutritionists recommend eating plenty of fresh fruit and vegetables on a daily basis. Antioxidants are also available in the form of supplements.

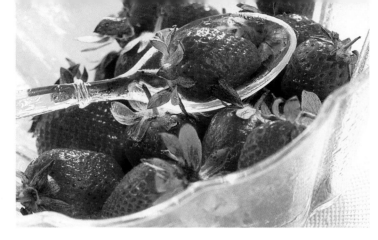

△ Strawberries contain a phytochemical called ellagic acid which is believed to fight against cancer.

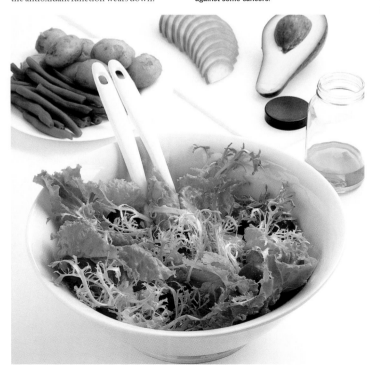

▽ The darker outer leaves of lettuce contain betacarotene, an antioxidant thought to protect against some cancers.

### WHERE TO FIND ANTIOXIDANTS

The main antioxidant nutrients are vitamins A, C, and E, and zinc and selenium. Foods containing these vitamins and minerals should be part of your daily diet. In addition to these vitamins and minerals, there are other substances known as phytochemicals, found in plants, that also have antioxidant properties. These include bioflavanoids (found in citrus fruit) and lycopene (found in tomatoes). Some amino acids, such as cysteine and glutamic acid also have antioxidant effects. Cysteine and glutamic acid are found in white meat, tuna, lentils, beans, nuts, seeds, onions and garlic.

### The following foods are excellent sources of antioxidants and can be eaten in abundance:

- Sweet potatoes
- Carrots
- Watercress
- Broccoli
- Peas
- Cauliflower
- Tomatoes
- Citrus fruit
- Watermelon
- Strawberries
- Seeds
- Nuts

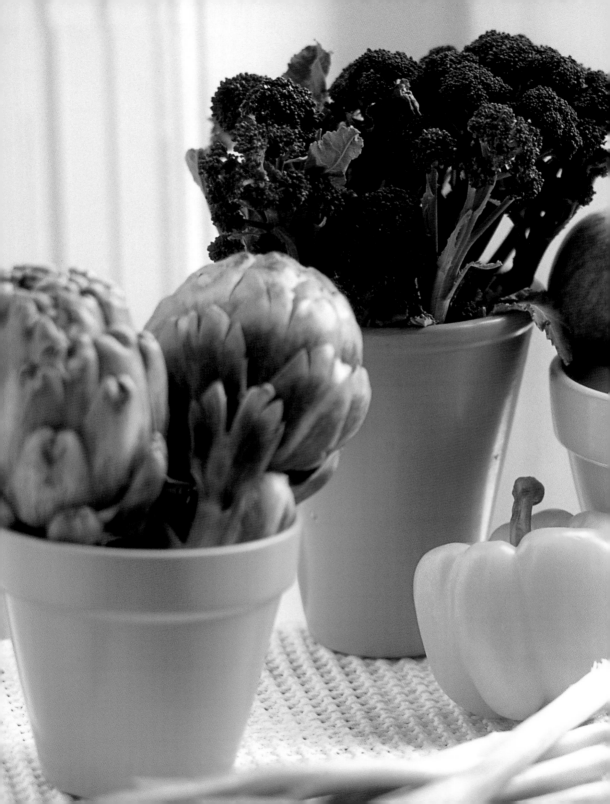

# Anti-aging Diet

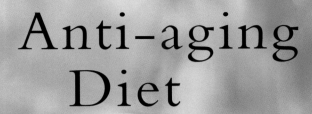

Through the leaps made in the science of
nutrition, we now know that the food we eat
can make a huge contribution to our health
and wellbeing. We can help prevent many
aging-related problems, such as heart disease,
by concentrating on some food groups in the
diet and limiting others.

# Revising your eating habits

Between the ages of 40 and 65, life becomes more sedentary for many of us. We may retire and have fewer personal obligations than before. A slower lifestyle means that the body needs fewer calories. Yet our vitamin and mineral requirements remain the same or increase in order to prevent cell aging and dietary deficiencies.

## healthy eating patterns

Since diet is so important as you get older, it is advisable to periodically alter your diet and eating patterns. Do you eat with health in mind or are your eating habits based on convenience? Are you prone to eating lots of "empty calories" in the form of fatty and sugary foods? Are you at risk of diet-related health problems such as osteoporosis (a chronic disease that weakens the bones)?

Nutritionists recommend a low-fat diet based on fresh fruit and vegetables, unrefined, complex carbohydrates and protein foods such as oily fish. This keeps the immune system in good working order and helps to prevent cell aging and degenerative diseases caused by free radicals (highly reactive molecules within our bodies). The World Cancer Research Fund estimates that 40 per cent of cancers (approximately 4 million cases worldwide) can be avoided by following a healthy diet and not smoking.

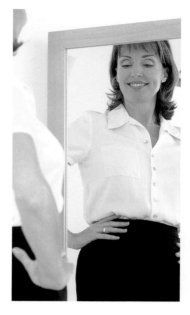

▷ Avoid elasticated waist bands on skirts and trousers since they allow clothes to remain comfortable, instead of giving early warning of creeping weight gain.

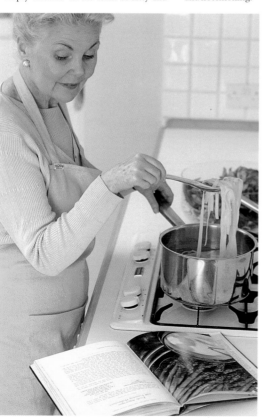

◁ White pasta offers less fibre, minerals and vitamins than wholemeal pasta, but is still a useful source of low-fat complex carbohydrate.

## do you need to lose weight?

Excessive weight gain is not inevitable as we age. In fact we should not weigh more than 9 kg/20 lbs more at the age of 50 than we did at 20, regardless of height. Many wieght charts are standardized to include age, height and sex; if your weight is 20 per cent above or below the standard, it is advisable to have a medical check up to ensure no problems exist.

In 1999, Dr Margaret Ashwell, a nutritionist, recommended a new and simple method of determining acceptable weight to the British Royal Society of Medicine. According to her method, if your waist measurement is less than half your height measurement, then your weight does not present a health hazard. If this method is applied to people in the UK, 15 per cent of men and 11 per cent of women can be considered dangerously overweight.

Another way of assessing weight is to calculate what percentage of your body consists of fat. This is a test that can be performed by some health centres and sports clinics. On average our bodies are composed of approximately: 63 per cent water, 22 per cent protein, 13 per cent fat and 2 per cent vitamins and minerals.

If your fat ratio is significantly higher than 13 per cent a doctor is likely to advise you to reduce your fat intake and increase the amount of aerobic exercise you do. These are important measures in the prevention of chronic health problems.

As you get older it is advisable to avoid foods that contain too many additives such as sugar and salt, which are implicated in health problems such as hypertension and diabetes. As part of your dietary reassessment, study the labels of the foods in your kitchen. Compare the additives and ingredients in different foods. Ideally, the food on your shelves should be low in calories, saturated fat, sodium and sugar, and high in fibre and vitamins and minerals. If you become familiar with the composition of different foods, you will quickly become adept at monitoring what you are eating.

**THROW AWAY UNHEALTHY RECIPES**
When you are revising your eating habits, it can help to throw away recipes for unhealthy foods such as cakes, puddings and rich dishes that contain a lot of cream. This way you will not be tempted to cook them. Start to build a collection of new recipes that are low in fat and high in fibre, vitamins and minerals. Buy yourself a new cookery book containing healthy recipes.

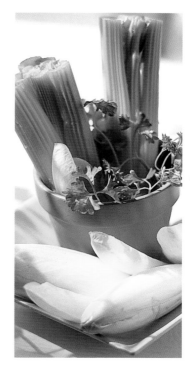

▷ **Keep a variety of easy-to-prepare raw fruit and vegetables as nibbles, and only buy cakes and biscuits for special occasions.**

▽ **Try to make time to sit down and enjoy meals, rather than grabbing a quick snack on the run.**

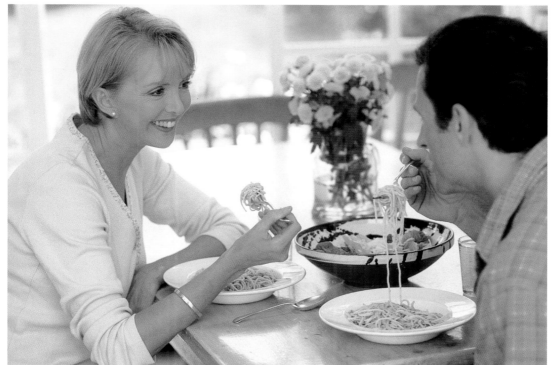

# How to eat a healthy diet

What we eat, and when, has a direct effect upon our body systems. By eating a balanced diet we can stay healthy, maintain energy levels, preserve healthy muscles and bones and help our brains to work efficiently, no matter how old we are. The guidelines for a balanced diet are straightforward and are based on eating the right amounts of foods from various different food groups.

## when to eat

Traditionally, people have eaten three meals a day: breakfast in the morning, lunch at midday and dinner in the evening. Although this is a useful template, people often develop the habit of eating a small breakfast and lunch, and a large evening meal. This has a detrimental effect on digestion, especially as our digestive systems become more

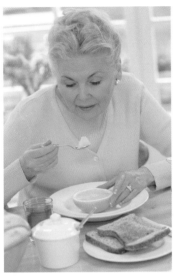

△ **Allow yourself time to enjoy a healthy breakfast each morning.**

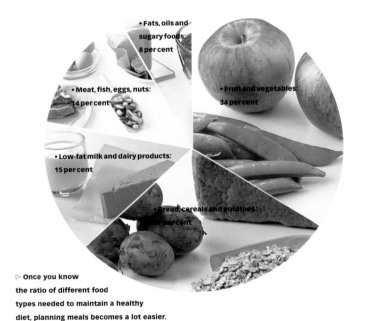

• **Fats, oils and sugary foods: 8 per cent**

• **Meat, fish, eggs, nuts: 14 per cent**

• **Fruit and vegetables: 34 per cent**

• **Low-fat milk and dairy products: 15 per cent**

• **Bread, cereals and potatoes: per cent**

▷ **Once you know the ratio of different food types needed to maintain a healthy diet, planning meals becomes a lot easier.**

## food groups

There is a broad consensus among doctors and nutritionists that foods fall into several discrete categories and that we should eat specific percentages of different types of foods. The breakdown of these food groups is shown in the pie chart above.

This breakdown exists as a rough guide and is not designed to be followed on a rigid daily basis. It does, however, show the emphasis that should be placed upon fruit, vegetables and complex carbohydrates.

sluggish with age. It also means that we have an inadequate supply of energy at the times of day when we are most active and a calorie overload at the end of the day when we are winding down.

A preferable eating pattern is a large breakfast, a substantial lunch and a comparatively small meal early in the evening. Alternatively, some people favour the grazing approach to eating in which they eat small quantities of food throughout the day. This prevents overloading the

digestive system and ensures a consistent supply of energy throughout the day. The grazing method is also a good way of stabilizing blood sugar levels in the body, which may be useful for people suffering from adult-onset diabetes.

## how healthy is meat?

Meat has had a lot of bad press in many countries in recent years for reasons such as infection with bovine spongiform encephalopathy (BSE) or the presence of antibiotics. Meat is high in saturated fat, which is implicated in the development of heart disease. It is also high in an amino acid called arachidonic acid, which increases levels of pro-inflammatory chemicals and should therefore be avoided by people of a rheumatic disposition. It does, however, still remain possible to eat meat safely. If you are concerned about the presence of antibiotics, choose organically produced meat, and cut away any visible fat on meat to avoid consuming too much saturated fat. Moderation is the key: the World Cancer Research Fund recommends that no more than 75g/3oz of meat should be eaten per day.

Eaten in moderation, meat is a useful source of antioxidant minerals such as zinc and selenium. Antioxidants can help prevent degenerative diseases, such as cancer. Beef is a good source of iron, zinc and B vitamins; choose lean cuts such as topside in which the fat content is only 2.7 per cent per 115g/4oz – minced beef can contain up to 25 per cent fat.

Pork supplies B vitamins, iron, zinc and selenium. Excess fat should be removed, and pork crackling should be avoided. Chicken supplies only about half the zinc and iron of red meats, but if the skin is removed prior to cooking it is very low in fat. It is also an excellent source of the antioxidant selenium.

Older people are advised to eat plenty of oily fish because they contain omega-3 fatty acids. These are essential fatty acids that are vital for health but cannot be made by the body. Omega-3 fatty acids can help to fight against heart disease, and are found in abundance in salmon, mackerel, sardines, pilchards, herrings, kippers and tuna.

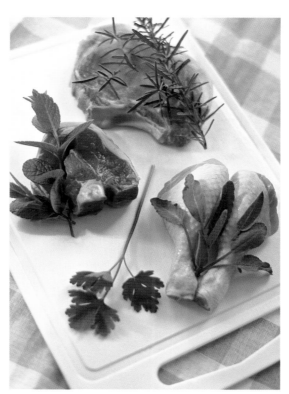

◁ Buying small, easy-to-prepare cuts of meat will help you to monitor the amount of saturated fat that you eat each day.

▽ Instead of using heavy, fattening sauces to liven up fish, try sprinkling it with herbs to help bring out the full flavour.

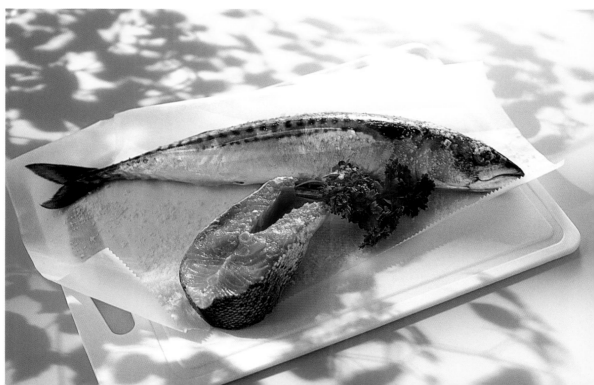

# Anti-aging foods

The general guidelines for the anti-aging diet are: keep your calorie consumption and saturated fat intake down; eat plenty of wholegrains, oily fish and fresh fruit and vegetables; and cut down on salt and sugar. In addition to these general guidelines, there are specific foods that have a role in anti-aging and that you should regularly include in your diet.

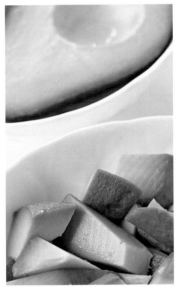

△ An avocado a is very versatile fruit that can be eaten either cooked or raw, and used in both savoury and sweet dishes.

## avocado

This fruit, which is usually eaten as a vegetable, is a good source of healthy monounsaturated fat that may help to reduce levels of a bad type of cholesterol in the body. Avocado is a good source of vitamin E and can help to maintain healthy skin and prevent skin aging (vitamin E may also help alleviate menopausal hot flushes). It is rich in potassium which helps prevent fluid retention and high blood pressure.

## berries

All black and blue berries such as blackberries, blueberries, blackcurrants and black grapes contain phytochemicals known as flavonoids – powerful antioxidants which help to protect the body against damage caused by free radicals and aging.

## cruciferous vegetables

The family of cruciferous vegetables includes cabbage, cauliflower, broccoli, kale, turnip, brussels sprouts, radish and watercress. Cruciferous vegetables assist the body in its fight against toxins and cancer. You should try to consume at least 115g/4oz (of any one or a combination) of these vegetables on a daily basis. If possible, eat them raw or very lightly cooked so that the important enzymes remain intact.

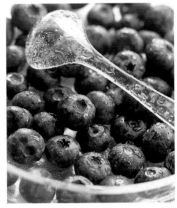

△ **Blueberries are rich in vitamin C and flavonoids which help to prevent cancer.**

▽ **Broccoli, cabbage and cauliflower contain high levels of cancer-fighting phytochemicals.**

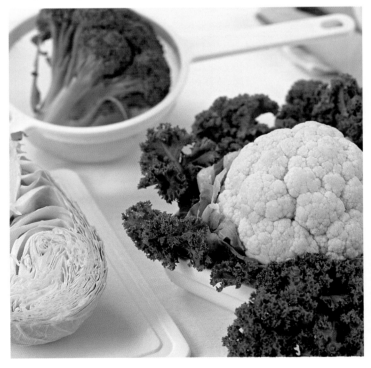

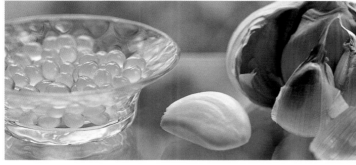

△ You can boost your garlic consumption by taking it as a supplement.

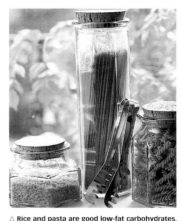

△ Rice and pasta are good low-fat carbohydrates.

## garlic

Eating a clove of garlic a day (raw or cooked) helps to protect the body against cancer and heart disease. The cardioprotective effects of garlic are well recorded. One 1994 study in Iowa, USA, of 41,837 women between the ages of 55 and 69 suggested that women who ate a clove of garlic at least once a week were 50 per cent less likely to develop colon cancer. Another study at Tasgore Medical College in India suggested that garlic reduced cholesterol levels and assisted blood thinning more effectively than aspirin, thus helping to reduce the risk of heart disease.

## ginger

This spicy root can boost the digestive and circulatory systems, which can be useful for older people. Ginger may also help to alleviate rheumatic aches and pains.

▽ A glass of hot water with a little ginger can alleviate nausea, especially car and sea sickness.

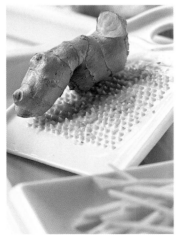

## nuts

Most varieties of nuts are good sources of minerals, particularly walnuts and brazil nuts. Walnuts, although high in calories, are rich in potassium, magnesium, iron, zinc, copper and selenium. Adding nuts to your diet (sprinkle them on salads and desserts) can enhance the functioning of your digestive and immune systems, improve your skin and help prevent cancer. Nuts may also help control cholesterol levels. Never eat rancid nuts, however, as they have been linked to a high incidence of free radicals.

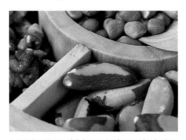

△ Brazil nuts are rich in magnesium and selenium.

## soya

Menopausal women might find that soya helps to maintain oestrogen levels. Soya may alleviate menopausal hot flushes and protect against Alzheimer's disease, osteoporosis and heart disease. Look out for fermented soya products, which are more easily digested, therefore more nutritional, and do not generally cause food intolerances. You may want to check that soya products have not been genetically modified. Soya should not be confused with soy sauce, which is full of salt and should be used sparingly, if at all.

▷ Chilled water melon is refreshing on hot days.

## wholemeal pasta and rice

Complex carbohydrates provide a consistent supply of energy throughout the day and should make up the bulk of your diet. Wholemeal pasta is an excellent complex carbohydrate. It is high in fibre and contains twice the amount of iron as normal pasta. Brown rice is another recommended complex carbohydrate, which is high in fibre and B vitamins.

## watermelon

Both the flesh and seeds of the watermelon are nutritious so try blending them together in a food processor and drinking as a juice. The flesh contains vitamins A, B and C; the seeds contain selenium, essential fats, zinc and vitamin E, all of which help against free radical damage and aging.

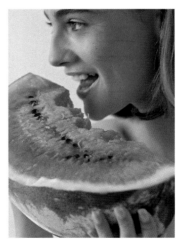

# Food intolerance

Many people find that they start to suffer from food intolerance as they grow older. This is partly due to long-term exposure to an irritating substance and partly due to the fact that the digestive system becomes less efficient with age. Eating foods to which you are intolerant is like continually stubbing your toe – the discomfort will become worse over a period of time and eventually the damage can become permanent.

## what is food intolerance?

A food intolerance should not be confused with an allergy. An intolerance occurs when the body finds a substance difficult to cope with, whereas an allergy to a substance is an active fight that involves the body's immune system.

Although there are many different types of food intolerance, some foods are more likely to cause intolerances than others. They include soya products, caffeine, chocolate, orange juice, tomatoes and food additives. Two foods that commonly cause intolerances are cow's milk and wheat (or other grains).

If you have an intolerance to cow's milk, this means that your body finds it difficult to digest lactose, the sugar found in milk. As a result, lactose moves through the

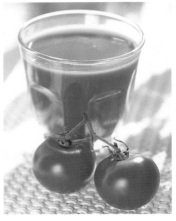

△ Tomatoes are a good source of disease-fighting antioxidants, but some people may find they develop an intolerance to them.

◁ By keeping a diary of foods ingested each day, it is often possible to detect small intolerances before they become too problematic.

intestines undigested and when it reaches the colon, bacteria start to ferment it, producing gas. The result may be abdominal discomfort, flatulence and diarrhoea.

An intolerance to wheat and grains means that you have difficulty digesting the protein gluten. Gluten intolerance can cause weight loss, loss of appetite, abdominal cramps and poor vitamin and mineral absorption from food.

## detecting food intolerances

You may already suspect that you have an intolerance to a particular food, simply because you suffer discomfort when you consume it. To confirm that this is the case, try eliminating the suspicious food for a month before re-introducing it to your diet. Keep a daily diary of your symptoms and note whether they return when you re-introduce the food. Alternatively, you can seek the professional advice of a doctor, dietician or naturopath.

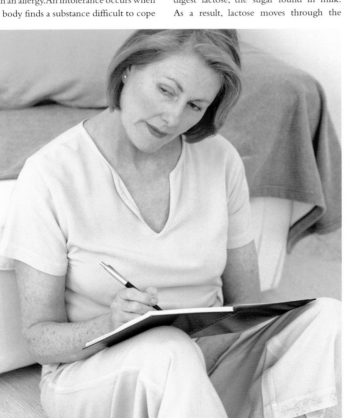

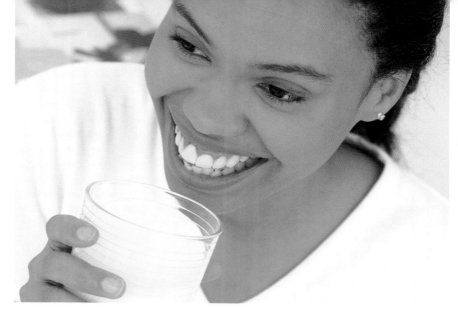

▷ Soya milk offers a good alternative to dairy products containing lactose. Although soya beans have a higher fat content than other pulses, the fat is mostly unsaturated and is considered to be non-harmful.

## dealing with food intolerances

There is no cure for food intolerance except simply avoiding the relevant foods. If you identify the foods that you cannot tolerate, you can look for alternatives that satisfy your nutritional needs and personal tastes. For example, if you cannot tolerate orange juice, drink

**SIGNS TO LOOK OUT FOR**

You may have a food intolerance if you suffer from any of the following symptoms on a regular basis:

• Anxiety
• Depression
• Fatigue
• Headaches
• Skin disorders
• Asthma
• Joint or muscle pain
• Rheumatoid arthritis
• Ulcers (mouth or stomach)
• Water retention
• Stomach bloating
• Nausea
• Vomiting
• Constipation
• Diarrhoea
• Irritable bowel syndrome

▽ For those suffering from lactose intolerance, live yogurt is easier to digest than milk, and is a good way to boost calcium levels.

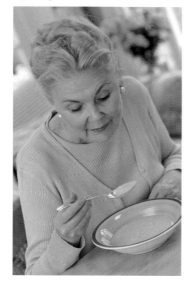

apple juice instead. It may not even be necessary to exclude foods completely. For example, if you have an intolerance to cow's milk you may still be able to tolerate a small amount of milk in one cup of tea a day.

If you are lactose intolerant try to avoid dairy products, and check food labels for the presence of lactose. Substitute soya milk for cow's milk. Women who need to exclude dairy products should ensure that they receive

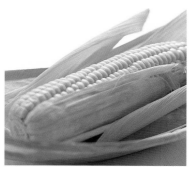

△ Corn is a good alternative to wheat for those with a gluten intolerance.

enough calcium from other sources to maintain healthy bones. Live yogurt is a good calcium source for people who are lactose intolerant (the bacteria present in the yogurt helps to break down lactose). Gluten intolerant people should avoid wheat, rye, and barley. Switching to corn, rice, soya, and potato starch can be helpful.

**WARNING**

If you are suffering from unusual digestive complaints such as nausea, diarrhoea or persistent indigestion, seek a diagnosis from your doctor before you make any dietary changes. A full elimination diet should be supervised by a medical professional.

# Dietary tips

Nutritionists and dietary therapists have now identified the eating habits that bring health and those that do not. The main guideline for a healthy diet as we grow older is to eat a diet rich in antioxidants – substances that actively fight the cell damage that leads to aging. Antioxidants are found in abundance in fruit and vegetables. There are a number of other guidelines that become especially important with age.

## good and bad fats

Some fats are necessary for health and others are harmful. Unsaturated fats are essential to our bodies for the transportation of vitamins A, D, E and K, lowering harmful cholesterol, and aiding the nervous system, cardiovascular system and brain. Good sources of unsaturated fat are olive oil, oily fish, nuts and seeds.

Saturated fats are linked to the build up of fatty deposits on artery walls leading to blocked arteries. There may also be an association between high saturated fat intake and certain cancers. Foods that contain saturated fat should be avoided or eaten in moderation. They include meat,

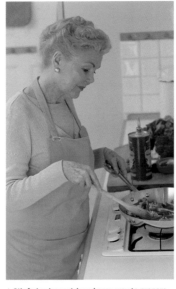

△ **Stir frying is a quick and easy way to prepare appetizing low-fat meals.**

dairy products and palm and coconut oils. Fried food and fat found in cakes, cookies and prepared meals should also be avoided.

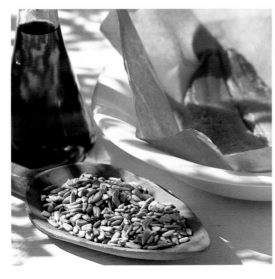

▷ **Sunflower seeds are a good source of vitamin B₃ (niacin) which can fight against depression, circulatory problems, high blood pressure and cholesterol, tinnitus, and breathing problems in asthmatics.**

**AVOIDING FATS**
- Check food labels for hidden fats.
- Choose low-fat cooking techniques, such as grilling or stir-frying.
- When cooking meat, place it on a rack so that excess fat drips off.
- Add yogurt rather than cream to your desserts.
- Buy canned fish in brine rather than in oil.

## understanding cholesterol

Not all cholesterol is unhealthy. There are two types of cholesterol: high density lipoprotein (HDL) which is popularly known as "good cholesterol", and low density lipoprotein (LDL), popularly known as "bad cholesterol".

Explained simply, HDL stops the build up of fatty deposits in the arteries and LDL creates them. If your HDL levels are high compared to your LDL levels, then you are at a low risk of cardiovascular disease. The ideal ratio is thought to be three parts HDL to one part LDL.

As you age it is important to maximize your cardiovascular health by keeping your LDL levels low and your HDL levels high. The best way to achieve this is to avoid fried foods and saturated and hydrogenated fats – the main sources of LDL. (Hydrogenation is a process that turns vegetable oil into hard fat.) Other ways to promote a healthy HDL/LDL balance include:
- eating plenty of garlic
- a diet rich in vitamin C
- eating foods rich in vitamin B₃
- including plenty of oily fish in your diet

## cut out sugar and salt

Although complex carbohydrates, such as whole grains and pulses, are good for us, simple carbohydrates such as refined sugar are not. All forms of sugar whether brown sugar, white sugar, honey or syrup cause our blood sugar levels to increase rapidly. If this instant supply of energy is not used, the body stores it and eventually it is converted into fat. Keep refined sugar intake to a minimum; it has no nutritional value and causes sudden highs in blood sugar levels, followed by slumps that can leave you feeling moody and irritable. If you have a sugar craving, eat a piece of fruit. Sugar, and the foods that it is found in (candy, cakes and many other processed foods), are said to contain "empty calories" because they offer short-lived energy without the benefit of nutrients such as vitamins and minerals.

Cut down on salt or eliminate it from your diet and never eat more than about a teaspoon a day. Too much salt causes fluid retention, places stress on the kidneys and heart, and lessens the amount of potassium absorbed by the body. High blood pressure becomes more likely as we get older, and a high-salt diet can contribute to its development. Check for the presence of salt or sodium chloride on food labels, and where possible avoid adding salt to food during cooking or at the dining table.

## fibre – nature's broom

Dietary fibre is essential for a healthy digestive system. It is sometimes referred to as "nature's broom" because it sweeps

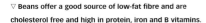

△ The membranes around orange segments contain a soluble fibre, pectin, which helps to lower levels of LDL cholesterol. Oranges also contain vitamin C and flavonoids, which maintain healthy skin and help in the fight against disease.

through the intestines transporting debris and residue out of the body. Fibre is not digested by the body so it retains its original mass and contributes to healthy, regular bowel movements. It may also decrease the amount of fat absorbed by the body and help to protect the arteries. Fibre absorbs water in the intestines so it is important to drink extra water if you include a lot of fibre in your diet. Try to eat plenty of natural sources of fibre such as lentils, dried beans, seeds, whole grains, fruit and vegetables.

## be sparing with protein

Protein is essential for life, but only a very small amount is needed each day. Too much can contribute to a variety of health problems, including osteoporosis. Most of us eat far more protein than we actually need and, contrary to popular belief, many plant foods are rich in protein. For example, a meal containing rice and lentils, but no meat or dairy products, is a source of good quality protein. Estimates for protein requirement vary, but range from 4.5 to 8 per cent of our total calorie intake. Try to eat less protein foods and replace animal proteins with plant proteins, such as tofu, spinach and pumpkin seeds. Plant proteins are advantageous in that they contain fibre but no saturated fat.

▽ Beans offer a good source of low-fat fibre and are cholesterol free and high in protein, iron and B vitamins.

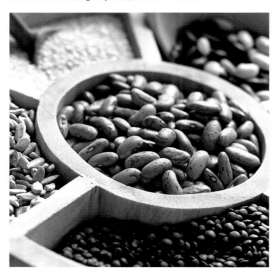

▽ Tofu is made from soya beans and is a valuable addition to vegan and dairy-free diets.

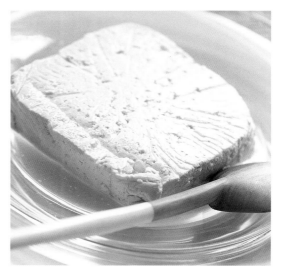

# Drinking fluids

Water is a vital nutrient and one that we cannot store in the body. We lose water all the time through sweat, urination, defecation and simply exhaling water vapour. It is essential to drink a minimum of 1.5 litres/2½ pints of water a day, preferably 2 litres/3½ pints. As we grow older our thirst mechanism becomes less reliable and we are more prone to dehydration.

## water – the healthiest drink

The best drink to keep the body hydrated is pure water. Fruit and vegetable juice and herbal teas are also good choices. Soft drinks that contain flavouring, preservatives and sugar can place stress on the body or add "empty calories" to your diet and should be drunk infrequently. If your diet is very high in fibre, you will need to drink extra water (fibre absorbs water in the intestines).

Carbonated water is an acceptable alternative to still water, but it should be drunk in moderation, as dietary therapists believe it raises the pH of the stomach and the reduced acidity makes it harder for the body to digest protein.

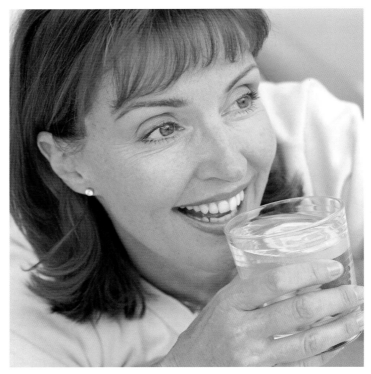
△ A glass of body-temperature water with a slice of lemon is a good drink to wake up the body each morning.

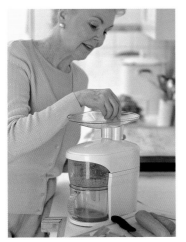
▽ Carrot juice is a tasty source of vitamin A, which fights against cancer and heart disease.

Apart from preventing dehydration, keeping up your fluid intake may help to prevent bladder cancer as you get older. This may be because a regular flow of fluid prevents prolonged exposure of the bladder tissue to potential carcinogens. Drinking water is also good for your appearance: if your skin is properly hydrated it will look younger and healthier.

## don't rely on thirst

As you grow older you should not rely on feeling thirsty to tell you when to drink. Instead, drink water throughout the day and monitor the colour of your urine. A pale golden colour means that you are probably getting enough to drink; dark amber means that you are not. Dehydration can be exacerbated by hot climates, exercise, alcohol, illness (especially vomiting and diarrhoea) and taking diuretic medications.

Most people do not drink enough fluid on a daily basis to keep the body fully hydrated, or they drink too many diuretic drinks, such as coffee, which increase the body's fluid loss. As a result, many of us suffer from symptoms of mild dehydration such as fatigue and headaches, and the body functions at a sub-optimum level. If you become seriously dehydrated, your skin becomes dry, your eyes appear sunken, your urine turns dark and you may suffer from constipation, dizziness, nausea, cramps, confusion, low blood pressure and itchiness.

vitamins and minerals from being used effectively by the body, raise blood pressure and cause an increase in the secretion of stress hormones. Different types of coffee contain different amounts of caffeine: instant coffee contains the least caffeine; ground, unfiltered coffee contains the most. A good alternative is steamed decaffeinated coffee, which unlike other decaffeination processes, does not involve the addition of toxic chemicals. For a healthier alternative try dandelion coffee or a cereal beverage made with barley or chicory.

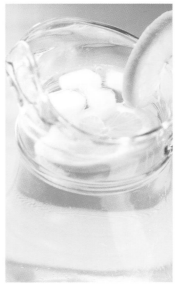

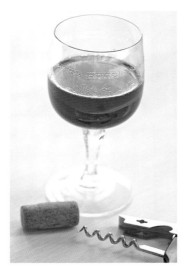

△ The flavonoids in red grape skins are thought to reduce arterial and immune system aging.

## alcohol

As you get older, alcohol can take its toll on the body. Drinking more than recommended guidelines places stress on the liver, hinders the absorption of nutrients, dehydrates the body, damages cells and causes the body to age prematurely. This is especially noticeable in the skin. Yet if alcohol is drunk in moderation, it can offer some benefits. Half to one unit per day for women and two units for men may help to reduce arterial aging and heart attacks. Scientists are not entirely certain how alcohol produces these beneficial effects, but some believe that it may prevent fat from oxidizing and forming deposits on artery walls.

Red wine may be beneficial if drunk in moderation. The flavonoids in red grape skins are thought to have antioxidant properties. Antioxidants help to prevent disease and the degeneration of body cells.

## caffeinated drinks

Some of our most popular drinks, such as tea, coffee and cola drinks, contain caffeine. Apart from its diuretic effect, opinions are mixed about whether caffeine constitutes a threat to health. It is therefore advisable to drink caffeinated drinks in moderation (no more than 2 or 3 cups a day). Overuse may cause sleep disturbances, prevent

**HOW TO STAY HYDRATED**

• Eat foods with a high water content such as fruit and soup.

• Drink a glass of water as soon as you get up in the morning.

• Drink a glass of water at least half-an-hour before each meal.

• Sip water at 10 to 15-minute intervals during exercise (many people underestimate how much they sweat; try weighing yourself before and after you sweat).

• Drink water at the first sign of a headache or muscle cramp.

• Choose low-caffeine or decaffeinated drinks that will not have a diuretic effect on the body.

• Buy a juicer and make your own fruit and vegetable juices. Alternatively, make fruit smoothies in a blender.

▷ **Readily available and easily prepared, mint tea is a good remedy for nausea, migraine, indigestion, flatulence and irritable bowel syndrome.**

△ Keeping the body hydrated helps to cleanse the body by ensuring the elimination of toxins.

## herbal teas

A great variety of herbal teas are available, and you can even make your own herbal infusions with medicinal benefits. Herbal teas have the benefit of hydrating the body while being caffeine free. To make a cup of camomile tea, place a handful of the fresh herb in a teapot, pour on boiling water, leave to infuse for 5 minutes, stir and pour through a strainer. Camomile can help to relieve anxiety and insomnia.

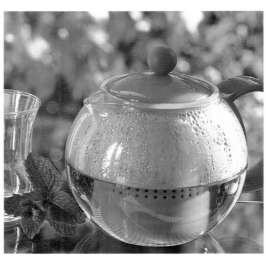

# Weight loss

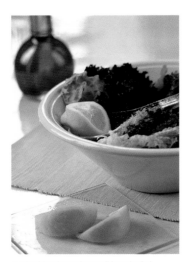

△ A healthy alternative to oil-based salad dressings is to squeeze fresh lemon juice onto the salad immediately before serving.

As you grow older, being overweight puts you at risk of a range of health problems including diabetes and hypertension. If you are overweight, changing your diet can significantly reduce your chances of illness (as well as raise your self-esteem). You do not have to go on a starvation diet to lose weight, but you do need to make long-term changes to your eating patterns by cutting out processed foods and full-fat products.

## consume fewer calories

The rate at which you burn energy or calories – your metabolic rate – slows down as you get older (a calorie is the amount of heat needed to raise the temperature of 1 litre/ $1^{3}/_{4}$ pints of water by one degree). You may find that continuing to eat the same amount that you did previously causes you to slowly gain weight. The way to lose weight is to consume fewer calories than you expend so that the body is forced to burn stored fat.

Daily calorie requirements vary according to your lifestyle, but, as a rough guide, women need approximately 2,000 calories

per day and men need 2,500. These figures increase if you have an active lifestyle. By eating 1,000 calories less than these energy requirements each day, you should be able to achieve a steady weight loss of about 1kg/$2^{1}/_{4}$ lbs a week, although the loss may be higher at first due to fluid losses. It is not advisable to lose more than 1kg/$2^{1}/_{4}$ lbs a week as you are likely to be losing fluid, and bone and muscle mass, all of which can accelerate the aging process.

Many foods are labelled with their calorie contents, so it is easy to become familiar with the energy values of different foods. You should, however, try not to count calories obsessively.

## types of food

The types of food that you should eat during a weight-loss diet are the same as those for a normal, well-balanced diet: concentrate on complex carbohydrates and fresh fruit and vegetables. Avoid fatty foods especially saturated fats (found in meat, dairy products

▽ Always strain herbal teas prior to drinking to allow the subtle fragrance and flavour through without any bitter aftertaste from the leaves.

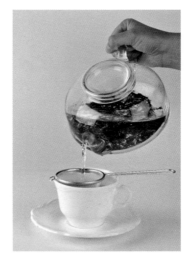

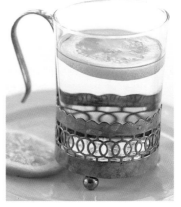

△ Rest a slice of lemon in a glass of boiling water for five minutes for a refreshing drink to enjoy at any time of day.

and coconut and palm oils). Remember that fats contain twice as many calories as carbohydrates and proteins:

1g carbohydrate = 4 calories
1g protein = 4 calories
1g fat = 9 calories

As well as eating low-fat foods, try to eat little and often. Start the day with a glass of warm (body temperature) water and a slice of lemon. Eat a breakfast of wholegrains – such as wholemeal toast or muesli – half an hour after getting up. Avoid butter and use skimmed instead of full-fat milk. Snack on raw vegetables until lunch time and then make lunch the main meal of the day. Drink fruit juices, smoothies made with low-fat yogurt and herbal teas in the afternoon. Try to eat a light dinner a minimum of 3 hours before going to bed. Eat raw fruit whenever you feel hungry. Keep meals under 350 calories and allow 250 calories for drinks and snacks such as apples and carrots.

## tips for losing weight

Before starting to diet, set yourself a target weight. If you are particularly overweight, you may want to decide this in conjunction

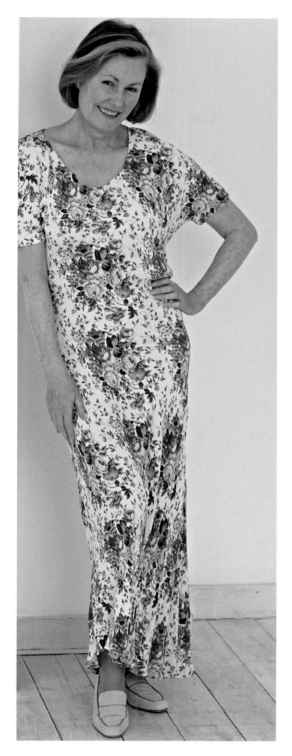

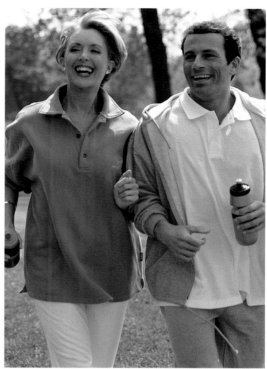

△ Many people find exercise easier to maintain if they undertake it as a routine social interaction, such as jogging with a partner each day, or exercising the dog.

◁ Fluid, longline clothing is more slimming than clothing that cuts the body in half or is more bulky.

with your doctor. If you are only slightly overweight, you may simply want to slim down until you can fit into a favourite item of clothing. If you have a lapse in your diet, do not see it as a reason to give up. Remember that you are only human.

Avoid alcohol: not only is it high in calories, but research in Holland has found that people who drank alcohol half an hour before a meal ate quicker and consumed more calories than those who remained alcohol free. Instead, drink a glass of water before a meal to help you feel full.

Avoid using dieting aids or diuretics to assist weight loss, since they will upset the body's natural balance, and can lead to problems such as vitamin deficiencies and digestive disorders.

Combine your weight-loss diet with regular aerobic exercise. This will help to speed up fat loss and develop firm muscles.

When you have reached your target weight, continue to eat sensibly. Try to keep meals to fewer than 500 calories so the body can break down each meal easily. This allows three meals of 500 calories as well as drinks and snacks of fruit.

# Dietary supplements

Although the diet can provide many essential nutrients as you grow older, there are some vitamins and minerals that you may need to take in supplement form. Some dietary therapists say that the modern Western diet and lifestyle exposes people to so many nutrient "depleters" that supplements are the best way to achieve optimum nutrition.

## your nutrient needs

Deficiency in fat, carbohydrate or protein is very rare in the West, but experts believe that many of us are lacking in vitamins and minerals. However, it is difficult to work out exactly which vitamins and minerals you receive in abundance and those that you may need to supplement. The best advice is to consult a naturopath or dietician who will carry out a detailed analysis of your personal nutritional needs. Both your hair and blood can be analyzed to provide information about the nutritional state of your body.

Even without professional assessment, you can make a reasonable estimate of your needs by looking at the foods you eat in your diet and examining your lifestyle and current health. For example, if your diet includes many substances, such as salt, sugar, caffeine and alcohol, that deplete the body of nutrients, then it may be advisable to take a

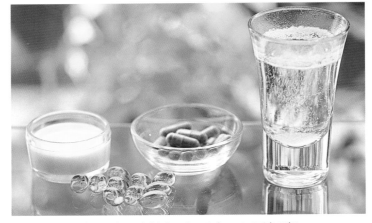

△ **Supplements come in many forms; chelated supplements, however, contain amino acids which make them more readily absorbed by the body for maximum benefit.**

multivitamin and mineral supplement. Diet can sometimes be misleading though; you may eat healthy foods but still have problems absorbing all the nutrients you need for health.

If you have a stressful lifestyle, smoke cigarettes, drink alcohol and are exposed to environmental pollution on a daily basis, then you are very unlikely to be getting all the vitamins and minerals that you need. If this is the case, taking daily supplements is probably advisable.

Your current health is often a good indication of whether you are suffering from sub-optimum nutrition or deficiency. Problems as diverse as mouth ulcers, muscle cramps, frequent colds, irritability and dry skin can often – but not always – be traced to a lack of essential vitamins and minerals.

### DAILY NUTRIENT INTAKE

Recommended daily allowances (RDAs) are standard amounts set by governments. They represent the daily amounts of a nutrient that we should consume in order to stay healthy. RDAs are criticized by some dietary therapists who say that they are far too low. It is argued that, although an RDA is high enough to prevent a deficiency disease such as scurvy (caused by insufficient vitamin C), it is not high enough to keep the body functioning at an optimum level for health and wellbeing. Critics say that RDAs should be increased to encourage people to eat healthier diets.

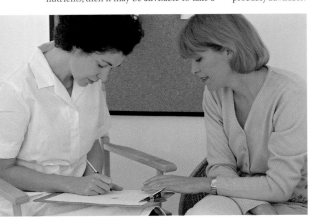

◁ **Many health problems can reduce the body's ability to absorb nutrients, and it may be worth visiting a nutritionist who can advise on your dietary requirements.**

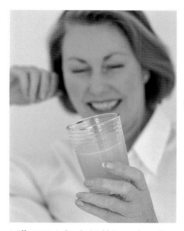

△ Effervescent vitamin C tablets are pleasant to take, but many of them contain artificial sweeteners and flavourings.

## what are supplements?

Supplements usually come in tablet form. They contain a stated amount of the essential nutrient plus other ingredients, such as fillers, bindings and coatings to give bulk, consistency and shape to the tablet. If you cannot tolerate cow's milk, check that supplements are lactose-free. Follow the instructions regarding dosage carefully.

Some supplements (usually vitamin C and B vitamins) work on a slow-release basis because they cannot be stored efficiently by the body. To avoid the product being excreted, slow release systems gradually release the nutrients, usually over a period of six hours, to allow maximum benefit.

Liquid supplements often contain sugars and sweeteners, but are easily assimilated into the body. Always take a liquid supplement in the dosage stated and do not drink it directly from the bottle or guess the amount taken.

## which supplements?

Some health problems become more common with age and they can be prevented or alleviated with supplements. Consult a nutritionist or dietary therapist if you are in any doubt which supplement to take in which dosage.

- **General prevention of aging and degenerative diseases:** Vitamin A, C, E, betacarotene, selenium, zinc or a general antioxidant supplement.

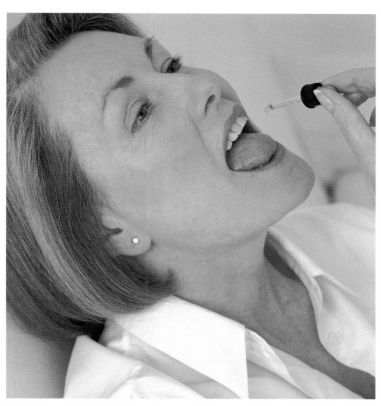

△ Tinctures should be dropped directly onto, or underneath, the tongue for easy absorption.

- **Menopausal symptoms:** Evening primrose oil, vitamin C with bioflavonoids, vitamin E, or a general multivitamin and mineral supplement.
- **Prostate problems:** Saw palmetto (for enlarged prostate), general antioxidant supplement, or a general multivitamin and mineral supplement.
- **Osteoporosis:** Bone mineral complex, vitamin C, or a general multivitamin and mineral supplement.
- **High blood pressure:** Vitamin C, general antioxidant, or a general multivitamin and mineral supplement.
- **Diabetes:** Vitamin C, B complex, zinc, chromium, or a general multivitamin and mineral supplement.
- **Arthritis:** Vitamin C, vitamin B5, gamma-linolenic acid (GLA), eicosapentaenoic acid (EPA), bone mineral complex, general antioxidant supplement, or a general multivitamin and mineral supplement.

▽ Gelatine capsules are unsuitable for vegetarians and vegans, who should look for seaweed alternatives.

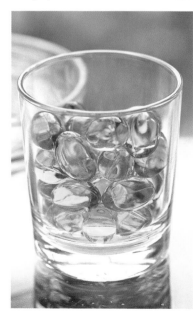

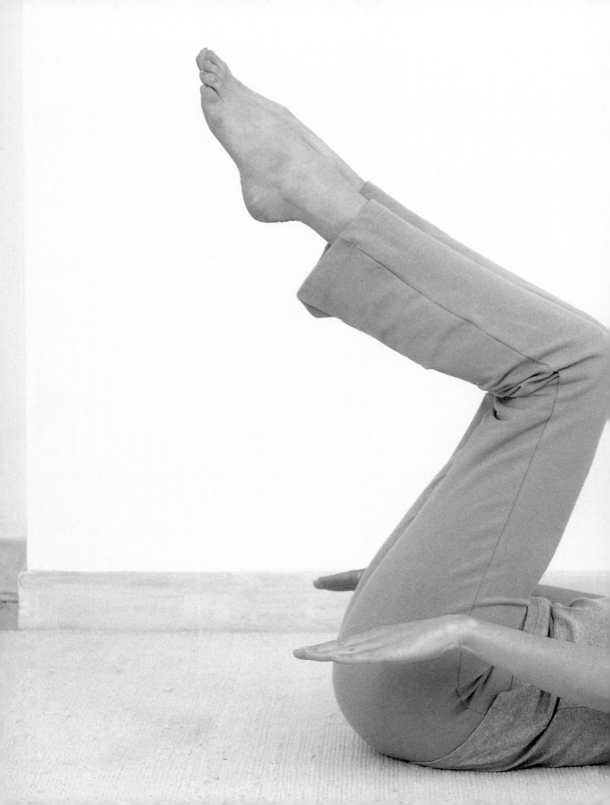

# Staying Fit Throughout Life

In conjunction with a healthy diet, exercise is the best way to stay well, slow down the aging process and keep your body fit, toned, agile and attractive. You can reap huge benefits from relatively small increases in your activity levels. For example, walking instead of driving, swimming once or twice a week and doing some weight-lifting exercises in front of the television will quickly increase your overall fitness levels. You are never too old to start exercising.

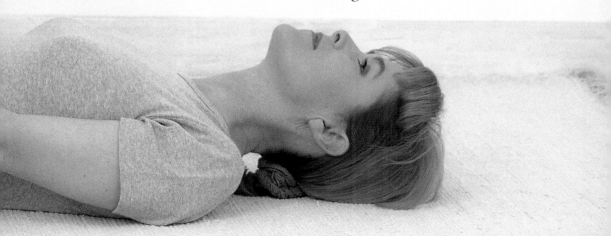

# Taking up exercise

Exercise is a vital part of preventative health care as you get older. By taking regular exercise you can prevent weight gain and keep all your organs and body systems healthy. You will also help to prevent cardiovascular disease, osteoporosis, arthritis and many other health problems.

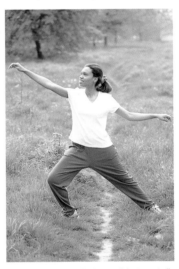

△ T'ai chi is a non-combative martial art reputedly practised by Taoist monks in 13th-century China. It uses fluid, graceful sequences along with controlled breathing to exercise the body, calm the mind and promote self healing.

## the effects of exercise

The heart is a muscle and needs to be exercised just like any other muscle in order to stay strong and healthy. Working the heart during exercise also maintains the health of the arteries and ensures that blood circulates to all the body's organs, keeping them supplied with oxygen and nutrients.

Exercise has a beneficial effect on every part of the body. It keeps the skin and hair in good condition, it makes you more energetic, it speeds up the passage of food through the digestive system, it speeds up metabolism (the rate at which the body

**STAYING MOTIVATED**

Enthusiasm and motivation may be high at the beginning of a new exercise campaign but typically wane as the weeks go by.

• Try to make exercising part of your normal everyday routine, like combing your hair or eating dinner.

• Make exercise sociable and enjoyable: exercise with a friend or in a group.

• Choose an exercise that's right for you. If you find the gym boring, try other forms of exercise: join an exercise class, play tennis or squash or go swimming.

• A sense of achievement can act as a motivating force. Whenever you reach a target, however small, set yourself a new one.

• Fit exercise into your day. If you are very busy, find opportunities for exercise in your existing schedule. For example, cycle to work, take the stairs instead of the elevator or use a manual lawnmower to mow the grass.

• Keep reminding yourself of the health benefits of exercise and the dangers of a sedentary life. Exercise is an investment in your current and future health.

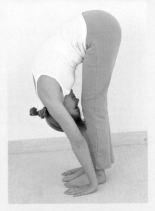

△ Touching your toes is a good way to improve flexibility in the hips and spine.

burns calories), it strengthens bones and muscles, it stabilizes blood sugar, it prevents weight gain and, if you are carrying surplus fat, it helps you to shed it. In other words, exercise prevents many of the physical changes that come with age. Exercise also has a positive effect on the mind and

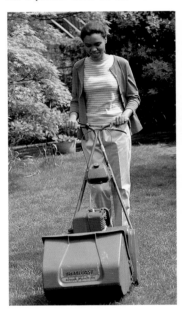

△ Gardening is a great way to keep your body in good shape while enjoying the outdoors.

emotions. It is an excellent way of alleviating stress, beating depression and raising your self-esteem.

## how fit are you?

Your resting heart rate provides a rough guide to your overall level of fitness. Generally, the lower your heart rate, the fitter you are. If you know that you are very unfit, you have not exercised for many years, you are overweight or you have health problems, you should consult your doctor before taking up exercise. To measure your heart rate, press your first two fingers

## FITNESS LEVELS INDICATED BY HEART BEATS PER MINUTE

### MEN

**Age 20–29**
Very fit: less than 60
Fit: 60–69
Moderate: 70–85
Unfit: over 85

**Age 30–39**
Very fit: less than 64
Fit: 64–71
Moderate: 72–85
Unfit: over 85

**Age 40–49**
Very fit: less than 65
Fit: 65–73
Moderate: 74–90
Unfit: over 90

**Age 50 +**
Very fit: less than 68
Fit: 68–75
Moderate: 76–90
Unfit: over 90

### WOMEN

**Age 20–29**
Very fit: less than 72
Fit: 72–77
Moderate: 78–95
Unfit: over 95

**Age 30–39**
Very fit: less than 72
Fit: 72–79
Moderate: 80–97
Unfit: over 97

**Age 40–49**
Very fit: less than 75
Fit: 75–79
Moderate: 80–98
Unfit: over 98

**Age 50+**
Very fit: less than 75
Fit: 75–85
Moderate: 85–102
Unfit: over 102

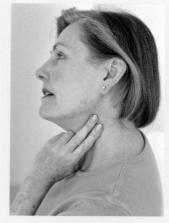

△ To calculate your pulse rate place the tips of your first two fingers on the pulse point at the side of your neck or on your inner wrist.

lightly on the pulse point in your neck and count the number of beats over a 15 second period, then multiply that number by 4 to calculate the number of beats per minute.

## how hard should I exercise?

While you are exercising, your optimum heart rate should always be between 60 and 80 per cent of the maximum heart rate (MHR) for your age. In order to calculate your MHR, you simply subtract your age from 220.

### 220–age = MHR

Next you should calculate 60 per cent of your MHR. This is the minimum elevation of your heart rate that you should aim for during exercise. Then calculate 80 per cent of your MHR. This is the maximum elevation of your heart rate that you should aim for during exercise. A heart rate that is between 60 per cent and 80 per cent of your MHR is said to be in your "training zone". If you are 50 years old, your MHR is 170, your minimum training heart rate is 102 and your maximum training heart rate is 136. If you stick to these guidelines, you will be able to burn body fat and exercise your cardiovascular system safely.

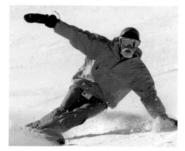

When you have finished exercising, you should check that your heart returns to its normal rate within 10 minutes. If it takes

◁ Once you become more agile through exercise you could try out an adventurous new sport.

longer than 10 minutes, it is advisable that you exercise at a slower pace until you become fitter. Another quick test to ascertain whether you are exerting yourself too hard is known as the "talking test". Make sure that you can always hold a conversation while you are exercising. If you find that you are too out of breath or fatigued to talk, then you are probably exercising too hard.

▽ Yoga tones muscles and stretches the spine.

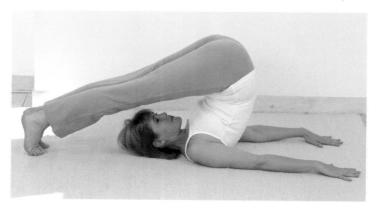

# The benefits of exercise

There are three broad categories of exercise: aerobic exercise, anaerobic exercise and flexibility exercise. These are also known as the three "Ss": stamina, strength and suppleness. As you grow older, your heart needs a regular aerobic workout to function efficiently, your muscles need strength training to prevent them from losing mass, and your joints need flexibility exercise to maintain a full range of movement.

## aerobic exercise

Aerobic exercises are those which bring your heart rate into the "training zone" (60 to 80 per cent of your maximum heart rate) and increase the body's circulation and respiratory rate. Aerobic exercise is sustained by oxygen and it is sometimes called fat-burning exercise, cardiovascular exercise or cardiowork. Aerobic exercise can be kept up for long periods of time; in fact the longer you exercise for, the greater the health benefits.

▽ For those without joint problems, cycling provides an enjoyable form of aerobic exercise as well as a pollutant-free form of transport.

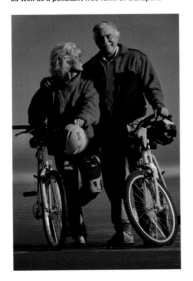

## benefits of aerobic exercise

Aerobic exercise gives the heart a good workout, burns up fat, boosts the immune system and helps to prevent the build-up of fatty deposits in the arteries. It enhances joint and muscle flexibility, stamina, sleep and digestion, and it normalizes hormone levels, helping to alleviate premenstrual syndrome and menopausal symptoms. Aerobic exercise that is also weight-bearing can help to prevent osteoporosis by strengthening and slowing down the loss of calcium in the bones.

## types of aerobic exercise

Walking, jogging, cycling, swimming and dancing are effective, cheap and fun ways of taking aerobic exercise. Most gyms hold a range of classes that teach aerobic routines. Some classes use steps and weights, some are high impact and others are low impact – choose a class that matches your fitness level.

Swimming is not a weight-bearing exercise and should be combined with another form of exercise, such as walking, in order to preserve healthy bones.

## getting started

Aerobic exercise can put stress on the heart if you are not accustomed to it and this is especially true for older people or those who are overweight. For this reason, it is essential to start slowly and build up gradually. As the fitness level of the body increases, the heart will slowly gain strength, until it reaches a point at which it does not need to work so hard to supply the body with sufficient oxygen to maintain exercise. At this point you will have made a positive change to your fitness levels and should start feeling the benefits of exercise.

Walking is a good way to get started on a programme of aerobic exercise: try walking to work or to the shops and walking upstairs whenever possible. As you become fitter, increase the challenge by walking faster and

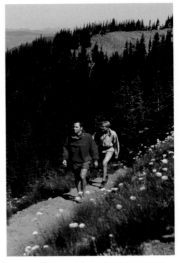

△ Walking helps to stabilize blood sugar levels, thus regulating mood swings and energy levels, as well as fighting osteoporosis, weight gain, and heart disease.

for longer periods, or try hill-walking. You can also join a low-impact aerobic class and work at your own pace. Cardiovascular equipment in gyms – such as treadmills and training bikes – is useful because it provides immediate feedback on your heart rate, allowing you to slow down if you are working too hard. Once you have reached a reasonable level of fitness, try to do at least 35 minutes of aerobic exercise (excluding warming up and cooling down) three or four times a week.

## anaerobic exercise

The term "anaerobic" means "without oxygen". During anaerobic exercise, muscles work at high intensity for a short period of time. Whereas oxygen enables long periods of exercise, anaerobic exercise is necessarily short in duration.

Anaerobic exercise results in the build up of a by-product known as lactic acid in the muscles. This causes discomfort and fatigue,

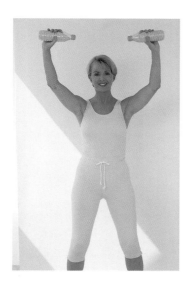

△ Regular use of arm lifts using hand weights will quickly show favourable results.

which is another reason why anaerobic exercise cannot be sustained over long periods of time. Lactic acid must leave the muscles before you can attempt further anaerobic exercise.

## benefits of taking anaerobic exercise

Anaerobic exercise has far-reaching benefits for your body and health. It will keep your muscles strong and prepare your body for quick bursts of activity, such as running to catch a train or fleeing from danger. Strong, toned muscles have a variety of health benefits. They improve your

posture, they give the body a lean and taut appearance, they make you physically stronger and more powerful, and the more muscle tissue you build up, the more calories you will burn off, even during periods of complete inactivity.

You lose muscle tissue as you age (up to a third by the age of 65). In fact, a significant cause of low energy levels, fatigue and immobility in middle and later life is the decline in the amount of skeletal muscle. You can reverse this by taking anaerobic exercise several times a week.

## types of anaerobic exercise

Examples of anaerobic exercise include weight lifting, sprinting, or any rapid burst of hard exercise. For example, squash is an anaerobic form of exercise because it involves short and intensive movements.

## getting started

There are several ways to get started on a regular programme of anaerobic exercise. Some people join a gym and use the weights and resistance machines; others take up swimming, squash or yoga. However, the easiest (and cheapest) way to get started is to lift some weights at home.

Remember, your first aim is to tone muscles, not increase their bulk. Start by lifting a small weight a few times and increase the weight and amount of repetitions when the exercises become easier.

You can also strengthen the muscles without using weights. The simplest muscle exercises involve repeatedly clenching and

relaxing muscles. This works best on muscles such as the buttocks that are easy to isolate. It is also the principle underlying Kegel exercises which strengthen the pubococcygeal muscles and help to support the pelvic organs. To practise Kegel exercises, simply contract the pelvic floor muscles, hold for 5 seconds and release. Repeat three times.

### FLEXIBILITY EXERCISE

Practising flexibility exercises on a regular basis helps to preserve the full range of motion in the joints, improves posture and helps to alleviate problems such as arthritis. Flexibility exercises are essentially stretching exercises, such as those performed in yoga and Pilates.

### GUIDELINES FOR EXERCISING

• Stop exercising at any time if you feel dizzy, faint, nauseous or in pain.

• Always warm up and cool down before and after exercise to allow a slow build up to your training zone heart rate and to avoid injury to muscles, tendons and ligaments.

• If you lift weights, do not train the same muscle groups on consecutive days. Allow at least one or two days of rest between training sessions.

• Always pay careful attention to your posture when lifting weights.

• Try to take moderate exercise three or four times a week rather than intensive exercise intermittently.

• If possible, get a personally tailored exercise programme from a doctor, fitness instructor or personal trainer.

• Always wear comfortable, well-fitting sneakers that cushion the feet and offer good ankle support.

• When swimming, avoid the breast stroke if you suffer from back problems.

• Take care when exercising outside. Try to avoid exercising in adverse weather conditions and do not exercise in deserted places. Wear sufficient layers (you can shed them if you need to) and make sure that you are visible to traffic.

• If you lack motivation, try exercising with a friend to encourage you along.

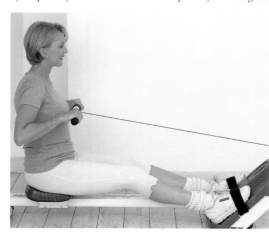

▷ A rowing machine can help to strengthen the spine and muscular system, but for those with back problems should only be used under supervision.

# yoga and Pilates

## the benefits of yoga

Yoga is a holistic system. It is based upon the believe that the physical, emotional, mental and spiritual levels of your being interact within the "energetic apsect" that is the invisible double of your physical body. This aspect has its own interconnecting pathways. The main channel passes, like a motorway, through the energetic aspect of the physical spine. Anything that influences the flow of energy through your body affects you at ever level.

Yoga is one of the best ways to keep the joints and muscles flexible as you grow older. It can also relieve problems such as stress, anxiety, depression, back pain, asthma, hormonal imbalances, insomnia and irritable bowel syndrome. Although it has been practised in India for thousands of years, yoga did not appear in the West until the 19th century, and only became popular during the 1960s.

## learning yoga

In the East, yoga is perceived as a route to spiritual enlightenment. In the West, however, the emphasis tends to be on yoga as a physical discipline. Western yoga classes usually focus on physical postures, known as asanas, and breathing techniques, known as pranayama.

The best way to learn yoga is from a trained teacher or therapist who will show you how to co-ordinate your breathing with your movement and help you to align your body correctly within the postures. There are also plenty of books available to help you practise yoga at home. When practising alone, make sure that you do not push your body further than is comfortable and remember to start slowly and build your flexibility gradually; the people you see in yoga books have practised for years to become flexible.

Yoga teachers recommend practising for 30 to 60 minutes a day to gain full benefit, but many people find this difficult, and 20 minutes on a regular basis is sufficient to enhance energy and stamina levels, muscle tone, digestion, flexibility, strength and general wellbeing.

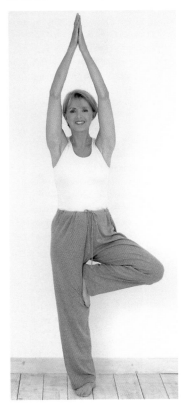

◁ **This basic yoga pose, the tree, is good for strengthening the pelvis, hip joints and shoulders.**

**TYPES OF YOGA**

There are many different types of yoga. The type most widely practised in the West is "Hatha" ("ha" meaning "sun" and "tha" meaning "moon") representing the balancing and harmonization of positive and negative forces, usually through breathing and postures. Hatha yoga is just one branch of yoga and within Hatha yoga there are various "sub-categories":

• Astanga Vinyasa: a fast series of challenging postures performed using synchronized breathing. This is probably the most aerobic form of yoga.

• Iyengar: alignment and precision of movement are used to enhance posture, breathing and flexibility.

• Kundalini: breathing techniques and prana ("life force") are worked on to balance the body's energy and achieve relaxation.

• Sivananda: breathing and meditation are practised to produce a feeling of calm and inner peace.

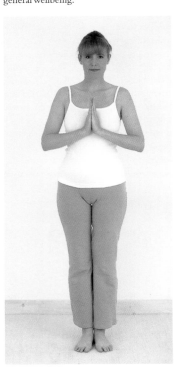

△ **The Namaste pose allows you to breathe more deeply in your upper and middle back and to build up inner strength in your open heart area.**

## the benefits of Pilates

The Pilates method was devised by Joseph Pilates during the 1920s and has evolved over the years to offer both mental and physical training. It aims to increase body awareness, gently realign the body, enable efficient movement and enhance control of both body and mind.

Pilates has something to offer everyone, of whatever age or current fitness level. Although overall strength is increased, one of the main benefits of Pilates is an increase in core strength. This is a phrase that is used over and over again in connection with Pilates, and it refers to the important abdominal and back muscles at your centre that support your whole body whether moving or at rest. As these muscles are strengthened, your posture will improve and you will find it easier to do daily tasks.

If you are completely new to Pilates, you will find the exercises different from others you might have tried, although there are some overlaps with yoga. First of all, Pilates is a series of movements that flow into one another without pauses. Most conventional exercise starts and stops: you might do 12 repetitions of a move, rest, and then start up again with the next sequence. Pilates concentrates on the body as a whole, stretching some muscles, strengthening others and, by helping you to function more

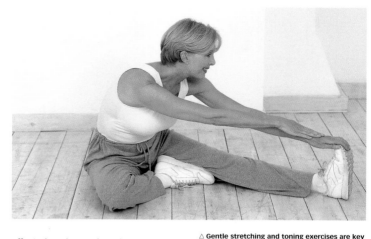

△ **Gentle stretching and toning exercises are key to the Pilates tradition. Never push yourself too far, stop if you feel in any pain whatsoever.**

effectively, reducing the risk of injury, not only while you are exercising but in everything you do.

## the importance of focus

Another distinguishing feature of Pilates is that to practise it you must be totally focused and concentrated, and this concentration creates a mind-body connection. This doesn't mean that conventional exercise can be done without thought of course, but it does mean that Pilates needs all your attention and focus in order to get the best results. If you sometimes feel overwhelmed by everday problems and stresses, giving all your attention to the movements of a Pilates sequence can help to still the insistent chatter of your daily life, acting like a meditation to calm your mind and help you see things more clearly. This total concentration and

attention to alignment and detail makes Pilates quite unique and very satisfying.

The best way to learn the Pilates method is in a class taught by an experienced teacher. As with yoga, breathing is an important part of the Pilates method. Try to breathe deeply into the lower ribcage during each exercise. Pilates is a very personal experience. Listen to your body and stop if anything feels uncomfortable or causes pain. As with any new exercise routine, seek the advise of a doctor before taking it up.

▽ **Start and end your Pilates sessions with a couple of minutes in the relaxation position. It will help you focus on your body, as well as making you feel relaxed and refreshed.**

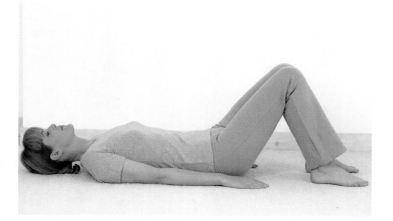

### CONTROLLED BREATHING

Learning to breathe correctly is an essential part of Pilates training. By breathing deeply into the lower ribcage and back out, you can ensure maximum use of your lung capacity. Try to breathe slowly, softly and rythmically to avoid any feeling of dizziness from overbreathing. The increase in oxygen supply provided by correct breathing will help the body replenish itself, while the exercise involved will help increase upper body flexibility. Never hold your breath during Pilates exercises as this will increase blood pressure, and waste energy in parts of the body where it is not needed.

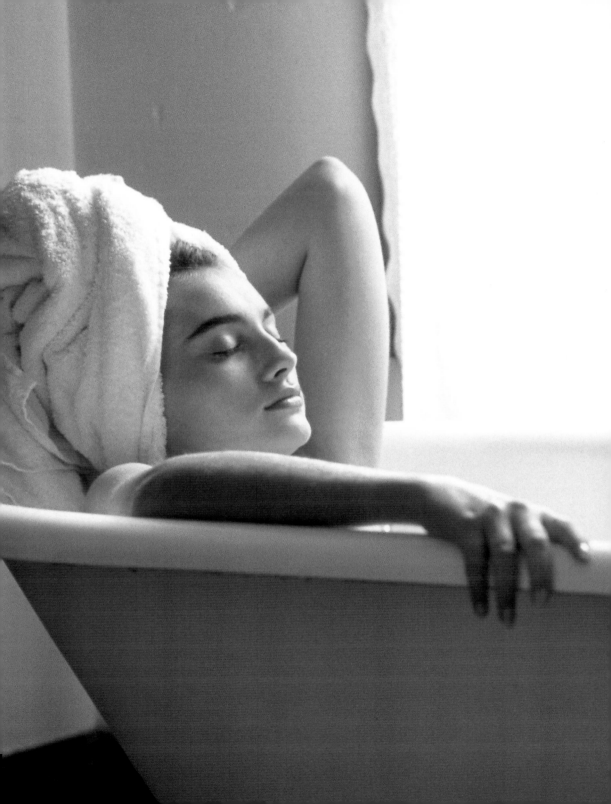

# Looking After the Body

Many of the signs of aging are invisible because they occur inside the body and do not cause external changes. Fortunately, if we look after ourselves as we enter our 40s, 50s and 60s, by eating a healthy diet and getting plenty of exercise many age-related changes can be prevented.

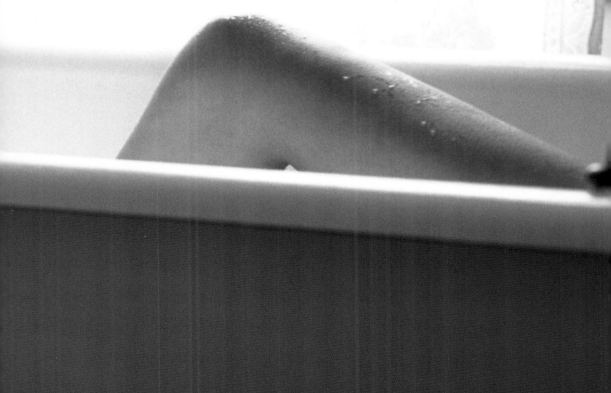

# The skeletal system

If you have healthy bones, the chances are that you will have an active and energetic later life. As you age, your mobility and range of movement depends largely on the health of your skeletal system. It is never too late to start looking after the health of your bones and by doing so you can help to prevent a range of problems including osteoporosis, arthritis and back pain.

## osteoporosis

From your 30s onwards your bones gradually start to become thinner, less dense and more porous. This loss of bone density accelerates in women after the menopause and some go on to develop osteoporosis – a disease in which the bones are so weak that they fracture even on minor impact. Men can suffer from osteoporosis too, but it tends not to appear until much later in life.

People who have osteoporosis may have a hunched appearance resulting from compression of the vertebrae in the upper spine. They may also suffer from fractures of the wrist, hip or vertebrae. Risk factors for osteoporosis include family history, poor diet, lack of weight-bearing exercise, lack of sunlight, early menopause, smoking, high alcohol, coffee or salt intake, digestive problems, eating disorders, overuse of laxatives or commercial bran products and being underweight.

Incidences of osteoporosis are increasing dramatically in Europe and the USA. In the UK approximately 200,000 bone fractures occur as a direct result of osteoporosis each year, and of these cases 80,000 people die as a result, usually due to lung or blood complications caused by immobilization.

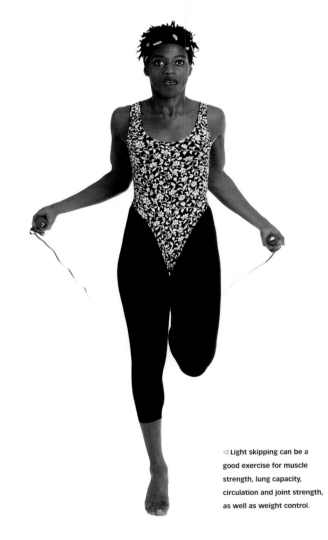

◁ Light skipping can be a good exercise for muscle strength, lung capacity, circulation and joint strength, as well as weight control.

## preventing osteoporosis

The key to prevention is diet. The most important mineral for healthy bones is calcium and it is important not only to include enough calcium in the diet but also to make sure that calcium absorption and uptake into the bones is maximized.

Good sources of calcium in the diet are dairy products, almonds, brewer's yeast, parsley, globe artichokes, prunes, pumpkin seeds, cooked dried beans and cabbage. Try not to rely on high-fat dairy products such as milk and cheese to supply all your calcium needs. However, if you do drink milk, remember that calcium is absorbed more efficiently in the presence of fat, so semi-skimmed milk is preferable to skimmed milk.

Factors that hinder calcium absorption include excess protein in the diet (over $40g/1^1/_2$ oz per day causes calcium to be excreted in the urine), excess caffeine

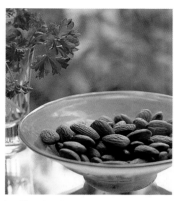

△ Adding almonds to your diet is a tasty way to boost your intake of copper, magnesium, potassium, calcium, iron and zinc.

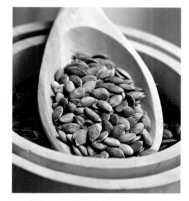

△ Sprinkle pumpkin seeds into dishes during cooking or on salads and cereals for added flavour and valuable nutrients such as zinc and iron.

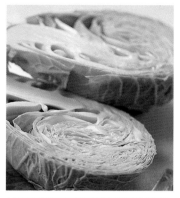

△ Most of the vitamins and minerals in cabbage are contained in the dark outer leaves; but the inner leaves are still an excellent source of fibre.

consumption and foods such as wheatbran, chocolate and rhubarb. Avoid these foods where possible.

Both cigarette smoking and drinking excessive amounts of alcohol can dramatically increase your risk of suffering from osteoporosis. As you grow older it is essential to quit smoking and restrict drinking to within government guidelines.

Since calcium is absorbed by the gut, it makes sense to look after your digestive system. Any form of bloating, flatulence or indigestion is a sign that the digestive system is not breaking down foods efficiently. If this is the case, consult a dietary therapist who may suggest taking digestive enzymes or going on an elimination diet to establish the cause of the problem.

If you know that you have a number of risk factors for osteoporosis, and you are a postmenopausal woman, ask your doctor about the possibility of having a bone density test and taking hormone replacement therapy (HRT). A course of HRT lasting a minimum of one year has been shown to improve bone density. You can also ask whether it is appropriate to take dietary supplements. There are some multivitamin and mineral combinations that are specially formulated for postmenopausal women and a magnesium/calcium compound (in a 2:1 ratio) may also be of benefit. Other useful supplements may include 15mg doses of zinc citrate and 50mg doses of vitamin B complex.

Weight-bearing exercise, such as walking, has a key role to play in the prevention of osteoporosis. Try to go for a brisk 30-minute walk at least every other day.

### THE VINEGAR DIET

Research at a Japanese University suggests that calcium absorption is facilitated in rats by giving them a diet rich in vinegar. Other research indicates that the amount of available calcium in chicken stock increases by 40 per cent when vinegar is added to the boiling liquid. It is thought that the acetic acid in vinegar breaks down the minerals in the bones in the stock. Dr Anthony Leeds of King's College, London suggests using vinegar as a condiment at meal times since it may enhance calcium uptake.

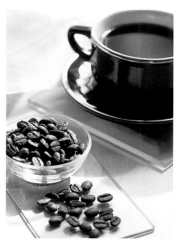

◁ Large quantities of coffee are known to leach vitamins and minerals from the digestive system, increasing the risk of dietary malfunctions, and contributing to conditions such as osteoporosis.

▷ Nowadays vinegars come in a variety of flavours, making them an appetizing addition to many dishes.

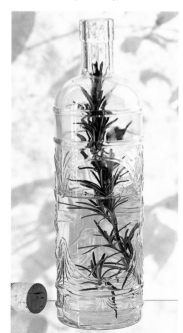

# Maintaining skeletal health

## rheumatoid arthritis

Although doctors do not know the precise cause of rheumatoid arthritis it is thought to be an auto-immune disease in which the immune system starts to attack its own tissues. The most commonly affected areas are the hands and feet, followed by the knees, wrists, neck and ankles, although the disease can affect any joint in the body. Initial symptoms may include fatigue and fever followed by stiffness and swelling in the joints. Joint pain can become so bad that it restricts movement and in severe cases, bones may fuse together, making movement in the joint impossible.

Rheumatoid arthritis affects more women than men (in a 3:1 ratio) and usually appears between the ages of 40 and 50, although it can also appear in younger people, and is often accompanied by mild aneamia.

## treating the symptoms of rheumatoid arthritis

You should always receive conventional medical diagnosis and treatment for rheumatoid arthritis. Doctors may recommend immuno-suppressant drugs or, in severe cases, joint replacement.

Complementary therapies can be useful for symptom relief. Dietary therapists may recommend limiting animal fats in the diet and taking supplements such as multivitamins, vitamin B complex, vitamin C, vitamin E (except when anti-coagulant drugs are being taken), glucosamine sulphate and zinc. An elimination diet may also be recommended if it is suspected that the disease is related to a food intolerance. Joint mobility can be helped by swimming, and pain can be eased by applying gentle heat to the area.

## osteoarthritis

As the joints age they become prone to osteoarthritis. The cartilage in the joint wears away and the ends of the bones may rub together and develop growths which are known as spurs. The symptoms include joint pain that is exacerbated by movement, stiffness in the morning and bony growths on the fingers.

Osteoarthritis usually affects joints that have been subjected to excessive wear and tear. It is common in weight-bearing joints that have been overused in the past. Too much kneeling, for example, may cause osteoarthritis in the knees. There is no

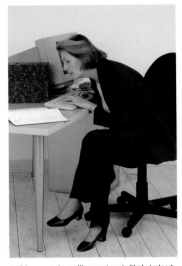

△ This woman's apalling posture is likely to lead to all sorts of health problems. When sitting you should always place both feet flat on the floor and ensure your back is straight in a chair which offers support to the small of the back.

definitive cure for osteoarthritis; treatment consists mainly of pain relief and, occasionally, joint replacement surgery. Being overweight places unnecessary stress on the joints, so an important part of preventative care is maintaining a healthy weight or losing weight if necessary. Try to keep joints as strong and as flexible as possible by taking regular exercise. A healthy diet that is low in saturated fats, and high in fish oils may also be helpful.

## supportive action for osteoarthritis

It is thought that damaging substances known as free radicals may play a major part in arthritis. Taking an antioxidant supplement can help combat free radical damage to the joints. Dietary therapists also recommend taking a daily supplement of gamma-linolenic acid (GLA). If you suffer from osteoarthritis, you should avoid tasks,

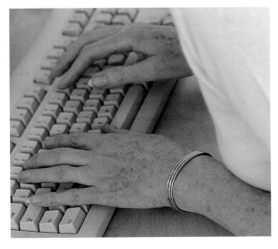

◁ Since copper can be absorbed by the skin, many people find wearing a copper bracelet to be of use in the fight against bone disease.

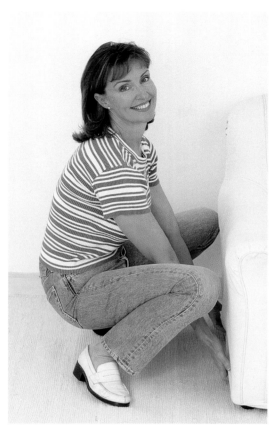

◁ Back problems are most commonly caused by lifting heavy objects incorrectly. Always bend at the knees and hips, taking the weight on your legs rather than your spine. Keep your back straight as you lift.

## preventing back complaints

The mainstay of preventative care is regular exercise that strengthens the back muscles. Both swimming and yoga are excellent. You should also pay careful attention to your posture when sitting, standing and lying. If you work at a desk make sure that it is at a comfortable height and that your chair offers lower back support. Be careful how you lift heavy items – always bend at the hips and knees, taking the weight on your legs and keeping your back straight. Never lift and twist at the same time.

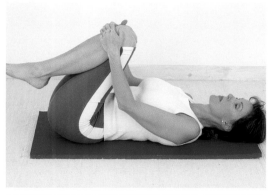

△ Lower back pain can be relieved by lying on your back, slowly lifting your knees and clasping them towards you. If you find this difficult, try lifting and clasping just one leg at a time and slowly build up to lifting both legs.

such as carrying heavy bags, which place unnecessary stresses and strains on the affected joints. Swim regularly and consult a physiotherapist about specific exercises to prevent muscle wasting around the affected joints. Useful complementary treatments that you may wish to try include osteopathy and chiropractic.

## back problems

As you grow older, everyday stresses and strains on the spine can build up and result in chronic back problems. The people most likely to suffer are manual workers, office workers, the overweight and the elderly. Back pain is usually caused by muscle or ligament strain or disc problems.

▷ Camomile, eucalyptus, lavender and rosemary essential oils can be used in a warm bath or hot compress to help relieve back pain.

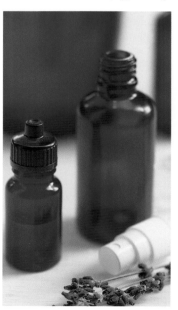

**EASING BACKACHE**

If you have back pain, there are a number of things that you can do to relieve the pain.

• Lie flat on your back with your knees bent.

• Apply a cold compress to the affected area.

• Make a hot compress, of camomile, rosemary, eucalyptus and lavender essential oils. Allow up to 8 drops of essential oil per 100ml of hot water. Soak muslin in the water and oil, squeeze out excess and apply to the back. Place a warm towel over the compress and leave for at least 2 hours. (Eucalyptus may cause skin irritation, so use sparingly.)

• Hot showers may ease pain.

• Make sure your back is adequately supported by your chair and mattress.

• Sleep on your side with your knees bent and a pillow between them (or on your back with pillows beneath your knees).

# The cardiovascular system

The chances of having a heart attack or a stroke increase with age and this is something that many people fear. You can help yourself by understanding the factors that put you at risk of problems and identifying those that are preventable. For example, although you cannot change your genetic predisposition, other risk factors such as poor diet, obesity and lack of exercise are within your control.

## cardiovascular disease

As we grow older we become more prone to disease of the arterial walls. Over a period of years fatty deposits build up on the inner layers of the arteries and they gradually harden into plaques known as atheroma. As a result the arteries become narrow and the flow of blood is impeded. Another age-related change that affects the arteries is a gradual thickening and loss of elasticity of the walls. In combination, these changes are known as atherosclerosis.

Damage to the arteries around the heart caused by atherosclerosis can lead to conditions such as angina, in which the blood flow to the heart is restricted. The main symptom of angina is chest pain during exertion. If blood flow to the heart is blocked, the result is a heart attack. This can be fatal or it can cause long-term damage to the heart.

A stroke happens when the brain is deprived of oxygen as a result of a blockage in a blood vessel. This causes damage to the brain, which can be fatal or cause serious impairment. Hypertension refers to abnormally high blood pressure in the arteries caused by a hardening of the walls.

## preventing cardiovascular disease

Since diet and lifestyle play such a major role in cardiovascular disease it is possible to make changes that drastically reduce your chances of becoming ill. The best preventative measures are:

• Eat a low-fat, high-fibre diet that includes plenty of oily fish, fruit and vegetables (*see* Anti-aging Diet). This should become your permanent diet.

• If you are overweight, go on a weight-reduction diet. Consult your doctor about how much weight you need to lose and what types of food you should eat.

• Take aerobic exercise on a regular basis.

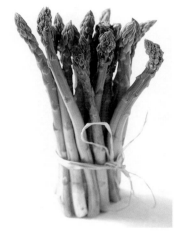

△ **Cook vegetables in a steamer to maintain the vitamins and minerals that are lost by boiling.**

Aerobic exercise gives your entire cardiovascular system a workout (*see* Staying Fit Throughout Life). A brisk 30-minute walk taken at least three times a week can dramatically lower the risk of premature death.

• Cut down the amount of alcohol you drink to within established guidelines.

• Reduce the amount of stress in your life. Practise relaxation techniques, particularly meditation and yoga.

• Give up smoking.

• If you are a postmenopausal woman with a history of cardiovascular disease in your family, consult your doctor about taking hormone replacement therapy (HRT).

• If you suffer from diabetes, make sure that it is meticulously controlled. Consult your doctor about this.

• You should have regular health checks, particularly cholesterol tests and blood pressure checks.

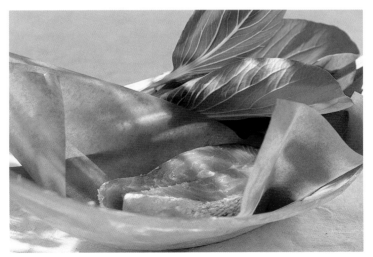

◁ **A low-fat Mediterranean diet consisting of fish, fresh fruit and vegetables, olive oil and a small amount of red wine promotes good circulation.**

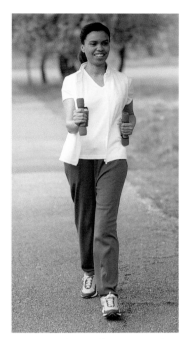

△ **Aerobic exercise taken three times a week strengthens the heart and increases blood flow.**

▽ **The shoulder rise stops blood from stagnating in the lower limbs of varicose vein sufferers.**

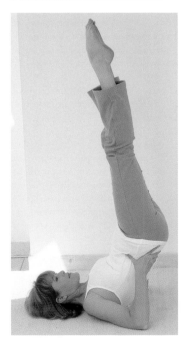

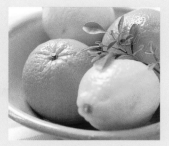

△ **Citrus fruit are rich in vitamin C.**

## varicose veins

When the valves in the veins are weakened, preventing the proper flow of blood back towards the heart, varicose veins occur. Blood then stagnates in veins, usually in the lower limbs. Varicose veins appear as swollen, twisted clusters of purple or blue veins. They are more common in women than in men, and usually worsen with age, especially during pregnancy and the menopause.

## fighting varicose veins

Preventative action against varicose veins includes taking regular exercise, eating a healthy and varied diet, weight control and avoiding long periods of standing. Complementary therapies that may be useful include aromatherapy, yoga, hydrotherapy, reflexology and naturopathy. A cold compress of witch hazel may be used to ease painful varicose veins.

Folic acid is another nutrient that is implicated in cardiovascular disease. It is thought to reduce the level of an amino acid, called homocysteine, which may cause arterial clogging and heart attacks. It is suggested that eating a bowl of cereal a day may be helpful. Apart from cereal, other good sources of folic acid include spinach, peanuts, broccoli, cauliflower, asparagus and sesame seeds.

Chocolate may have hidden health benefits. Research by scientists suggests that chocolate consumption can increase blood antioxidants. Drinking cocoa in moderation may have cardioprotective properties. However, most chocolate products are also high in fat and sugar.

▽ **Research in the US and Brazil has shown that moderate chocolate consumption increases blood antioxidants within two hours of ingestion.**

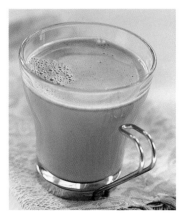

# The digestive system

Some people find that the digestive system becomes sluggish and less efficient with age. If your diet has always been low in fibre and high in refined foods, digestive problems may make their first appearance in middle age. Some women first experience digestive disturbances around the time of the menopause.

## digestive problems

Complaints that become more common with age are indigestion, bloating, constipation, flatulence and a condition known as diverticulosis. Diverticulosis occurs when pockets form in the intestinal wall. Food can become lodged in these pockets where it ferments, producing large amounts of gas. The sufferer typically experiences flatulence, bloating and abdominal discomfort. If the pockets become infected, this gives rise to a condition known as diverticulitis. The symptoms of this are abdominal cramping, nausea and fever.

Apart from poor dietary habits, one reason why older people may suffer from digestive problems is that hydrochloric acid production declines with age. Hydrochloric acid is released from the stomach wall and it begins the breakdown of protein in the stomach. If you notice that you are prone to indigestion after eating high-protein foods, you may not be producing enough stomach acid. One solution to this is to take a digestive supplement containing betaine hydrochloride.

## preventing digestive problems

The best way to prevent digestive problems is to eat a high-fibre diet. Fibre is not digested by the body so it passes through the gut intact, effectively "exercising" the intestines and adding bulk to stools. It is important to remember that if you increase the amount of fibre in your diet you should also increase the

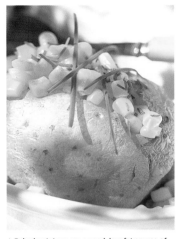
△ **Baked potatoes are a good, low-fat source of dietary fibre when eaten with the skin.**

amount of water that you drink. This is because fibre swells and absorbs water in the intestines.

Foods that are rich in fibre include oats, baked potatoes, lentils, brown rice, beans, fruit, wholegrain bread and wholewheat cereals. Eating cruciferous vegetables, such as broccoli and cabbage, several times a week may help to reduce the risk of colon cancer. Getting plenty of exercise is another important way of ensuring digestive health.

## supportive action for digestive problems

One way of testing how well your digestive system is working is by timing how long it takes for food to pass through your system. This is known as "transit time".

To do the transit test, include a test food in your diet that you would not normally eat. It should be a food, such as beetroot, that will be visible in your stools. Alternatively, you can use charcoal tablets from a pharmacy. The time between eating the food and its first appearance in your stools should be 12–14 hours. The colour should disappear from your stools after

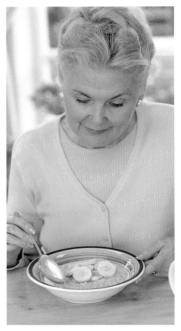
△ **Commercial bran and laxatives should be avoided where possible. Instead eat oats, which hold water and stimulate bowel movements.**

36–48 hours (this is called the retention time). If the transit time is significantly longer than 14 hours and retention time is 72 hours or more, then this is a sign that your bowel function is sluggish.

Sluggish bowel function can be treated by a wide range of complementary therapies such as massage, acupuncture, acupressure, homeopathy, herbalism and naturopathy. Naturopaths may recommend going on a cleansing diet that gives your gut a chance to clear itself. The best self-help treatment is gradually including more fibre in your diet. You should avoid taking commercial laxatives and bran products, which do not allow the body to assimilate nutrients fully, and can be harsh on the body. Specific problems may be alleviated by a number of herbal or dietary remedies.

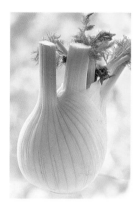

△ Fennel can be useful in controlling flatulence.

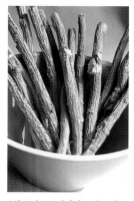

△ Liquorice can help keep bowel movements regular.

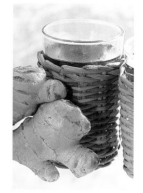

△ Eating ginger is an excellent remedy for nausea.

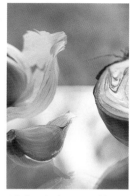

△ Garlic and onion are good for cleansing the digestive system.

• Garlic, peppermint, camomile and fennel may relieve flatulence.

• Linseed, prunes, rhubarb, ginger, chilli, liquorice, olive oil and honey may help to relieve mild constipation.

• Tea made with ginger root may help to alleviate nausea.

• Garlic and onions may help to cleanse the digestive system.

• Psyllium husks may help to relieve constipation. They are available in capsule form from health food shops.

▷ Advances in dental care mean that dentures will soon be a thing of the past.

Colon cleansing formulas are also available.

• Broad spectrum digestive enzymes, which can be bought from health food shops, may be helpful in the treatment of indigestion.

• A supplement containing acidophilus and bifidus bacteria can ensure a healthy bacterial environment in the gut.

**EARLY WARNING SIGNS**

If you have any unusual or persistent digestive symptoms, such as a sudden, inexplicable change in bowel movements, blood in the stools or pain in the abdomen, consult your doctor.

**MAINTAINING HEALTHY TEETH**

The process of digestion begins in the mouth when we chew our food. Chewing has a valuable function: it increases the surface area of the food so that it is easier for enzymes to break down nutrients into their basic components. If your teeth are in poor health, they cannot perform their function properly and you will be restricted in the types of food you can eat. Pay meticulous attention to dental hygiene as you get older, visit a dentist regularly and use disclosing tablets and floss after brushing to identify and remove plaque. Gum recession, which can cause teeth to become loose in their sockets, is one of the main problems that arises with age. Try not to encourage this process: use a soft toothbrush and avoid brushing the gums.

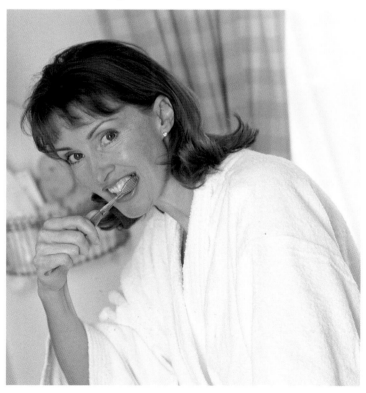

# Looking after your eyesight

The senses often become blunted with age. Changes tend to take place very gradually. If you experience a sudden change in your ability to see or hear, consult a doctor as it may be a sign of underlying illness.

## vision problems

The eyes undergo a number of changes as you grow older. The lens becomes more opaque and loses its flexibility, the iris becomes sluggish, the retina can become less sensitive to light, and a condition called glaucoma – in which pressure builds up inside the eye – becomes more likely. On average, the eye of a 60-year-old person lets in half as much light as a younger person's. The most common type of age-related vision change is long-sightedness.

Warning signs of eye problems are as follows:

• difficulty seeing objects close-up (this may be caused by long sightedness)
• hazy vision, a blur around lights and the sensation of looking through fog (this may be caused by cataracts)
• loss of peripheral vision, flashes of light and floating shapes (this may be caused by retinal detachment)

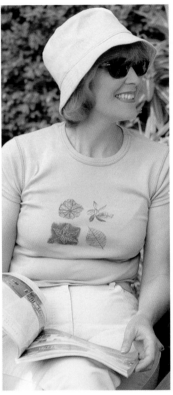

△ You should always ensure that your sunglass lenses are scratch free, otherwise they may do more harm to your eyesight than good.

• rapid or gradual vision loss and distorted vision when reading (this may be caused by macular degeneration)
• blurred vision, sudden and severe eye pain, teary, aching eyes, halos around lights, headache, nausea and vomiting (this may be caused by glaucoma).

You should have your eyesight tested yearly as you get older, and consult your doctor or ophthalmologist about any

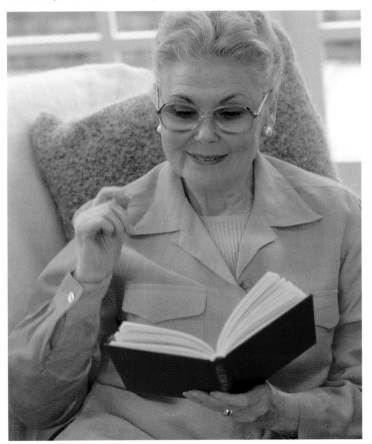

◁ Glaucoma may occur in people over the age of 40. Nutritionists suggest a diet rich in vitamin A may be of assistance in protecting sight.

## THE BATES METHOD

This is a series of eye exercises that may help to improve vision.

• splash the eyes with warm water 10 times and then cold water 10 times to increase blood circulation to the eyes.

• twice a day, rest your elbows on a table and cup your hands over your eyes. Allow yourself to relax for 10 minutes. If you do a lot of close up or computer work try to do this for one minute on a regular basis.

• try not to stare rigidly at any object for a long period of time. Every five minutes look away briefly and focus on something else for a few seconds.

• to strengthen the eye muscles, hold one index finger 10cm/4in in front of your eyes, and place the other index finger at arm's length behind it. Focus with both eyes on the nearest finger for a few seconds, blink, and then focus on the distant finger. Repeat this exercise 10 times, blinking between each change of focus to lubricate and clean the eyes.

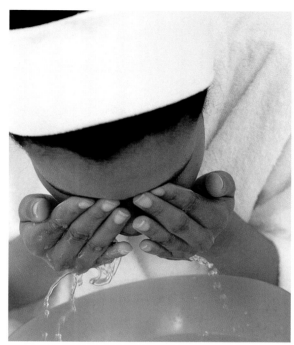

▷ By splashing the eyes with warm and then cold water, circulation can be increased which may help against sight degeneration.

changes in your vision. The treatment for eye problems ranges from reading glasses for long-sightedness to surgery for cataracts. If you have adult-onset diabetes, you should be particularly vigilant about having regular eye checks – diabetes is one of the main causes of blindness.

Try to protect your eyes as much as possible by not working in poor light, avoiding spending hours in front of a computer, learning some basic Bates method exercises, eating a healthy diet and taking regular exercise to increase the blood supply to the eyes. You should also wear sunglasses in bright light.

▽ **Always remove contact lenses or glasses before practising any eye exercises.**

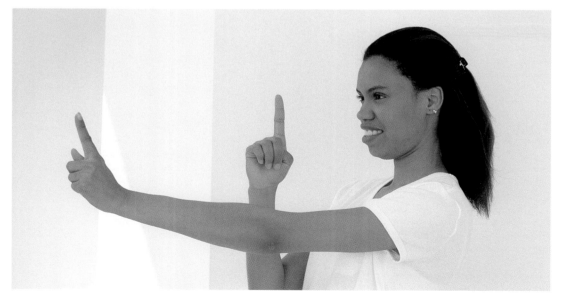

# Smell, taste and hearing

## hearing problems

Problems with hearing may occur as we age due to deterioration of the sensory nerve cells and the minuscule hairs within the inner ear. Loss of hearing is a very gradual process that actually starts at the beginning of life: from the moment we are born the tiny hairs in the inner ear start to die. All of us, as we age, lose the ability to hear high-pitched sounds as clearly as when we were young. Rumbling base sounds, on the other hand, become clearer.

Age-related hearing loss is known as presbycusis. It is common in men over 40 and may be genetically influenced. Because it can be accelerated by exposure to loud noise, it is very important to avoid exposure to repetitive noise, such as music or drilling. Hearing loss is gradual and you should look out for the following warning signs:
• difficulty hearing high frequencies
• difficulty understanding speech
• difficulty hearing in noisy places
• being unable to hear sounds you used to
Consult your doctor at the first sign of hearing loss. The main treatment for age-related deafness is a hearing aid. Some people benefit from learning lip reading and sign language. Complementary treatments that may help to improve hearing include reflexology and osteopathy.

Tinnitus is another age-related problem. It presents itself as a continuous high-pitched ringing, buzzing, humming, hissing or whistling that only the sufferer can hear. There are various causes including prolonged exposure to loud noise, high blood pressure, blockage with wax, ear infection and a perforated eardrum. Some drugs cause tinnitus as a side-effect.

The best way to prevent tinnitus is to wear ear plugs in noisy situations. You should also get plenty of rest, minimize stress and limit your salt intake. Playing soft music,

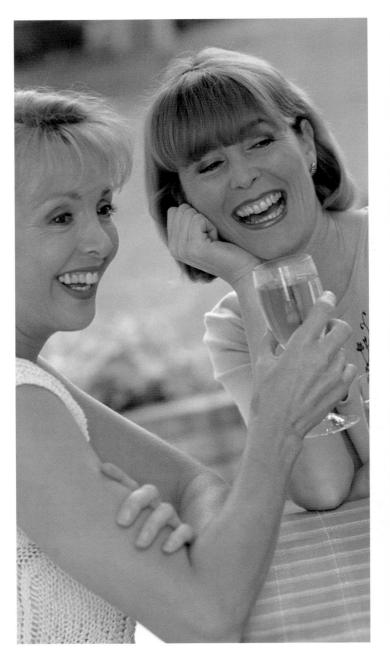

▷ **Consult your doctor if you begin to have difficulty following conversations.**

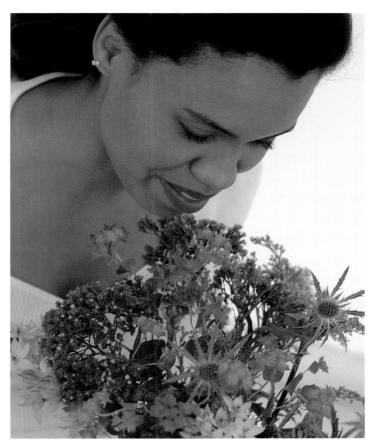

▷Your sense of smell may be heightened by eating zinc-rich foods such as peanuts or ginger root.

exercising regularly, practising relaxation techniques and avoiding smoking and alcohol may ease symptoms.

## smell

Our sense of smell is a much neglected asset. As well as protecting us in dangerous situations – alerting us to a fire, for example – it can also influence mood. Aromatherapists rely heavily on the olfactory system for their work. Receptors in the nose absorb smells that stimulate the olfactory bulb. Signals are then transmitted to the limbic system – part of the brain involved in the control of emotions. As you age your sense of smell is blunted and it becomes harder to differentiate between smells. Combined with a loss of taste this can mean that food becomes less appetizing

## taste

There are an average of 10,000 taste buds on the tongue, the roof of the mouth, the pharynx and the oesophagus. When you are young these taste buds are replaced on a regular basis but, with age, the replacement process becomes less efficient. This means that food may not taste as interesting or diverse as it used to as you get older. Smoking, drinking alcohol and certain medications can exacerbate this. People who wear dentures may suffer additionally because the taste receptors in the palate are covered. Women may not notice any decline in their ability to taste until after menopause when oestrogen levels decline.

Although a decline in sense of taste and smell may not seem to present a serious problem, it can mean that older people start to compensate by eating different foods. For example, they may start to avoid fruit and vegetables because they taste bland, and concentrate instead on salty food, sauces and strongly flavoured cheese and meat. This can have serious implications for health. A diet with a high salt content is associated with high blood pressure, and a diet rich in saturated fat is linked to cardiovascular disease. Dietary therapists say that a decline in taste and smell may be due to a lack of zinc and that, when

zinc-rich foods are eaten in the diet, taste and smell become more acute. Examples of zinc-rich food are oysters, ginger root, pecan nuts, brazil nuts, peanuts, wholewheat grains, dry split peas and egg yolk. If you want to add flavour to foods, try to use herbs and spices rather than salt.

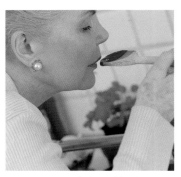

△ To avoid overuse of salt, try adding herbs and spices to enhance flavour.

▽ Pecan nuts are a source of zinc which is thought to improve taste and smell.

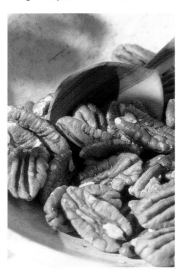

# Sexual health

The sexual role models that we see in the media are usually between the ages of 18 and 30. Older people are rarely depicted in a sexual way. One result of this is that we may start to feel marginalized sexually. However, most of us keep our sexual vigour as we age and many of us can look forward to staying sexually active for the rest of our lives.

## age related changes

Many people enjoy sex more as they grow older because they have gained considerable sexual experience and confidence. They know what sort of sexual activities arouse them and they may feel relaxed about communicating their sexual needs and desires.

How people change in their physical responses as they age varies from person to person. Most people in their 40s do not notice any significant sexual changes. People in their 50s may begin to notice that their sexual responses are slower than before and some people may begin to suffer problems related to medication, disability or underlying illness.

## women's sexuality

The main changes that affect women's sexuality are those that take place around the time of the menopause and afterwards. Menopausal symptoms such as hot flushes, night sweats, fatigue and mood swings may have a negative impact on a woman's sex drive. More specifically, the decline in oestrogen that happens at menopause can affect the urogenital tract itself, causing dryness and itchiness of the vagina and vulva. Women may find that they no longer produce so much vaginal lubrication during sexual arousal as they once did. This can be solved by using a lubricating gel or spending longer on foreplay.

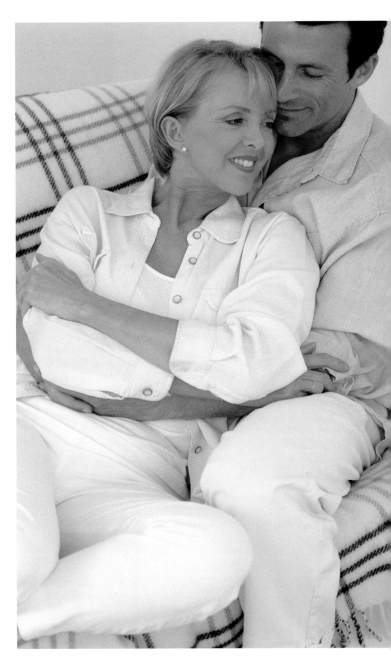

▷ **Once the children have grown up and left home, partners are often able to revitalize the intimate side of their relationship.**

If you are suffering from menopausal problems that affect your enjoyment of sex, seek the help of a doctor or complementary therapist (a wide range of herbal and homeopathic remedies is available).

Although women's fertility declines around the time of the menopause, women who do not want to conceive should use contraception for at least a year after their last menstrual period. Barrier methods such as the condom or diaphragm are recommended and they do not interfere with hormone replacement therapy should you decide to take it. The natural, or "rhythm", method of contraception is not appropriate because ovulation becomes very erratic around the time of the menopause.

## men's sexuality

Men may notice that their sex drive is lower in their 40s and 50s than it was when they were younger. They may also notice that that their erections are softer or smaller and at a less upright angle than they used to be. Ejaculation may be less intense and less forceful and the refractory period (the length of time before a man can have an erection after he has ejaculated) may increase.

Feelings of arousal are more likely to come from direct touch than, for example, visual cues such as the sight of a partner undressing. Sometimes these changes can have a positive effect on your sex life: because your sexual responses are slower and more focused on tactile stimulation you may be more sexually synchronized with your partner.

If you experience problems achieving or maintaining an erection, it is important to seek a medical opinion. Sometimes erectile problems are a warning sign of blocked arteries. Erection of the penis occurs because blood is actively pumped into the penile tissues – if your arteries are blocked then the blood is pumped less efficiently into the penis. Having said this, erectile problems can also result from stress or emotional problems. Try to reduce stress levels by giving your partner a soothing massage prior to sex and making the bedroom look as relaxing and welcoming as possible.

**HEALTH PROBLEMS THAT AFFECT SEX**

Some health problems become more common with age. These are the ones that can affect sexual function:
• Cardiovascular disease
• Diabetes
• Multiple sclerosis
• Alzheimer's disease
• Parkinson's disease
Sexual function may be affected by taking certain drugs including antidepressants, antipsychotics, beta-blockers and diuretic drugs. Occasionally, men who have prostate gland surgery may also experience changes in sexual function. You should consult your doctor about all of these issues.

▽ **Massage is a good way to rediscover the areas of your partner's body which enjoy attention the most.**

**SEX TIPS FOR OLDER PEOPLE**

Accept the changes that take place in your body and accommodate them. Spend longer on foreplay and make sex into a long, sensual encounter. Use massage oils and a lubricant if you need to. Introduce variety into your lovemaking by making love at unusual times in unusual places. Be experimental in whatever ways you like: use erotica, swap roles during sex, share sexual fantasies and read sex books together. The saying "use it or lose it" is particularly pertinent to sex as you get older. Staying sexually active keeps your sex organs functioning and maintains sexual desire. Remember that sexual activity does not have to mean intercourse; it can also mean extended foreplay, oral sex, masturbation (with or without a partner) or kissing and cuddling that makes you feel aroused.

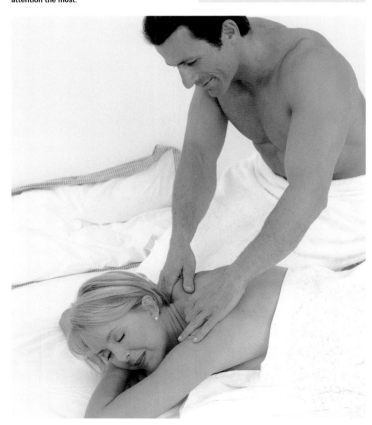

# Overcoming stress

looking after the body

Research shows that your stress levels can have a profound effect on your health. If you suffer from chronic stress you may exist in a permanent state of physiological arousal: your heart beat and blood pressure are constantly elevated and stress hormones such as adrenaline are circulating in your bloodstream. Chronic stress is implicated in a number of age-related health problems, the main one being cardiovascular disease.

## what is stress?

Stress is a physiological survival mechanism. When you sense that you are under threat, the brain responds by sending a message to the adrenal glands on top of your kidneys, which, in turn, respond by releasing adrenaline. Adrenaline has effects on various body systems that, in combination, enable you to take action: to either run away from the source of the threat or to stay and fight it. This is known as the "fight or flight response".

Although this physiological response may have been useful in primitive times, when humans needed to literally fight or run away from sources of danger, it is less useful in modern society, where sources of threat are mainly psychological. For example, a contemporary source of stress might be travelling to work on crowded public transport when you are already late for a meeting. Your brain registers stress but you will not be able to take advantage of the subsequent adrenaline rush because no physical action is necessary.

When instances of stress are occasional and short-lived, the body can cope (some degree of stress helps us to stay motivated and to meet our goals), but when they are frequent and long-lasting the body may be perpetually in a state of high alert. This is when your vulnerability to problems such as cardiovascular disease increases. For this reason, it is essential to find ways to overcome chronic stress as you get older.

## dietary support

People often turn to "quick fixes" when they are under stress. They feel tired, irritable and lacking in energy and they often turn to chocolate, caffeine or alcohol for stress relief, or a quick energy burst. Unfortunately, these substances deplete the body of energy and make you feel worse.

The most important nutrients to include in the diet when you are under stress are the B vitamins, vitamin C, zinc, chromium and magnesium. Dietary therapists may recommend taking a multivitamin and

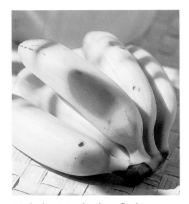

△ Eating bananas rather than refined-sugar products can boost natural sugar levels, which helps to combat stress.

mineral supplement that supplies these nutrients. It is also very important to avoid sugary foods when under stress because they stimulate the stress hormone cortisol. Instead, eat foods such as bananas, wholegrains, seeds, beans and lentils.

## yoga, meditation and breathing

Learning relaxation techniques is a powerful antidote to stress. Yoga and meditation teach you how to still the mind

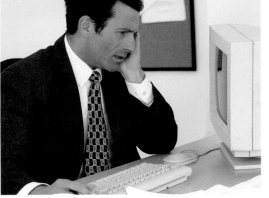

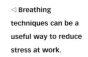

◁ Breathing techniques can be a useful way to reduce stress at work.

▷ Relaxation techniques can help in the fight against stress-induced digestive disorders such as ulcers and indigestion.

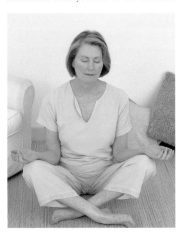

and focus on something simple such as the breath flowing in and out of your body. When you are stressed your breathing is usually fast and shallow. Making a conscious effort to relax your muscles and breathe deeply can help you to overcome stress. Yoga and meditation techniques are best learned from a trained therapist or teacher, but there are also plenty of books available.

One useful meditation technique is the humming bee practice. Sit in a comfortable position and close your eyes. Focus on the breath entering and leaving your nostrils. Say to yourself: "I am aware of breathing in. I am aware of breathing out". Use your fingers to close your ear flaps and imagine the sound of a humming bee inside your head. Breathe in and, as you breathe out, make the sound of a humming bee. Breathe in and repeat. Try to concentrate on the sound and on your breathing. Regular practice of this exercise should help to still your mind.

## aromatherapy and massage

A range of complementary therapies can help to ease stress: acupuncture, reflexology, hypnotherapy, homeopathy and flower remedies. Aromatherapy and massage are very widely used in the treatment of stress and aromatherapists recommend the following essential oils: basil, bergamot, clary sage, camomile, geranium, hyssop, juniper, lavender, marjoram, thyme, cedar, neroli, rose and sandalwood. Massage can help to ease stress by relieving muscle tension and enhancing circulation.

Try a stress-relieving bath consisting of 2 drops each of camomile and marjoram, and 4 drops of juniper. Alternatively, try a drop each of camomile, juniper and marjoram dropped onto a tea bag and put in a large cup of hot water during times of stress.

## personal stress-beaters

Everyone has their own ways of overcoming stress and it is important to cultivate methods that work for you. Some people unwind by talking to friends or a partner or by being sociable, others relax by spending time on their own. Exercise is a stress-beating technique that works for many people as it uses up adrenaline. The

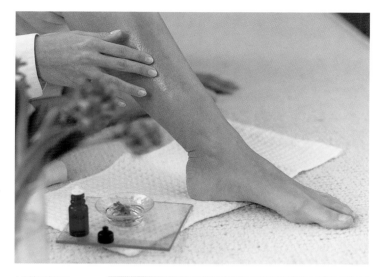

△ Taking time to massage yourself with stress-relieving essential oils can be a good antidote to stress.

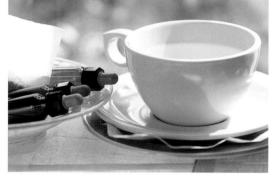

▷ Herbal teas and Bach Flower Remedies are quick and effective cures for stress.

endorphin rush that exercise brings can also provide a sense of well-being.

Sometimes a change of attitude can turn a stressful situation into a non-stressful one: ask yourself if a situation can be turned to your advantage in any way. Some people decide that, rather than trying to relieve the symptoms of stress, they will tackle the underlying cause. This may involve leaving a stressful job or ridding yourself of other responsibilities you can no longer manage.

Pet ownership can have a remarkable effect on stress levels. Pets act as morale boosters by offering unconditional loyalty. They can provide a valuable outlet for people who find it difficult to express their emotions – this in itself is cathartic.

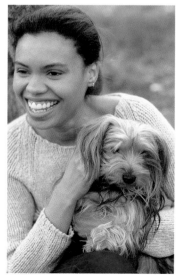

▷ By allowing us to care for them, pets can make us feel needed and appreciated.

# understanding depression

Many psychologists make a distinction between depressed mood and depression. Depressed mood describes the temporary sensation of "feeling down" that you have when something goes wrong in your life. Depression, on the other hand, is more intense and long-lasting. It can affect your behaviour, your relationships, your eating and sleeping patterns and your entire world view. The likelihood of depression may increase as you grow older. Elderly people, in particular, are more prone to suffering from depression.

## recognizing the signs

Feelings of dejection, hopelessness and inadequacy are the most common signs of depression. But depression can manifest itself in a variety of ways and it is important to be aware of the signs, both in yourself and in others.

- Loss of interest in everyday activities
- Excessive sleeping or insomnia
- Fatigue and lack of energy
- Feelings of hopelessness and worthlessness
- Loss of sexual interest
- Apathy
- Excessive overeating or undereating
- Dejection, sadness and crying
- Problems with concentration and remembering things
- Difficulty making decisions
- Indifference to the world around you
- Suicidal thoughts and urges

## what causes depression?

Depression can be triggered by a specific event. Life events that are associated with depression include divorce, separation, bereavement (particularly of a close family member), or being fired or made redundant. Sometimes depression has no specific or obvious cause. Depression that occurs in older people may result from a perceived loss of control in life. The prospect of growing older may in itself be depressing,

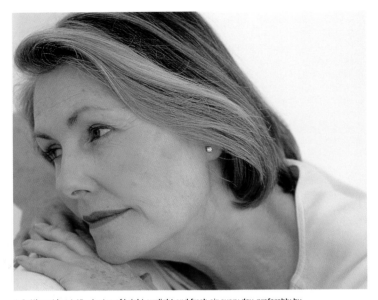

△ Getting at least 15 minutes of bright sunlight and fresh air every day, preferably by taking a brisk walk in full daylight, can help to banish feelings of depression.

especially given the fact that many societies tend to devalue aging and equate power and sexuality with youthfulness.

## self-help for depression

If you feel depressed, try to make sure that you continue to eat and sleep properly. Avoid resorting to destructive props such as alcohol, cigarettes or drugs. Make sure that your diet is high in vitamin C, B vitamins, essential fatty acids and unrefined carbohydrates. Avoid refined, sugary foods.

If possible, stay active, exercise regularly (the endorphins released during exercise can help to combat depression) and seek the support of friends and family. Speak about how you are feeling and do not be afraid to express negative emotions such as fear, guilt, anger or sadness. Complementary therapies may help to combat depression. Herbalists

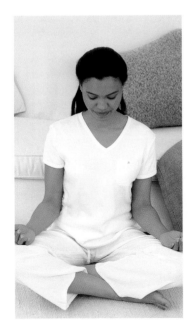

▷ Taking time out to practise meditation may help you to relax and forget your worries.

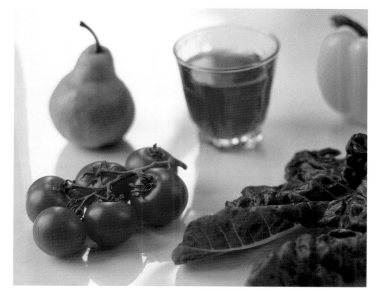

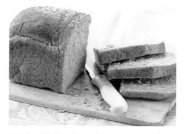

△ A sluggish digestive system can cause and increase feelings of depression, so ensure a high fibre intake is maintained.

◁ Vitamin C is essential in the fight against depression, yet it is depleted by stress.

recommend taking St. John's wort for depression, although long-term use of the herb may cause sensitivity to light. Aromatherapists say that essential oils such as basil, bergamot, clary sage, camomile, geranium, lavender, thyme, jasmine, neroli (orange blossom), rose, sandalwood and ylang ylang can help to lift mood, especially if used in combination with massage.

Understanding some of the cognitive processes that underpin depression can be helpful. The cognitive psychologist, Aaron Beck, says that depressed people often make "errors" in their thinking. If possible, try to challenge the following thought processes when they happen to you:
• Overgeneralization: the depressed person makes sweeping, negative generalizations. For example, "my whole life is pointless".
• Selective abstraction: the depressed person focuses on small negative details. For example, from a list of compliments, the depressed person remembers a chance remark that could be construed as negative.
• Magnification and minimization: the depressed person dramatizes the importance of negative events and downplays the importance of positive events. For example, a man who is not invited to a party sees himself as a social failure despite the fact that he has recently had an enjoyable meeting with some old friends.

• Personalization: the depressed person takes responsibility for things beyond his control. For example, "Today's train strike has happened because I need to get somewhere urgently".
• Arbitrary inference: the depressed person infers something without justification. For example, a woman infers from her husband's angry expression that she has done something wrong. If she had enquired further she would have discovered that her husband was angry about something unrelated to her.

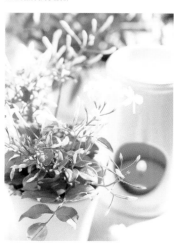

△ Time spent making your surroundings more enjoyable can enhance your appreciation of life.

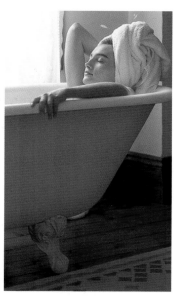

△ A warm, relaxing bath using uplifting aromatherapy oils can help against depression.

## seeking professional help for depression

If you are suffering from depression you should consult your doctor. Treatment for depression consists of anti-depressant medication or psychotherapy, sometimes a combination of the two. There are different types of psychotherapy ranging from counselling to cognitive therapy to psychoanalysis. Discuss with your doctor which type meets your needs. If you are taking any complementary medicine, inform your doctor.

# Thinking positively

Optimism, enthusiasm and a refusal to tolerate boredom are characteristics that are often associated with young people. There is no reason why this should be the case, however, and one of the best ways to remain psychologically young is to cultivate the art of positive thinking.

## foster a sense of optimism

Life brings many experiences: some positive and some negative. As people get older they may fall into the trap of focusing on negative experiences and unwittingly cultivating a sense of pessimism about the future.

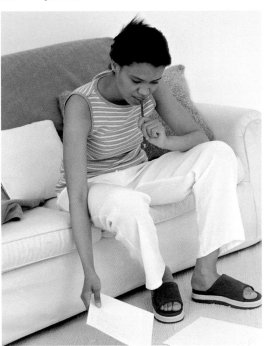

◁ **By making a list of positive and negative aspects of our lives, we enable ourselves to see the areas needing attention.**

Pessimism can be further encouraged by media messages that value youth and denigrate aging.

Resolve to clear out your emotional baggage and foster a sense of optimism about the present and the future. Optimism has huge benefits for both psychological

and physical health – it can even boost your immunity to illness. Make a list of the life experiences that have affected you positively and negatively. Compare the positive list with the negative list. Ask yourself if anything from the negative list can be discarded or turned into a positive situation. Congratulate yourself on your achievements in life and concentrate on the future rather than the past.

Optimism is cultivated by keeping busy and active. Take up activities that make you feel good about yourself such as yoga, walking or swimming. Learn something

completely new. Make sure that you are always working towards new goals and challenges. Set up a timetable in which to meet these goals. For example: "by the end of the year I will have converted one room of the house into a studio for painting, reading and music practice".

## distance yourself from problems

If there are situations and problems in your life that you find inescapable, try to distance yourself from them. Take an overview: tell yourself that this is one episode in your life and it will not last indefinitely. If possible, try to see humour in difficult situations. Imagine that you are a stranger walking past the window of your own house. What would the stranger see? What would the stranger make of the events going on?

Ask yourself whether your current problems will still affect you in a year's time

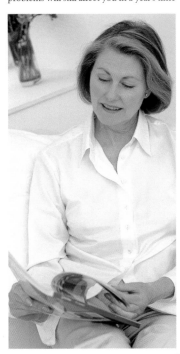

▷ **Planning a holiday can cheer you up by giving you something to look forward to.**

or in five or ten years? If you can, let go of things that you cannot change and concentrate on the things that you can. Remember that, even if you cannot change a situation, you always have the option of changing the way that you think about it. Cultivate a sense of control.

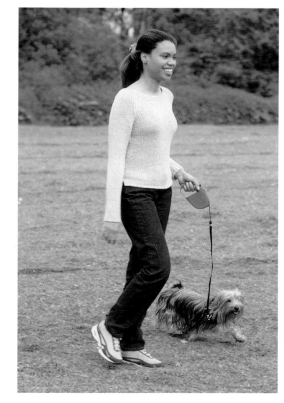

▷ Dogs have an unlimited capacity for enjoyment which can be infectious.

## have a mental clear-out

One negative stereotype of aging is that our beliefs become more rigid and inflexible as we get older. Challenge this assumption by discarding old beliefs and values. A belief that you have held for years may no longer be useful to you, it may be outdated or experience may have taught you new lessons. Question your beliefs about everything from gender roles to politics. Also question your beliefs about yourself. If you find yourself thinking you are incapable of doing something, ask yourself why.

Have a physical clear out as well as a mental and emotional one. If you make the symbolic gesture of throwing out clothes and other possessions that you have not used for years, this will reinforce your feelings of positivity and change.

## enjoy the simple things

Think positively about small things in life as well as big things. Derive pleasure from everyday activities such as cooking meals, bathing and reading a book or newspaper. Immerse yourself in whatever you are doing. Take the time to look at your surroundings. If you always travel by public transport, try making the effort to walk once in a while.

Friendships are important in helping us to think positively. Friends provide support, companionship, humour and affection, as well as a valuable buffer against stress.

▽ Taking time to enjoy the company of a good friend can change a dull day into a good one.

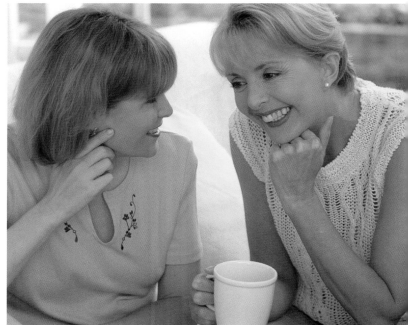

# The importance of sleep

Sleep is essential to your mental and physical well-being. If you do not have sufficient sleep, you are likely to become moody and bad-tempered. If your insomnia is chronic, you may be permanently tired, lacking in energy and depressed. Although sleeping patterns change as you grow older, getting a good night's sleep remains essential for the regular rejuvenation of the body.

## why do we need sleep?

Sleep experts are not sure about the precise functions of sleep but it is thought that the body needs a period of rest every night to allow it to recuperate from the day and to repair cellular damage and maintain the immune system. Cells all over the body have the chance to regenerate and the brain consolidates what has happened during the day into long-term memory. People who are deprived of sleep may suffer from mood swings, irritability and psychoses.

## sleep and aging

There is a popular misconception that people need less sleep as they grow older. In fact, your sleep requirements remain fairly constant throughout adulthood. Most people need approximately eight hours a night whether they are young or old. However, a variety of changes take place in sleeping patterns as people grow older and these changes conspire to make the overall duration of sleep shorter than before.

Sleep experts say that the "architecture" of sleep changes with age. Older people spend less time in deep sleep or "delta sleep" than younger people, although they continue to spend the same amount of time in dream or "rapid eye movement" (REM) sleep as younger people.

People may find it more difficult to get to sleep as they grow older and this may be because they produce less of the chemicals that control the sleep/waking cycle. For

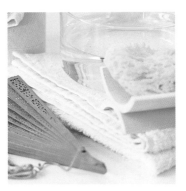

△ **If menopausal hot flushes keep you awake during the night, keep a fan, sponge and water beside your bed, so that you can easily cool yourself down.**

example, older people secrete less melatonin, a sleep-promoting substance produced by the pineal gland in the brain.

Other age-related changes to sleeping patterns include waking up more frequently and spending more time awake during the night. Generally, people adapt to these natural changes and do not find them debilitating.

## problems with sleep

There are a number of specific problems that affect people's sleep as they grow older. For example, menopausal women may find their sleep is disrupted by hot flushes or night sweats. Typically, women wake up at intervals throughout the night feeling hot, feverish and drenched in sweat. They may need to change their bed clothes and bed linen, which adds to sleep disruption. In the long term this can lead to poor concentration, irritability, depression and reduced immune system efficiency. If your sleep is severely disrupted by night sweats, you should consult your doctor.

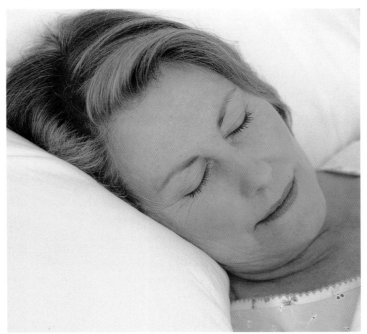

◁ **Skin cells regenerate at a much faster rate during sleep, so a good night's rest is important to a healthy body.**

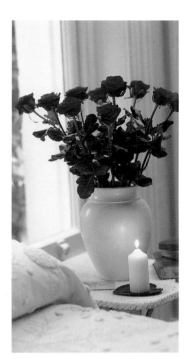

△ Making your bedroom welcoming and relaxing can help to induce sleep.

Immediate self-help measures include keeping a bowl of water, a sponge, a hand-held fan and a towel by your bedside. Always wear night clothes made of natural fibres and keep a change of night clothes beside the bed.

Some age-related illnesses may interfere with sleep patterns. The aches and pains associated with arthritis can make it difficult to get to sleep and can disrupt sleep throughout the night. Digestive problems such as gastro-oesophageal reflux can abbreviate sleep. This is a disorder where

there is a backflow of stomach acid into the oesophagus. Sufferers may find that sleep problems can be resolved simply by raising their heads up off the bed.

Other age-related illnesses that can interfere with sleep patterns include cancer, osteoporosis, Parkinson's disease, bladder problems and cardiovascular disease. Some prescribed medications may also be responsible for disrupting your sleep. Diuretic drugs may cause you to get up frequently during the night to visit the bathroom.

Insomnia can sometimes have a psychological origin. If you are depressed, upset or anxious, for example, then sleep is likely to be elusive. You should consult your doctor if you frequently suffer from chronic insomnia – it is important that the underlying cause is diagnosed and treated correctly.

On the other hand, a daytime nap can be a valuable way to relieve fatigue and sleepiness. If your night sleep is temporarily being disrupted and you are not usually an insomnia sufferer, a short nap during the day (before 3:00 pm if possible) can revive and refresh you, and give you the energy to keep going through the remainder of the day.

▽ Try to take cat naps before 3:00 pm to avoid disturbing your ability to fall asleep at night-time.

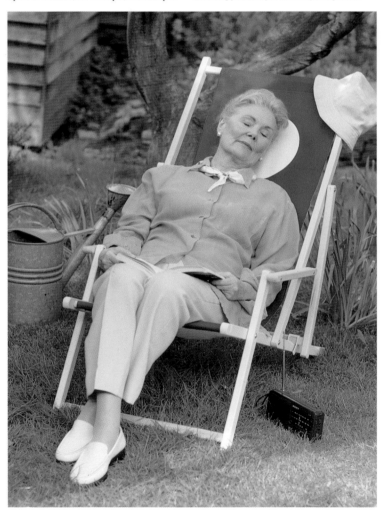

### DAYTIME NAPPING

Opinions are mixed about the value of napping during the day. If you are suffering from insomnia, it can exacerbate it. Also, rather than compensating for insomnia, you should try to discover and treat the underlying cause. On the other hand, by training our bodies to accept short periods of sleep when we need it we can avoid overstretching our systems during the day.

# Quality sleep

## coping with snoring

Snoring increases with age. It is not usually a sign of a serious problem, although it can disrupt the sleep of a partner. Snoring results when the airways are obstructed, usually because the muscles that keep them open are too lax or because there is a build up of fatty tissue around the airways. Anything that encourages muscle relaxation, from lying on your back to drinking alcohol, may make snoring worse. The noise of snoring comes from the air rattling over the relaxed tissues of the palate and throat.

Snoring is most common in middle-aged people who are overweight. There are several preventative measures:
• Lose weight.
• Avoid drinking alcohol or eating heavily before you go to bed.
• Sleep without a pillow.
• Quit smoking. Smoking is a major cause of airway congestion.
• Sleep on your side rather than on your back. You can force yourself to do this by sewing a tennis ball into the back of your nightclothes.

## sleep apnea

Occasionally, snoring may be associated with a serious disorder known as sleep apnea which becomes more common in middle and later life. Sleep apnea occurs when the upper airway becomes blocked and prevents you from breathing. In severe cases, sleep apnea may result in high blood pressure and increase your risk of heart attack and stroke.

During the night the apnea sufferer stops breathing, levels of oxygen in the bloodstream fall rapidly and the sufferer wakes up briefly, gasps for breath and then falls asleep again. This happens over and over again throughout the night and often means that the sufferer feels extremely sleepy during the day. Sleep apnea may be accompanied by loud snoring and is most common in overweight or obese people. If sleep apnea is mild, it may be overcome by

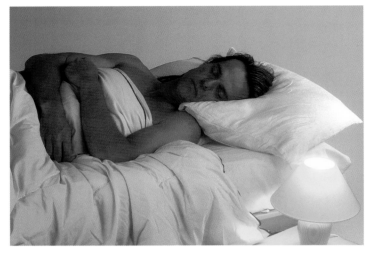

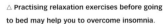

△ Practising relaxation exercises before going to bed may help you to overcome insomnia.

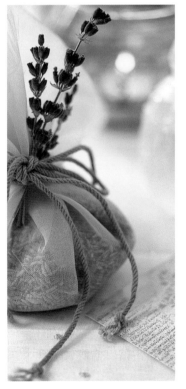

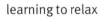

◁ A lavender sachet beside the bed, or a few drops of lavender oil on your pillow may enduce sleep.

weight loss, lying on your side and avoiding smoking, alcohol and sedative medications. If it is severe, a doctor may recommend keeping the airways open with a special device or, sometimes, with surgery.

## learning to relax

One of the best ways of enhancing sleep is learning an effective method of relaxation. Complementary therapies, such as aromatherapy, massage, acupuncture and flower remedies, can help you to relax and overcome insomnia. T'ai chi and yoga are also very useful. Or you can try the following creative visualization exercise.

Lie flat on your back with your arms by your sides, palms up, and your legs straight and hip-width apart. Breathe in and out deeply. Try to draw the breath down into your abdomen so that your lungs are taking in the maximum amount of oxygen to replenish your body. Close your eyes and focus your thoughts on a single item that

▷ A warm aromatherapy bath before bedtime can relax muscles and emotions.

▽ Leave an aromatherapy burner alight whilst you prepare for bed to help your body and mind relax.

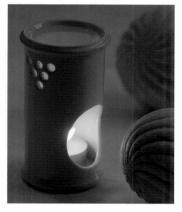

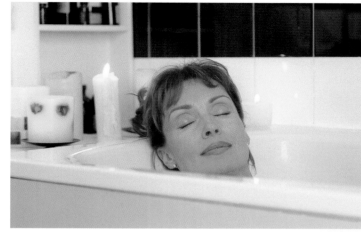

you find relaxing, such as a cloud, a tree, a lake or the sea. Concentrate on the qualities – the texture, depth, colour and movement – of the image you have chosen. If any distracting thoughts come into your head, acknowledge them and then visualize them as leaves being gently blown away. Keep breathing deeply into your abdomen. When you are ready to finish your relaxation session, do so slowly. Let your thoughts return to the room you are in and gently move your toes and fingers. Roll onto one side and get up. Alternatively, you can do this exercise in bed before you go to sleep.

## ENHANCING SLEEP QUALITY

Try to maximize your sleep quality by making your environment as comfortable as possible and by developing good sleeping habits.

• Make sure your bedroom is relaxing, warm and well aired.

• Burn lavender essential oil in an aromatherapy burner in your bedroom. Or put a handkerchief with a few drops of lavender oil under your pillow.

• Avoid eating a heavy meal immediately before going to bed.

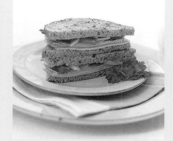

△ Some foods, such as turkey, avocado, cottage cheese, milk and bananas contain tryptophan which may assist healthy sleep.

• Avoid caffeinated drinks or alcohol before you go to bed. Although alcohol can speed up the onset of sleep, it disrupts the pattern of sleep at a later stage in the night.

• Go to bed at roughly the same time every night (preferably earlier rather than later).

• Get up at roughly the same time every morning, even if you go to bed later than usual.

• If possible, use your bedroom for sleep only (rather than for work, watching television or talking on the telephone, for example). This way your brain will learn to associate the bedroom with sleep.

• Make sure your bed is comfortable and supports your spine. If you have a back problem, try sleeping on your side with your knees bent and a pillow between them.

• Cut out any sources of light that may keep you awake.

• Eliminate irritating noises. Fix dripping taps and noisy plumbing or radiators. Alternatively, buy some good quality ear plugs.

• Wear night clothes made from natural fibres.

• Have a warm bath and a milky drink before going to bed. Try the following essential oils in your bath: 2 drops each of camomile and rose with 4 drops each of juniper and marjoram, or 2 drops each of camomile and juniper and 4 drops of neroli.

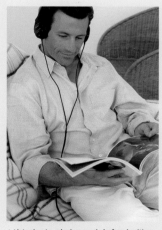

△ Listening to relaxing music before bedtime helps many people to switch from an active to a passive state of mind.

• Eating foods that contain the amino acid tryptophan may help you to sleep. These include avocado, turkey, cottage cheese, milk and bananas.

• Do something relaxing and enjoyable, such as reading a book or listening to soothing music, before you go to bed.

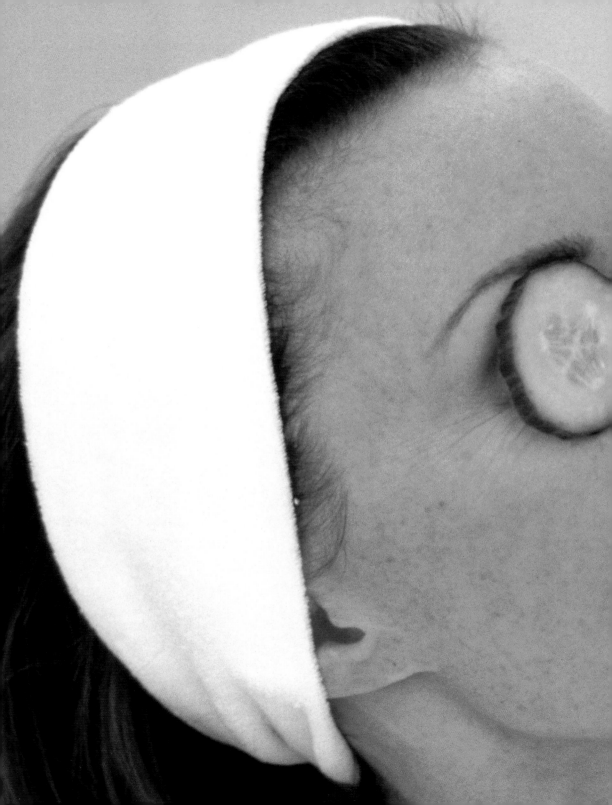

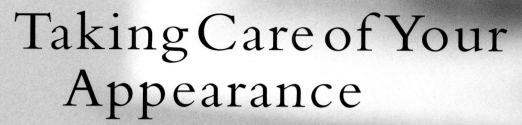

# Taking Care of Your Appearance

As you grow older the skin loses its natural elasticity and the hair becomes prone to greying and thinning – for many people these are the first visible signs of aging. There are some good techniques for preventing or accommodating changes in your appearance. It is worth remembering that if you are happy about the way you look this has an inspiring effect on your mood, making you feel more positive, confident and sociable.

# Protecting the skin

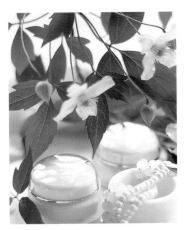

△ Add evening primrose oil or vitamin E to face cream to help rejuvinate mature skin.

The skin is our largest organ and it serves as a protective barrier against bacteria and other invaders. As you age, your skin loses its elasticity, it gets thinner and it starts to wrinkle. In fact, the appearance of the skin is one of the main criterion that we use to judge a person's age. But, although the aging process results in skin wrinkling, it is only partly responsible: ultraviolet light from the sun also plays a large role.

## how the skin ages

A protein called collagen is responsible for keeping the skin supple, elastic and youthful. When the skin is exposed to ultraviolet light from the sun, collagen fibres are attacked and destroyed. Although you lose collagen naturally with age, exposure to the sun greatly accelerates this process (so does cigarette smoking). Ultraviolet rays also damage the layer of skin where new cells are formed. The shape of the cells changes and they become smaller. This causes the skin to lose its thickness and become more translucent. Skin ages at a different rate on different areas of the body. Two of the first places that wrinkles appear are the hands and the face because both are constantly exposed to the elements. The skin on the neck, which is very mobile, is also prone to visible loosening and sagging with age.

Sebaceous glands, which secrete a lubricating substance onto the surface of the skin, become less active with age, resulting in dryness and flakiness.

## common skin problems

Apart from wrinkling and sagging, there are some specific skin problems that are more likely to occur with age. These include broken veins and itchiness.

Broken veins become more visible as the skin ages and becomes translucent. As with age spots, broken veins do not require any special treatment. If broken veins are particularly unsightly, however, they can be removed using techniques such as electrocautery.

Itchiness of the skin may sometimes be associated with the menopause. A persistent sensation of tingling or itchiness around this time is known as formication. Some doctors may recommend hormone replacement therapy (HRT) to treat this irritating condition, as well as other menopausal symptoms.

## taking care of your skin

The single most effective way to prevent premature skin aging is to protect your skin from the ultraviolet rays of the sun. This means avoiding exposure to intense sunlight whenever possible, covering your skin and wearing a sun hat on sunny days, and getting into the habit of always wearing a high protection sunscreen or sunblock.

Another way to protect your skin is to minimize free radical damage to body cells (free radicals are highly reactive substances produced during oxidation) from cigarette smoking and pollution. Avoid exposure to cigarette smoke (or quit smoking yourself) and environmental pollution, and eat foods that are rich in vitamins A, C, and E, betacarotene and selenium or zinc. These nutrients help to fight free radicals in the body; you can also take them in supplement form. Skin health can also be enhanced by making sure that you always have sufficient quality sleep.

Other dietary habits that will keep your skin youthful include the following:
• Limit your intake of tea, coffee, alcohol, sugar and saturated fat.
• Take an evening primrose oil supplement. This contains essential fatty acids that are needed by skin cell membranes.
• Drink plenty of pure water. Dehydration affects the skin and makes it dry.
• Increase the amount of fruit and vegetables in your diet, especially red, orange and yellow ones.

There are some "external" habits that you can adopt to preserve your skin. Try not to wash your skin too often and avoid harsh soaps that strip the skin of oil. Add oil to bath water and use good quality moisturizers (preferably containing sunscreen) on your body, hands and face. Moisturizers prevent the top layer of the skin from drying out but they cannot restore lost collagen.

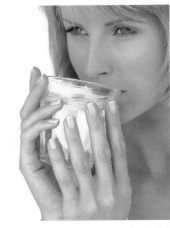

△ Drinking water not only hydrates the skin but also helps to flush away toxins.

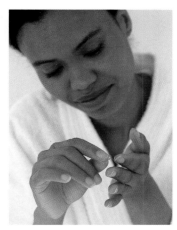

△ Applying the contents of a vitamin E capsule to your face once a week can help to soften aging skin.

## beauty tips

Cosmetic products and procedures – and even cosmetic surgery – are frequently presented as a panacea for age-related problems. Unfortunately, they are often expensive and do not yield any long-term benefits. The alternative to shop-bought products are safe and simple techniques and practices evolved over hundreds of years from complementary therapies such as herbalism and aromatherapy.

## stay moisturized

Even if moisturizers cannot restore lost skin tone, they can rehydrate the top layer of your skin, making it look firmer and healthier. To optimize absorption of moisturizer, apply it immediately after a bath when your skin is still warm and damp. Do not forget to moisturize your neck, an area which is much neglected and that is prone to sun damage.

Vitamin E is an important anti-aging vitamin for the skin which can be applied externally or ingested. Massage the contents of a vitamin E capsule into your face or, if you prefer to include vitamin E in the foods you eat, good sources include unrefined corn oil, sunflower seeds, sesame seeds, beans, wheatgerm and tuna.

Try the following recipe for calendula (marigold) cream. Mix 55g/2oz lanolin with 50ml/2fl oz wheatgerm oil. Add a handful of fresh or dried calendula flowers and heat for approximately two hours. Strain the liquid, add two capsules of vitam in E and leave to set in a jar. Use as an everyday moisturizer.

You can also use essential oils to lubricate your skin. Use 15ml/1tbsp of a base oil, such as evening primrose or sweet almond oil, and add 1 drop of an essential oil such as frankincense, geranium, lavender, neroli (orange blossom), or sandalwood. Massage gently into the skin taking care to avoid the eyes.

## take herbal baths

You can improve the way you look and feel by taking a relaxing and therapeutic herbal bath. Turn out the lights and place some lit candles around the bath. Make sure that the water is the right temperature. There are a wide variety of commercial aromatherapy and herbal products that you can add to a bath or you can try making your own. To make a herbal tea bag, place the herbs in the centre of a coffee filter. Fold it and sew the open edges closed with a needle and cotton. Alternatively, place the herbs into a piece of muslin and tie the material with ribbon. Hang the bag onto the bath and let the hot water run through it. For a calming bath, use equal parts of camomile, hops and passion flower. For a stimulating bath, use equal parts of peppermint, eucalyptus and lavender.

Aromatherapists recommend that you add essential oils to your bath water to benefit from their therapeutic effects. For a calming bath use four drops of lavender, four drops of neroli and two drops of geranium For a stimulating bath use two drops of lemon, three drops of peppermint and three drops of rosemary.

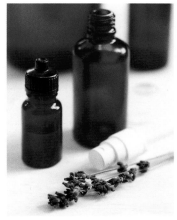

△ Add different essential oils to your bath water to achieve calming or invigorating baths; Lavender and camomile are very relaxing.

While you are in the bath you can give your eyes a treat by covering them with cold, damp teabags, cucumber slices, or cotton wool.

## have a massage

Having a regular massage is an excellent way to increase circulation, calm the nervous system, relieve muscle tension, promote sleep and improve posture, vitality and mood. These, in turn, have a knock on effect on your appearance. If you can, have an aromatherapy massage on a regular basis. Alternatively, give and receive a massage with a friend or partner

When you give a massage, you should always lubricate your hands with a base oil, such as almond, wheatgerm or olive, first. Avoid giving massage to people who suffer from skin problems or health problems such as osteoporosis.

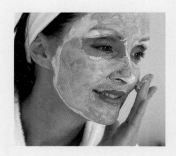

**A NATURAL FACE PACK**

As your skin ages, you may find that commercial face packs strip your skin of oils, especially if they contain clay. To make a natural face pack that will help to moisturize and condition older skin, mash together half an avocado (or one raw egg yolk) with a small amount of honey. Apply to the face avoiding the eye area, and leave on for approximately 10 minutes. Use this face pack every week.

# Hand and foot care

Hands are a good indication of the state of the body and many therapists use them as diagnostic tools when judging general health. Dry or brittle nails, for example, may reveal a lack of B vitamins, white flecks may indicate a lack of zinc, and weak nails could be caused by a calcium deficiency.

## how the hands age

As you age, the skin on your hands tends to become dry and fragile, the nails may thicken and become ridged or they may get brittle and prone to breaking. Veins become more pronounced, age spots appear and the hand becomes thinner and less fleshy.

## common hand problems

As you grow older it is common for age spots to appear on the backs of the hands. Age spots, sometimes known as liver spots, are due to melanin-producing cells clumping together with age. Melanin is a pigment produced by the skin that gives rise to the characteristic brown colour of a suntan. When melanin-producing cells clump together they produce distinctive brown spots or patches. Although age spots are not thought to be harmful, they can be

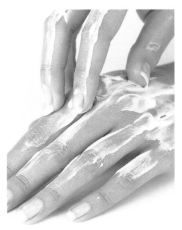

△ You should try to remember to moisturize your hands at least twice a day.

removed using laser or chemical treatment. Massaging the hands with saffron oil may also be helpful. Age spots may be worsened by cold weather and exposure to the ultraviolet rays of the sun, so always wear sunscreen on the hands in summer and gloves in winter.

Arthritis can cause problems such as pain, restricted movement and dexterity and even disfigurement in the hands as you grow older. Arthritis should receive medical diagnosis and treatment, but self-help measures include taking painkillers and applying alternate hot or cold compresses to the hands. Hand massage can also be helpful.

To give a massage, lubricate your hands with base oil mixed with a few drops of marjoram essential oil and gently sandwich one of the sufferer's hands in between both of yours. Gently stroke the length of the hand from the wrist to the fingertips. The warmth of your hands will ease the pain. Now gently rub and stroke the thumb.

## looking after your hands

Moisturize your hands as often as possible, but at least once in the morning and evening, and after immersing your hands in water. Moisturizer is absorbed into the skin most quickly when it is warm, so apply it to warm hands or keep a bottle near to a source of heat.

Cleaning dishes in hot water that contains detergent can take its toll on your hands over many years. A good way to prevent skin damage is to cover your hands in handcream and put rubber gloves on before washing up. The warmth of the water will enhance the skin's absorption of the moisturizer.

Once a week, soak your fingertips in warm olive oil (or cider vinegar if you have weak nails) for 10 minutes. Then gently rub a teaspoon of salt into your hands. The abrasive action of the salt will remove dead skin cells. Now trim your nails using a pair of nail scissors, and file them into shape. Use an

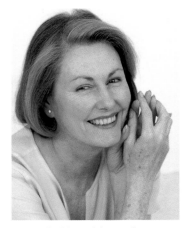

△ Light nail polishes and shorter nails are more flattering for older hands.

emery board and sweep from the outer corner of the nail inwards. Push the cuticles back with an orange stick wrapped in cotton wool. Now buff your nails to smooth away ridges and give them a natural shine.

Always try to wear at least a clear nail polish to protect your nails against everyday wear and tear. If you are applying a coloured nail varnish, always use an undercoat first to prevent the pigment from sinking into the nails and causing staining. A top coat can double the length of time required between manicures by preventing chipping.

### SKIN AGING ON THE HANDS

The backs of the hands are often the first place where skin starts to age. Try pinching the skin on the back of your hand for a few seconds and then release it. The rate at which it falls back into place varies according to age.

Under 30: 1 second
30–40 years: 1–2 seconds
40–50 years: 2–5 seconds
50–60 years: 10–15 seconds

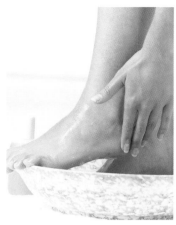

△ Add a few drops of peppermint essential oil to baby oil and massage to relieve tired feet.

## foot care

Years of wear and tear combined with badly fitting or poorly designed shoes can have an adverse effect on the feet as you grow older. You can also add to the burden by trimming the toenails badly or neglecting problems such as dry skin, corns and bunions. Good foot care is an important investment in your mobility – present and future.

## common foot complaints

Corns and calluses are caused by friction between shoes and the bony areas of the foot. The bony parts of the foot become less padded with age, making corns and calluses

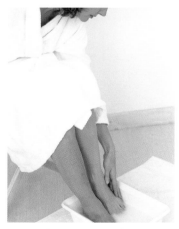

△ To nourish the skin add a handful of dried milk to a warm footbath and soak your feet for at least 15 minutes.

more likely. Prevention consists of wearing padded insoles, padding vulnerable areas of the feet and wearing well-fitting shoes. You can treat corns and calluses using over-the-counter medication.

Ingrown toenails occur when the toenail pierces the skin of the foot, and are most common on the big toes. This problem is usually caused by trimming the toenails in the wrong way. To prevent ingrown toenails, always cut the nail square across and level with the top of the toe. Never taper the sides of the nails or poke scissors or other implements underneath the nail. If you suspect that you have an ingrown toenail, visit a doctor or chiropodist (podiatrist).

Bunions are painful and severely retard mobility. They are caused by the overgrowth of bone tissue, and although the problem is often hereditary, it can be exacerbated by wearing ill-fitting shoes. A bunion is characterized by a swollen, tender big toe joint that protrudes from the foot. In mild cases, the bunion can be accommodated by wearing wide-fitting shoes or a protective pad on the toe joint. In severe cases, the foot can become misaligned and medical attention is necessary. Your doctor may recommend drug treatment or surgery.

Skin cracking around the heel becomes common with age. A self-help treatment is to soak your feet in warm water, then cover them with petroleum jelly, and put on a pair of cotton socks before going to bed. You can also alleviate dry skin by increasing the amount of essential fatty acids in your diet. Essential fatty acids are found in extra virgin olive oil, sunflower seeds and oily fish. You may also benefit from taking a vitamin E supplement or a tablespoon of linseed oil every day. If cracking is severe, dietary therapists may recommend taking 30mg of zinc twice a day over an eight-week period.

Even if you do not suffer from cracked skin, moisturize your feet after bathing. Skin on the foot is drier than elsewhere on the body, so try to use specially designed foot care products. If your feet sweat excessively, soak them in a bowl of warm water mixed with a handful of dried milk instead of applying moisturizer. Another useful remedy for dry, tired feet is a few drops of peppermint oil, added to some baby lotion and rubbed into the skin after bathing.

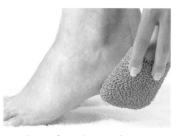

△ Regular use of a pumice stone after bathing can stop hard skin building up.

## looking after your feet

Babies are born with fat, padded feet, but as you grow and your bones form, the feet become leaner and more defined. As you age the padding on the feet lessens still further and the feet become wider. Because your feet change throughout life, it is essential to have your feet measured periodically so that you can buy shoes that fit correctly. Choose socks that are the right size for your feet and whenever you have the chance, go barefoot. Another aspect of good foot care is a regular visit to a chiropodist (podiatrist).

The following tips can help to maintain the health of the feet and prevent problems.
• Give yourself a foot massage using essential oils mixed with a base oil.
• Avoid exposure to cold temperatures.
• Make sure that your socks do not impede circulation.
• Avoid sitting with one leg crossed over the other.
• Promote circulation by flexing and pointing your toes and circling your ankles, especially if you sit still for long periods of time.
• Sit with your feet raised if possible.
• Treat your feet to a warm foot bath and apply a special foot moisturizer afterwards.

**FOOTCARE FOR DIABETICS**

The feet are particularly vulnerable to infection in people who suffer from diabetes (adult-onset diabetes becomes more common as you age). If you have diabetes, pay careful attention to foot care and consult your doctor about any foot problems, even minor ones such as corns and calluses. Avoid self-help treatment and visit a chiropodist regularly.

# Healthy hair

As we age our hair tends to get thinner and turn grey. These tangible signs of aging are ones that many people try to prevent or conceal. As a result we spend much time and money on styling, colouring, treating and transplanting hair. Ultimately, many age-related hair changes are hard to prevent because they are genetically controlled. But this does not prevent us from having hair that is healthy and attractive.

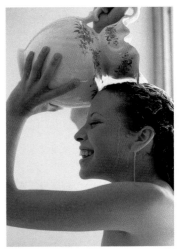

△ After shampooing, rinse your hair with warm water until the water runs clear and clean.

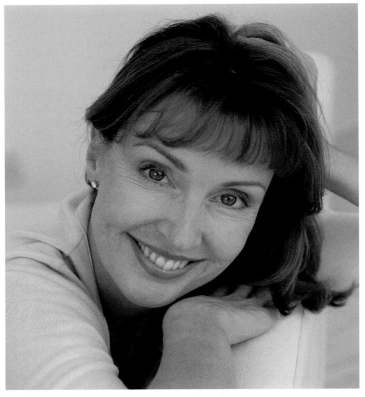

△ Having a fringe is flattering on older people as it can often soften their appearance as well as help to hide forehead lines.

## how the hair ages

On average we lose between 70 and 100 hairs per day. When we are young we replace these lost hairs with new ones but, as we grow older, hair loss speeds up and new growth slows down. Some hair follicles become sluggish and have long resting phases, other hair follicles appear to be completely deactivated. The result of these changes is fewer hairs and the overall appearance of thinning. Women may notice that their hair starts to thin out around the time of the menopause. However, if you suffer from sudden or severe hair loss, consult your doctor.

Men are prone to a particular type of hair thinning known as "male pattern baldness". This is distinct from age-related thinning and it is genetically controlled. Hair follicles that are affected by male pattern baldness start to produce a new type of hair known as a vellus hair. These are thin and delicate and they only grow to a short length. Because they are difficult to see, vellus hairs may give the impression of baldness. Eventually, true baldness occurs as the follicles die completely. Men can usually predict whether they will go bald simply by looking at older male members of their family. Although men may suffer from thinning and baldness of head hair, they may find that nasal and eyebrow hair begins to grow more vigorously with age.

Hair that turns grey does so because of the loss of a pigment called melanin. As a hair shaft is produced, the hair follicle secretes melanin giving hair its characteristic colour. As pigment cells start to die – but some melanin is still produced – the hair has a grey colour. When the pigment cells die completely, the hair is white. Unpigmented hair has a characteristic coarse, wiry texture. Many people start to develop grey hairs in their 30s and 40s and hair becomes progressively more grey with age.

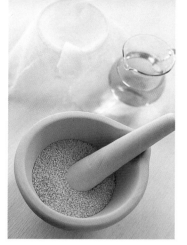

△ Use as few chemicals as possible, instead opt for natural products such as sesame conditioner.

## looking after your hair

The key to having attractive and healthy hair as you get older is to wear it in a style that suits you and to keep it in optimum condition. This does not mean buying expensive hair products; in fact, the major determinants of hair health are regular exercise, a well-balanced diet and adequate sleep.

• Grey hair can be concealed with temporary or permanent colouring. Choose a shade that is lighter than your original colour. You may need to experiment with different products – the way in which your hair responds to colorants depends on how porous your hair shafts are.

• To condition dry, brittle hair, boil 3 tablespoons of ground sesame seeds in a little water for 10 minutes, strain through muslin and allow to cool. Massage the mixture into the hair and leave for 10 minutes before rinsing thoroughly.

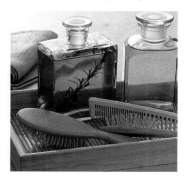

▷ Always gently comb conditioner through the hair to ensure it is evenly distributed and reaches as many hairs as possible.

• Aromatherapists recommend the following tonic to revitalize hair: mix 10 drops of cedarwood essential oil, 10 drops of juniper essential oil and 15 drops of rosemary essential oil in 50ml/2fl oz of surgical spirit (alcohol). Massage a small amount of this mixture into damp hair and leave to dry naturally. Wash your hands afterwards.

• Dietary therapists recommend eliminating coffee, tea and sugar from the diet in order to promote hair health. Useful nutrients include essential fatty acids for dry or brittle hair, zinc for poor hair growth and a general multivitamin and mineral supplement for overall hair health.

• Avoid drying out your hair using hot hair dryers or styling tools, and try not to use bleach – it strips the hair of natural oils. Use an intensive conditioning treatment on your hair once a month.

### MENOPAUSAL CHANGES TO HAIR

Oestrogen receptors are present in hair follicles and when oestrogen levels fall at the time of the menopause the growth and rest cycle of the hair is disrupted. Many women notice for the first time that their hair is thin, fine and difficult to style. This change is completely natural. Although you cannot reverse hormonally-related hair thinning (except with hormone replacement therapy) you can help to minimize hair loss by treating your hair gently. When you wash your hair, mix a mild shampoo with some water and then pour the mixture over your head. Leave it for a minute and then massage very gently and rinse off with warm water. Dab your hair rather than rubbing and comb with a wide-toothed comb. Leave your hair to dry naturally.

◁ Herbal hair rinses use natural ingredients to leave your hair shining and well conditioned.

▷ Comb wet hair with a wide-toothed comb to gently free any tangles.

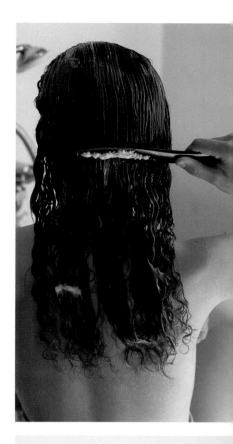

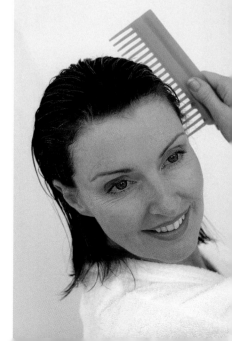

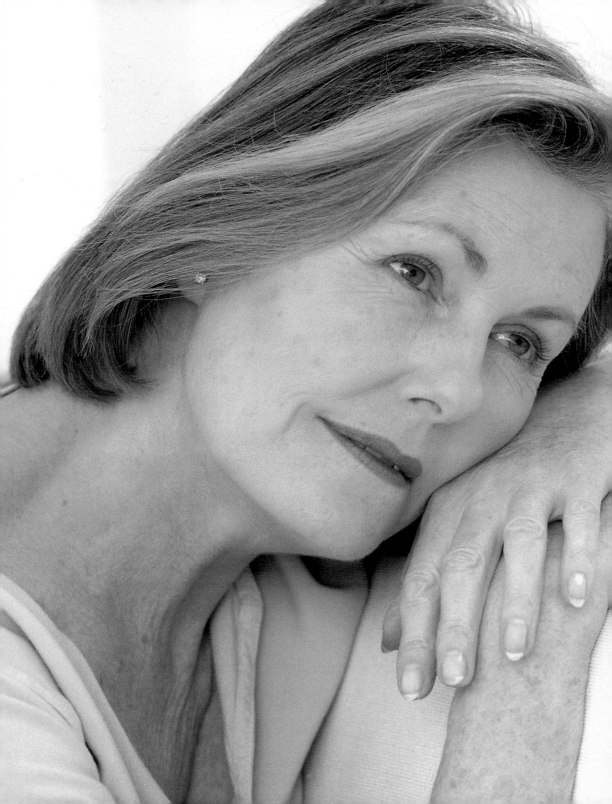

# Menopause

The menopause is the permanent cessation of the
menstrual cycle, bringing to a close the period of
life in which it was possible to bear children.
It usually occurs between the ages of 45 and 50,
although both early and late menopause are not
unusual. While the prospect of the menopause
may seem daunting, you should try to not
to worry unduly. You can reduce the
likelihood of suffering physical or
psychological problems by adopting a positive
attitude towards this new stage in your life.

# The changing menstrual cycle

To understand what happens during menopause, it is important to know about the sequence of finely tuned hormonal events that takes place in the normal menstrual cycle.

## the menstrual cycle

At the beginning of every menstrual cycle, a hormone is released from the brain called follicle-stimulating hormone (FSH). It stimulates the development of egg follicles in the ovary. As the follicles develop they produce the hormone oestrogen. One egg follicle eventually becomes dominant and releases an egg – a process known as ovulation – which travels down the fallopian tube. The follicle that produced the egg is left behind on the ovary where it starts to secrete the hormone progesterone.

As the egg travels down along the fallopian tube, the uterus, under hormonal direction, is preparing itself for a possible pregnancy. Oestrogen makes the uterine lining thicken and progesterone stimulates the growth of blood vessels so that the uterus is ready to receive a fertilized egg. If fertilization does not happen then the egg and uterine lining are simply shed from the body in a process known as menstruation.

In most healthy young women, the menstrual cycle takes place on a fairly regular basis – about every 28 days on

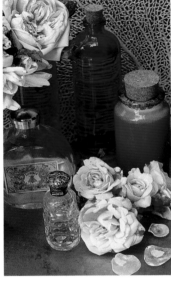

△ Irregular periods may be stabilized by adding 4 drops each of rose, camomile and melissa to a warm bath.

average. Several factors can change or disrupt the menstrual cycle, such as stress, illness, losing an excessive amount of weight or taking the contraceptive pill. The biggest changes, however, come with menopause.

## changes to the cycle

As women grow older the brain releases follicle-stimulating hormone (FSH) in the way that it always has done, but the ovary does not respond in the usual way. With age there are less follicles left in the ovary to be stimulated, and the ones that remain may be of insufficient quality to make it to ovulation. This has several results: the brain increases the amount of FSH to "force" the ovary to respond, the remaining follicles

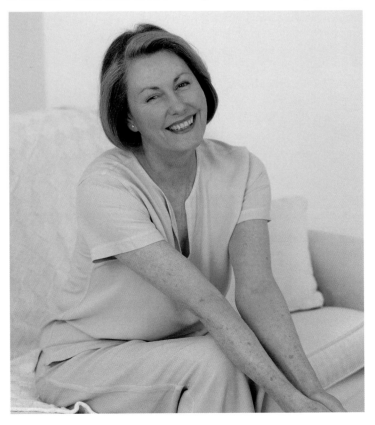

◁ The menopause usually occurs between the ages of 45 and 50, although both early and late menopause are not unusal.

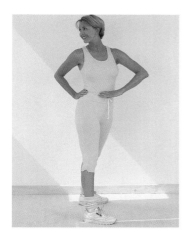

△ Regular exercise helps keep the body in balance by regulating body fluids and reducing fluid retention.

produce less oestrogen than normal and, if ovulation does not happen, no progesterone is secreted.

These are the kinds of disruptions that take place in the menstrual cycle during the build up to the menopause. Ultimately, oestrogen levels go into permanent decline and ovulation becomes erratic and ceases, causing progesterone production and periods to stop as well.

## the menopause timetable

Menopausal changes rarely happen suddenly. They usually take place over years. You may notice that your periods become more frequent and longer in duration. Or you may notice that your periods become infrequent with less blood loss than usual. Or you may alternate between both patterns. It is difficult to know what to expect. Some women skip periods for several months and then suddenly start menstruating again.

The word "menopause" refers to a single event rather than a series of ongoing changes: it is a woman's last ever menstrual period. This cannot be identified when it is happening – it can only be identified retrospectively. A more accurate word to describe the ongoing hormonal changes of midlife is the "perimenopause". Or some doctors use the word "climacteric". The postmenopause describes the years between the last period and the end of a woman's life.

• Premenopause: periods are still regular but symptoms may start to appear.
• Perimenopause: periods become unpredictable and symptoms may worsen.
• Postmenopause: periods stop permanently and, in time, the body adjusts to low hormone levels.

## the age of menopause

Most women become menopausal in their 40s and 50s. The average age of menopause is about 51 years, although perimenopausal signs may be apparent before this age. Premature menopause takes place before the age of 35 and delayed menopause takes place after the age of 55.

It is likely that, as individuals, we are biologically programmed to reach menopause at a certain age. There is no link between the age of menopause and age of first menstruation or first pregnancy. Taking

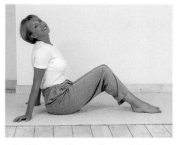

△ Practising relaxation exercises can help to harmonize your body and alleviate symptoms of the menopause.

the contraceptive pill is not thought to influence the age of menopause. The age at which your mother was menopausal may affect the age of your menopause, but this is not conclusive. Smoking and low body weight, however, have been found to bring on the menopause earlier.

▽ The more positive an outlook you have on life, the fewer physical and psychological problems are likely to occur at the time of the menopause.

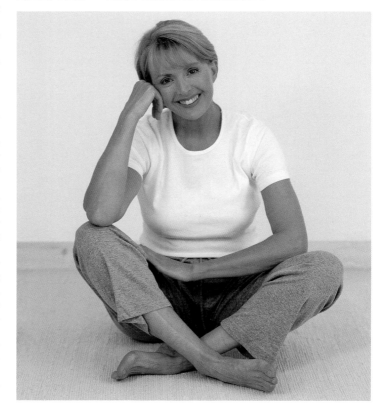

# Symptoms of the menopause

Although some women experience very few problems at menopause, others begin to experience an array of symptoms that affect both the body and mind. One of the main reasons for this is the fact that oestrogen influences many different body functions. In fact, special receptor cells for oestrogen are present all over the body and in the brain.

## why the menopause causes symptoms

Some experts have compared the symptoms of oestrogen decline to drug withdrawal: when supplies of oestrogen start to become erratic the body reacts negatively; if oestrogen levels are restored, the body gets its "fix" and returns to normal. Eventually, the body adapts to low oestrogen levels but this is something that may take years. Problems may also result from the fact that hormones released in the brain such as follicle stimulating hormone (FSH) can become unusually high.

Much research focuses on the importance of oestrogen but it is now thought that progesterone (or its absence) may also be important. After menopause, progesterone production stops completely whereas small amounts of oestrogen are still produced (fat cells produce oestrogen). This relative imbalance, coupled with progesterone deficiency, is thought to be a cause of troubling symptoms.

**WARNING SIGNS**

Menstrual upheavals are common around the time of the menopause but you should consult your doctor if you experience any of the following:
• Bleeding between periods
• Heavy bleeding with clots
• Bleeding after sex
• Bleeding following a year without periods

**COMMON SYMPTOMS**

Symptoms are many and varied as the hormone levels in the body fluctuate. Some of the most common symptoms are:
• Hot flushes and night sweats
• Palpitations
• Breast changes
• Mood swings
• Depression
• Poor memory
• Insomnia
• Tiredness
• Poor concentration
• Loss of sex drive
• Vaginal dryness
• Urinary problems
• Fluid retention
• Weight gain and shape change

▽ **Wearing cotton clothes, drinking iced water and using a battery-operated fan can help to ease the symptoms of hot flushes.**

## hot flushes and night sweats

The most easily identifiable symptoms of the menopause are hot flushes and night sweats. Blood rushes to the face, neck and chest and you become hot, flushed and sweaty. Afterwards you may feel very cold. This can happen very frequently, sometimes several times an hour. When it happens at night, you may wake up drenched in sweat and feeling hot and feverish. Self-help measures:
• Find effective ways of cooling down. Carry a battery-operated fan or an insulated flask of iced water with you.
• Wear cotton or other natural fibres.
• Wear clothes that can be unbuttoned at the neck.
• Keep a record of when you have hot flushes and see if you can recognize a pattern. Are there any specific triggers?
• Avoid spicy food, caffeine and alcohol.
• Learn to relax and practise creative visualization techniques.

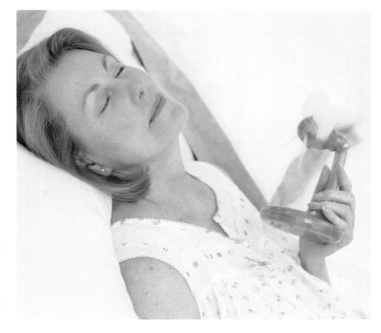

## palpitations

Many women experience palpitations at the same time as they have a hot flush. However, they can also appear independently of hot flushes. The heart feels as though it is racing or beating irregularly and some women feel as though they are having a panic attack. Self-help measures:
• Take a break and sit or lie down.
• Close your eyes, inhale deeply through your nose and take the breath down into your abdomen.
• Tell yourself that the feeling is temporary and will soon pass.

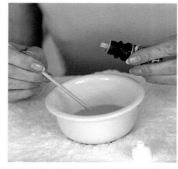

△ **Aromatherapists recommend the use of clary sage against hot flushes and night sweats.**

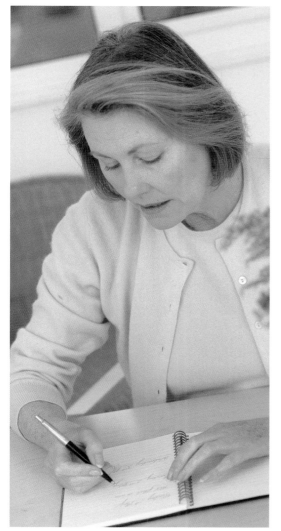

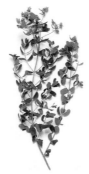

△ **St John's Wort, recommended for lifting depression and stabilizing mood swings, can be taken as a tea, a tincture or a supplement.**

◁ **Keep a diary of menopausal symptoms – there may be a pattern to hot flushes and palpitations.**

▷ **Creating a relaxing atmosphere can help to ease palpitations, mood swings and depression.**

## breast changes

The most common type of menopausal breast change is mastalgia. The breasts typically feel swollen, tender and painful to the touch. Self-help measures:
• Wear a good quality bra that supports your breasts. Wear a bra in bed if necessary.
• Cut down on the amount of saturated fat that you eat.

## mood swings and depression

Fluctuating hormone levels may give rise to emotional problems such as irritability, crying fits, angry outbursts and anxiety. This is because oestrogen receptors in the parts of the brain that control mood are deprived of oestrogen. Disrupted sleep due to night sweats may give rise to mood swings. Feeling tired all the time will lessen your ability to cope. Self-help measures:
• Seek the support of your friends, family and partner. Explain to them how you are feeling.
• Talk to other menopausal women about their feelings or read the experiences of others. Join a self-help group.
• Learn relaxation and mood-lifting techniques that work for you.
• Try taking flower remedies or herbal remedies such as St. John's wort or kava kava (stop if you experience any side effects and if you are taking prescribed medications, consult your doctor).

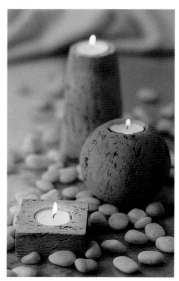

# More menopausal symptoms

## poor memory

Forgetfulness often becomes a problem around the time of menopause. You may find yourself missing appointments or forgetting where you put things. The hippocampus, the part of the brain that is associated with memory, contains oestrogen receptors and may be less efficient at storing information when oestrogen levels start to decline.

Self-help measures:

• Teach yourself to rely on diaries and lists. Keep exhaustive lists of everything that you need to remember.

• Keep a pen and a piece of paper by your bed and in your car.

• Highlight the most essential daily tasks that you must do. Tick them off at the end of the day.

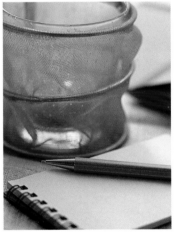

△ Keep a pen and paper beside the bed so that you can easily jot down important things that you remember during the night.

## insomnia

The inability to fall asleep, waking frequently during the night and waking up too early are all classified as signs of insomnia. Suffering from insomnia may be a menopausal symptom in its own right or it may be caused by night sweats.

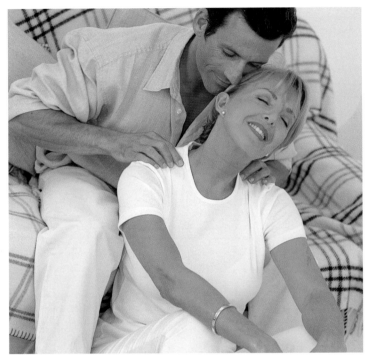

△ Massage relaxes the muscles and releases sleep-inducing chemicals in the brain.

## tiredness

Feeling sleepy, apathetic or fatigued during the day can exacerbate other menopausal symptoms such as poor memory and concentration. Muscle fatigue is common during the menopause. Self-help measures:

• Accept your limitations: if you feel tired, try to rest rather than keep going.

• Avoid artificial stimulants such as coffee, chocolate and alcohol.

• Practise good sleeping habits (see Looking after the body).

## poor concentration

Like poor memory, poor concentration is another cognitive deficit caused by declining or fluctuating levels of oestrogen in the body. Some people also find decision making more difficult than previously.

Self-help measures:

• Be lenient on yourself. Find out what your attention span is and work around it.

• Do not resign yourself to diminishing brain power. Stay mentally active.

## loss of sex drive

Women notice that their sex drive decreases or even disappears around the time of menopause. This may happen spontaneously or it may be the result of an underlying problem such as vaginal dryness, breast pain, tiredness or depression.

Self-help measures:

• Establish the underlying cause of the problem and, if possible, treat it.

• Remember that sex does not always have to be penetrative. Try being sexually intimate with a partner by cuddling or

giving each other a massage.
• Remember that postmenopausal women often experience renewed sexual interest.

## vaginal dryness

Declining levels of oestrogen cause the urogenital tract to become thin and dry. The vaginal tissues shrink and less lubrication is produced than previously. This can make sex difficult and painful. Menopausal women may also be prone to vaginal soreness and minor infection.
Self-help measures:
• Insert a vitamin E capsule into the vagina nightly for a month and then whenever you need to.
• Use a natural lubricating gel, such as aloe vera or comfrey cream.
• Spend longer on foreplay during sex – the vagina may just be slower to lubricate than before.
• You should try and remain sexually active, as this will keep your reproductive system in good shape.

## urinary problems

The urinary tract lies very close to the vagina and it also responds to declining oestrogen levels by becoming thin. The result of this may be discomfort on passing urine and frequent and urgent urination. Some women suffer from stress incontinence in which small amounts of urine escape from the body on laughing,

coughing or picking up a heavy object.
Self-help measures:
• Drink 2 litres/3¹/₂ pints of water a day to keep the bladder flushed out.
• Practise Kegel exercises. These involve tensing the pelvic floor muscles (those used to stop urination) for a count of five. Repeat throughout the day.

## fluid retention

A common feature of premenstrual syndrome, fluid retention, can become worse in the build-up to the menopause. You may feel bloated, swollen and heavy. If your weight fluctuates substantially, you should seek a professional diagnosis as you may have developed a food intolerance.
Self-help measures:
• Cut out salt, processed food and junk food.
• Eat foods that act as natural diuretics such as celery, parsley, chicory and dandelion.
• Avoid standing for long periods.
• Take plenty of exercise.

## weight gain and shape change

Many women find that they put on weight during the menopause due to a lowered metabolism and a change in the way that fat is deposited in the body. Long-term low oestrogen levels also cause the body to change shape. The waist-to-hip ratio alters so that the waist thickens and comes out to meet the hips.

Self-help measures:
• Avoid faddish diets and calorie restriction at the time of the menopause. You need calcium and all the other nutrients that a normal diet supplies.
• Use exercise to control your weight and increase muscle tone.

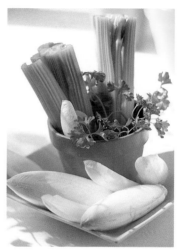

△ Natural diuretics such as celery, chicory, parsley and dandelion can help fight against fluid retention.

▽ Tightening and relaxing the muscles used to stop urination helps to prevent stress and incontinence.

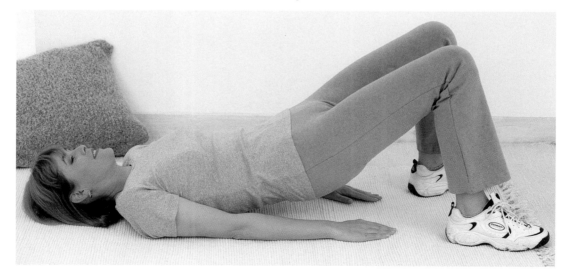

# hormone replacement therapy

Hormone replacement therapy (HRT) is a type of medication that is designed to return a menopausal women's hormone levels back to her premenopausal levels. Doctors often prescribe HRT to treat debilitating menopausal symptoms such as hot flushes, insomnia and depression. HRT may also have a role in protecting women against the long-term health problems that are most frequently associated with the postmenopause such as osteoporosis and cardiovascular disease.

## what is HRT?

HRT consists of the hormones oestrogen and progestogen (the synthetic form of progesterone). Oestrogen is widely considered to be the most important hormone in HRT; the role of progestogen is to induce a monthly bleed and to protect the uterus from cancer. Women who have had a hysterectomy may be prescribed oestrogen only.

The main advantage of HRT is that it may reverse many of the changes associated with menopause. This means that premenopausal body shape, skin and hair condition, sex drive and cardiovascular health can all be preserved and the classic menopausal symptoms are alleviated. The disadvantages are that women continue to bleed on a monthly basis (this is a withdrawal bleed rather than a proper period) and that HRT can cause side effects. HRT is also unsuitable for some women because of their medical history.

Some women feel that the menopause is medicalized in Western cultures and that taking medication during this time simply adds to the perception that the menopause is an illness or disease. This is a matter for debate: some people argue that women are suffering from a hormone deficiency disease that deserves medical treatment; others say that menopause is a natural rite of passage and the view that women are ill should not be encouraged.

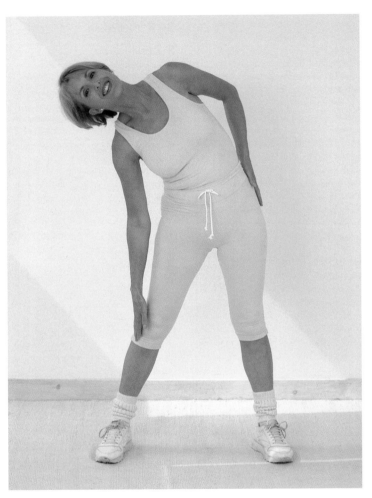

△ **Weight bearing exercise can help to prevent osteoporosis, as well as promote good circulation.**

## types of HRT

HRT is usually taken in pill form. The pills often come in calendar packs and you take one pill a day. All the pills usually contain oestrogen, whereas progestogen is only included in 10–14 pills in the latter half of the pill cycle.

Hormones can be absorbed through the skin and are available in the form of skin patches. The fact that hormones do not have to pass through the liver means that dosages are comparatively low and this may be an advantage for some women. The patches should be changed every three or four days.

HRT is also available in implant form. The implant is inserted under the skin in a minor surgical procedure carried out by your doctor. Although implants are convenient, in that you do not need to take pills or change patches, it is difficult to control the dosage. Localized symptoms of low oestrogen levels, such as vaginal dryness, may be treated with oestrogen cream or pessaries. However, this form of HRT does not ease other menopausal symptoms, such as hot flushes, and it does not have the long-term benefits of other types of HRT.

## the possible side effects

It may take the body a while to adjust to the hormones in HRT and some women find that they are troubled by side effects even after several months of taking hormones. There are lots of different types, products, doses and regimes in hormonal medication and, ideally, HRT should be tailored to suit every woman's individual needs. If you are taking HRT and you experience side effects, consult your doctor about trying a different brand or type of HRT or changing the dose or regime. It may be necessary for you to take HRT for at least four months before your body adapts.

Your doctor may decide that HRT is not appropriate for you if you have any of the following:
• High blood pressure
• Endometriosis (in which the lining of the uterus grows outside the uterus)
• Benign breast disease, such as cysts
• Benign uterus disease, such as fibroids
• A history of thrombosis
• Migraine
• Ovarian or uterine cancer
• Pancreatic disease
• Liver disease
• Recent cardiovascular disease
• Breast cancer or a family history of breast cancer.

Research shows that taking oestrogen and progestogen may be associated with an increased risk of breast cancer. This does not rule out taking HRT altogether but the risks and benefits for each woman need to be assessed carefully by a doctor.

▷ **You should discuss any menopausal symptoms with your doctor to make sure that you receive the advice and treatment that you require during the menopause.**

**SIDE EFFECTS OF HRT**
Some women may find that they suffer from side effects while taking HRT. These side effects may include:
• Headaches
• Nausea
• Impaired eyesight
• Breathlessness
• Premenstrual syndrome
• Heavy or irregular bleeding
• Breast tenderness
• Skin problems such as acne and itchiness
• Weight gain
• An increased or decreased sexual drive
• Muscular pains and backache

▷ **Some women find HRT patches more beneficial than tablets. Since the hormone does not have to travel through the liver, side effects are reduced.**

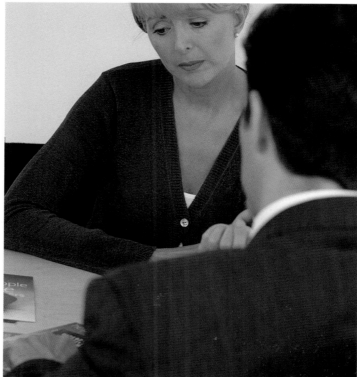

# Natural alternatives to HRT

More and more women are turning to complementary therapies to help them through the menopausal years. A range of therapies offer gentle but effective ways to overcome symptoms and increase overall well-being. Although many therapies can be practised safely in the home, it can be helpful to seek the guidance of a therapist, at least in the first instance.

## herbalism

There are many herbal treatments for menopausal symptoms and the best advice is to visit a medical herbalist who will tailor treatments to your individual needs. Herbal remedies come in a variety of forms including infusions, decoctions and tinctures – these can be made with fresh or dried herbs. There are also many commercial herbal supplements in the form of pills or capsules that are available in health food shops or some pharmacies.

Herbs that contain oestrogen-like substances – known as phyto-oestrogens – may compensate for declining oestrogen levels at menopause and ease many menopausal symptoms. Such herbs include panax ginseng, black cohosh, dong quai, alfalfa, liquorice and red clover. Remedies that are recommended for specific menopausal symptoms are as follows:
• Hot flushes and night sweats: agnus castus, sage, yarrow, motherwort
• Poor memory or concentration: ginkgo biloba
• Depression: St John's wort
• Anxiety: vervain
• Breast pain and pre-menstrual syndrome: evening primrose oil
• Insomnia: valerian, passionflower

Stop taking herbs if you experience any side effects. Consult your doctor before taking herbs if you suffer from high blood pressure or cardiovascular disease.

## aromatherapy

The essential oils that are therapeutic at the menopause include sage, camomile, geranium, rose, jasmine, neroli, ylang ylang, bergamot and sandalwood. You can use these essential oils in the bath, in a massage (mixed with a base oil), you can burn them in an aromatherapy burner or you can put a few drops on a tissue or a pillow. Sage essential oil is thought to be good for hot flushes and ylang ylang is recommended for reviving the libido.

## flower remedies

There is a wide choice of flower remedies available and you do not need to consult an expert before taking them. There is a range of flower remedies to suit various emotions and you can combine remedies to achieve the mixture that is right for your specific emotional symptoms.

## homeopathy

A homeopath can assess your symptoms and choose the most suitable remedy and potency for you. Health food shops and some pharmacies also sell a standard range of homeopathic remedies. The remedies that are most frequently recommended for menopausal symptoms are as follows:
• Hot flushes: Lachesis, Sepia, Belladonna
• Breast pain: Bryonia
• Mood swings and irritability: Lachesis, Sepia, Pulsatilla
• Insomnia: Pulsatilla
• Premenstrual syndrome: Bryonia, Pulsatilla
• Vaginal dryness: Sepia, Natrum muriaticum

## traditional Chinese medicine

Practitioners of Chinese medicine aim to restore the flow of energy, or Qi, through the body using acupuncture, acupressure and Chinese herbalism. Both herbs and acupuncture may be recommended for hot flushes. Always consult a registered doctor of Chinese medicine.

## massage

Receiving massage can have a relaxing and therapeutic effect on both the mind and the body. If possible, visit a massage therapist and explain your symptoms. Regular massage can help to relieve insomnia, anxiety, depression and muscle and joint pain.

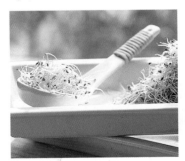
△ Sprinkle alfalfa shoots onto salads for a tasty and nutritious source of phyto-oestrogens.

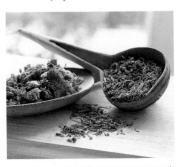
△ The storage methods for herbs can vary greatly so always read the instructions carefully.

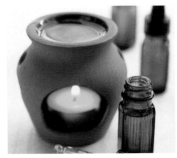
△ Essential oils, such as sandalwood, clary sage, or camomile, can have an uplifting effect.

## yoga

A core benefit of yoga during the menopause is that it teaches you relaxation techniques that you can use at any time in your day-to-day life. The practice of breathing techniques (pranayama) can still the mind and relieve stress and anxiety. Meditation can also be of great benefit. The physical postures of yoga (asanas) can help to maintain flexibility and strength in the joints and muscles and bring balance to the body and mind. If possible, join a class and learn yoga from an experienced teacher.

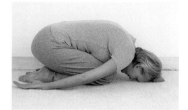

△ **This yoga position, known as the Child's pose, is an excellent relaxer for the body and mind.**

## dietary therapy

Research suggests that Asian women do not suffer as badly as Western women from menopausal problems and this is believed to be due to their soya-based diet, rich in phyto-oestrogens and calcium. It is worth experimenting by drinking two glasses of soya milk per day for a period of a month to see if you experience a lessening of symptoms. Other foodstuffs rich in phyto-oestrogens include oats, barley, wild rice, brown rice, wholewheat, celery (which is also useful against fluid retention), sprouts and green beans. Recommended supplements during menopause include evening primrose oil, vitamin C with bioflavonoids, vitamin E, and a general multivitamin and mineral supplement.

It is advisable to avoid the following in your diet around the time of the menopause:
• Caffeine
• Hot spicy foods
• Alcohol
• High sugar consumption
• High salt consumption
• High animal fat consumption
• Bran-based foods that may strip the body of nutrients such as calcium.

**"NATURAL HRT" CAKE (7 DAY SUPPLY)**
The following recipe for a natural HRT cake contains ingredients that are rich in phyto-oestrogens and vitamin E. It is low in fat and high in fibre and may help to alleviate symptoms of the menopause.
115g/4oz soya flour
115g/4oz wholewheat flour
115g/4oz porridge oats
5cm/2in chopped stem ginger
2.5ml/¹/₂ tsp ground ginger
2.5ml/¹/₂ tsp nutmeg
2.5ml/¹/₂ tsp cinnamon
200g/7oz raisins
115g/4oz linseeds
50g/2oz sunflower seeds
50g/2oz sesame seeds
50g/2oz sliced almonds
15ml/1tbsp malt extract
600ml/1pint soya milk

Sift the flour and add all the dry ingredients. Mix well before slowly adding the milk and malt extract. Cover and leave to soak for an hour. Spoon mixture into a cake tin lined with waxed paper and bake for up to 75 minutes on 190°C/370°F/gas 5. Allow to cool and eat one slice per day.

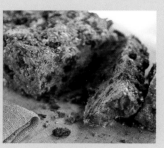

△ **Store your HRT cake in an airtight container, and eat within seven days.**

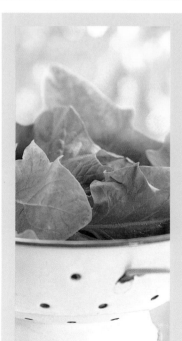

△ **You should always wash fresh fruit and vegetables thoroughly before eating in order to rinse off any traces of pesticides.**

**ESSENTIAL NUTRIENT GUIDE FOR THE MENOPAUSE**
Take plenty of the following:
• Phyto-oestrogens: replace your usual milk and flour with soya milk and flour.
• Selenium-rich foods: wheatgerm, wheatbran, tuna, tomatoes and onions.
• Vitamin E-rich foods: sunflower oil, sun-dried tomatoes, seeds, almonds, unsalted peanuts, leafy green vegetables and eggs.
• Calcium-rich foods: tofu, cheese, leafy green vegetables, root vegetables, nuts and salmon.
• Magnesium-rich foods: brown rice, nuts, wholegrains and legumes.
• Potassium-rich foods: avocados, leafy green vegetables, bananas, nuts and potatoes.
• Zinc-rich foods: meat, mushrooms, eggs, wholegrains, nuts and seeds.
• Foods rich in vitamin B-complex: wholegrains, brown rice, milk, cereals, leafy green vegetables, fish, meat, eggs, avocados, seeds and yogurt.
• Vitamin D-rich foods: oily fish such as sardines, mackerel and tuna (vitamin D can also be obtained from exposure to bright sunlight).
• Water, juices and herbal teas to keep the body sufficiently hydrated.

# Health checks

You should start to have regular health checks in middle age. Some, such as blood pressure tests, may be practised routinely by your doctor as you get older. Others, such as bone density scans, are specialized tests that may be performed if you are thought to be at particular risk of disease.

## self checks

As you approach the menopause, keeping a diary of your periods and any physical and emotional symptoms you experience enables you to look for patterns and develop coping strategies. This information is also useful to your doctor. You should also perform a breast self-examination once a month and weigh yourself on a weekly basis to check that you are not gaining weight. If you are, you can take steps to lose it quickly.

## blood cholesterol tests

Testing the blood for cholesterol is one way to assess your vulnerability to cardiovascular disease. If your blood cholesterol is too high, you can try to reduce it by making dietary changes. Blood cholesterol checks can be carried out by your doctor or it is possible to buy home-test kits.

## blood pressure checks

Checking your blood pressure is a routine test that most doctors will carry out at regular intervals as you grow older. If your blood pressure is too high, you can try to reduce it through dietary changes, or your doctor may prescribe medication.

## bone density scans

Postmenopausal women become more vulnerable to osteoporosis as they get older. Although it is not a routine health check, the best way to gain a picture of bone health is a specialized type of x-ray, known as a bone density scan. If you have already been diagnosed with osteoporosis, doctors may recommend bone density scans to assess the efficacy of any treatment you are having.

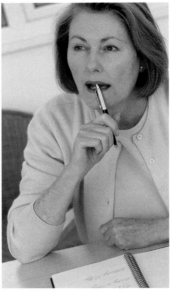

△ **By keeping a diary of health changes you may be able to give your doctor valuable information should their help be required.**

## cervical smear tests

Cancer of the cervix affects younger women more than older women but, nevertheless, the cervical smear test remains an important diagnostic tool. It can show up precancerous changes in the cervix in women of all ages and action can be taken to prevent the cancer developing. You should have a cervical smear test every two or three years; more frequently if you have a history of genital warts.

If any abnormalities are detected during a cervical smear test, a doctor may perform a colposcopy. This is a technique that permits close-up inspection of the cervix at a microscopic level.

## electrocardiograms

An electrocardiogram (ECG) is a specialized test that may be performed if your doctor suspects heart problems.

Electrodes applied to your body transmit electrical signals to a monitor. The signals appear as a trace on the monitor screen and provide detailed information about the contractions of the heart muscle.

## eye tests

Because you become more susceptible to eye problems as you get older, it is important for you to visit an ophthalmologist annually. Eyesight problems can have serious repercussions with age and, when combined with weak bones, can increase the chances of falls and fractures.

## hormone level tests

Testing the blood for the presence of elevated hormone levels can provide valuable information about the stage you are at in the menopause. For example, when the aging ovary fails to respond to follicle-stimulating hormone (FSH) the brain responds by releasing higher-than-usual amounts of FSH into the bloodstream. Hormone level tests are most likely to be performed by a gynaecologist.

## mammography

The cure rate for breast cancer depends on the stage at which it is detected and whether or not it has spread. Mammography makes the early detection of breast cancer possible by providing an x-ray-type image that shows up changes in breast tissue. Mammograms are recommended every two years from the age of 45 (earlier if you have a family history of breast cancer).

## other tests

There are other tests that your doctor may perform based on your individual medical history and current health. Both adult-onset diabetes and ovarian cancer, for example, can be detected by a blood test. You should try to keep abreast of the health tests that are available and ask your doctor about them.

▽ Weighing yourself once a week, at the same time of day, not only checks against weight gain, but also detects weight loss which can be an early sign of some illnesses.

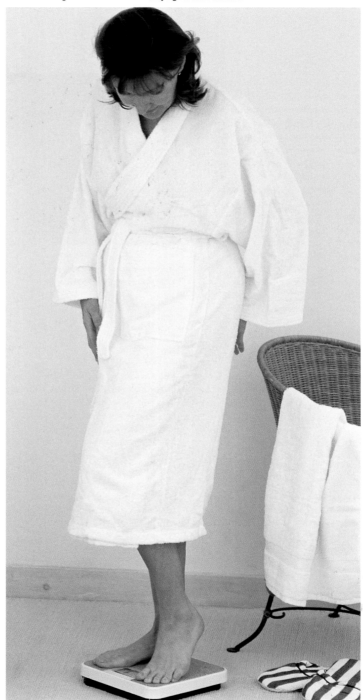

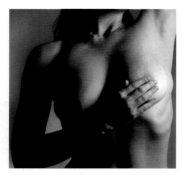

△ **By performing breast examinations once a month, at the same point of the menstrual cycle, you will be able to detect any changes in the tissue at an early stage.**

## breast self-examination

It is important that you examine your breasts regularly, once a month at the end of your cycle if you are still menstruating, and at any time if you have ceased menstruation. Standing in front of a mirror, look for any changes in shape or texture of the breast tissue or around the nipples. Do this first with your arms by your sides and then with your hands raised behind you head.

Lie on your back with your shoulders slightly raised. With the fingers of your right hand gently examine your left breast in widening circles from the nipple outwards. Then, using your left hand, repeat the examination on your right breast. Finally, raise each arm behind your head in turn and check the armpits.

Consult your doctor if you notice any unusual lumps, dimples, nipple discharge, or the inversion of a previously normal nipple.

### COMPLEMENTARY HEALTH

Practitioners of complementary health use a variety of diagnostic tools and techniques to assess health and detect illness. Some are the same as those used by conventional medical practitioners, others may be less familiar. For example, naturopaths use x-rays and blood tests in the diagnostic process. Practitioners of Chinese medicine are more likely to look at the colour of your skin, the colour and coating of your tongue and feel the rhythm and strength of the pulses at the wrists.

# Herbs for health

Most people are familiar with herbs that are commonly used in cooking, such as basil, bay, chives, mint, oregano, parsley, sage and thyme. But taking into account the broader definition of the term "herb", one can include plants such as aloe vera, spices such as ginger, flowers such as marigolds and roses, and fruits such as lemons and rose-hips.

As well as adding aroma and delicious flavour to food, culinary herbs have some nutritional value, often containing appreciable amounts of vitamins, minerals and trace elements. Adding herbs to your food on a daily basis actively promotes good health. Many herbs have excellent digestive qualities, helping the body to process and eliminate oily, fatty or gas-producing foods. But adding a generous sprinkling of fresh or dried herbs to your food is not the only way to benefit from these versatile plants.

## herbal medicine

Many herbs have a therapeutic and medicinal value and can be taken in a variety of forms to prevent and cure illness and to promote health. Taken internally they can be made into herbal teas, decoctions, tinctures and inhalations. Externally they can be applied as compresses, poultices, ointments, creams or infused oils. Herbs add

▽ Pot marigolds, dried in the summer when they are plentiful, can be made into healing salves and ointments.

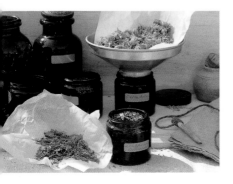

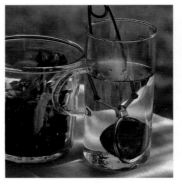

△ A tea infuser, available from health or cookware stores, is a useful gadget for making a single cup of tea from dried herbs.

their aroma to bath water for a therapeutic soak and essential oils distilled from the flowers can be used for a massage.

## harvesting herbs

The best time to harvest the arial parts of herbs is after their flower buds have formed but before they are in full bloom. Roots should be dug up in the autumn, cleaned and chopped into small pieces. Never pick herbs without being able to correctly identify them, or pick so many that you reduce next year's growth.

Spread the herbs out to dry in an airy position out of direct sunlight – an airing cupboard is an ideal place. Leafy bunches can be tied into little bundles and hung up. Spread flower heads on tissue or newspaper and dry them flat. It can take a week for them to dry. The volatile oils in herbs start to deteriorate quickly once the herbs are put in the light. Store dried herbs in separate, airtight containers away from the light and they will keep for up to six months.

## herbal teas

Herbal infusions make wonderfully refreshing drinks and can be drunk as caffeine-free alternatives to ordinary tea and coffee. Herbal teas can be taken to help ward

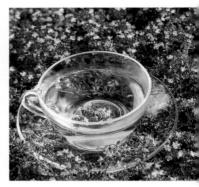

△ The antiseptic and antibacterial properties of thyme make it a first-choice tea for sore throats, colds and chest infections.

off colds and flu, to aid digestion, promote sleep, to relieve headaches, anxiety and stress, even to promote energy.

To make a herbal infusion, allow 30ml/ 2 tbsp fresh or 15ml/1 tbsp dried herb to each 600ml/1 pint/2½ cups water. For a single cup (250ml/8fl oz), use two small sprigs of fresh or 5ml/1 tsp dried herb. If you are using fresh herbs, wash them first, especially if they have been picked from the wild. Put the herbs into a warmed pot. Pour on boiling water. Replace the lid to prevent vapour dissipation. Leave to brew for three or four minutes, then strain the tea into a cup for a refreshing drink.

Drink a cupful of the appropriate tea no more than three times a day, and for sleep disturbances, drink a cup before going to bed. Teas can be stored for up to 24 hours in the refrigerator. Herb teas can be sweetened with honey to taste, but never add milk.

**CAUTION**

Herbs are powerful and can be harmful if taken in excess. Do not make teas stronger or drink them more frequently than recommended. Seek medical advice before taking herbal remedies when pregnant.

# Herbal tea remedies

| HERB | TREATMENT |
|---|---|

## Teas for coughs and colds

**Horehound**
*Marrubium vulgare*

chesty cold.

Make with the fresh or dried herb. Sweeten to taste with honey and add a dash of lemon juice. Take it for a

**Purple Sage and Thyme**
*Salvia officinalis* and *Thymus vulgaris*

Use in equal quantities in a tea to ease a sore throat. For a more powerful effect, add 1.5ml/¼ tsp cayenne pepper, which has antibacterial properties.

**Peppermint, Elderflower, Chamomile and Lavender** *Mentha x piperita, Sambucus nigra, Chamaemelum nobile* and *Lavandula officinalis*

At the onset of a cold, use 2.5ml/½ tsp of each of the first three, with a pinch of lavender, per cupful of water. Add a sprinkling of ground ginger, 5ml/1 tsp honey and a slice of lemon.

**Hyssop**
*Hyssopus officinalis*

For a cough, use the fresh or dried leaf, or the leaf and flowers. Hyssop is quite bitter, so sweeten this tea with honey and a little freshly squeezed orange juice, which adds valuable vitamin C.

**Thyme** *Thymus vulgaris*

Its antiseptic properties are good for chest infections. use 5ml/1 tsp dried thyme, or 10ml/2 tsp fresh, per cup. It has a warming effect and can also be used for digestive problems and stomach chills.

## Teas for digestive troubles

**Chamomile**
*Chamaemelum nobile*

For digestive upsets, brew tea from the dried flowers. For a change, substitute half the chamomile for dried peppermint.

**Peppermint and Lemon Balm** *Mentha x piperita* and *Melissa officinalis*

Use fresh herbs in equal quantities for a pleasantly flavoured digestive tea to drink after a meal.

**Fennel Seed**
*Foeniculum vulgare*

For flatulence and indigestion. Crush the seeds and simmer in an enamel saucepan for 10 minutes before straining. This is also a traditional slimming aid and can help relieve hunger pangs. Caraway seeds can be prepared in the same way.

▷ **Limeflowers and elderflowers have a gentle soporific action as a nighttime drink. Sweeten with honey to taste.**

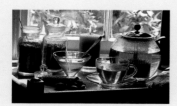

## Teas as tonics

**Stinging Nettles**
*Urtica Dioica*

A tonic tea to cleanse the system. It may also help alleviate rheumatism and arthritic pains. Chop up a small handful of young, fresh nettle leaves and infuse in 600ml/1 pint/2½ cups boiling water before straining.

**Spearmint** *Mentha spicata*

The tea has a zingy, uplifting taste. Use 15ml/1 tbsp chopped, fresh leaves per cup and sweeten to taste.

**Basil** *Ocimum basilicum var. album*

Calming to the nervous system, it also helps relieve nausea. Add 3–4 fresh leaves per cup.

## Teas for disturbed sleep

**Chamomile**
*Chamaemelum nobile*

One of the best bedtime drinks for those who have difficulty getting to sleep. It is calming to the nervous system, as well as a digestive. Make it with 5ml/1 tsp dried chamomile to a cup and try adding a pinch of lavender for extra relaxation.

**Limeflower and elderflower** *Citrus aurantiifolia* and *Sambucus nigra*

A pleasant bedtime tea. Add a dash of grated nutmeg and sweeten with honey.

**Valerian**
*Valeriana officinalis*

Use the dried and shredded root for a tea to calm the nerves. Using 10ml/1 tsp to a cup of water, simmer gently for 20 minutes in an enamel pan with a lid. Let it cool, then strain, re-heat and drink.

## Teas for headaches, anxiety and depression

**Rosemary**
*Rosmarinus officinalis*

One of the more pleasant tasting teas when made with the fresh herb. Put one or two small sprigs per person into a teapot or cup and add boiling water. Rosemary is invigorating and refreshing. It clears the head and helps to ease headaches. Add a few betony leaves to relieve nervous tension if you prefer.

**Lemon Balm**
*Melissa Officinalis*

For tea, always use the freshly gathered herb. It has a long tradition as an anti-depressant.

**St John's Wort**
*Hypericum perforatum*

Use fresh or dried leaves and flowers. It helps to relieve nervous tension, anxiety and depression.

# Herbal beauty treatments

Many of the old herbals included advice on using herbs for beauty, and making prefumed preparations was part of the apothecary's art. The following recipes are not solely cosmetic but are directed towards therapeutic beauty treatments and will promote general health through an enhanced sense of well-being.

## dry skin moisturizer

Moisturizing cream prevents dryness of the skin, keeps wrinkles at bay and protects your skin from the weather. If you prefer, substitute dried elderflowers for the pot marigolds. Splash a little tonic on to your face first to feel refreshed.

### ingredients

- 120ml/4fl oz/ ½ cup water
- 20ml/4 tsp fresh or 10ml/2 tsp dried marigold petals
- 30ml/2 tbsp emulsifying ointment
- 5ml/1 tsp beeswax
- 30ml/2 tbsp almond oil
- 2.5ml/ ½ tsp borax

Boil the water and pour over the dried marigold petals in a jar. Leave to stand for 30 minutes then strain.

Put the emulsifying ointment, beeswax and almond oil into one bowl and the

▽ **Pot marigolds are recognized for their ability to soothe all manner of skin irritations.**

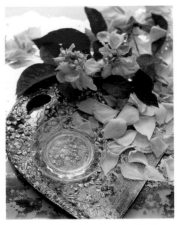

△ **There can be few pleasanter ways of dealing with stress and anxiety than sitting back and breathing in the therapeutic fragrance of essential oils.**

elderflower infusion and borax into another. Set both over hot water and stir until the oils melt and the borax dissolves.

Remove from the heat and pour the elderflower mixture into the oils. Stir gently until incorporated. Leave to cool, stirring at intervals. Pour into a jar before it sets.

## Rose petal toner

Infusions of flowers and herbs make excellent skin toners. Apply with cotton wool (cotton balls) after removing a face mask or make-up, or use at any time to freshen the skin. These toners must be kept chilled and used up within a few days as they

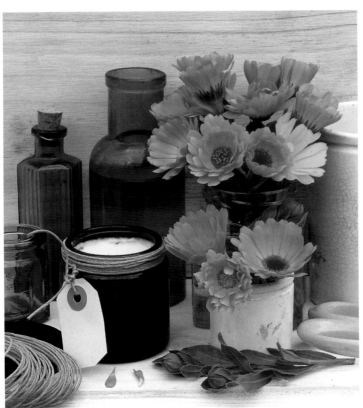

**CAUTION**

Be aware that herbs are a potent source of medicine, containing essential oils and potentially therapeutic properties that can be harmful if misused, or used in larger quantities than specified. Pregnant women should avoid all kinds of herbal remedies unless under professional supervision.

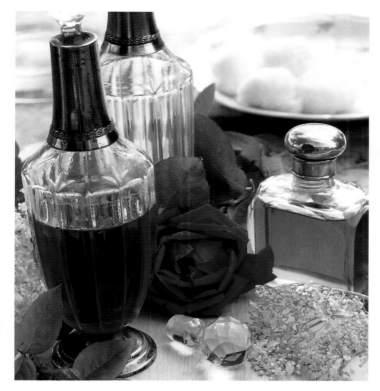

△ Use dark red roses for the best colour.

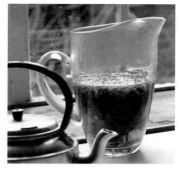

▽ A herbal foot bath restores and revitalizes the whole body.

cover both head and basin with a towel for about 30 seconds. Take a short break and then repeat two or three times.

## herbal foot bath

There is nothing like a fragrant foot bath for refreshing tired feet. At the same time, it revitalizes the whole being, its warmth relaxes the body and the scent of the herbs calms the mind. Foot baths are also comforting if you have a cold.

### ingredients

- 50g/2oz mixed fresh herbs: peppermint, yarrow, pine needles, chamomile flowers, rosemary, houseleek
- 1 litre/1¾ pints/4 cups boiling water
- 15ml/1 tbsp borax
- 15ml/1 tbsp Epsom salts

Roughly chop the herbs, put them in a large bowl and pour in the boiling water. Leave to stand for 1 hour. Strain, and add to a basin containing about 1.75 litres/3 pints/7½ cups hot water – the final temperature of the foot bath should be comfortably warm. Stir in the borax and Epsom salts. Immerse the feet and soak for 15–20 minutes.

---

**VARIATION**

For a quick alternative foot bath, instead of making an infusion float fresh chamomile flowers and leaves in hot water. You could also use mint, marjoram, marigolds or rose petals. Or, for extra fragrance, try adding a few drops of an essential oil such as lavender to the water.

---

soon deteriorate. Any fragrant roses are suitable for this recipe, as long as they have not been sprayed with pesticide. Pink or red ones are best.

### ingredients

- 40g/1½oz fresh rose petals
- 600ml/1 pint/2½ cups boiling water
- 15ml/1 tbsp cider vinegar

▽ A steam treatment relaxes and softens the skin. Make it with an infusion of dried herbs, or simply float fresh herbs in boiling water.

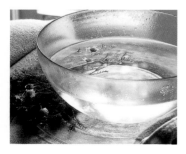

Put the rose petals in a bowl, pour over the boiling water and add the vinegar. Cover and leave to stand for 2 hours, then strain into a clean bottle.

## chamomile steam facial

An occasional facial steam treatment deep cleans the skin. The heat relaxes the pores and boosts blood circulation. With the addition of herbs, the stimulating and cleansing action of the steam is increased. Always close the pores afterwards by dabbing with a cooled skin toner appropriate to your skin type or by using a face mask. Steam facials should be avoided by those with a tendency to thread veins.

### ingredients

- 40g/1½oz fresh or 15g/ ½oz dried chamomile flowers
- 600ml/1 pint/2½ cups boiling water

Make a strong infusion of the fresh or dried flowers in boiling water. Leave to stand for 30 minutes, then strain. Re-heat the infusion, pour into a bowl and, keeping your face about 30cm/12in above the steam,

# glossary

*agni* fire, transformative force that drives metabolic processes such as digestion.

*akhrot* walnut.

*ama* a toxin that can be formed by both physical and non-physical causes, such as indigestible food or painful experiences.

*amla/amala/amalaki* the Indian gooseberry (*Emblica officinalis*).

*analgesic* reduces sensitivity to pain.

*anaphrodisiac* diminishes sexual drive.

*antiallergic* reduces sensitivity to various substances.

*anticoagulant* agent which stops blood from clotting.

*antidiabetic* prevents the development of diabetes.

*antifungal* prevents the development of fungus.

*antilactogenic* prevents or slows down the secretion of milk in nursing mothers.

*antimigraine* reduces or prevents migraines.

*antiparasitic* prevents the development of parasites.

*antipruritic* prevents itching.

*antipyretic* counteracts inflammation or fever.

*antisclerotic* anti-aging; prevents hardening of tissues.

*antiseptic* prevents the development of bacteria.

*antispasmodic* prevents muscle spasm, convulsion.

*antitussive* relieves or prevents coughing.

*antiviral* prevents the development of viruses.

*arjun/arjuna* extract from the bark of the arjun tree (*Terminalia arjuna*).

*aromatology* the study of essential oils for health, including intensive and internal use.

*astringent* causes contraction of living tissue.

*badam* almond.

*baingan* aubergine, eggplant or brinjal.

*balsamic* fragrant substance that softens phlegm.

*besan* chickpea or gram flour.

*bhasmas* medicines traditionally made from precious stones.

*bibhitaki* extract from the fruit of the beleric myrobalan tree (*Terminalia belerica*).

*bindi* decorative mark worn on the forehead.

*brahmi* oil infused with the Indian herb gotu kola (*Centella asiatica*).

*capillary dilator* dilates the capillaries, aids circulation.

*cardiotonic* has a tonic effect on the heart.

*carminative* relieves flatulence (wind).

*chemotype* visually identical plants with significantly different chemical components

and properties, e.g. *Thymus vulgaris* phenol and alcohol chemotypes.

*choleretic* stimulages bile production in the liver.

*cicatrizant* healing; promotes scar tissue

*dalchini* cinnamon.

*depurative* purifying or cleansing.

*dhania* coriander or cilantro.

*diaphoretic* *see* sudorific.

*dinacharya* the Ayurvedic daily routine.

*diuretic* promotes the secretion of urine.

*diya* traditional ghee-burning lamp with a cotton wick.

*emmenagogic* induces or regularizes menstruation.

*febrifuge* reduces temperature, antipyretic.

*fixed oil* non-volatile vegetable oil.

*gram flour* chickpea flour or besan.

*gulab* rose petals.

*gunas* sattva, rajas and tamas, the three inner qualities of all things.

*haritaki* extract from the fruit of the Indian gall nut (*Terminalia chebula*).

*hatha yoga* the physical exercises that form a part of yoga.

*hypertensor* increases blood pressure in hypotensive person.

*hypotensor* reduces blood pressure in hypertensive person.

*kapha* dosha representing earth and water.

*karma* the result of our actions in this and previous lives.

*kesar* saffron.

*kokum* a sour fruit native to the west coast of southern India, usually available dried.

*lactogen* promotes the secretion of milk.

*litholytic* breaks down sand or small kidney or urinary stones.

*lypolytic* breaks down fat.

*maceration* the extraction of components from plants by steeping in fixed oil.

*mahabhutas* the five "great elements": earth, water, fire, air and ether (space).

*manjishtha/manjista* extract from the root of Indian madder (*Rubia cordifolia*).

*margosa* *see* neem.

*marma point* place where two kinds of bodily tissue or two different energies meet; prana may become blocked at these points.

*mehendi* the art of painting the hands and feet with henna.

*methi* fenugreek.

*mucolytic* breaks down mucus and catarrh.

*multani mitti/mati* fuller's earth.

*neem* Indian tree (*Azadirachta indica*), also known as margosa; all parts are used therapeutically.

*neurotonic* stimulates and tones the nervous system.

*oestrogenic* stimulates the action of the female hormone, oestrogen.

*ojas* the substance that holds body, mind and spiritual levels together.

*panchakarma* detoxifying procedure that may include enemas and nasal washes.

*phlebotonic* improves or stimulates lymph circulation; lymph tonic.

*pitta* the dosha representing fire and water.

*prakruti* the constitution at birth, with all the doshas present in the right balance.

*purvakarma* preparatory treatments before panchakarma, including steam baths and herbal oil massages.

*rasayana* treatments aimed at rejuvenation or regeneration.

*rubefacient* increases local blood circulation causing redness of the skin.

*shatavari* extract from the tuber of wild asparagus (*Asparagus recemosus*).

*shikakai* Indian soap nut; the ground pods of *Acacia concinna*, used to treat the hair.

*shodhana* the full detoxifying process, including purvakarma and panchakarma.

*sindoor* vermilion powder applied to a woman's hair parting during her wedding.

*stomachic* stimulates secretory activity in the stomach.

*styptic* arrests haemorrhage by means of astringent quality; haemostatic.

*sudorific* induces or increases perspiration.

*swedana* sweat therapy.

*tadrak* ginger.

*tamas/the tamasic state* the lowest state of mind: greedy, selfish, violent and dull.

*triphala* blend of three herbs, amla, haritaki and bibhitaki, to balance the doshas.

*tulsi/tulasi* holy basil (*Ocimum sanctum*).

*ubtan* a powder used for skin cleansing.

*vasodilator* causes blood vessels to increase in lumen (the hollow inside of the blood vessel)

*vata* the dosha representing space and air.

*vikruti* a person's current state, in which health and feelings are affected by the changing balance of the three doshas.

*vulnerary* promotes the healing of wounds.

*yoga* literally "union", a set of spiritual and mind–body practices, including the physical exercises called hatha yoga.

# Useful addresses

## United Kingdom
*Aromatherapy associations*
Aromatherapy Organizations Council
(AOC), P. O. Box 19834, London SE25 6WF
Tel: 020 8251 7912

International Society of Professional
Aromatherapists (ISPA)
ISPA House, 82 Ashby Road, Hinckley
Leics LE10 1SN Tel: 01455 647 987

International Federation of Aromatherapists
(IFA)
Stamford House, 2–4 Chiswick High Street,
London W4 1TH Tel: 020 8742 2605

*Aromatherapy products*
Shirley Price Aromatherapy Limited
Essentia House, Upper Bond Street
Hinckley, Leics LE10 1RS Tel: 01455 615 466

*Specialized short courses in aromatherapy*
Penny Price
Sketchley Manor, Burbage, Leics LE10 2LQ
Fax: 01455 617 972

*Aromatic medicine and aromatology*
Dr Robert Stephen
4 Woodland Road, Hinckley
Leics LE10 1JG Fax: 01455 611 829

*Ayurvedic remedies and treatments*
The Ayurvedic Shop, 299 King Street, London
W6 9NH Tel: (020) 8563 0303

*Neem products*
Bioforce (UK) Ltd, Brewster Place, Irvine
Ayrshire KA11 5DD www.neemco.co.uk

British Wheel of Yoga
25 Jermyn Street, Sleaford, Lincs NG34 7RU
Tel: (01529) 306 851 www.bwy.org.uk

*Ayurvedic facelift*
Savita Patel, 151 Drummond Street, London
NW1 2PB Tel: (020) 7388 9795
e-mail: savita@facelift.fsnet.co.uk

Transcendental Meditation
Freepost, London SW1P 4YY, Tel: (08705) 143
733 www.t-m.org.uk
e-mail: mail@tm-london.org.uk

*Ayurvedic therapies and beauty treatments*
Pinka Yusupoff, 95 Kenbrook House, Leighton
Road, London NW5 2QW Tel: (020) 7284
4883. e-mail: pinkayusupoff@aol.com

## United States
*Aromatherapy associations*
National Association for Holistic
Aromatherapy
2000 2nd Avenue, Suite 206
Seattle, WA 98121 Tel: (888)-ASK-NAHA

*Aromatherapy products*
Adriaflor
188 Lancaster Road, Walnut Creek
CA 94595 Tel: (925) 935-3601

All Aroma
1324 Sinloa Drive, Glendale
CA 91207 Tel: (077) 81-AROMA

Aromatherapy Outlet
666 West 84th Steet, Hialeah
FL 33014 Tel: (35) 828-7655

American Yoga Association
P. O. Box 1998, Sarasota, FL 34276
Tel: (941) 927 4977
www.americanyogaassociation.org

*Aromatherapy teaching*
Aroma Studio
4 Taylor Road, Warwick, NY 10990

Nordbloom Swedish Healthcare Center
178 Mill Creek Road, Livingstone
Montana 59047, Tel: 406 333 4216

The Australasian College of Herbal Studies
P. O. Box 57, Lake Oswego, Oregon 97034
Tel: 503 635 6652

*Ayurvedic treatments, products and training*
Ganesha Institute for Ayurveda and
Vedic Studies
4898 El Camino Real, suite 203, Los Altos, CA
94022 Tel: (650) 961 8316
e-mail: info@healingmission.com

## Australia
*Aromatherapy products*
Nature's Energies
P. O. Box 112, Upper Ferntree Gully
Victoria 3156. Tel: (03) 9779-4369

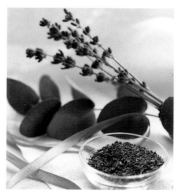

International Yoga Teachers Association
P. O. Box 31, Thornleigh, New South Wales
2120
Tel: (02) 9484 9848 e-mail: info@iyta.org.au

*Ayurvedic consultations, products and training*
OmVeda Beauty and Health Centre
P. O. Box 248, Rozelle, New South Wales 2039
Tel: (02) 9810 1830 www.omveda.com.au

## France
*Ayurvedic products and training*
Vedicare, 7 Impasse St Pierre, 75020 Paris
Tel: 33 (0) 1 44 93 91 26 www.vedicare.net

## India
*Ayurvedic treatments after personal consultations,
products, online courses*
Jiva Ayurvedic Research Institute
1144 Sector 19, Faridabad 121002, Haryana
www.ayurvedic.org

## Northern Ireland
*Aromatherapy products*
Angela Hills, 32 Russell Park
Belfast BT5 7QW

## Republic of Ireland
*Aromatherapy products*
Chritine Courtney, Oban Aromatherapy
53 Beech Grove, Lucan, County Dublin

## Norway
*Aromatherapy products*
Margareth Thomte, Nedreslottsgate 25
0157 Oslo, Tel: 22 170017

# index

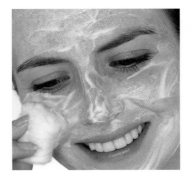

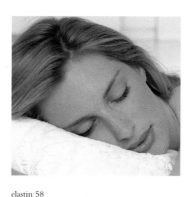

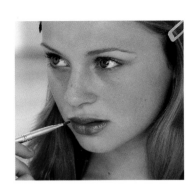

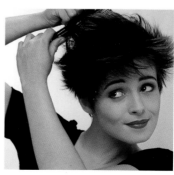

index

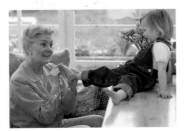

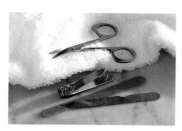

# ACKNOWLEDGEMENTS

### MAKE-UP AND HAIRSTYLING PRODUCTS

With many thanks to the following companies. **Beauty products** from The Body Shop, Boots, Bourjois, Crabtree & Evelyn, Cutex, Elancyl, L'Oréal, Rimmel and Sensiq. **Hair products** from Aveda, Bain de Terre, The Body Shop, Citre, Clynol, Daniel Gavin, Dome, Goldwell, John Frieda, Joico, KMS, Lamaur, Lazartigue, L'Oréal, Matrix Essentials, Neal's Yard Remedies, Nicky Clarke, Ore-an, Paul Mitchell, Phytologie, Poly, Redken, Revlon, Schwarzkopf, Silvikrin, St Ives, Trevor Sorbie, Wella and Vidal Sassoon and Zotos. **Electrical styling products** from Babyliss, Braun, Clairol, Carmen, Hair Tools, Philips, Rowenta and Vidal Sassoon. **Clothing and accessories** from Adrian Man, Bhs, Debenhams, Descamps, Empire, Fenwicks, Freemans, French Connection, Knickerbox, Marks & Spencer and Whistles.

### HAIR PHOTOGRAPHY CREDITS

The Publishers are grateful for the following photographers and companies for permission to reproduce their photographs:

p105b: Silvikrin; p107tl: Braun; p107tm: Taylor Ferguson, Glasgow; p107tr: Antoinette Beenders at Trevor Sorbie, London for Denman, photography Simon Bottomley; p108bl and br: Regis; p109tr: Joseph and Jane Harling, Avon; p109ml: Paul Falltricks, Essex; p109mr: Regis; p109bl: Nicky Clarke, London; p109br: Essanelle Salons, Britain; p112l: Trevor Sorbie; p112r: L'Oréal; p114 all: Carlos Calico, Madrid; p114t: Silvikrin; p116: Daniel Galvin for L'Oréal, photography Iain Philpott; p120: Daniel Galvin,

London; p122t: Bain de Terre Spa Therapy; p122bl & br: Daniel Galvin; p123tl: Bain de Terre Spa Therapy; p123br: Daniel Galvin; p124: Nicky Clarke; p125tl: Babyliss; p125tr: Yosh Toya, San Francisco, photography Gen; p125br: Daniel Galvin; p127tl: Daniel Galvin; p127tr: Wella, photography Mark Hill; p128: Clynol; p129tl: Terence Renati, London and Melbourne; p129tm: Patrick Cameron for Alan Paul, Wirral; p129tr: Regis; p130 bl: Richard M. F. Mendleson of David's Hair Designers, Maryland, USA; p130bm and br: Eugene at Xtension Masters, London; p131br: Macmillan, London; p131tr: Richard M. F. Mendleson; p135l: Sam Mcknight for Silvikrin; p135tr: Paul Falltrick, photography Iain Philpott; p135br: Jed Hamill of Graham Webb International for Clynol, photography Ian Hooton; p136tl & br: Regis, photography John Swannel; p136tm: Yosh Toya, photography Gen; p136bl and br: Regis, Europe, photography John Swannel; p137tr: Paul Fattrick, for Clynol, photography Alistair Hughes; p137tm: Yosh Toya, photography Gen; p137tr: Alan Edwards for L'Oréal. p137ml: Daniel Galvin; p137mr: Nicky Clarke, photography Paul Cox; p137bl: Frank Hession, Dublin, for L'Oréal; p137bm: Neville Daniel, London, photography Will White; p137br: Neville Daniel for Lamaur; p138tl: Charles Worthington, London for L'Oréal; p138tr: L'Oréal; p138bl: Trevor Sorbie, photography Mark Havrilliak; p138bml: Umberto Giannino, Kidderminster for L'Oréal; p138bml: Stuart Kirby of Eaton Hair Group, Portsmouth, for L'Oréal; p138bl: Anthony Mascolo, Toni & Guy, for L'Oréal; p139tl & tm: Yosh Toya, photography Gen; p139ml & mr: Regis, photography John Swannel; p139bl: Barbara Daley Hair Studio, Birmingham, for L'Oréal; p139bml: L'Oréal; p139bmr & br: Mod Hair, France, for Schwarzkopf; p140tl: Steven Carey, London; p140bl & r: Neville Daniel, for Lamaur; p141tl: Daniel Galvin; p141tm & tr: Nicky Clarke; p141ml & mr: Silvikrin; p141bl: John Frieda, London and New York; p141bm & br: Daniel Galvin; p142tl: Adam Lyons, Grays, for L'Oréal; p142tm: Taylor Ferguson; p142tr: Paul Falltricks, for Clynol, photography Alistair Hughes; p142b (all): Taylor Ferguson; p143tl: Zotos International; p143tm: Steven Carey, photography Alistair Hughes; p143tr: Schwarzkopf; p143bl: Regis, photography Mark York; p143bml: Steven Carey, photography Alistair Hughes; p143bmr: Partners, London; p143br: Keith Harris for Braun; p146bl: Silvikrin; p146tr: Clynol; p147tr: Babyliss; p148tr: Babyliss; p149tr: Silvikrin.

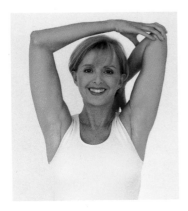